D0499451

Preface

This dictionary is intended to be a quick and ready reference to the common terms used in those medical and healing practices that lie outside of conventional medical venues. It is our hope that it will provide a resource for improving communication among practitioners of various disciplines and between patients using those practices and their conventional health care providers. With this in mind, we have selected the most common concepts and terms in use around the world and have provided both definitions and descriptions of their meaning.

Complementary and alternative medicine (CAM), which includes diagnostic and treatment practices that lie outside the fields of modern Western biomedicine, is steadily growing in use. Various surveys have shown that 30% to 60% of the public in the West now use CAM practices or products in any given year, and in the United States there are more visits to CAM practitioners than to conventional primary care doctors. Many CAM practices are a major part of healing traditions from around the world. More than 80% of populations outside the West use herbal and other traditional medicines. As the world becomes smaller, with increasing communication, travel, and migration, concepts and terms in these traditional practices are becoming commonplace in the vernacular of people across the globe. Many people, however, are unfamiliar with the meanings of these terms and concepts. For example, traditional Chinese, Indian, Native American, Japanese, African, and South American practices employ concepts and terms that are unfamiliar to conventional health care practitioners and to providers of other CAM practices.

Of concern is that 60% to 70% of patients who use CAM do not discuss these practices with their conventional health care practitioners. Although fear of ridicule is sometimes the cause, many patients believe that their doctors do not know much about CAM and so cannot give them informed advice. Although medical, nursing, and allied health schools are beginning to introduce CAM concepts during training, most conventional health care practitioners are unfamiliar with CAM terms and concepts. For example, practitioners often confuse homeopathy with herbal medicine, and Kampo with Chinese medicine. This book is a ready reference for clarifying such confusion. Although practitioners cannot be familiar with all of the concepts in CAM and conventional medicine, this dictionary provides them with quick and ready access to many unfamiliar terms. Thus, it can be a valuable resource for improving communication about CAM with patients.

In selecting and defining the terms in this dictionary, we have not attempted to be comprehensive, but rather to provide those terms most commonly used in CAM practices, in the CAM literature, and also by patients in areas of the world where conventional medicine predominates. As such, we have not always followed standard dictionary format, frequently opting instead to provide descriptive information about the term and practice. This dictionary should be most useful for conventional practitioners who need to find definitions and descriptions of common CAM terms quickly, and as a reference for those in introductory courses on CAM in medical, nursing, and allied health schools. Our hope is also that all libraries, medical and otherwise, will have copies available for ready access to the public.

With the globalization of medicine, it is not only Western biomedicine that is spreading around the world. Traditional practices formerly restricted to certain regions of the world are now spreading beyond their previous boundaries. Medicine of the future, much of it already here, will draw from many of these traditions as it evolves and integrates the best of healing practices from around the world. It is our hope that this dictionary will become a resource to facilitate this integrated, global medicine.

Wayne B. Jonas, MD

Contents

Introduction, ix
Pronunciation Guide, xi
Alphabetic Listing of Terms, 1
Appendices

A	Acupuncture, 469	
B	Aromatherapy, 471	
C	Ayurveda, 472	
D	Biofeedback, 473	
E	Bodywork, 475	
F	Chiropractic, 477	
G	Energy Medicine, 478	
H	Environmental Medicine, 479	
I	The Health Insurance Portability and Accountability Act (HIPAA) of 1996, 480	
J	Homeopathy, 483	
K	Hypnotherapy, 485	
L	Latin American Medicine, 486	
M	Magnetic Field Therapy, 487	
N	Massage Therapy, 488	
O	Native American Medicine, 490	
P	Naturopathic Medicine, 491	
Q	Orthomolecular Medicine, 493	
R	Osteopathic Medicine, 494	
S	Reflexology, 495	
T	Relaxation Therapies, 497	
U	Spiritual Healing and Subtle Energy Medicine, 498	
V	Tibetan Medicine, 499	
W	Traditional Chinese Medicine (TCM), 501	
X	Yoga, 503	

Illustration Credits, 504
Bibliography, 506

Introduction

Complementary and alternative medicine (CAM) continues to grow in popularity, introducing a host of new terms and concepts to health care providers and laypeople alike. As a result, modern healthcare professionals must have a basic understanding of the various concepts and healing modalities comprising CAM in order to effectively respond to patient questions and concerns. As well, for the medical professional and the layperson alike, this profusion of new terminology may be bewildering. It is our hope and intention that this dictionary will facilitate communication about CAM between patients and their healthcare providers.

Mosby's Dictionary of Complementary and Alternative Medicine contains approximately 6600 definitions that cover the five major areas of CAM as outlined by the National Center for Complementary and Alternative Medicine of the National Institutes of Health:

1. Alternative healthcare systems
2. Mind-body interventions
3. Biologically based therapies
4. Manipulative and body-based healing methods
5. Energy therapies.

Alternative healthcare systems are those integrated systems of therapeutic theory and practice that include homeopathy and traditional Chinese medicine (TCM). *Mind-body interventions* use the mind—ideation, emotions, imagery, etc.—to produce healing changes in the body. *Biologically based therapies* use naturally occurring therapeutic substances such as vitamins and herbs. *Manipulative and body-based healing methods* include chiropractic, osteopathy, massage, and bodywork. Finally, *energy therapies* are those therapeutic methods that work with energy fields, including those that are bioelectromagnetic in origin and those purported to exist but for which little scientific evidence currently exists.

In addition, the dictionary provides expanded pronunciations, illustrations, and appendices. Exhaustive descriptions of commonly used herbal supplements and definitions for terminology used in chiropractic, TCM, homeopathy, naturopathy, and Ayurveda, as well as in conventional medicine, have been included to make the text a valuable reference for today's healthcare professional. More than 500 diagrams, photographs, and line drawings visually illustrate the concepts discussed.

Finally, 24 appendices explore the history, theory, and practice of the following systems of CAM: acupuncture, aromatherapy, Ayurveda, biofeedback, bodywork, chiropractic, energy medicine, environmental medicine, homeopathy, hypnotherapy, Latin American medicine, magnetic field therapy, massage therapy, Native American medicine, naturopathy, orthomolecular medicine, osteopathy, reflexology, relaxation therapy, spiritual healing, Tibetan medicine, TCM, and yoga.

Pronunciation Guide

VOWEL SOUNDS

Print	Key words
a	hat
ä	father
ā	play, fate, feign
e	flesh
ē	she, sweet
er	air, ferry
i	sit
ī	eye, kind, mine
ir	ear, weird
o	proper
ō	nose, coal
ô	saw, fawn
ōi	coin, (German) feuer
o͞o	moon, move
o͝o	put, book
ou	out
u	cup, love
Y	(German) grün, Führer; (French) tu
ur	fur, first
ə	ago, career
œ	(German) schön, Goethe
N	This symbol does not represent a sound but indicates that the preceding vowel is nasal, as in (French) bon.

CONSONANTS

Print	Key words
b	book
čh	chew, watch
d	day, dead
f	fast, phone, enough
g	good
h	happy
j	jump, gem
k	cook, quick
l	late
m	mammal
n	noon
ng	sing, drink
ng-g	finger
p	pulp
r	ready, rely

s	**sassy**
sh	**sh**ine, **s**ure, lo**ti**on
t	**to**
th	**th**in (voiceless)
th	**th**an, wi**th** (voiced)
v	**v**al**v**e
w	**w**ork
y	**y**es
z	**z**eal, ha**s**
zh	a**z**ure, vi**si**on
(h)w	**wh**en, **wh**ile
kh	(Scottish) lo**ch**, (German) Ba**ch**
kh	(German) i**ch**
nyə	o**ni**on, (Spanish) se**ñ**or, (French) Boulo**gne**

A, *adj* See alveolar.

a, *adj* See arterial.

AACP, *n.pr* See Acupuncture Association of Chartered Physiotherapists.

AAFP, *n.pr* See American Academy of Family Physicians.

AATA, *n.pr* See American Art Therapy Association.

abduct, *v* to move in the direction away from the center line of the body.

abduction (ab·duk'·shən), *n* joint movement away from the body along the horizontal plane.

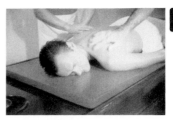

Abhyanga. (Sharma and Clarke, 1998)

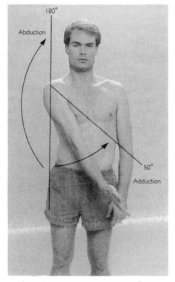

Abduction. (Seidel et al, 1995; Patrick Watson)

abhyanga (əbh·yän'·gə), *n* in Ayurveda, an oil massage, recommended for increasing flexibility of muscles and joints, rejuvenating skin, and keeping impurities from accumulating in the body by stimulating various tissues.

abortifacient, *adj/n* an instrument or material capable of terminating a pregnancy.

abreaction (a'·brē·ak'·shən), *n* the remembrance and release of emotions relating to a repressed experience or trauma that can occur on its own or be induced artificially, as through hypnosis. See also catharsis.

Abrus precatorius, *n* See Indian licorice.

absolute, *n* a residue obtained from aromatic plant material via the methods of solvent extraction or enfleurage. The residue will only contain those volatile oils from the plant that are alcohol soluble. See also enfleurage.

absolute concentration, *n* a state of mind held by a practitioner of Tibetan medicine during a session with a patient. As a result of continual instruction and training, the practitioner can focus on the patient without being distracted by thoughts of anticipated future or past occurrences. Working in this frame of mind allows the practitioner to gain the patient's confidence, which is of principal significance to the practitioner.

ACA, *n.pr* See American Chiropractic Association.

***Acacia catechu* (ä·kä·sēə kä·tä·chōō),** *n* parts used: bark, heartwood extract, gum, shoots, fruits; uses: in Ayurveda balances kapha and pitta doshas (bitter, astringent, light, dry); heartwood: asthma, bronchitis, diarrhea, dysentery, liver protection, antiinflammatory; bark: ulcers, psoriasis, gum conditions; precautions: none known. Also called *black* *catechu, cutch tree, khadira, khair,* or *terra japonica.*

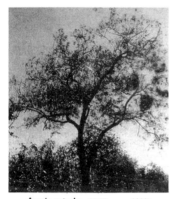

Acacia catechu. (Williamson, 2002)

Acacia senegal, *n* See gum Arabic.

Acanthopanax senticosus, *n* See ginseng, Siberian.

acardia (ā·kär´·dē·ə), *n* an extremely rare condition in which an individual is born without a heart. Occurs occasionally in conjoined twins; the circulatory system of one twin supports the survival of the other.

acausal, *n* **1.** lacking a causal principle. **2.** not following the principles of final causation or linear direction.

acceleration, *n* in osteopathy, the process of increasing speed or velocity of a manipulative technique.

accessory movements, *n.pl* movements within a joint and the surrounding tissue that are necessary for the full range of motion but that can be performed actively.

accommodation, *n* an impermanent adjustment or adaptation that automatically reverses when whatever is being accommodated is removed.

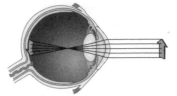

Distant image: lens is flattened

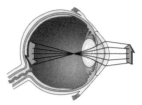

Close image: lens is rounded

Accommodation of lens. (Thibodeau and Patton, 2003)

ACE, *n.pr* See angiotensin-converting enzyme.

acetabulum (a·sə·ta´·byə·ləm), *n* the bowl-shaped cavity that houses the rounded tip of the femur, where the ischium, pubis, and ilium join.

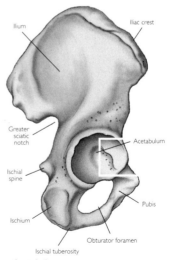

Acetabulum. (Herlihy and Maebius, 2000)

acetonuria (a·sə·tōn'·yōō·rē·ə), *n* condition in which diacetic bodies and acetone are present in the urine. Often found in individuals who are fasting or have diabetes.

acetract (ās'·trakt), *n* an herbal extract obtained by using acetic acid as the solvent.

acetyl cholinesterase (a·sē'·t əl kō'·lə·ne'·stə·rās), *n* enzyme found at both voluntary and parasympathetic nerve endings that hydrolyzes the acetylcholine byproduct of nerve impulses into acetate and choline.

acetylation (əsē·tə·lā·shən), *n* a phase II detoxification pathway occurring in the liver in which acetyl-CoA combines with metabolic products.

acetylcholine (ə·sē'·təl·kō'·lēn), *n* neurotransmitter that is produced in the central and parasympathetic autonomic nervous systems. It is the most prevalent neurotransmitter in the body and is crucial to arousal, learning, memory, and motor function.

Ach, *n* See acetylcholine.

AChE, *n.pr* See acetyl cholinesterase.

Achillea millefolium, *n* See yarrow.

acid, *n* a compound able to form hydrogen ions (H) when dissolved in aqueous solutions.

acid, alpha-linolenic, *n* a polyunsaturated fatty acid found in the blood. Deficiencies and imbalances can affect blood pressure, blood cholesterol, premenstrual symptoms, and skin conditions.

acid, alpha-lipoic, *n* a sulfurous antioxidant that is produced within the body as a constituent of multiple enzymatic systems and is also derived from food sources. Has been used to treat hypertension and as an adjunct to diabetes treatment and may benefit patients with cataracts or cardiovascular conditions. Also called *thioctic acid.*

acid, arachidic (ar·ə·ki·dik a'·sid), *n* a saturated fatty acid that provides energy.

acid, arachidonic (ar·ə·kə·dô'·nik a'·sid), *n* an omega-6 polyunsaturated fatty acid prevalent in red meats and a key component of many metabolic processes.

acid, ascorbic, *n* See vitamin C.

acid, azelaic (a'·zə·lā'·ik a'·sid), *n* a naturally occurring dicarboxylic acid commonly used as a topical treatment for acne.

acid, behenic (bə·he'·nik a'·sid), *n* a saturated fatty acid associated with degenerative neural diseases and some genetic disorders.

acid, capric (ka'·prik a'·sid), *n* a saturated fatty acid that has been linked to multiple aryl-coenzyme and dehydrogenation disorders.

acid, caprylic (kə·pri'·lik a'·sid), *n* a naturally occurring fatty acid used as an antifungal agent for treating candidiasis caused by the yeast *Candida albicans.*

acid, carboxylic (kär·bôk'·sə·lik a'·sid), *n* an organic compound that contains at least one carboxyl group; it is weaker than a mineral acid such as hydrochloric acid.

acid, conjugated linoleic, *n* a mixture of fatty acids (specifically mixed isomers of linoleic acid) obtained through diet or supplementation. Claimed to be useful as a weight loss aid and as a treatment for adult-onset diabetes. No known precautions with this substance exist.

acid, dihomogammalinolenic (dī'·hō'·mō·gya'·məti'·nəlē'·nik a'·sid), *n* a fatty acid necessary for proper cell and tissue functions.

acid, docosadienoic (dō·kō'·sə·dī'·ē·nō'·ik a'·sid), *n* omega-6 polyunsaturated fatty acid include in a typical fatty acid profile to study serum triglyceride analysis.

acid, docosahexaenoic (dō'·kō'·sə·hek·sə·ē·nō'·ik a'·sid), *n* an unsaturated fatty acid important in early neurological development.

acid, docosapentaenoic (dō'·kō'·sə·pen·t əē'·nō'·ik a'·sid), *n* an unsaturated fatty acid important in early neurological development.

acid, docosatetraenoic (dō·kō'·sə·te'·trə·ē·nō'·ik a'·sid), *n* omega-6 polyunsaturated fatty acid stored in adipose tissue and mobilized during fasting. High levels of this fatty acid in the blood are associated with obesity.

A

acid, eicosapentaenoic (ī'·kō'·sə·pen'·tə·ē'·nō'·ik a'·sid), *n* fatty acid found in fish oils. Deficiency has been linked to arthritis, depression, heart disease, and high cholesterol.

acid, eicosatrenoic (ī'·kō·sa'·tr ə·nō'·ik a'·sid), *n* an omega-3 series polyunsaturated fatty acid; represents less than 0.25% of serum phospholipid fatty acids in a normal individual.

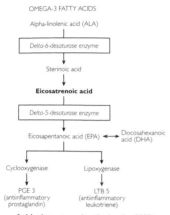

OMEGA-3 FATTY ACIDS

Alpha-linolenic acid (ALA)

↓

Delta-6-desaturase enzyme

↓

Sterinoic acid

↓

Eicosatrenoic acid

↓

Delta-5-desaturase enzyme

↓

Eicosapentanoic acid (EPA) ⟷ Docosahexanoic acid (DHA)

↓ ↓

Cyclooxygenase   Lipoxygenase

↓ ↓

PGE 3   LTB 5
(antiinflammatory   (antiinflammatory
prostaglandin)   leukotriene)

Acid, eicosatrenoic. (Leskowitz, 2003)

acid, elaidic (ē·lā'·dik a'·sid), *n* a trans-fatty acid found in hydrogenated oils. Elevated amounts have been linked to high cholesterol levels.

acid, erucic (i·rōō'·sik a'·sid), *n* a fatty acid found in rapeseed (canola), mustard seed, and wallflower seed. This compound is linked to elevated levels of fatty acids and is being studied as a possible treatment for degenerative neurologic disorders. See also Lorenzo's oil.

acid, folic, *n* See folate.

acid, gamma linolenic (gya'·mə li·nə·lē'·nik a'·sid), *n* an omega-6 polyunsaturated fatty acid found in black currant, borage, evening primrose oils, and hemp. It is a precursor of DGLA and arachidonic acid and is linked to reduced symptoms of rheumatoid arthritis and zinc deficiency but may also enhance tumor growth and formation if not supplemented by an omega-3 fatty acid.

acid, gamma-aminobutyric (gya'·mə-ə-mē'·nō·byōō·tir'·ik a'·sid), *n* amino acid that serves as the governing neurotransmitter in the spinal cord and brain. Also present in the lungs, heart, kidneys, and some plants.

acid, heneicosanoic (he'·nā·ē·kō'·sə·nō'·ik a'·sid), *n* fatty acid formed from propionic acid under conditions of vitamin B$_{12}$ deficiency.

acid, heptadecanoic (hep'·tə·de'·kə·nō'·ik a'·sid), *n* colorless, crystalline fatty acid which accumulates because of a deficiency of vitamin B$_{12}$. Also called *margaric acid.*

acid, hexacosanoic (hek'·sə kō'·sə nō'·ik a'·sid), *n* long-chain fatty acid whose elevated numbers in a fatty acid profile are associated with genetic disorders characteristic of sphingolipid accumulation. Also called *cerotic acid.*

acid, hydroxycitric (hī·drōk'·sē·si trik a'·sid), *n* an organic acid derived from the Malabar tamarind *(Garcinia cambogia)* fruit and used in appetite suppression and weight loss. Also called *gorikapuli, hydroxycitrate,* or *Malabar tamarind.*

acid, lauric (lô'·rik a'·sid), *n* a medium-chain fatty acid, the levels of which have been shown to rise in fatty acid catabolic disorders known as multiple acyl–coenzyme A dehydrogenation disorders.

acid, lignoceric (lig·nō·se'·rik a'·sid), *n* a long-chain fatty acid that has been linked to degenerative neural diseases and certain genetic disorders.

acid, linolenic (li'·nō·lē'·nik a'·sid), *n* an essential omega-6 polyunsaturated fatty acid found in corn, safflower, and other oils. Deficiencies have been linked to a number of health problems, including behavioral difficulties, cardiovascular disease, hair loss, infections, kidney degeneration, liver degeneration, miscarriage, and sterility.

acid, lipoic (**lī'·pō·ik a'·sid**), *n* a vitamin-like antioxidant found in leafy greens, brewer's yeast, red meat, and organ meats, used intravenously to treat diabetic polyneuropathy and orally to treat autonomic neuropathy and for preventing diabetic cataracts. No known precautions exist, but caution is advised for patients who use insulin. Also called *alphalipoic acid* or *thioctic acid.*

acid, malic (**ma'·lik a'·sid**), *n* an organic acid involved in the Krebs cycle. Used for treating fibromyalgia. No known precautions exist. Also called *apple acid.*

acid, myristic (**mə·ri'·stik a'·sid**), *n* a medium-chain fatty acid that has been linked to fatty acid catabolic disorders known as multiple acylcoenzyme A dehydrogenation disorders.

acid, myristoleic (**mə·ri·stō·lē'·ik a'·sid**), *n* a mono-unsaturated fatty acid involved in maintaining membrane fluidity.

acid, nonadecanoic (**nô·nə·de·kə·nō'·ik a'·sid**), *n* an odd-numbered fatty acid that accumulates with deficiency of vitamin B_{12} and accumulates in the membrane lipids of neural tissue.

acid, oleic (**ō·lā'·ik a'·sid**), *n* a mono-unsaturated fatty acid found in all fat-containing foods. Involved in maintaining membrane fluidity.

acid, palmitelaidic (**päl·mi·tə·lā'·dik a'·sid**), *n* a trans-fatty acid found in hydrogenated oils.

acid, palmitic (**pal·mi'·tik a'·sid**), *n* a saturated fatty acid converted into cholesterol by the liver. High levels have been linked to cardiovascular disease, atherosclerosis, and stroke.

acid, palmitoleic (**pal·mi·tə·lā'·ik a'·sid**), *n* a mono-unsaturated fatty acid involved in maintaining membrane fluidity.

acid, pentadecanoic (**pen·tə·de·kə·nō'·ik a'·sid**), *n* an odd-numbered fatty acid that accumulates with deficiency of vitamin B_{12} and accumulates in the membrane lipids of neural tissue.

acid, phytic (**fī'·tik a'·sid**), *n* dietary fiber found in cereals and legumes that has antioxidant and antitumor properties.

acid, p-aminobenzoic (**a·mē'·nō·ben·zō'·ik a'·sid**), *n* commonly abbreviated as PAB or PABA, it is a substance essential for the absorption of folic acid in many organisms. It is used in topical sun-screen because it absorbs ultraviolet light.

acid, stearic (**stē·ar'·ik a'·sid**), *n* a saturated fatty acid that can be converted into cholesterol. High levels have been linked to atherosclerosis, and low levels may increase the growth or spread of tumors.

acid, tricosanoic (**trī·kō'·sə·nō'·ik a'·sid**), *n* fatty acid with odd number of carbon atoms which accumulates because of vitamin B_{12} deficiency.

acid, uric (**yōō'·rik a'·sid**), *n* waste product of purine metabolism, high levels of which can be found in plasma. The kidneys produce the majority of uric acid in the body.

acid, usnic (**us'·nik a'·sid**), *n* compound found in the lichen *Usnea barbata,* which is used as an antibiotic.

acid, vaccenic (**vak·sen'·ik a'·sid**), *n* a crystalline unsaturated acid whose ratio to palmitoleic acid in a fatty acid profile may influence biotin needs.

acid profile, organic, *n* an analysis of organic acids (other than amino acids) excreted in the urine, used to assess metabolic disorders and nutrient deficiencies.

acids, amino (**ə·mē'·nō a'·sidz**), *n.pl* the 22 identified building blocks of proteins essential for growth and maintenance.

acids, branched-chain amino, *n.pl* a combination of three amino acids: leucine, isoleucine, and valine. It has been used for anorexia associated with chronic illness, amyotrophic lateral sclerosis, tardive dyskinesia, and muscular dystrophy and to increase athletic performance. Precaution suggested for patients taking levodopa.

acids, essential fatty, *n.pl* fatty acids (structural components of larger, nutritional fat molecules) that cannot be synthesized by the body and that must be obtained through dietary sources. They are components of cell membranes, contribute to the development and function of the nervous system, are stored for energy, and are used in the synthesis of important biomolecules. The two main types of essential fatty acids are omega-3 and omega-6. See also acids, omega-3 fatty and acids, omega-6 fatty.

acids, long-chain fatty, *n.pl* fatty acids with a basic structure of 12 or more carbon atoms. Essential fatty acids are typically long-chain fatty acids. Certain disorders, including intestinal lymphangiectasia and short bowel syndrome, may interfere with the ability to absorb long-chain fatty acids. See also acids, essential fatty; acids, omega-3 fatty acids; and acids, omega-6 fatty.

acids, omega-3 fatty, *n.pl* essential fatty acids found in flaxseeds, pumpkin seeds, walnuts, salmon, trout, tuna, and other sources. Omega-3 fatty acids include alpha linolenic acid, eicosapentaenoic acid (EPA), and docosahexaenoic acid (DHA). See also Acid, alpha linolenic; acid, eicosapentaenoic; and acid, docosahexaenoic.

acids, omega-6 fatty, *n.pl* essential fatty acids found in many cooking oils, such as corn, soy, and sunflower oils. Omega-6 fatty acids include linoleic acid, arachidonic acid, gamma linolenic acid, and dihomogamma linolenic acid.

acids, trans-fatty, *n.pl* a particular configuration of any of the unsaturated fats that have been hydrogenated. Hydrogenation can change a naturally occurring fatty acid from a *cis-* to a *trans-* configuration, which cannot be used by the body.

acids, unsaturated fatty, *n* fatty acids in which the carbon atoms in the hydrocarbon chain are joined by double or triple bonds. Monounsaturated fatty acids have one double bond or triple bond, whereas polyunsaturated fatty acids have more than one double or triple bond. Diets rich in polyunsaturated fatty acids and low

in saturated fatty acid levels are correlated with low levels of serum cholesterol. See also acids, omega-3 fatty; acids, omega-6 fatty; and polyunsaturated.

acidophilus, *n* Latin names: *Lactobacillus acidophilus, Lactobacillus bulgaricus;* part used: entire organism; uses: stimulates growth of bacteria in digestive tract; treats urinary tract infections, yeast infections, thrush in babies; also claimed to encourage nonspecific immunity and to prevent cancerous growths in breast and colon; precautions: lactose intolerance. Also called *Bacid, Lactinex, MoreDophilus, Probiata, Probiotics, Superdolphilus,* or *yogurt.*

acidosis (a·sə·dō'·sis), *n* an imbalance in the acid-base balance in the body, in which blood pH falls below the normal range (7.35–7.45) as the result of a build-up of acid or a depletion of a base, thus resulting in elevated hydrogen ion levels.

acne, *n* a condition of the skin characterized by various inflammatory lesions caused by a combination of bacteria and increased skin oil (sebum) production.

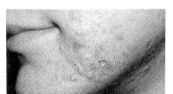

Acne. (White, 1994)

aconite (a´·kə·nīt), *n* **I.** Latin names: *Aconitum napellus, Aconitum columbianum, Aconitum chinense, Aconitum carmichaeli;* parts used: leaves, roots; uses: fever, arthritis, rheumatism, poor digestion; precautions: extremely toxic; cardiotoxic. Also called *blue rocket, bushi, friar's* cap, helmet flower, monkshood, soldier's cap, or wolfsbane. **2.** a homeopathic preparation of *Aconitum napellus,* used to treat colds, inflammatory conditions, and fevers accompanied with anxiety and restlessness.

Aconitum carmichaeli, *n* See aconite.

Aconitum chinense, *n* See aconite.

Aconitum columbianum, *n* See aconite.

Aconitum napellus L., *n* See aconite.

Acorus calamus, *n* See sweet flag.

acquired immunity, *n* noninnate immunity obtained during a person's lifetime either by developing antibodies in response to an infection (naturally acquired immunity) or by vaccination (artificially acquired immunity).

acrid, *adj* bitter, harsh, and persistently unpleasant in taste or smell.

acrodynia (a·krō·dī'·nē-ə), *n* pediatric disease possibly linked to mercury poisoning. Symptoms include generalized skin rash, pruritus, edema, painful extremities that appear pink, profuse sweating, clammy skin, scarlet-colored cheeks and nose, photophobia, polyneuritis, digestive problems, irritable episodes that alternate with apathetic attitudes, and general failure to thrive. Also called *erythredema polyneuropathy, Feer's disease, pink disease,* or *Swift's disease.*

acromegaly (a·krō·me'·gə·lē), *n* chronic metabolic disorder of middle-aged and older individuals, in which excessive growth hormone secretion results in the progressive thickening and enlargement of the facial bones and jaw. Also called *acromeglia.*

act, *n* decision by a legislative body that results in a law.

Actaea alba, *n* See cohosh, white.

Actaea racemosa, *n* See cohosh, black.

ACTH, *n.pr* See adrenocorticotropic hormone.

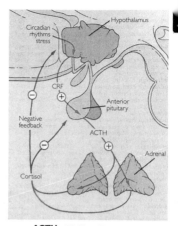

ACTH. (Zitelli and Davis, 1997)

actin (ak'·tin), *n* one of a pair of myofilaments involved in muscle contractions. See also myosin.

actionable per se, *n* a lawsuit in which the aggrieved party need not show loss in order to receive monetary compensation.

activator (ak·ti·vā'·ter), *n* a chiropractic technique that employs a device that, when applied to joints, muscles, and soft tissues, conveys a powerful impulse to correct subluxations.

active assisted movement, *n* a therapist-assisted client movement throughout the range of motion.

active end range, *n* the distance a joint can be moved by a person's own muscles. The first of the three barriers that end joint movement.

active joint movement, *n* a therapeutic technique in which the client moves a joint around its range of motion unassisted by the therapist.

active meditation, *n* meditation process which uses various techniques to help individuals improve self-awareness. The techniques include breathing, movement, visualization, and exercises. Exercises may be instructor-guided, and feedback between student and instructor is considered important to the process.

active motion, *n* See motion, active.

active range of motion, *n* any unassisted movement of a joint.

active resistive movement, *n* a therapeutic technique in which the therapist provides resistance against which the client moves a joint.

activity, *n* **1.** the modification brought about by a remedy in a living organism. **2.** the ability of a medicine to bring about modification in a living organism. See also drug action, reactivity, and receptivity.

acture (ak'·chər), *n* term coined by Moshe Feldenkrais to describe the minute adjustments that individuals make to maintain correct posture during day-to-day activities.

actus reus (ak·'təs rē·əs), *n* a physical, criminal act that must be undoubtedly established as having occurred in order to convict a defendant of a crime.

acumoxa (a'·kyōō·mäk'·sə), *n* treatment that incorporates acupuncture and moxibustion. See also acupuncture and moxibustion.

acuology (a·kyōō·ô'·lə·gē), *n* the ancient theories on which acupuncture is based.

acupoints, *n.pl* particular bodily locations that allow practitioners to balance client's qi to affect therapeutic changes with acupuncture or acupressure. See also acupressure, acupuncture, meridians, qi, and tsubo.

acupressure, *n* in acupuncture, a technique used to release blocked qi by applying finger pressure to points on meridians. Although pain relief tends to be short-lived, this treatment can be used for patients who want to avoid needles.

acupunctural treatment area, *n* any suitable sites of needle insertion that affect a therapeutic change. Also called *ATA.*

acupuncture, *n* a practice in Chinese medicine in which the skin, at various points along meridians, is punctured with needles to remove energetic blockages and stimulate the flow of qi. Often used to relieve pain. See also acupoints, meridians, and qi.

acupuncture analgesia, *n* the pain-reducing effect brought about by inserting tiny needles into key points of the human body, sometimes augmented by the use of low-frequency or high-frequency electrically charged needles.

acupuncture energetics **(a'·kyōō·pəngk'·chər e·ner·je'·tiks),** *n* in medical acupuncture, a fusion model of therapy that brings together local treatment with energy assessment throughout the body's channels. Primarily used in the United States, this model of therapy is derived from the European interpretations of the traditional Chinese methods and blends segmental innervation for pain therapies and neuromuscular anatomy of trigger points.

acupuncture, auricular, *n* therapy in which acupuncture points on the outer ear are treated to alleviate symptoms such as depression, insomnia, sexual dysfunction, and withdrawal symptoms.

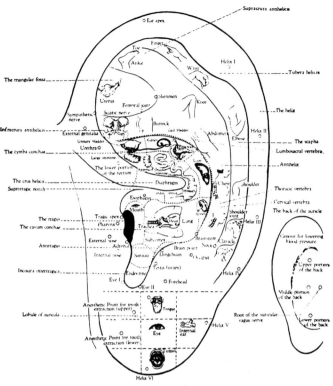

Auricular acupuncture. (Leskowitz, 2003)

acupuncture, chakra (shä'·lə ə·kyōō'·pəŋk·chə), *n* a hybridization of Chinese acupuncture and the Vedic chakra system in which the chakras are stimulated and energetic blockages are released through the needling of chakra points.

acupuncture, classical, n a variant of acupuncture in which practitioners translate and refer to original texts and rely on the philosophical as well as medical, aspects of those texts.

acupuncture, deep, n acupuncture in which the needles are inserted through the skin and subcutaneous tissues and into the muscles. Also called *intramuscular acupuncture.*

acupuncture, ear (EA), n therapy that treats and prevents disease by stimulating certain points on the ear. Standardized ear acupuncture is used to treat substance abuse in the United States.

acupuncture, five-element, n.pr a variant of acupuncture in which diagnosis is based upon the patient's unique relationship to the five elements (wood, fire, earth, metal, and water). The acupuncturist determines the patient's constitutional element and works to return this element to a state of balance.

acupuncture, formula, n technique in which the specific acupuncture points are fixed to promote uniformity for determining efficacy of a technique. See also acupuncture.

acupuncture, Japanese, n a gentle, minimally invasive type of acupuncture developed in Japan. Also called *toyohari.*

acupuncture, Korean hand, n method in which needles are inserted into the hands at points that correspond to the traditional Chinese meridians.

acupuncture, medical, n healing system based on Western views of neurophysiology, neuroanatomy, and trigger points in combination with European interpretation of Chinese classic medicine texts.

acupuncture, micro, n **I.** system of acupuncture in which the body is reflected in miniature on different parts of the body, as with reflexology. **2.** a term used by Felix Mann to describe his techniques of minimalist acupuncture. See also acupuncture, minimalist and acupuncture, new concept.

acupuncture, minimalist (**mi'·nə·məl·ist a'·kyōō·punk'·cher**), *n* a form of acupuncture in which the needles are placed just into the subcutaneous tissue, with little or no manual stimulation, and removed after a brief period to affect relief from pain. Also called *micro acupuncture.*

acupuncture, neuroanatomic, n a Western variant of acupuncture with a modern neurological orientation. Includes the use of electroacupuncture and is predominantly performed by medical doctors for pain relief.

acupuncture, new concept, n a form of acupuncture in which meridians and classical points are eschewed and instead local tenderness and the pattern of radiation are used to locate proper sites for needle insertion. This school of acupuncture also uses micro acupuncture and periosteal

needling. See also micro acupuncture.

acupuncture, periosteal (**per'·ē·äs'·tē·əl a'·kyōō·punk'·chər**), *n* method of acu-puncture in which the needle is inserted all the way into the periosteum (fibrous tissue which encases bone). Special care is taken in the vicinity of organs.

acupuncture, scalp, n the insertion of fine needles into meridians located throughout the scalp to restore health and balance to the body.

acupuncture, superficial, n method of acupuncture in which the needles are inserted into the skin and subcutaneous tissues only.

acupuncture, symptomatic, n a form of acupuncture applied as a first-aid technique for its analgesic properties.

acupuncture, trigger point, n a form of acupuncture that uses trigger points for needle insertion instead of the classical acupuncture points. See also points, trigger.

acupuncture, Yamamoto new scalp, n.pr technique developed by Toshikatsu Yamamoto in which filiform needles are inserted into meridians located on the scalp.

Acupuncture Association of Chartered Physiotherapists, *n.pr* the major British professional association for physiotherapists who incorporate acupuncture into their practices. It is responsible for professional acupuncture accreditation of physiotherapists.

acute, *adj* characterizing a rapid onset of signs or symptoms of short duration.

acute intracranial hemorrhage, *n* severe bleeding inside the skull.

acute myocardial infarction (ə·kyōōt' mī·ō·kar'·dē·əl in·fark'·shən), *n* early stage of heart muscle mortification caused by blockage in a coronary artery.

acute somatic dysfunction, *n* an immediate or short-duration impairment or alteration in function of interrelated parts of the musculoskeletal system.

acyclovir (a'·sī'·klō·vir'), *n* antiviral medication used topically to combat herpes virus types 1 and 2 as well as the varicella zoster and other viruses.

adaptogen (ə·dap´·tə·jen), *n* a substance that helps the body regenerate after being fatigued or stressed.

adaptogenic, *adj* generating a substance that balances the body, particularly when the body is under stress, by either stimulating or relaxing.

adduct, *v* movement toward the center line of the body.

adduction (ə·duk´·shən), *n* joint movement toward the body along the horizontal plane.

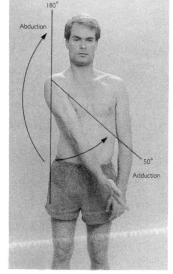

Adduction. (Seidel et al, 1995; Patrick Watson)

A-delta fibers, *n* small myelinated fibers that transmit information to the brain about the emotional effects of tissue damage and pain. In acupuncture, stimulation of the A-delta system is used to inhibit pain transmission.

adenalgia (a·də·nal´·gē·ə), *n* pain or discomfort in any of the glands.

adenectomy (a·də·nek´·tō·mē), *n* the surgical extraction of the andenoid glands.

adenosine diphosphate (ə·de´·nə·sēn dī·fôs´·fāt), *n* the compound produced when adenosine triphosphate (ATP) is hydrolyzed and energy is released. It is also used in the synthesis of ATP. Also called *ADP.*

adenosine triphosphate (ə·de´·nə·sēn trī·fôs´·fāt), *n* the compound that is hydrolyzed to produce the energy necessary for metabolic processes. Also called *ATP.*

ADH, *n.pr* See antidiuretic hormone.

Adhatoda vasica, *n* See vasaka.

ADHD, *n.pr* See disorder, attention deficit hyperactivity.

adhesion, *n* a lumpy scar that forms when at least two layers of soft tissue adhere as a result of trauma, thus interfering with free movement between and within the layers.

adhibhautika (ä·dhē·bhä·ōō·tē´·kə), *n* in Ayurveda, the category of diseases that originate outside the body and that are caused by germs, bacteria, viruses, and accidents or mishaps.

adhidaivika (a·dhē·dä·ē·vē´·kə), *n* in Ayurveda, diseases that cannot be explained and that originate from supernatural sources, including curses, planetary influences, and seasonal changes.

adhyatmika (a·dhyät·mē´·kə), *n* in Ayurveda, the category of diseases that originate within the body and that include hereditary diseases, congenital diseases, and diseases caused by an imbalance of doshas. See also doshas.

adjuvant, *n* a substance that improves the effectiveness of a medicine or enhances the ability to produce an immune response.

adoration, *n* a prayer of worship and praise.

ADR, *n.pr* See adverse drug reaction.

adrenal gland, *n* one of the two organs that secrete cortisol and androgens; located just above the kidneys.

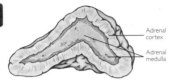

Adrenal gland. (Herlihy and Maebius, 2000)

Labels: Adrenal cortex, Adrenal medulla

adrenaline, *n* See epinephrine.

adrenocorticotropic hormone (ə·drē¯'·nō·kôr'·ti·kō·trō¯'·pik hôr'·mōn), *n* anterior pituitary gland secretion that encourages growth of the adrenal cortex as well as corticosteroid secretion. Increased levels of the hormone occur in response to stress, low cortisol levels, fever, acute hypoglycemia, and major surgery.

adrenoleukodystrophy (ə·drē¯'·nō·lōō'·kō·dis'·trō·fē), *n* rare childhood disease that affects boys; an inherited metabolic disorder in which patients often die within one to five years of diagnosis. Symptoms include cerebral nerve damage, mental decline, apraxia, aphasia, blindness, and quadriplegia.

adriamycin, *n* an antineoplastic agent used in cancer treatment.

adsorption, *n* a process in which gaseous material builds up on the outermost layer of a solid and forms a light film.

ADTA, *n.pr* See American Dance Therapy Association.

adulteration, *n* an accidental or purposeful addition of an impure substance to a product. This results in an alteration of properties and composition of the substance, thereby diminishing its quality.

advanced certified music therapist, *n* music therapists with advanced training and clinical experience, certified by the American Association for Music Therapy. Therapists with this designation are listed on the National Music Therapy Registry.

adverse drug reaction, *n* a detrimental outcome from a drug. Two types of ADRs exist: Type 1 results from dosage mismatch and Type 2

from rare conditions often as a consequence of a small dose. See also risk or sensitive type.

adverse events, *n.pl* the negative, health-diminishing side effects or secondary illnesses that can occur as a result of treatment.

advocate, *n* **1.** in the medical field, a person who focuses on bolstering the patient's role and rights in making decisions about his or her health care. **2.** one who assists another in legal matters; can be a professional or a layperson; may or may not work for a fee.

Aegle marmelos, *n* See bael.

aerobic exercise, *n* sustained repetitive physical activity, such as walking, dancing, cycling, and swimming, that elevates the heart rate and increases oxygen consumption resulting in improved functioning of cardiovascular and respiratory systems.

aerobic respiration, *n* an energy-yielding cellular process that efficiently breaks down glucose molecules by combining oxygen with hydrogen ions to produce large amounts of ATP and carbon dioxide.

Aesculus california, *n* See horse chestnut.

Aesculus glabra, *n* See horse chestnut.

Aesculus hippocastanum, *n* See horse chestnut.

aesthenic states (es·the¯'·nik stāts'), *n.pl* in medical acupuncture, a loose categorization for premorbid medical conditions. These dysfunctions typically are seen by conventional medicine practitioners but have not been associated with a definitive laboratory finding or diagnosis. Specifically, medical conditions fitting into this category will be indicated by a vague definition of fatigue, a mild form of depression, a myofascial indication related to stress or a disturbance in function. Circulating the appropriate amount of energy through the body is thought to treat successfully these types of conditions.

affirmation, *n* **1.** in psychotherapy, reflection on one's positive qualities when confronted with a challenge to self-esteem. **2.** a verbal component of yoga practice in which positive words are spoken by an instructor in order to assist an individual to leave behind subconscious negativity.

African trypanosomiasis (a·ˈfri·kən tri·paˈˈnə·sə·mīˈ·sis), *n.pr* parasite-induced blood and neurological disease contracted by the tsetse fly bite. Often fatal if not treated.

agammaglobulinemia (āˈ·gaˈ·mə·glôˈ·byəⁿ·ⁿnēˈ·mē·ə), *n* condition in which the serum immunoglobulin gamma globulin is absent, thus increasing risk of infection. Can be fleeting, hereditary, or acquired.

agar (ə·ˈgär'), *n* Latin names: *Gelidium cartilagineum, Gracilaria confervoides;* part used: thallus; uses: laxative, neonatal hyperbilirubinemia (debated); precautions: pregnancy, lactation, children, can cause coma, gastrointestinal blockage, weakens the body's ability to absorb minerals and vitamins. Also called *agar-agar, Chinese gelatin, colle du japon, E406, gelose, Japanese gelatin, Japanese isinglass, layer carang,* or *vegetable gelatin.*

Agency for Healthcare Research and Quality, *n.pr* formerly known as the Agency for Health Care Policy and Research, this agency researches the quality of medical care and health services.

agent, pathogenic, *n* any substance or condition that causes disease, including genetic defects, negative emotional states, toxins, and others.

aggravating factors, *n.pl* postures or movements that produce or intensify the symptoms of a patient and are used to establish the severity, irritability, and nature of the condition.

aggravation, *n* in homeopathy, a healing reaction induced by therapeutic stimulation.

aggressive, *adj* in Chinese medicine, pertaining to behavior associated with hot energy, excess energy, and restlessness. This may be a normal aspect of a person's character, or it may indicate an illness or imbalance. See also energy, hot.

agnis (əg·ˈnēs'), *n.pl* in Ayurveda, the elements that aid digestion. There are 13 types of agnis: five bhutagnis, which metabolize the five mahabhutas; seven dhatu agnis, which aid in tissue metabolism; and jatharagni, responsible for primary metabolism of food. See also mahabhutas and dhatus.

agonist (a·ˈgə·nist), *n* a muscle that, upon contraction, is balanced by the contraction of a different muscle. Also called *prime mover.*

agranulocytes, *n.pl* white blood cells with no cytoplasmic granules, including lymphocytes and monocytes.

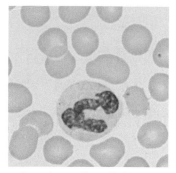

Agranulocyte. (Carr and Rodak, 1999)

agreement, *n* consent of two parties to a binding contract. If one party desires to change the contract, an agreement must be obtained from the other party in order to proceed.

Agrimonia eupatoria, *n* See agrimony.

Agrimonia japonica, *n* See agrimony.

Agrimonia pilosa var., *n* See agrimony.

agrimony, *n* Latin names: *Agrimonia eupatoria, Agrimonia pilosa* var., *Agrimonia japonica;* parts used: stems, leaves, buds; uses: hemostatic, sore throat, cuts, abrasions, cancer, (other claims: antiasthmatic, antiinflammatory, sedative, decongestant, diuretic); precautions: pregnancy, lactation, children, can cause flushing, palpitations, rash, photosensitivity, and photodermatitis. Also called *church steeples, cocklebur, langya-*

A

cao, liverwort, longyacao, philanthropos, potter's piletabs, sticklewort, or *stickwort.*

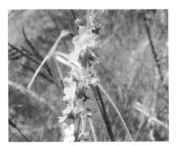

Agrimony. (Scott and Barlow, 2003)

Agropyron repens, *n* See couchgrass.

ahamkara (ä·häm'·kä·rə), *n* in Sanskrit, egotism or pride.

AHCPR, *n.pr* See Agency for Healthcare Research and Quality.

AHI, *n.pr* See Aviation Health Institute.

AHNA Holistic Nurse Certification Program, *n.pr* an educational curriculum established by the American Holistic Nursing Association (AHNA) that provides credentialing for nurses in holistic practice. The course of study is divided into four parts, and components of the course include learning about caring-healing modalities and holistic nursing. See also American Holistic Nursing Association.

AHRQ, *n.pr* See Agency for Healthcare Research and Quality.

ai ye (ä·ē yē), *n* Chinese name for the plant *Artemesia vulgaris,* the leaves of which are used in moxibustion to affect movement of qi in the body. See also moxibustion and qi.

AIDS (ādz), *n.pr* See syndrome, acquired immune deficiency.

AIH, *n.pr* See American Institute of Homeopathy.

AIS, *n* active isolated stretching; a sequence of stretching exercises that encourages flexibility by combining active stretching and reciprocal inhibition (RI) methods. The movements are performed repetitively until adequate progress has been made.

Unlike muscle energy techniques, these exercises do not make use of the numerous benefits of postisometric relaxation (PIR). See also MET and PIR.

Aje-Mutin trap (ä'·jā-mōō'·tēn trap'), *n* the difficulty in recognition of adverse reactions to herbal medicines because they are uncommon, develop gradually, or have an extended latency period.

ajowan (ä·jō'·wän), *n* Latin name: *Trachyspermum ammi;* parts used: seeds, oil; uses: in Ayurveda promotes pitta dosha and pacifies vata and kapaha doshas (pungent, bitter, light, dry, sharp), hypotensive, insecticide, molluscicide, antifungal, antibacterial, inhibits hepatitis C virus; seeds: carminative, stimulant, antispasmodic, flatulence, sore throats, bronchitis, decongestant, colds, coughs, influenza, rheumatism; oil: stomach ache, liver tonic, cholera, antiseptic, pain relief; precautions: pregnancy, membrane irritant. Also called *agnivardhana, ajwain, bishop's weed, omum,* or *yavanika.*

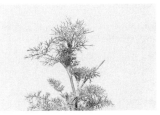

Ajowan. (Williamson, 2002)

AK, *n.pr* See applied kinesiology.

akasha (ä'·kä·shä), *n* in Ayurveda, space, which is one of the mahabhutas. See also mahabhutas.

akashi (ä·kä·shē), *n* a Japanese term for an acupuncture diagnosis achieved by thoroughly examining and interviewing a patient.

al kohl (äl kōl'), *n* a traditional preparation originating from Kuwait; used for cosmetic purposes and to provide strength and protection for the eyes from disease. Available in a black or gray powder, it is applied to the inner surface of the eyelid. There have been reports of lead poisoning from using al kohl. Also called *Kohl.* See also surma.

ALA, *n.pr* See acid, alpha-linolenic.

albinism, *n* hereditary condition present at birth in which the skin partially or totally lacks melanin.

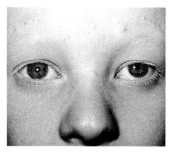

Albinism. (Zitelli and Davis, 1997)

Alchemilla mollis, *n* See lady's mantle.

Alchemilla vulgaris, *n* See lady's mantle.

alcohol, *n* a chemical compound formed when a hydroxyl radical connects to an aliphatic chain carbon, thus replacing a hydrogen molecule. Has the basic formula $C_nH_{2n+1}OH$. Ethanol and methanol are examples of alcohols.

alcohols, terpenic **(tur·pe´·nik al´·kə·hôlz´),** *n.pl* compounds consisting of terpene chains attached to hydroxyl groups, may exist as monoterpenols, diterpenols, or sesquiterpenols. Responsible for the gentle floral smells of certain essential oils. See also diterpenols, monoterpenols, and sesquiterpenols.

Alcoholics Anonymous (AA), *n.pr* a 12-step program designed to assist those addicted to alcohol; participants aim to achieve and maintain sobriety through personal and group accountability relationships.

alcoholism, *n* a chronic condition characterized by dependence on

alcohol, often accompanied by its behavioral and health consequences.

ALD, *n.pr* See adrenoleukodystrophy.

aldehyde, *n* hydrocarbon characterized by strong scent; antiviral, antiinflammatory, and soothing properties. Can irritate skin if administered improperly.

Aldehyde. (Clarke, 2002)

alder buckthorn, *n* Latin name: *Rhamnus frangula;* parts used: fruit, bark; uses: laxative; precautions: pregnancy; lactation; children; individuals with colitis, irritable bowel syndrome, abdominal pain, or gastrointestinal bleeding.

aldosterone (al·dôs´·tə·rōn), *n* an adrenal hormone that causes elevation of blood pressure through the retention of sodium and the resultant increase in blood plasma volume.

alfalfa, *n* Latin name: *Medicago sativa* L.; parts used: buds, seeds (budding), entire plant; uses: diuretic, stomach disorders, arthritis, increase blood clotting, treat boils and bites; precautions: pregnancy, patients with lupus erythematosus; can cause hypotension, photosensitivity, and bleeding. Also called *buffalo herb, lucerne, purple medic,* or *purple medick.*

algal polysaccharides, *n.pl* noncellulose polysaccharides that are found in food additives and provide dietary fiber. These include algin, agar, and carrageenan.

algometer (al·gô´·mə·ter), *n* tool used to determine the minimum amount of pressure required to locate and reproduce an area of discomfort in a patient's body. Helpful in training practitioners in the correct methods of applying pressure. Also called *pressure meter.*

algotomes (al´·gō·tōmz), *n.pl* areas to which pain from particular trigger points is consistently referred.

aliphatic chains, *n.pl* hydrocarbons consisting of two to four isoprene units that are joined together from top to bottom. See also isoprene.

alkali, *n* a compound able to form hydroxyl ions (OH) when dissolved in aqueous solutions. See also base.

alkaloids, *n* alkaline phytochemicals that contain nitrogen in a heterocyclic ring structure. They can have powerful pharmacological effects and are more often used in traditional medicine than in herbal treatments.

alkane (al'·kān'), *n* water-insoluble, saturated hydrocarbon compound, with the general chemical formula C_nH_{2n+2}. Hexane (C_6H_{14}) is used in the solvent extraction or enfleurage process. See also enfleurage.

alkene (al'·kēn'), *n* unsaturated hydrocarbon compound that has double covalent bonds with C_nH_{2n} as the general chemical formula. Terpenes, found in essential oils, are members of this functional group.

alkylglycerols (al·kəl·gli·ser·ôlz), *n.pl* biological compounds mostly derived from shark liver oil. May inhibit bacterial growth, promote blood cell production, and counteract radiation damage.

alkyne (al'·kīn'), *n* unsaturated hydrocarbon compound that has triple covalent bonds and C_nH_{2n-2} as the general chemical formula. This functional group is not common in components of essential oils.

ALL, *n.pr* See leukemia, acute lymphocytic.

allelopathy (əl·lē'·lə·pa·thē), *n* the system of natural defenses that protects one plant species from others around it.

allergen, *n* allergy-producing foreign substance.

allergenic load, *n* an individual's total allergic or chemical burden from exposure. Also called *allergen load.*

allergic reaction, *n* aggravated immune system response to a variety of environmental and other substances, both chemical or organic. Reactions may be mild to life-threatening and include urticaria, eczema, dyspnea, bronchospasm, diar-

rhea, rhinitis, sinusitis, laryngospasm, and anaphlaxis.

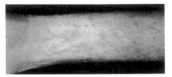

Allergic reaction. (Goldstein and Goldstein, 1997)

allergic threshold, *n* an individual's level of tolerance to allergens.

allergode (a'·lur·gōd), *n* a homeopathic preparation created from an allergen. See also isopathy.

allersodes (al'·ler·sōdz), *n.pl* in homeopathy, highly diluted formulations of antigens that are used to induce an immune response.

allicin (al'·lə·sin), *n* an active ingredient in garlic, thought to lower blood pressure.

allied health, *n* the domain of medical practices that support medical professionals.

Allium sativum, *n* See garlic.

All My Relations (äl' mī' rē·lā'·shə nz), *n.pr* an expression that asserts the basic philosophy of many Native Americans, according to which plants, stones, two-leggeds, animals, sky, earth, moon, spirit helpers, ancestors and—most significantly—the Great Spirit are related; good health results from harmony between all beings.

allodynia (al'·lō·dī'·nē·ə), *n* a condition in which pain arises from a stimulus that would not normally be experienced as painful.

allopathy (al'·lō·pa'·thē), *n* method of medical treatment in which drugs are administered to antagonize the disease.

all-or-none response, *n* the threshold response of each particular nerve cell and muscle fiber to a stimulus. A nerve cell will fire completely or not at all, and a muscle fiber will contract to its limit with a stimulus; both rest fully in the absence of stimulus.

allspice, *n* Latin names: *Pimento offic-inalis, Eugenia pimenta;* parts used: berries (dried, unripened), fruit (powdered); uses: gas, muscle aches, indigestion, toothaches; precautions: pregnancy; lactation; children; patients with colon disease, cancer, irritable bowel syndrome, Crohn's disease, diverticulitis. Also called *clove pepper, Jamaica pepper,* or *pimento.*

Alocasia macrorrhiza (al·ō·kā'·shə ma·krō·rī'·zə), *n* part used: root; uses: topical rubefacient; precautions: if taken internally—numbness and pain in throat, abdominal pain, nausea, vomiting. Also called *ape, cunjevoi, giant alocasia, giant taro, pai, alocasie, alokasie, mankachu* and *malanga.*

aloe, *n* Latin names: *Aloe vera* L., *Aloe perryi, Aloe barbadensis* Miller, *Aloe ferox, Aloe spicata;* parts used: leaves, secretory cells; uses: laxative, minor burns, sunburn, cuts, acne, stomatitis, (dried aloe juice currently under research: diabetes, HIV, cancer, ulcers, colon disease, bleeding, asthma, cold), precautions: (dried aloe juice) pregnancy; lactation; children younger than age 12; patients with renal disease, heart disease, or stomach blockage; not to be used topically by those hypersensitive to garlic, onions, or tulips; not for deep lacerations; can cause irreversible intestinal lining damage, hemorrhagic diarrhea, red urine, nephrotoxicity, contact dermatitis. Also called *Barbados, aloe, burn plant, Cape aloe, Curacao aloe, elephant's gall, hsiang-dan, lily of the desert, lu-hai,*

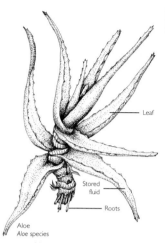

Aloe
Aloe species

Aloe. (Skidmore-Roth, 2004)

socotrine aloe, Venezuela aloe, and *Zanzibar aloe.*

Aloe ferox, *n* See aloe.

Aloe perryi, *n* See aloe.

Aloe spicata, *n* See aloe.

aloetic (al'·ō·et'·ik), *adj* containing or relating to aloe.

aloin (al'·ō·in), *n* an extract of aloe that consists of several active chemical components, primarily barbaloin, and has cathartic properties. See also barbaloin.

alopecia (a'·lə·pē'·shə), *n* Partial or total hair loss caused by a number of possible factors, including old age, drug reaction, endocrine disorder, skin disease, or cancer treatment.

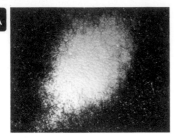

Alopecia. areata. (Courtesy Stephen B. Tucker; Thompson, 2002)

alpha, *n* a Greek letter symbolized by α. See also Greek letters.

alterative, *n* a class of herbs with several different but related functions. In the 19th century, alteratives were understood as *blood purifiers*. Alteratives are currently used to promote lymphatic flow and to stimulate the detoxifying functions of the liver.

altered states of consciousness, *n.pl* the various states in which the mind can be aware but is not in its usual wakeful condition, such as during hypnosis, meditation, hallucination, trance, and the dream stage. See also alternative states of consciousness.

alternate nostril breathing, *n* See nadi shodhanam and pranayama.

alternative states of consciousness, *n.pl* states of consciousness whose form and/or content are primarily determined through factors different from normal waking awareness. Includes those states of consciousness engendered through dreams, meditation, use of mind-altering substances, or mystical/transpersonal experience. The use of "alternative" connotes a nonnormative approach to waking consciousness. Also called *ASC.* See also altered states of consciousness.

ALTEs, *n.pr* See apparent life-threatening events.

Althaea officinalis, *n* See marshmallow.

aluminum, *n* toxic metal sometimes found in drinking water, medications, and cookware.

alveolar, *adj* pertaining to the air sacs where gases are exchanged during the process of respiration.

alzoon (al·zōōn'), *n* concoction of herbs used mostly in Switzerland for supportive measures in treating cancer. Juniper, ferns, dandelions, and other plants suffused with ultraviolet light and oxygen have shown some effectiveness in improving how the patient feels as well as in increasing apetite.

AMA, *n.pr* See American Medical Association.

amarga cascara (ä·mär'·gə kas·kär'·ə) *n* Latin name: *Sweetia panamensis*; part used: bark; uses: tonic; contradictions: none known. Also known as *guayacan corriente, huesillo, huesito, malvecino, rejo, vera de agua, visapolollo, almendra, balsamo amarillo, balsamo oloroso,* and *carboncillo.*

amaroid (a'·mə·roid), *n* any of a class of chemical constituents found in some bitter-tasting vegetables; stimulates the production of gastric fluid and saliva.

amautas (ä·mä·ōō'·täs), *n.pl* See yatiris.

amavata (ä·mä·vä'·tə) *n* in Ayurveda, arthritis; caused by an imbalance of vata dosha, which leads to accumulation of ama in the joints. See also vata and ama.

amaya (ä·mä'·yə), *n* in Ayurveda, a synonym for *disease,* which means "caused by ama." See also ama.

ambulatory blood pressure monitoring, *n* measurement of a patient's blood pressure at regular intervals while the patient carries out daily activities.

amebiasis (a·me·bī'·ə·sis), *n* intestinal infection caused by fecally contaminated food or water that contains the pathogenic protozoan *Entamoeba histolytica.* Symptoms range from absent to severe; infants and elderly most at risk if infected. Treated with amebicides, such as iodoquinole and paromycin.

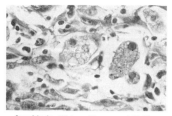

Amebiasis. (Cotran, Kumar, and Collins, 1999)

amelia (ə·mē·lē·ə), *n* **1.** missing a limb, or limbs. **2.** psychotic symptom characterized by extreme indifference or apathy in certain mental illnesses.

American Academy of Family Physicians, *n.pr* a national medical organization established in 1947 to promote the practice of family medicine.

American Academy of Medical Acupuncture (AAMA), *n.pr* U.S. organization of practicing acupuncturists who hold medical degrees. Membership requirements include two hundred and twenty hours of academy-approved training and two years of practical acupuncture experience.

American Art Therapy Association, *n.pr* a national organization of professionals who believe that creative process involved in the making of art can help heal and enhance the quality of life.

American Association of Naturopathic Physicians, *n.pr* an organization founded in 1905 that serves as the professional society representing naturopathic practitioners. The group promotes the development of the Naturopathic Physicians Licensing Examination (NPLEx), recognizes needs for research within the profession, develops professional standards for practicing naturopathic medicine, and promotes the development and progression of naturopathy. On a quarterly basis, it publishes the newsletter *The Naturopathic Physician.* Also called *AANP.* See also NPLEx.

American Association of Oriental Medicine (AAOM), *n.pr* umbrella organization of American professional acupuncturists founded in 1981 as the American Association of Acupuncture and Oriental Medicine (AAAOM). Assisted in establishing educational and professional standards for the practice of acupuncture and oriental medicine in the U.S.

American Board of Hypnosis in Dentistry, *n.pr* a professional organization that assesses and certifies practitioners' level of competence in dental hypnosis.

American Board of Medical Hypnosis, *n.pr* a professional organization that assesses and certifies practitioners' level of competence in medical hypnosis.

American Board of Psychological Hypnosis, *n.pr* a professional organization that assesses and certifies practitioners' level of competence in either experimental or clinical hypnosis. Recognized by the American Psychological Association (APA). Also called *ABPH.*

American Botanical Council, *n.pr* a nonprofit educational and research organization that provides information and promotes the safe and effective use of medicinal plants and phytomedicines. Also called *ABC.*

American Cancer Society, *n.pr* established in 1913, this national volunteer-based health organization is committed to the elimination of cancer through prevention and treatment and to diminishing cancer suffering through advocacy, scholarship, research, and ministration.

American Chiropractic Association, *n.pr* professional organization established in 1922 to represent doctors of chiropractic and to maintain, promote, and protect chiropractic as a healing profession.

American Dance Therapy Association, *n.pr* a national organization of professionals with training in dance and movement therapy, the goal of which is to use movement for therapeutic use that enhances the physical, cognitive, and social integration of an individual.

A

American hellebore, *n.pr* Latin name: *Veratrum viride* parts used: rhizomes (dried), roots; uses: anticonvulsant, pneumonia, nerve pain, (under research: myasthenia gravis, hypertensive crisis, hypertension caused by pregnancy); precautions: pregnancy, lactation, children, patients with heart disorders; can cause hypertension, hypotension, bradycardia, arrthythmias, dizziness, paresthesia, convulsions, nausea, stomach cramps, hampered breathing, diarrhea, burning throat, coma, paralysis. Also called *false hellebore, green hellebore, Indian poke, itchweed,* and *swamp hellebore.*

American Holistic Medical Association, Founded in 1978, the AHMA's mission is to support practitioners in their personal and professional development as healers and to educate physicians about holistic medicine.

American Holistic Nursing Association (ə·mer´·i·kən hō·li´·stik ner´·sing əsō´·sē·ā´·shən), *n. pr* an organization founded in 1981 that promotes the development and progression of holistic nursing. It focuses on holistic principles associated with preventive education and health as well as integrating complementary and alternative medicine with concepts of allopathic medicine to provide healing. The *AHNA Standards of Holistic Nursing* defines and determines the scope of holistic practices. Other key publications includes the *Journal of Holistic Nursing, The American Holistic Nurses' Association Core Curriculum for Holistic Nursing* and the *IPAKHN (Inventory of Professional Activities and Knowledge Statements of a Holistic Nurse) Survey.* Also called *AHNA.*

American Institute of Homeopathy, *n.pr* founded in 1844 in the United States for physicians practicing homeopathy and to enhance and restructure the material medica. The AMA was formed the next year partially in response to this organization. See also Flexner report.

American Medical Association, *n.pr* the largest organization of medical professionals made up of U.S. licensed physicians. Missions include the advancement of its members' professional concerns; advising the U.S. government on drug policy and healthcare legislation; and publishing journals with the latest medical, social, and economic studies.

American Medical Association Council on Scientific Affairs, *n.pr* committee of the American Medical Association that provides information and recommendations on medical and public health issues.

American Medical Student Association, *n.pr* the largest independent organization of medical students in the United States. Local and national initiatives led by this group involve medical education, patient and student advocacy, health policy, public health, and global health. The organization also acts as an advocate for humanistic, complementary, and alternative medicine education. Also called *AMSA.*

American Music Therapy Association, *n.pr* a national association of professionals who integrate music with conventional healing practices for therapeutic benefits.

American naprapathy (ə·mer´·ə·kən nə·pra·pə·the), *n* manual therapy that focuses on evaluation and treatment of neuromusculoskeletal disorders.

American Nurses Association, *n.pr* professional organization of registered nurses created to encourage high standards in nursing care, promote nursing as a profession, and lobby Congress for issues of concern to nurses.

American Osteopathic Association, *n.pr* an organization that promotes the development and progression of osteopathic medicine and serves as a professional society for osteopathic practitioners within the United States. It also provides accreditation for Colleges of Osteopathic Medicine, osteopathic internship and residency programs, and healthcare facilities. The organization annually publishes the comprehensive

Glossary of Osteopathic Terminology. Also called *AOA.*

American Society for Clinical Nutrition, *n.pr* a division of the American Society for Nutritional Sciences, the ASCN works to provide and implement educational and training programs for health professionals and students in the area of clinical nutrition. It provides support for current and ongoing research activities related to human nutrition. It also acts as an advocate for issues related to clinical nutrition and research, and promotes the professional use of nutrition science in disease prevention, health promotion, and patient care. The organization also publishes the *American Journal of Clinical Nutrition* monthly. Also called *ASCN.*

American Society of Clinical Hypnosis, *n.pr* Founded in 1957 by Milton H. Erickson, M.D., an organization that supports development of hypnosis as a clinical therapeutic approach. It establishes codes of ethics that define and limit persons who are eligible to learn hypnosis. It also serves as a professional society for practitioners who use clinical hypnosis, including psychiatrists, psychologists, marriage and family therapists, mental health counselors, clinical social workers, medical doctors, dentists, and nurses. Also called *ASCH.*

AMI, *n.pr* See acute myocardial infarction.

amino acid conjugation, *n* a phase II detoxification pathway that occurs in the liver in which amino acids including arginine, glutamine, glycine, ornithine, and taurine, combine with toxins and other substances.

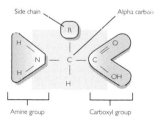

Amino acids. (Mosby's Medical, Nursing & Allied Health Dictionary, ed 6, 2002)

AML, *n.pr* See leukemia, acute myelocytic.

amla (äm´·lə), *n* Latin name: *Phyllanthus emblica;* parts used: fruit, flowers, leaves, root bark, seeds; uses: in Ayurveda—pacifies tridosha (heavy, dry), ingredient in triphala, hypolipidemic, antiviral, immunomodulator, hepatoprotection, antioxidant, antimicrobial; fruit—tonic, constipation, headache, diabetes, anxiety, memory; leaves—conjunctivitis, bronchitis; precautions: none known. Also called *amalaki, amlaki* or *Emblica officinalis.* See also triphala.

amlaki, *n* See amla.

Ammi majus **(äm´·mē mä´·jəs),** *n* part used: seeds; uses: prevent fertilization in females, diuretic, tonic, calm digestive system, angina, asthma, toothache, psoriasis, vitiligo; precautions: dizziness, nausea, headache, appetite loss, sleeping disorders, and pruritus. Also called *bishop's weed, akkerscherm, ameo bastardo, ameus, ammi commun, bishop's flower, bishopsweed, bullwort, false queen's anne lace, ghurair, groot akkerscherm, grosse knoropelmohre, khillah, laceflower, large bullwort, rindomolo,* and *toothpick ammi.*

Ammi visnaga, n See khella.

Ammi visnaga **(äm´·mē viz·nä´·gə),** *n* part used: seeds; uses: asthma, diuretic, litholytic, vasodilator, relieve pain associated with kidney stones, spasmolytic, angina, coronary arteriosclerosis; precautions: dermatitis, phototoxic reactions. Also called *anmi, bishop's flower, bisnaga das searas, biznaga, busnaga, fijn akkerscherm, greater ammi, khaizaran, khellakraut, khillah, pick tooth, toothpickweed, visnaga,* and *viznaga.*

amnesia, *n* memory loss; may be due to brain trauma, acute emotional distress, stroke, or other causes.

amnesia, sensorimotor, n concept explored in the Feldenkrais method in which students lie on the floor and scan their own bodies, discovering disconnections in terms of kinesthetic linking. See also method, Feldenkrais.

amniocentesis (am´·nē·ō·sen·tē´·sis), *n* procedure in obstetrics in which a needle is inserted into a pregnant woman's uterus in order to draw out a sample of amniotic fluid for laboratory analysis. Often used in older mothers to detect possible birth defects before birth.

amnion (am'·nē·ən), *n* membrane covering the placenta on the side that faces the fetus; also forms the outer layer of the umbilical cord.

Amorphophallus konjac, *n* See glucomannan.

Ampuku (äm·pōō·kōō), *n.pr* a form of abdominal massage developed in Japan from Chinese sources, in which palpation of the abdomen (hara) is used for both the diagnosis and treatment of health complaints. Also called *Japanese abdominal massage.*

amputation, *n* the removal of all or part of a limb through surgical means.

amrit kalash (əm·rit kä·ləsh), *n* in Ayurveda, a food supplement and rasayana based on an ancient recipe that comprises over 24 fruits and herbs. The formula used within Maharishi Ayurveda, Maharishi amrit kalash, consists of a fruit and herb paste called *nectar* and herbal tablets called *ambrosia*. Also called *amrit* or *chywanprash*. See also rasayana.

amrita (äm'·rë·tä), *n* Latin name: *Tinospora cordifolia*; parts used: stem, roots, leaves; uses: in Ayurveda pacifies tridosha (bitter, astringent, heavy, oily), antiallergic, anticancer, antineoplastic, antioxidant, antistress, antiulcer, immunomodulator, hepatoprotective, hypoglycemic, leprosy, tonic, stimulant, diuretic, stomachic, asthma, fever, jaundice, inflammation, sores, rheumatism, tuberculosis, liver conditions, malaria; leaves: gout; roots: emetic; precautions: nausea with large doses. Also called *gulancha tinospora guluchi* or *guruchi*.

AMTA, *n* See American Music Therapy Association.

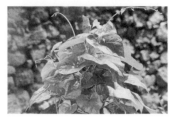

Amrita. (Williamson, 2002)

amygdala (ə·mig'·də·lə), *n* a key component of the limbic system in the brain, involved in the experience of anxiety, distress, and fear.

amygdalin (ə·mig'·də·lin), *n* drug derived from fruit pits and used as an anticancer medication under the name Laetrile. See also laetrile.

amyloidosis (a'·mə·loi'·dō'·sis), *n* disease of unknown origin in which a waxlike, sticky, glycoprotein (amyloid) collects in organs and tissues, thus inhibiting normal function.

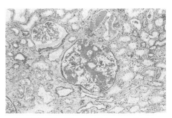

Amyloidosis. (Kumar, Cotran, and Robbins, 1997)

amyotrophic lateral sclerosis (ā·mī·ə·trō·fik la'·tə·rəl sklə·rō'·sis), *n* a fatal neurological condition in which the motor neurons in the anterior horns of the spinal cord and the corticospinal tracts degenerate, leading to weakness, muscle atrophy, and death, usually in 2 to 5 years. There is no known cure. Also called *Lou Gehrig's disease* or *wasting palsy*.

ANA, *n.pr* See American Nurses Association.

anabolism (ə·na·ˈbə·li·ˈzəm), *n* constructive metabolism in which complex substances are synthesized from simple ones.

anaerobic exercise, *n* physical activity, which instigates a metabolism that does not depend on oxygen. Examples include isotonics, in which the muscles contract against an object of resistance with movement (e.g., weight lifting); isometrics, in which muscles contract against resistance but without movement; and calisthenics (e.g., sit-ups and knee-bends), which increase flexibility and improve joint mobility.

anaerobic respiration, *n* a cellular process that occurs in the absence of free oxygen to partially break down glucose molecules and provide a small net gain of ATP.

anaerobic threshold (an·ˈə·rō·ˈbik thresh·ˈhōld), *n* at increasing speeds or intensity levels, the point above which the muscles derive their energy from nonoxygenic rather than oxygenic sources during exercise. The body can only operate above this threshold for a short period of time, such as when sprinting, before lactic acid builds up in the muscles.

analgesic, *adj* **I.** pain relieving. *n* **2.** medication used to manage mild to moderate pain, usually by acting on the central nervous system.

analysis, *n* the process of identifying a substance's composition. May include chromatography, mass spectrometry, infrared spectroscopy, optical rotation, specific gravity, and refractive index. See also qualitative analysis and quantitative analysis.

analysis, behavioral, *n* in behavioral medicine, the study of an association between an individual's behavior and the environmental conditions that influence the behavior and actions.

analysis, case, *n* **I.** procedure for recommending case management options. **2.** method for selecting the optimal homeopathic remedy; considers the evolution and set of symptoms involved in the course of the disease.

See also anamnesis, case taking, and patient history.

analysis, evidence–based, *n* critical analysis and appraisal of published research studies, using systematic, predefined criteria and approaches.

analysis, hair mineral, *n* an analysis of the mineral content of hair; used to assess metabolic disorders and mineral toxicity or deficiencies.

analysis, instrumental (in·ˈstrə·men·ˈtəl ə·nal·ˈ·ə·sis), *n* use of a device, such as a mass spectrometer or gas chromatograph, for chemical analysis.

analysis, intention-to-treat, *n* analysis of the data obtained from an investigational method that includes all the participants involved in the study from the beginning. This prevents bias caused by participants dropping out of the study.

analysis, Laban movement, *n* diagnostic measure in dance/movement therapy.

analysis, qualitative, *n* **I.** method for evaluating qualitative, rather than quantitative data, making it more amenable to assessment and communication. **2.** identification of the components that make up a substance.

analysis, quantitative, *n* **I.** method for evaluating data using a system of numerical measurement. **2.** measurement of the amounts of specific components that constitute a substance.

anamnesis (a·nam·nē·ˈsəs), *n* **I.** the historical circumstances of a patient's illness from a personal perspective. **2.** the practice of acquiring a patient's description of the course of illness. See also case-taking.

Ananas comosus, *n* See pineapple.

ananda (ä·nän·ˈdə), *n* Sanskrit term for bliss, an aspect of pure consciousness.

anaphrodisiac, *adj/n* a substance that tends to lessen sexual desire.

anatomic position, *n* a reference posture of the human body, in which the anterior view of the human body is shown standing with legs slightly apart, feet forward, palms facing forward.

A

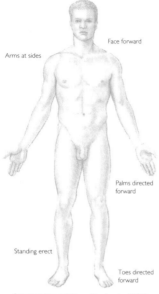

Face forward

Arms at sides

Palms directed forward

Standing erect

Toes directed forward

Anatomic position. (Applegate, 2000)

anatomical end range, *n* the distance a joint can be moved from the passive end range before the ligaments of the joint tear. The third of the three barriers that end joint movement. Also called *paraphysiologic joint space.*

anatomy, *n* **1.** the study of the structure and parts of the body. **2.** in chiropractic, a component of the vertebral subluxation complex that refers to the specific structural implications present when subluxation has occurred.

anatomy trains, *n.pl* lines of bone and connective tissue that run throughout the body, organize the structural forces required for motion, and link all parts of the body. May act as conduits for acupuncture stimulation and other energetic modalities.

androgens (an'·drə·jenz), *n.pl* hormones produced in the adrenal cortex

that maintain secondary male characteristics.

Andrographis paniculata, *n* See kalmegh.

andrographolide (an'·drō·gra'·fə·līd), *n* the primary component of a traditional medicinal herb, *Andrographis paniculata,* found in Asia and India. It has been used in traditional Chinese and Indian medicine to treat a variety of viral infections and has been found to have an inhibitory effect on HIV. See also *Andrographis paniculata.*

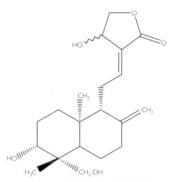

Andrographolide. (Standish, 2002)

androstenedione (an'·drō·ste'·nə·dī'·ōn), *n* a biochemical precursor to both estrogen and testosterone. Used as a dietary supplement because it is believed to boost testosterone levels and claimed to increase athletic performance and muscle mass. It increases estrogen levels more than testosterone, may interfere with hormone levels, and may heighten the risk of hormone-sensitive cancers or cancers of the liver.

anecdotal evidence, *n* information obtained from personal accounts, examples, and observations. Usually not considered scientifically valid but may indicate areas for further investigation and research.

anecdotal health reports (a'·nik·dō'·təl helth'·rəpōrts'), *n.pl* information about the usefulness of a health intervention based on impressionistic experience or personal history.

anecdote, *n* in medicine, an interesting fact or story, typically unpublished, about a treatment or healing modality.

anemia, *n* condition marked by low hemoglobin levels in the blood; below 12–16 g/dL for women and below 13.5–18 g/dL for men.

anemia, megaloblastic **(meg'·ə·lō·blas'·tik ə·nē'·mē·ə),** *n* a disorder of blood characterized by large, nonfunctioning, immature red blood cells in the bone marrow known as megaloblasts; typically associated with folic acid deficiency anemia or pernicious anemia.

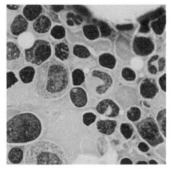

Anemia, megaloblastic. (Carr and Rodak, 1999)

Anemone pulsatilla, *n* See pulsatilla.

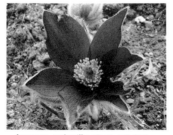

Anemone pulsatilla. (Scott and Barlow, 2003)

anesthesia, *n* absence of physical sensation, particularly pain. May occur from trauma, mental illness, with acupuncture and hypnosis, by topical, regional, local, or general drug applications.

Anethum graveolens, *n* See dill.

aneurysm (an·yə·ri'·zəm), *n* bulging area of a blood vessel wall caused by weakness, or thinning in the wall's structure.

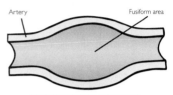

True fusiform abdominal aortic aneurysm

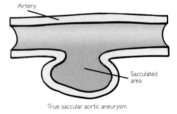

True saccular aortic aneurysm

Aneurysm. (Lewis, Heitkemper, and Dirksen, 2000)

angelica, *n* Latin names: *Angelica sinensis, Angelica acutiloba, Angelica archangelica, Angelica atropurpurea, Angelica dahurica, Angelica edulis, Angelica gigas, Angelica keiskei, Angelica koreana, Angelica polymorpha, Angelica pubescens, Angelica radix;* parts used: entire plant, fruit, roots, seeds; uses: antiseptic, expectorant, diuretic, antispasmodic, cholagogue, circulation aid, stomach cancer, bronchitis, epidermal maladies, headaches, back pain, asthma, allergies, osteoporosis; precautions: pregnancy; patients with diabetes, ulcers, liver disease, or bleeding disorders; can cause hypotension, anorexia, gas, dyspepsia, photosensitivity, photodermatitis, phototoxicity. See also dong quai.

angelica, Chinese (chī'·nës an·je'·li·kə), *n* Latin name: *Angelica sinensis;* part used: oils taken out of roots; uses: relaxes blood vessels, heart rate regulation, malaria, changes urine process, gynecological conditions, circulation problems; precautions: bleeding, sensitivity to light, interaction with anticlotting drugs. Also called *dong quai.*

Angelica acutiloba, *n* See angelica.

Angelica archangelica, *n* See angelica.

Angelica atropurpurea, *n* See angelica.

Angelica dahurica, *n* See angelica.

Angelica edulis, *n* See angelica.

Angelica gigas, *n* See angelica.

Angelica keiskei, *n* See angelica.

Angelica koreana, *n* See angelica.

Angelica polymorphia var. sinesis, *n* See dong quai and angelica.

Angelica pubescens, *n* See angelica.

Angelica radix, *n* See angelica.

Angelica sinensis, *n* See angelica.

angina (an·jī'·nə), *n* heart pain characterized by spasm, cramping, pressure, or choking.

angina pectoris (an·jī'·nə pek·tōr'·is), *n* chest pain, often caused by myocardial anoxia and arterial constriction.

angiogenesis (an'·jē·ō·je'·nə·sis), *n* the formation and growth of new blood vessels.

angiology (an·jē·ô'·l ə·jē), *n* the branch of anatomical study that focuses on the blood and lymph vessels.

angioma (an·jē·ō'·m ə), *n* benign tumor that contains blood or lymph vessels; some disappear with no treatment; most are congenital.

angiotensin-converting enzyme (an'·jē·ō·ten·sin kon·ver'·ting en'·zīm), *n* glycoprotein that converts angiotensin I to angiotensin II by dividing two terminal amino acids.

Angioma. (Christiansen, 1993)

angiotensin II (an'·jē·ō·ten'·sin tōō), *n* a powerful stimulant used to raise blood pressure by stimulating the release of aldosterone while concurrently causing vasoconstriction.

angle, *n* the divergence of two lines or planes from a common point of origin. *angle of the sacrum, inferior lateral,* *n* the point on the lateral surface of the sacrum as it curves toward the middle of the fifth sacral vertebra.

angle, Ferguson, *n.pr* See angle, lumbosacral.

angle, lumbolumbar lordotic, *n* the angle between the top (superior surface) of the second lumbar vertebra and the bottom (inferior surface) of the fifth lumbar vertebra, used as a measurement of the curve of the lumbar spine.

angle, lumbosacral, *n* the angle between a horizontal line (drawn through the sacrum) and the top (superior surface) of the first sacral vertebra. This angle is used to assess possible musculoskeletal contributions to lower back pain. Also called *sacral base angle.*

angle, lumbosacral lordotic, *n* the angle between the top (superior surface) of the second lumbar vertebra and the top (superior surface) of the first sacral vertebra, used as a measurement of the curve of the lumbar spine.

anima (an'·ə·mə), *n* sensitive soul; term coined by George Ernest Stahl

(1659–1734) to explain human vitality beyond the basic mechanics of the body.

animal magnetism, *n* theory advanced and practiced by Dr. Franz Anton Mesmer in the late 18th century as a healing technique, according to which a natural fluid exists throughout the universe, in and between all people and earthly and heavenly bodies. An imbalance of this fluid in the human body is believed to cause disease, but the fluid can be made to flow from one person to another, as from doctor to patient, to restore equilibrium and thereby cure illness.

anion (a·̇nē¹·ən), *n* a negatively charged ion that is formed when an atom or a molecule gains one or more electrons. See also ion.

anise (a·̇nəs), *n* Latin name: *Pimpinella anisum;* part used: fruit; uses: antibacterial, stimulant, antispasmodic, diuretic, diaphoretic, pulmonary ailments and disorders, sinus infections, colic, cancer, cholera, dysmenorrhea, sleep disorders, upset stomachs, nausea, lice, migraines, neuralgia, rashes; precautions: pregnancy, (essential oil) children, patients with liver or kidney disease; can cause seizures, edema in the lungs, hypermineralocorticism, stomatitis, nausea, and contact dermatitis. Also called *aniseed* and *sweet cumin.*

ankle, *n* **1.** anatomical area (joint) just above the foot. **2.** in craniosacral therapy, one of two places on the body where the caregiver lays both hands and determines the vitality and bounty of cerebrospinal fluid. See also listening posts.

anklyoglossia (an·klī¹·ō·glôs¹·sē·ə), *n* tongue anomaly in which movement is inhibited because of partial or complete fusion of the tongue to the mouth floor.

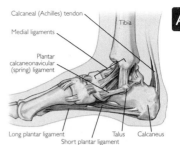

Ankle joint of the right foot: medial view

Ankle. (Mosby's Medical, Nursing & Allied Health Dictionary, ed 6, 2002)

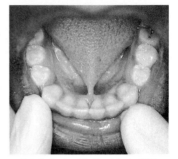

Ankyloglossia. (Zitelli and Davis, 1997)

ankylosing spondylitis (ang·ki·lō¹·sing spän·də·lī¹·təs), *n* a painful, progressive, arthritic condition in which some (or, rarely, all) of the spinal joints and vertebrae fuse together. It may also affect other joints and ligaments. Administration of antiinflammatory drugs and regular exercise help control inflammation and reduce pain. Also called *AS.*

anma (än·mä), *n* traditional Japanese massage.

anmo (än·mō), *n* traditional Chinese massage.

A

annavahasrotas (än′·nä·vä′·häs·rō′· täs), *n* in Ayurveda, channels that originate in the stomach and function to convey food from outside. See also srotas.

anodyne, *n* a substance with pain-relieving properties.

anomalous cognition (ə·nô′·mə·lis kôg·ni′·shən), *n* a term used for such phenomena as clairvoyance, precognition, remote viewing, and telepathy.

anomie (a′·nə·mē), *n* a sociological phenomenon in which individuals display profound lack of expected social behaviors, often seen when people are uprooted from their places of origin.

anorexia, *n* absence of the desire to eat, induced by psychological drugs or by social, environmental, or other factors.

anosmia, *n* the inability to smell; may be short-term, selective (only affecting certain aromas), or total and permanent.

antacid, *n* a substance that can counteract or neutralize acidity in the stomach.

antagonism, *n* situation that occurs when an intervention brings about an opposite effect.

antagonists, *n* muscles that counterbalance agonists during specific movements.

anterior component, *n* a description of the position of one side of a vertebra after it has rotated. In left rotation of the spine, the anterior component is the right side and vice-versa.

anterior innominate rotation (an·tir′·ē·or in·nô′·mə·nət rō·tā′· shən), *n* a condition in which the movement of the hipbone is restricted in upward and rearward directions and unrestricted in downward and forward directions, because the anterior superior iliac spine (ASIS) is positioned in front of and below the contralateral point.

anterior pubic shear, *n* a condition in which one pubic bone is displaced in front of its normal mate.

anterior sacrum, *n* condition in which forward rotation of the sacrum and side-bending to the side opposite the rotation have occurred. Resulting tissue changes may be located at the deep sulcus.

anterior translated sacrum, *n* condition in which the whole sacrum has moved forward between the ilia. Forward motion is freer; backward motion is restricted.

anthelmintic, *adj/n* eradicating intestinal worms.

Anthemis nobile, *n* See chamomile.

Anthemis nobilis (an′·thə·mis nō· bi′·lis), *n* Latin name: *Chamaemelum nobile*; part used: flower; uses: antiinflammatory, antispasmodic, antibacterial, sedative; precautions: ragweed allergy; patients being administered sedatives, tranquilizers, or antidepressants. Also called *chamomile* or *Roman chamomile.*

anthocyanidin (an′·thō·sī·an′·ə·din), *n* plant pigment thought to have antioxidant, antiplatelet, and wound-healing properties.

anthraquinones (an·trə·kwā′· nōōnz), *n.pl* plant chemicals formed on anthracene (a triple benzene ring) skeleton. Used as short-term laxative. Extensive use can cause electrolyte imbalance.

anthropometric measurements (an′·thrō·pə·me′·trik me′·zhər· mənts), *n.pl* a set of noninvasive, quantitative techniques for determining an individual's body fat composition by measuring, recording, and analyzing specific dimensions of the body, such as height and weight; skinfold thickness; and bodily circumference at the waist, hip, and chest.

Test	Gender	Normal values	Values showing malnutrition
Triceps skinfold	Male	11-12.5 mm	7.5-11 mm
(TSF)	Female	15-16.5 mm	10-15 mm
Mid upper arm	Male	26-29 cm	20-26 cm
circumference	Female	26-28.5 cm	20-26 cm
(MUAC)			
Arm muscle	Male	23-25 cm	16-23 cm
circumference	Female	20-23 cm	14-20 cm
(AMC)			
		AMC = MUAC − 0.314 = TSF	

Anthropometric measurements. (Mosby's Medical, Nursing & Allied Health Dictionary, ed 6, 2002)

antianginal (an·tī·an·jī'·nəl), *n* a drug used to treat angina pectoris, a symptom of ischemic heart disease. Such drugs include beta blockers, Ca^{++} antagonists, and nitrates that facilitate vasodilation. See also angina pectoris.

antiangiogenic (an'·tī·an'·jē·ō·jen'·ik), *n* a drug or substance used to stop the growth of tumors and progression of cancers by limiting the pathologic formation of new blood vessels (angiogenesis).

antianxiety, *n* See anxiolytic.

antibacterial peptides, *n.pl* natural bactericidal peptides produced in the body and skin and by neutrophils and natural killer cells.

antibiogram (an'·tē·bī'·ō·gram), *n* method of testing the efficacy of antibiotics by introducing an antibiotic into the middle of a bacteria-laden petri dish. A clear zone indicates the bactericidal activity. The greater the diameter of the zone, the higher the efficacy of the antibiotic.

antibiotic, *n* a substance that combats bacterial infection by killing bacteria or stopping bacterial growth.

antibiotic resistance, *n* the ability of certain strains of microorganisms to develop resistance to antibiotics.

antibody, *n* any of a wide assortment of glycoproteins typically present in the bloodstream that attack antigens during an immune response.

antibody–dependent cytotoxic hypersensitivity, *n* an exaggerated immune response in which antibodies attack cellular antigens and thereby destroy cells or tissue.

anticancer, *n* a medicine or substance used to treat cancer.

anticipation stress, *n* the anxiety and emotional fatigue suffered before meaningful life experiences, whether positive or negative.

anticoagulant (an'·tē·kō·ag'·yə·lə nt), *n* a substance that inhibits blood clotting.

antidepressant, *n/adj* a substance that can alleviate depression.

antidiuretic hormone, *n* hormone secreted by the hypothalamus that decreases urine production by causing renal tubules to reabsorb water.

antidontalgic (an'·tē·dôn·tal'·jik), *n* a substance that has the ability to relieve toothache.

antidote, *n* a substance that relieves, prevents, or opposes the action of a poison.

antidrugs, *n.pl* a term used for vitamins and minerals used by practitioners of orthomolecular medicine in an effort to use chemicals that are natural to the body without resorting to synthetic drugs.

antiemetic (an'·tē·e·me'·tik), *n* a substance that can prevent or lessen the feeling of nausea and vomiting.

antifungal, *adj/n* effective against fungi in the body; beneficial property of some essential oils, such as fennel, cinnamon, clove, and thyme.

antigen, *n* any substance regarded by the body as foreign that provokes an immune system response.

antigenic load (an'·ti·jen·ik lōd'), *n* total exposure to substances, usually foreign proteins, that may trigger an immune response.

antihypertensive, *n* a medicine or substance that reduces blood pressure.

antiinflammatory, *adj/n* serves to relieve inflammation in cases, such as injury or infection; beneficial trait of some essential oils.

antiinflammatory leukotriene (LTB5) (an'·tī-in·fla'·mə·tō·rē lōō'·kō·trēn), *n* a lipid that suppresses inflammatory tissue reactions in the body.

OMEGA-3 FATTY ACIDS

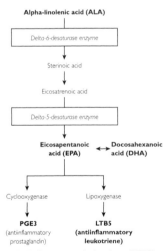

Antiinflammatory leukotriene (LTB5). (Leskowitz, 2003)

antimicrobial (an'·tē·mī·krō'·bē·əl), *n* a substance that combats microbial infection by killing microorganisms or inhibiting their replication or growth.

antimony, *n* a toxic metal sometimes found in alloys, semiconductors, and local pollution. Exposure has been linked to anemia, bleeding gums, conjunctivitis, headaches, laryngitis, skin disease, and weight loss.

antineoplastons (an'·tī·nē'·ō·plas'·tənz), *n.pl* chemicals derived from phenylacetate salts, phenylacetate, glutamine, and isoglutamine; claimed to have anticancer effects.

antinociceptive peptides (an'·tī·nō'·si·sep'·tiv pep'·tīdz), *n.pl* endogenous peptides, such as enkephalins, endorphins, and dynorphins, that possess pain-reducing (analgesic) properties.

antinuclear antibody, *n* an autoantibody that reacts with nuclear material and is present in individuals with autoimmune disorders; detectable by immunoflourescent assay technique.

antioxidants, *n.pl* substances that protect the body from free radicals and reactive oxygen species by converting the free radicals into more stable substances.

antipathic (an·te·path'·ik), *adj* in opposition to the disease. Describes a method of treatment whose main consequence is the antithesis of the malady. The drugs used in this technique contrast those used in the homeopathic method where the consequences of the remedies are the same as the disease. Also called *enantiopathic*. See also allopathic.

antiphlogistic, *adj/n* a substance that functions to relieve inflammation and fever.

antipraxy (an·te·prak'·sē), *n* a theory about the effects of homeopathic remedies that states that all medicines produce opposite results depending on dose. See also law, Arndt-Schultz; dose-dependent reverse effect; and hormesis.

antipsoric (an·tip·sōr'·ik), *adj* remedy for healing itchy skin eruption (or the psoric miasm) within a homeopathic framework. Also called *homeopsoric*. See psoric miasm.

antipyretic, *adj/n* a drug that reduces fever. Also known as *febrifuge*.

antiseptic (an'·tə·sep'·tik), *n/adj* a substance that controls infection by inhibiting growth and replication of the causative agent.

antispasmodic (an'·tē·spaz·mô'·dik), *n/adj* a substance that relieves cramping and spasms.

antisudorific (an'·tē·sōō·dō·ri'·fik), *n/adj* a substance that reduces sweating.

antisycotic, *n/adj* remedy to offset the effects of gonorrhea or sycosis. Also known as *homeosycotic.*

antisyphilitic, *n/adj* homeopathic remedy to thwart a condition characteristic of syphilitic miasm. Also known as *antiluetic* or *homeosyphilitic.* See miasm.

antitaxic drug action, *n* the effect of a medicine that in dilution achieves the antithesis of its effect at standard dosage. See also law, Arndt-Schulz; biphasic activity; dose-dependent reverse effect; hormesis; and simillimum.

antithermic, *n/adj* a substance that manages fever and temperature.

antitoxic, *adj* having the capacity to render bacterial toxins inert

antitoxin, *n* a substance used to counter directly the effects of a toxin. May be produced by the body or administered from outside the body.

antitussive, *adj/n* a substance with cough-suppressing properties.

antiviral (an'·tē·vī'·rəl), *n* a substance that combats viral infection.

anuloma viloma, *n* See nadi shodhanam.

anuria (an·yōō·rē'·ə), *n* lack of urination or urine production of less than 100 ml per day.

anxiety, *n* emotional tension, generally accompanied by increased sympathetic nervous system response.

Anxiety Sensitivity Index, *n* a psychological questionnaire used to identify whether a patient is experiencing a general sense of worry or has specific concerns relating to symptoms of stress.

anxiolytic, *adj/n* the ability of a substance to alleviate emotional anxiety and stress.

AOC, *n* an acronym for the Aromatherapy Organizations Council.

aortic glycosaminoglycans (ā·ôr'·tik glī·kō'·s ə·mē·nō·glī'·kanz), *n.pl* orally administered extracts of bovine aorta.

aperient, *n* a substance with the ability to purge the digestive system of a given agent.

aperitif (ə·per'·ə·tēf'), *n* an appetite stimulant. Also called *aperitive.*

aphagia (a·fə·jē'·ə), *n* inability to swallow; may be psychological or physical.

Aphanes arvensis, *n* See parsley piert.

aphasia (ə·fā'·zhə), *n* inability to speak or express oneself in words. Often caused by stroke.

apheresis (əfer'·ə·sis), *n* process in which blood is drawn from a donor, followed by selective separation of one or more constituents and then reinfused back into the body.

aphrodisiac (a'·frədē'·zē·ak), *n/adj* substance that enhances sexual desire.

aphthous stomatitis (af'·thōs stō'·mə·tī'·tis), *n* a common condition that affects the oral cavity; indicated by the appearance of painful, shallow lesions found alone or in clustered groups. A reddish border surrounds the small ulcers, and a pseudomembrane covers them. Injury to the mouth, sensitivity to certain foods, nutrient deficiency, and/or stress may cause it. The lesions typically heal within one to three weeks of appearance. Also called *common canker sore* or *ulcerative stomatitis.*

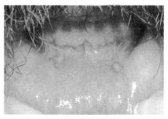

Aphthous stomatitis. (Michelson and Friedlaender, 1996)

A

apitherapy (ā'·pə·the'·rə·pē), *n* the use of products produced by honeybees, such as pollen, honey, royal jelly, propolis, and bee venom, for therapeutic and pharmacologic purposes. See also royal jelly, propolis, and bee venom.

Apium graveolens, *n* See celery.

apnea (ap'·nē·ə), *n* cessation of breathing; arrested respiration.

apoplexy (a'·pə·plek'·sē), *n* reduced circulation in the brain. It occurs when a blood vessel bursts spontaneously or is blocked or by physical injury to the head, arteriosclerosis (hardening of the arteries), atherosclerosis (excess cholesterol in the blood), and high blood pressure. Also called *stroke, cerebral embolism, cerebral hemorrhage, cerebral infarction,* and *cerebral thrombosis.*

apoptosis (a·pəp·tō'·sis), *n* programmed destruction of cells; mechanism that keeps cell numbers in check by eliminating senescent cells or those without useful cell function.

apothecary, *n* precursor to the present-day pharmacy.

apparent life-threatening events, *n.pl* conditions or episodes that could result in the termination of the life of the patient.

applied kinesiology, *n* **1.** a physical therapy model that draws on varied therapeutic schools of thought. The goal of this therapy is the recovery of muscles that are functionally inhibited with respect to the normal range of motion and strength. Also addressed in the framework are functional weaknesses due to disturbances in the nervous and neuromuscular systems that can manifest as fatigue, autoimmune problems, back and neck pain, anxiety, and depression. Also called *AK.* **2.** a technique used to test for the suitability of treatments or the cause of diseases in which the practitioner checks muscle strength of the patient when touching those substances or their symbols.

applied psychophysiology, *n* the practical understanding of the mind-body interrelationship with regard to therapeutic treatments of various kinds.

Applied Spinal Biomechanical Engineering (ASBE), *n* a chiropractic course of treatment developed to strengthen the intrinsic muscles of the spine.

approach, *n* in medicine, the method or procedure used to address a situation, such as surgery or other treatment plan.

approved indication, *n* **1.** reliable signs that a certain remedy should be used. Not synonymous with "authorized." **2.** FDA-approved condition for a drug or other treatment that allows labeling.

approximation, *n* a massage technique in which muscle fibers are pressed together along the direction of the fibers in order to relieve cramping.

apsoric (ap·sō'·rik), *adj* unrelated to itching or to the psoric miasm; term used in homeopathy.

aquapuncture (ä'·kwə·punk'·chər), *n* injecting water beneath the skin to ease or relieve pain.

aqueous, *adj* relating to water.

araha-vabhedaka (ä·rä'·hə·vä·bhā'·dä·kə), *n* Ayurvedic term for migraine headache.

Aran-Duchenne Muscular Dystrophy, *n.pr* a muscular disease that first affects the arms, hands, legs, and shoulders before progressing to the rest of the body.

arava (ä'·rə·və), *n* in Ayurveda, a method of medicine preparation in which an alcohol-based herbal tincture is created through natural fermentation. Herbal juices are mixed with raw sugar (jaggery) and dried forest-flame bush flowers (which contain yeast). Also called *asava.* See also arista.

archaeus (är·kā'·əs), *n* the luminous, radiating healing energy that surrounds and permeates human beings, as described by the 16th-century alchemist Paracelsus.

arcing, *n* a diagnostic technique used in craniosacral therapy in which the practitioner traces energy waves back to the source of the pain. See also therapy, craniosacral.

Arctium lappa, *n* See burdock.

Arctium minus, *n* See burdock.

Arctostaphylos adenotricha, *n* See bearberry.

Arctostaphylos coactylis, *n* See bearberry.

Arctostaphylos uva-ursi, *n* See bearberry.

Areca catechu, *n* See betel palm.

areca nut (ə·rē´·kə nut´), *n* Latin Name: *Areca catechu;* part used: seed; uses: astringent, teeth-cleaning, anthelmintic, pupil contraction, salivary gland and bowel movement stimulation; precautions: can cause intoxication, oral cancers, bronchoconstriction, not to be used with anticholinergic agents. Also called *betel nut* and *pinang.*

arginine (är´·jə·nēn), *n* an essential amino acid that has been used as an adjunct therapy in congestive heart failure, erectile dysfunction, peripheral vascular disease (PVD), and angina pectoris. It may also be useful in the treatment of upper respiratory ailments, type II diabetes, and various hematologic conditions. Precaution advised for those with gastritis, peptic ulcers, and acid reflux disease as well as for those taking NSAIDs, antiplatelet medications, theophylline medications, corticosteroids, postassium-sparing diuretics, or ACE inhibitors.

aril (ar´·əl), *n* a fleshy, often colorful and edible covering that surrounds immature seeds in many plant species.

arista (ä·ri´·stə), *n* Ayurvedic method of medicine preparation that uses natural fermentation, similar to arava. Instead of using herbal juice, however, the herbs are infused or decocted in water; to this aqueous extract are added jaggery (raw cane sugar) and dried forest-flame bush flowers (containing yeast). See also arava.

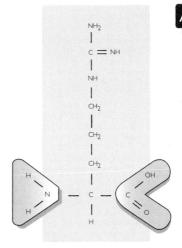

Chemical structure of arginine

Arginine. (Mosby's Medical, Nursing & Allied Health Dictionary, ed 6, 2002)

Aristolochia indica, *n* See Indian birthwort.

arjuna (är·jōō´·nə), *n* Latin name: *Terminalia arjuna;* parts used: bark, fruit; uses: in Ayurveda pacifies kapha and pitta doshas (astringent, light, dry), hypolipidemic, hepatoprotection, antineoplastic, antimutagenic, antibacterial, antiviral, cardiotonic, angina, hypertension, coronary artery conditions, myocardial infarction, liver conditions, urogenital diseases, STDs, colic, dysentery, poisoning, wounds;

precautions: none known. Also called *arjun* or *kakubha*.

arka (är'·kə), *n* in Ayurveda, a method of medicine preparation in which aqueous herbal extracts are distilled to produce herbal essences.

arm levitation, *n* a type of suggestion sometimes used in hypnosis whereby the patient is induced to think that the mind has complete control over the body, thus causing the patient's arm to become weightless and rise.

Armoracia rusticana, *n* See horseradish.

armoring (är'·mə·ring), *n* according to jin shin do, a form of acupressure in which tension is built up by repeated stress at a point where excess energy is accumulated as the result of various stimuli.

Arnica montana **L.,** *n* See arnica.

arnica (ôr'·ni·kə), *n* Latin name: *Arnica montana* L.; part used: flowers; uses: antiinflammatory, antimicrobial, antiecchymotic, analgesic, bruises, strains, sprains, muscle aches, varicose veins, hemorrhoids, insect bites, dandruff, baldness; precautions: patients with open wounds; can cause contact dermatitis, eczema, toxic if ingested (unless at homeopathic dosages).

aroma chemical, *n* an odorous chemical with useful properties that is also legal and safe to use as a flavor or fragrance.

aromatherapy, *n* controlled use of essential oils to promote the vitality and health of spirit, mind, and body. It involves external application of essential oils via full-body massage, inhalation, topical application, steam, and compresses.

aromatic, *n* an organic compound derived from benzene. Also called an *aromatic compound.*

aromatic ring, *n* closed ring structure formed by six carbon atoms, with a single hydrogen atom attached to each one. Also called a *phenyl ring* or a *benzene ring.*

aromatogram (er·ō·mat'·ō·gram), *n* a test used to determine the antibacterial activity of essential oils in which the oil is introduced into the center of a bacteria-laden petri dish. A clear zone indicates the bactericidal activity of the oil. The greater the diameter of the zone, the higher the efficacy of the oil.

aromatologist (ə·rō'·mə·tä'·lə·jist), *n* term used in some European countries for practitioners of aromatherapy.

aromatology (ə·rōm·ə·tô'·lə·gē), *n* the managed use of essential oils to elevate and sustain the health of an individual's mind, body, and spirit through various means of administration, including but not limited to inhalation, massage of various types, compresses, and baths.

arousal, *n* a state of being responsive to sensory stimulation. Also called *termination* and *return to everyday activity.*

arrythmia (ə·rith'·mē·ə), *n* an irregularity in heart rate.

arsenic, *n* toxic metal found in some cereals and Chinese and Ayurvedic herbal remedies. Exposure has been linked to anemia, bladder cancer, jaundice, muscular weakness, and other ailments.

arsenicum alba (ar·se'·ni·kəm al'·bə), *n* a white-colored oxide of arsenic, used in homeopathy to treat anxiety, gastric upset, asthma, sore throat, and skin conditions. Also called *Ars, arsenicum, arsenicum album,* or *white arsenic trioxide.*

artav (är'·təv), *n* in Ayurveda, semen and reproductive tissues as a fundamental tissue (dhatu). See also dhatus.

Artemesia annua **(är'·tə·mē'·zē·ə an·nōō'·ə),** *n* parts used: dried aerial portions; uses: fever, malaria, parasites; precautions: possible neurotoxicity in high doses. Also called *annual wormwood, qinghao, sweet annie* or *sweet wormwood.*

Artemisia absinthium, *n* See wormwood.

Artemisia cina, *n* See levant wormseed.

Artemisia vulgaris, *n* See mugwort.

arteparon (är'·tə·pa'·rôn), *n* derived from bovine tracheal and lung cartilage, an agent used to prevent the destruction of cartilage and/or facilitate repair of damaged cartilage; improper use can cause serious thromboembolic complications like pulmonary embolus, myocardial infarction, cerebral hemorrhage, and hemiplegic apoplexia. Reported side effects also include serious allergic reactions, subcutaneous fat necrosis, reversible alopecia, and arthropathy.

arterial, *adj* of the arteries, the vessels through which oxygenated blood flows.

arterioles, *n* small blood vessels that branch from the arteries and transport blood from the heart to the body tissues.

arthritis, *n* a condition characterized by inflammation of the joints.

arthritis, degenerative, *n* painful joint disease marked by lack of mobility caused by degeneration of the articular cartilage.

arthritis, inflammatory, *n* disease marked by swollen joints, often painful; may be the result of trauma, infection, metabolic disturbances, or other causes.

arthrokinematic movement (är·thrŏ·ki·nə·ma'·tik mōōv'·mənt), *n* small, involuntary movements within a joint; caused by the natural laxity of the articulate parts.

artichoke, *n* Latin name: *Cynara scolymus;* part used: leaves; uses: lowers cholesterol, treats nonulcer dyspepsia, provides hepatoprotection; precautions: patients with gallstones or other gallbladder conditions. Also called *globe artichoke.*

articular pillar, *n* columnar structure created by the flexible junction of the articular processes of the cervical vertebrae.

articulation, *n* **1.** a juncture between two bones that moves. **2.** a massage technique in which a joint is passively moved, repetitively, through its range of motion.

articulatory pop, *n* the sound that results from gas bubbles being released from a joint, as when "cracking" the knuckles.

articulatory treatment system, *n* a low velocity/high amplitude osteopathic technique that carries a joint through the full range of motion in order to increase the free range of motion.

artifact, *n* **1.** anything made by human hands or activities. **2.** a product that may develop during an analysis performed to identify the composition of a substance. Mainly a consequence of the conditions of the analysis.

artificial somnambulism, *n* an induced state in which subjects exhibit behavior similar to that displayed by sleepwalkers. A precursor to the Freudian psychotherapeutic techniques of catharsis and free association; evolved from the practice of animal magnetism, so named in the early 19th century by the Marquis de Puysegur. See also catharsis and animal magnetism.

ARTT, *n.pr* See asymmetry/range of motion alteration/tissue texture alteration/tenderness.

arumalon (ə·rōō'·mə·lôn), *n* an agent used to prevent the destruction of cartilage and/or facilitate repair of damaged cartilage that is derived from red bone marrow of calves and a cartilage extract. Administration of the agent via parenteral means has been linked with allergic reactions, fatal dermatomyositis, and myositis.

asafetida (a·sə·fe'·tə·də), *n* Latin name: *Ferrula ass-afoetida;* part used: an oleogum-resin obtained from the root; uses: relieves cramps, spasms, promotes digestion, relieves and removes gas, promotes bowel evacuation, induces relaxation, induces removal of mucous secretions within the lungs, relieves pain, increases sexual desire, removes intestinal worms; precautions: can cause methemoglobinemia. Also called *a wei, devil's dung, ferula, food of the gods,* and *hingu.*

asanas (ä'·se·näs'), *n.pl* in Ayurveda, exercises based on stretching, deep breathing, and concentration. Promote rejuvenation of specific organs, glands, and the spine.

ascariasis (as'·kə·rī'·ə·sis), *n* an infection caused by the common parasitic roundworm *Ascaris lumbricoides.* Symptoms include temporary cough, labored respiration, wheezing, distension, and discomfort in the abdomen and sporadic vomiting. In rare cases, the infected individual may develop a blockage in the intestines.

ascending reticular activating system (ARAS) (ə·sen'·ding rə·ti'·kyə·ler ak'·tə·vā'·ting sis'·təm), *n* system that transmits messages to the limbic system and hypothalamus, triggers release of hormones and neurotransmitters, and facilitates functions such as learning, memory, and wakefulness.

asepsis (a'·sep'·sis), *n* lack of germs and germ activity; sterile.

ashwagandha (äsh·wä·gän·dhə), *n* Latin name: *Withania somnifera;* parts used: leaves, roots, whole plant; uses: in Ayurveda, balances kapha and vata doshas (bitter, pungent, light, oily), general tonic herb, adaptogen, antiinflammatory, antiviral, hepato-protection, antioxidant, antitumor, antistress effects, memory improve-ment, immunomodulator, lowers high blood pressure; precautions: none known. Also called *asagandh.*

ASI, *n* See Anxiety Sensitivity Index.

asiaticoside (ā'·zhē·a'·ti·kō'·sīd), *n* the active chemical component of the plant *Centella asiatica.* Has been used to treat wounds and burns.

ASIS, *n* anterior superior iliac spine; the hip bones located towards the front of the body. During evaluation, a practitioner examines the right and left bones to determine the presence and type of dysfunction.

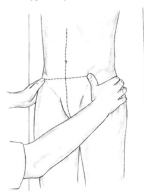

ASIS. (Chaitow, 2003)

asparagus (ə·spar'·ə·gəs), *n* Latin name: *Asparagus officinalis;* part used: roots; uses: diuretic, laxative, clearing of sediment from the bladder, urinary tract irritation; precautions: allergies.

Asparagus racemosus, *n* See shatavari.

asphyxia (as·fiks'·ē· ə), *n* obstruction of air flow resulting in hypoxia severe enough to cause unconsciousness, hypercapnia, hypoxemia, and death, if not immediately treated.

aspidium (as·pi'·dē·əm), *n* Latin name: *Dryopteris filix-mas* L; parts used: leaves, oil, resin, roots; uses: in topical preparations for circulatory, respiratory, and skin conditions, joint or muscle pain, internal preparation for tapeworm; precautions; preg-nancy; poisonous when ingested.

assault and battery, *n* bodily injury; encompasses an offense in which one person intimidates another into believing personal injury is imminent.

assault occasioning actual bodily harm, *n* an offense in which physi-cal injury to another person is the result.

assessment, *n* **1.** in clinical medicine, evaluation of the patient for the purposes of forming a diagnosis and plan of treatment. **2.** in research, evaluation of a treatment or diagnos-tic test through experiment and measurement.

assistant ingredient (ə·sis'·tənt in·grē'·dē·ənt), *n* one of the four components in a typical Chinese herbal formula used to enhance the result produced by the chief ingredi-ent and also to lessen or remove the toxicity associated with the chief and the deputy ingredients. See also chief ingredient, deputy ingredient, and envoy ingredient.

Association for Applied Psy-chophysiology and Biofeedback, *n.pr* an organization founded in 1969 to promote development of biofeed-back and applied psychophysiology. It encourages expansion of educational and clinical applications of biofeed-back and applied psychophysiology; promotes scientific research; works to integrate biofeedback and other types of self-regulatory methods; encourages higher level of standards associated with professional education, practice, and ethics; fosters educational opportunities for members; and increases knowledge of biofeedback to the public. Members represent a variety of fields, including medicine, psychology, social work, nursing, physical therapy, counseling, and education. The group was initially formed

hospitals, promoting research in the health sciences, and integrating education into the provision of effective health care. Also called *AAMC.*

assumption of risk, *n* the voluntary acceptance of the potential hazards associated with a particular form of treatment by a patient.

asterion, *n* point on the skull where the lambdoid, occipitotemporal, and parietotemporal sutures meet.

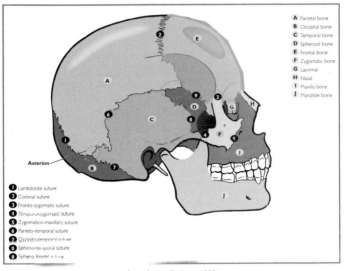

Asterion. (Chaitow, 1999)

as the Biofeedback Research Society. Also called *AAPB.*

Association of American Medical Colleges, *n.pr* a nonprofit organization founded in 1876 to reform medical education and represent medical schools, major teaching hospitals, scientific and academic faculty, medical students, and residents. Its mission is to improve public health by improving education and training provided in medical schools and teaching

asthavahasrotas **(äs'·thä·vä'·häs·rō'·täs)**, *n* in Ayurveda, channels that originate in the hip bone and convey components for bone tissue. See also srotas.

asthi (äs·thē), *n* in Ayurveda, bone as a fundamental tissue (dhatu). See also dhatus.

asthma, *n* respiratory illness in which constricted bronchi and sticky bronchoid secretions cause wheezing and paroxysmal dyspnea.

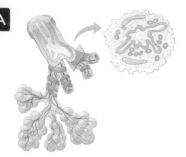

Asthma. (Thibodeau, 1999)

Aston arthrokinetics (as·'tən är'· thrō·kə·ne·'tiks), *n.pr* a form of Aston patterning that works very deeply along bones, with joints and with abnormally hardened tissues. Requires advanced training. See also Aston patterning.

Aston ergonomics (as·'tən er·gə· nô·'miks), *n.pr* the arrangement or modification of objects such as tools or furniture to support healthy biomechanics. Considered essential to support and maintain Aston work. See also Aston patterning.

Aston facial fitness, *n.pr* a form of Aston patterning focused on facial expression and tone; includes arthrokinetic and myokinetic forms, isometric exercises, massage, and lymphatic drainage. See also Aston patterning.

Aston fitness training, *n.pr* individually designed program of exercises to loosen, stretch, and tone specific muscle groups; emphasizes whole-body cooperation and honoring asymmetry. See also Aston patterning.

Aston movement education, *n.pr* progressive teachings of Aston based body mechanics from very basic movements to complex, specialized actions. See also Aston patterning.

Aston myokinetics (as·'tən mī'·ō· kə·ne·'tiks), *n.pr* a form of Aston patterning focused on strategic myofascial release of tissues ingrained by overuse or trauma. See also Aston Patterning.

Aston paradigm (as·'tən par'·ə· dīm), *n.pr* ideas about human movement, structure, learning, and self-expression developed by Judith Aston. Key features of this paradigm are the assertions that every body is asymmetrical, unique, three-dimensional, and spiraling in motion and form. See also Aston patterning.

Aston mechanics, *n.pr* the applied theories and observations of the Aston paradigm. Applications include bodywork and fitness techniques, and ergonomic movement and design. See also Aston patterning.

Aston patterning, *n.pr* a somatic education process developed by Judith Aston; based on asymmetry as a key characteristic of the human body; aimed at developing patterns of alignment and movement comfortable for the individual.

astragalus (a·'strə·gä·ləs), *n* Latin names: *Astragalus membranaceus, Astragalus gummifer*; part used: roots; uses: cold, fatigue, bronchitis, flu, immune system stimulant, reduction of side effects of chemotherapy; precautions: none known. Also called *huang-qi* or *tragacanth*.

Astragalus gummifer, *n* See astragalus.

Astragalus membranaceus, *n* See astragalus.

Astragalus membranaceus, *n* See Mongolian milk-vetch.

astral force (as·'tr əl fōrs'), *n* term used by theosophists to describe cosmic fluid with which humans should attempt to be in balance for good health. Also called *auric force, psychic force* and *subtle energy.*

astral travel, *n* the belief in or experience of disembodied consciousness (i.e., the "astral body") moving into other nonphysical realms (i.e., the "astral plane"). Also called *astral projection, mind projection, OBE,* or *out-of-body experience.*

astringent, *n* a substance that contracts or tightens tissue, thereby alleviating conditions such as diarrhea, hemorrhages, and secretions.

asymmetric carbon atom, *n* a carbon atom attached to four functional groups or four different atoms. See also isomerism and optical isomers.

asymmetry, *n* lack of symmetry, particularly in situations where some form of symmetry is to be expected.

ATA, *n.pr* See acupuncture treatment area.

ataxia (ə·taks'·ē·ə), *n* postural imbalance and a staggering ambulatory style.

atherosclerosis (a'·thrō·sklə·rō'·sis), *n* degenerative disease characterized by plaques of cholesterol and lipids in the arterial walls, leading to thickening of arteries and ultimately to coronary heart disease, angina, and other cardiac diseases.

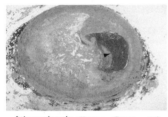

Atherosclerosis. (Kumar, Cotran, and Robbins, 1997; Dr. Sid Murphree, Department of Pathology, University of Texas Southwestern Medical School, Dallas, TX)

atlas, *n* C1, the first cervical vertebra. The skull sits upon this vertebra, which allows the head to tilt forward and backward. The atlas rests on the axis, allowing for rotation. See also axis.

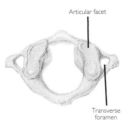

Articular facet

Transverse foramen

Atlas. (Applegate, 2000)

ATM, *n.pr* See Awareness Through Movement.

atman (ät'·m ən), *n* according to Vedic tradition, the "self" or the "individual soul." Unification of atman with Brahman leads to enlightenment of an individual. Also called *atma*. See also Brahman.

atom, *n* the smallest component of an element that retains the element's chemical properties. Atoms comprise molecules and are themselves divisible into electrons, neutrons, and protons.

atomic number, *n* the number of protons within an atom's nucleus.

atomic weight, *n* the total number of protons and neutrons within an atom's nucleus. This number represents the atom's approximate mass.

atopic dermatitis (ā·tô'·pik der'·mə·tī'·tis), *n* a common chronic skin condition that is a variant of the skin disease eczema and is characterized by thick, leathery skin, and dry rectangular-shaped scales. Hives, lesions, and small bumps with a rough texture may also indicate the condition. Often runs in families.

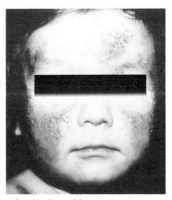

Atopic dermatitis. (Zitelli and Davis, 1997)

atopic eczema (ā'·tô'·pik eg'·zə·mə), *n* chronic skin disease marked by thickened, scaly, inflamed, and itchy rashes often seen in individuals with familial history of allergic conditions, such as hay fever or asthma. Often treated with emollients, antihistamines, and steroid creams. Also called *atopic dermatitis* or *infantile eczema.*

atrial fibrillation (ā'·trē·əl fi·bri·lā'·shən), *n* quick uncoordinated twitching movements of the muscles of the atria of the heart; may result in a lack of regular pulse and lowered circulation.

atrophy, *n* shrinking or wasting of a body part as a result of lack of use or disease.

attention–focusing, *n* a psychological technique for controlling pain by averting the concentration. Focus can be averted to any number of things, such as a particular point on the body.

attention placebo control group, *n* a group of persons that serves as a baseline for comparison for assessment of the effects of a particular intervention. While persons in the treatment group receive the experimental treatment being studied, the attention placebo control group receives a treatment that mimics the amount of time and attention received by the treatment group but is thought not to have a specific effect upon the subjects.

attenuation, *n* **1.** reduction in concentration. **2.** decrease in the ability of a pathogenic organism to cause disease.

attics (a'·tiks), *n* the sinus passages connected to the nose where cool air is warmed and filtered.

attunements (ət·tōōn'·mənts), *n.pl* in Reiki, ceremonial procedures in which a practitioner's energy field is aligned to access the universal life energy and transferred to others through the hands. Also called *alignments* or *initiations.* See also Reiki.

audit, *n* a process used to determine whether existing standards of care are being met.

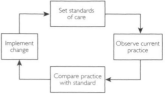

Audit. (Rankin-Box, 2001)

Aum (ä·ōōm'), *n.pr* **1.** in Ayurveda, the subtle, noiseless cosmic vibration in which consciousness existed in the beginning, before the elements appeared. Also called *Om.* **2.** mantra seed syllable often used in meditation.

auras (ōr'·əz), *n.pl* energies that are believed to surround the surface of an object, reflecting the life force that permeates all living beings.

auric force (ô'·rik fōrs'), *n* See astral force.

auricle, *n* the external part of the ear that is treated in ear acupuncture.

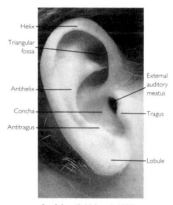

Auricle. (Seidel et al, 1999)

auriculotherapy (ə·rik·yə·lō·the·rə·pē), *n* a form of acupuncture in which needles are placed in various portions of the ear to affect the person. It postulates body correlates on the ear, so a treatment performed upon the ear will have effects on the reflected body part. See also acupuncture and reflexology.

auscultation (ô·skəl·tā´·shən), v listening to body sounds—especially the heart, lungs, intestines, pleura, blood, and vessels—for diagnostic purposes or to find a fetal heartbeat.

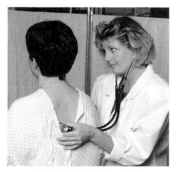

Auscultation. (Belcher, 1992)

authentic movement, n See movement-in-depth.

authoritarian hypnotists (əthôr´·ə·te´·rē·ən hip´·nətists), n.pl practitioners of a school of hypnotherapy who impose both the trance states and the solution to the problem. Also called *paternal hypnotists.*

authoritative suggestion, n a type of instruction more on the order of a command, which may be used by therapists in hypnotic sessions with compliant subjects.

autism, n mental disorder in which language and social and relational skills are undeveloped. Individuals can be abnormally socially withdrawn.

autocrine (ô´·tō·krin), adj affecting the cells of origin, used in describing glandular and hormonal action.

autogenic training, n an outgrowth of self-hypnosis, a method of achieving a self-induced state of trance by passive concentration and awareness of body sensations to induce relaxation.

autoimmunity, n abnormal immune response where the body attacks its own tissue constituents. Also called *acute immune disease.*

autointoxication, n disease caused by the accrual of contaminants produced inside the living organism.

autoisopathy (ô·tō·ī·sô´·pə·thē), n medical method that uses remedies produced from bodily substances that are byproducts of the patient's disease. Also called *autopathy.*

automatic thoughts, n.pl internalized perceptions involuntarily generated by an individual. These impressions may be triggered by becoming aware of a situation or circumstance, may develop quickly, and are not subject to detailed inquiry or logical examination.

autonomic nervous system (ô·tō·nô´·mik ner´·vəs si´·stəm), n involuntary nervous system consisting of the sympathetic and the parasympathetic subsystems.

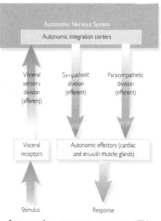

Autonomic nervous system. (Thibodeau and Patton, 1999 [modified])

autonomy (ô·tô´·nə·mē), n a principle of medical ethics according to which a person should respect the rights of other individuals to freely determine their own choices and decisions.

autonosode (ô'·tō·nə·sōd), *n* homeopathic remedy created from the patient's own disease-causing material, such as bodily fluids or warts. See also autoisopathy and nosode.

autopsy, *n* a surgical examination of a corpse performed to ascertain the cause of death.

autoregulation, *n* **1.** self-adjustment. **2.** inherent capability to adjust one's own physiology. See also homeostasis and naturopathy.

autumn nutrition, *n* in Tibetan medicine, the purposeful adjustment of an individual's eating habits to autumn weather. Between the winter and the summer solstice, it is traditionally thought that, as the amount of energy exerted by the sun decreases, digestive processes associated with badahan and schara begin a transitional period to prepare themselves for the peak level of activity that occurs during the winter. During this time, these digestive functions become quite vulnerable to errors in dietary habits. As a rule, the selection of foods during meals becomes more and more limited. Individuals are encouraged to consume foods that are light with—in this specific order—predominantly sour, salty, astringent, and sweet taste. While the performance of the gastrointestinal tract progressively increases, it is best to avoid foods that are heavy, have a strong taste, and stimulate. The individual should consume meals frequently, but small quantities are encouraged so as to keep the digestive processes reasonably occupied. However, these processes should not become overwhelmed. Establishing a specific place and time for meals is a priority throughout autumn. See also schara and badahan.

auxiliary substance, *n* inert substance added to a remedy to stabilize it. See also vehicle.

avaleha (ä·və·lā'·hə), *n* in Ayurveda, a method of medicine preparation in which herbs and/or herbal extracts are mixed into a syrup.

Avena sativa, *n* See oats.

avens (a'·vənz), *n* Latin name: *Geum urbannum;* parts used: plant (dried), rhizome, roots; uses: astringent, antiinflammatory, antiseptic, diarrhea, sore throat, fever, headache; precautions: none known. Also called *Benedict's herb, bennet's root, blessed herb, city avens, clove root, colewort, geum, goldy star, herb bennet, way bennet, wild rye,* or *wood avens.*

Aviation Health Institute, *n.pr* a British foundation that concerns itself with the quality of air travel conditions and the resultant effects on passenger health.

avila (ä·vē̄·lə), *adj* in Ayurveda, "cloudy" as a guna, one of the qualities characterizing all substances. Its complement is vishada. See also gunas and vishada.

avocado-soybean unsaponifiables (ä'·v ə·kä'·dō-soi'·bēn un'·sə·pôn'·ə·fī'·ə·bəlz), *n.pl* compounds extracted from avocado and soybean oils; believed to affect the development and repair of cartilage that protects the ends of the bones; used to treat osteoarthritis of knee and hip.

Avogadro's law, *n.pr* Avogadro advanced the principle that equal volumes of all gases under identical temperature and pressure contain the same number of molecules.

Avogadro's number, *n.pr* the number of molecules that exist in one mole: 6.0225×10^{23}.

awareness, *n* **1.** the faculty of attention, of being conscious. **2.** in the Alexander technique, a heightened sense of proprioception that allows one to recognize unbalanced habits of posture and bearing and to undo these harmful habitual patterns. See also technique, Alexander.

Awareness Through Movement, *n.pr* the Feldenkrais method, especially when taught to a group of students, as opposed to a one-on-one session. Students learn to focus on forgotten or poorly used body parts to recover full functionality. Also called *ATM.* See also method, Feldenkrais.

axis, *n* **1.** an imaginary line around which motion occurs, as in an axis of rotation. **2.** C2, the second cervical vertebra, around whose odontoid process the atlas rotates. See also atlas.

axes, transverse, *n* axes located at the junctions of the frontal and horizontal planes, around which nutation and counternutation occur. Also called *z axes.*

axis of rib motion, *n* an imaginary line through the costovertebral and costotransverse rib articulations.

axis, anterior-posterior, *n* axis located at the junction of the horizontal and sagittal planes. Also called the *x axis.*

axis, anteroposterior rib (an¹·tə·rō·pô·stē¹·rē·ôr rib¹ a¹·ksis), *n* the imaginary line crossing between the sternum and the spinal column, about which the ribs rotate in bucket handle rib motion. See also axis of rib motion and bucket handle rib motion.

axis, hypothalamic-pituitary adrenal *(HPA axis)* (hī·pō·thə·la¹·mik pi·tōō¹·i·ta·rē ə·drē¹·nəl a¹·ksis), *n* major component of the neuroendocrine system that controls reactions to stress and manages metabolic function; involves interactions of the hypothalamus, pituitary gland, and adrenal glands.

axis, inferior transverse, *n* a hypothetical axis passing from side to side through the lower auricular surface of the ilia and sacrum, describing iliac motion on the sacrum. Proposed by osteopathic physician Fred Mitchell, Sr. Also called the *innominate axis.*

axis, longitudinal, *n* a hypothetical axis located at the junction of a frontal and the median-sagittal planes. See also vertical axis.

axis, middle transverse, *n* hypothetical axis for the nutation/counternutation of the sacrum, located horizontally through the front of the sacrum at the second segment. Proposed by osteopathic physician Fred Mitchell, Sr.

axis, postural, *n* See axis, middle transverse.

axis, respiratory, *n* See axis, superior transverse.

axis, sacral motion, *n* movement of the sacrum around any of its axes.

axis, superior transverse, *n* hypothetical axis around which involuntary sacral movement is believed to occur during the craniosacral cycle. The axis passes through the articular processes behind the dura mater's attachment point in the second vertebral segment of the sacrum. Proposed by osteopathic physician Fred Mitchell, Sr.

axis, vertical, *n* axis located at the junction of the frontal and sagittal planes. Also called the *y axis.* See also axis, longitudinal.

axonopathies (aks·ə·nô¹·pə·thēs), *n.pl* forms of encephalopathy in which a particular part of the axon is damaged by a toxin. Includes proximal axonopathy and distal axonopathy.

axoplasmic transport (a·ksō·plas¹·mik tran¹·spōrt), *n* the simultaneous movement of proteins and other materials from the cell body of the neuron to the nerve fiber terminals and from the nerve fiber terminals to the cell body. Also called *axoplasmic flow.*

ayapana (ä¹·yä·pä¹·nə), *n* Latin name: *Eupatorium ayapana;* part used: leaves; uses: aromatic, diaphoretic, skin protectant, stimulant, stomachic, wound healing, and as a household remedy for assorted ailments; precautions: none known

aynI (T¹·nē), *n* in the Kallawaya system of healing practiced in Bolivia, the communal act of bringing music, money, food, and other supportive items to sustain the motivation, faith, and recovery efforts of a person affected with disease.

Ayurveda (ä¹·yurr·wā¹·də), *n.pr* the science (veda) of life (ayu); ancient Indian health system that uses Vedic knowledge to reestablish the balance between body and mind.

Azadirachta indica, *n* See neem.

B

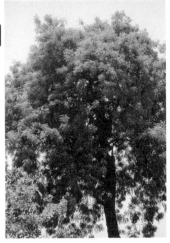

Azadirachta indica. (Williamson, 2002)

azarcón (ä·sär·kōn´), *n* a traditional preparation originating from Mexico used to relieve empacho, an infection thought to be related to the obstruction of gastrointestinal tract in children. There have been reports of lead poisoning and fatal encephalopathy from using azarcón. Also called *alacorn, coral, luiga, maria luisa,* or *rueda.*

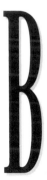

ba gang bian zheng system (pä·gäng pē·än dzəng sis´·təm), *n* eight-parameter pattern diagnostic system in modern Chinese acupuncture that focuses on the functions and dysfunctions of the organs. See also acupuncture.

babalawo (bä´·bä·lä´·wō), *n* spiritual leader of the Yoruba people of Nigeria who is believed to have healing powers.

Bachelor of Ayurvedic Medicine and Surgery, *n* a degree awarded after completion of an undergraduate program in Ayurveda. To earn this degree, one must complete a course of study related to the foundations of Ayurveda and participate in a clinical setting under the direction of an experienced Ayurvedic practitioner.

bacille Calmette-Guérin (bə·sēl´ kôl·mət-ger´·ən), *n.pr* an inactive strain of tubercle bacilli, used as a vaccine against tuberculosis in many countries; also has been used as a treatment for bladder cancer and leprosy.

backward bending, *n* extension of the spine.

backward torsion, *n* condition in which the sacrum rotates about an oblique axis so that sacral base side opposite to the axis involved rotates to the posterior.

backward upward laterally, *adv* the directions in which a bone structure or cavity may extend in the body—in this case specifically backward, upward, and to the side.

backward upward medially, *adv* the directions in which a bone structure or cavity may extend in the body; in this case specifically backward, upward, and toward the middle.

Bacopa monniera, *n* See brahmi.

bacteremia (bak·tə·rē´·mē·ə), *n* condition marked by the presence of bacteria in the bloodstream.

bacterial endocarditis (bak·tē´· rē·əl en´·dō·kar·dī´·tis), *n* bacterial infection in the heart valves, the endocardium, or both. May be acute or subacute. Symptoms can include heart murmur, embolic phenomena, splenomegaly, bacteremia, extended fever, and heart failure.

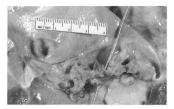

Bacterial endocarditis. (Kumar, Cotran, and Robbins, 1997)

bacterial sinusitis (bak·tē′·rē·əl sī′·nə·sī′·tis), *n* an inflammation of the sinus cavities, open air passageways within the human body, caused by bacteria such as streptococci, staphylococci, pneumococci, or *Haemophilus influenzae.* Prevalent symptoms include congestion in the nasal passages and pain, tenderness, and swelling in the approximate area of the affected cavity. Headaches, chills, and fever may also occur. In some cases, it may develop immediately after a viral infection in the upper respiratory tract.

bacteriotherapy (bak·tē′·rē·ō·the′·rə·pē), *n* a treatment for recurrent group A betahemolytic streptococci pharyngitis that involves colonizing group A nonbetahemolytic streptococci in the throat.

badahan (bä·dä·hän), *n* in Tibetan medicine, compassion (one of the three functions of the mind), which is the state of being in which an individual is at peace with himself or herself. It is a feeling of being devoid of attachment, anger, pride, and jealousy. According to the philosophy of Tibetan Vajrayana Buddhism, it is only from this state of complete openness and peace that one is able to experience fully the suffering of others and to work toward alleviating it. The embodiment of this feeling or state that is conducive to one's health is acknowledged as the high level of vitality or "living warmth." See also chi and schara.

badahan type (bä·dä·hän tīp), *n* in Tibetan medicine, a unique psychosomatic set of characteristics; on a physical level, a person possessing this set of characteristics will have a figure that is apt to be overweight; a muscular, short-size neck; a wide, overdeveloped chest; firm, broad shoulders; large-sized abdomen; disproportionately short legs and arms; large-sized feet and hands; large-sized, broad, white nails; and smooth, moist, thick, and pale-colored skin. On a psychological level, the person possesses a sense of compassion, love, stability, a pleasing personality, and strong listening abilities. See also chi type and schara type.

baduanjin (bä·dōō·ən·jēn), *n* "eight pieces of brocade," a millennia-old variation of qi gong characterized by eight pairs of simple movements. Also called *pa tuan chin* or *pa tuan tsin.* See also qi gong.

bael (bāl), *n* Latin name: *Aegle marmelos;* parts used. fruit (ripe and unripe), pulp, bark, roots; uses: in Ayurveda considered a rasayana, pacifies kapha and vata doshas, increases pitta dosha (bitter, astringent, light, dry); unripe fruit: astringents, digestive problems; ripe fruit: diarrhea, dysentery; roots: melancholia, fevers, cardiac tonic; leaves: cardiac tonic, skin ulcers, eye disorders; precautions: large doses may cause liver abnormalities. Also called *bel, beli, Bengal quince, bilva,* or *shivadruma.*

B

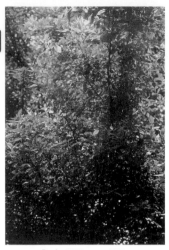

Bael. (Williamson, 2002)

bai zhu (pô dzōō), *n* Latin name: *Atractylodes macrocephala;* part used: rhizomes; uses: digestion, diuretic, eating disorders, diarrhea; precautions: none known.

baking soda, *n* Scientific name: *NaCHO₃*; uses: counter excessive acidity in the stomach; precautions: overdose. Also called *bicarb, bicarbonate of soda, sodium acid bicarbonate,* and *sodium bicarbonate.*

bala (bə·lä), *n* in Ayurveda, strength or life force indicative of general well-being.

balanced antagonism, *n* the continual fluctuation between the actions of the parasympathetic and sympathetic nervous systems to create a dynamic homeostasis in the organism.

balancing, *adj* referring to the adaptability of some substances with which a given dosage may have a stimulating effect on the body in one instance and a soothing effect in another instance.

ball mill, *n* porcelain jar containing rollers spun on larger rollers, used to grind substances, such as homeopathic remedies, to a fine powder.

balloon flower, *n* Latin name: *Platycodon grandiflorum;* part used: roots; uses: cough aid, antiinflammatory, expectorant, infections of the upper respiratory area; precautions: none known.

balm, *n* a healing or comforting ointment.

balneology (bal'·nē·ô'·lə·gē), *n* the study and practice of therapeutic bathing.

balneotherapy (bäl'·nē·ō·the'·rə·pē), *n* the practice of administering medicinal baths in order to treat injuries or disease.

balsam of Gilead (bôl'·səm əv gil'·ē·ad), *n* Latin name: *Populus candicans* L; parts used: buds, oil, resin; uses: antiscorbutic, aromatic, expectorant, joint and muscle pain, respiratory disorders, skin conditions, stimulant, tonic; precautions: aspirin sensitivity, anticoagulant therapy, IUD usage, kidney disease. Also called *balm of Gilead* and *Mecca balsam.*

balsam of Peru, *n* Latin names: *Myroxylon balsamum, Myroxylon pereirae;* parts used: oleo-resin, essential oil; uses: (suppositories) hemorrhoids, (internally) cough, respiratory illnesses, burns, fever, scabies (topical), circulation booster, arthritis; precautions: patients with kidney disease or febrile conditions, can cause kidney necrosis if taken internally. Also called *balsam of tolu, balsam tree, opobalsam, Peruvian balsam, resina tolutana, resin tolu,* or *Thomas balsam.*

balsamic (bäl·säm'·ik), *n* a substance that can soften and reduce mucus.

BAMS, *n.pr* See Bachelor of Ayurvedic Medicine and Surgery.

banxia (pän·zhē·ä), *n* Latin name: *Pinellia ternata;* part used: rhizomes; uses: expectorant, prevents vomiting, cough, asthma; precautions: pregnancy.

bao (pä·ö), *n* preciousness, one of the five virtues in Chinese medicine, for which po is responsible. See also po.

baptisia **(bap·ti'·zhyǝ)**, *n* Latin name: *Baptisia tinctoria* (L.) R.Br. ex Ait. f.; parts used: whole plant, roots; uses: antimicrobial, immunostimulant, systemic lymph infections, infections of the ears, nose, throat, mouth sores, catarrh; precautions: theoretically teratogenic, theoretically mutagenic, avoid long-term usage. Also called *indigoweed* or *wild indigo*.

Baptisia tinctoria (L.) R.Br. ex Ait. f., *n* See baptisia.

baquet (bǝ·ket'), *n* a wooden container filled with water, glass, and magnetized iron filings and iron rods protruding from it, which was used in group animal magnetism treatments. Patients simultaneously touch the rods to facilitate the flow of a healing magnetic energy among them. See also animal magnetism.

barbaloin (bar'·bǝ·lō'·in), *n* an active chemical component of aloes that has purgative properties.

barberry **(bär'·ber·ē)**, *n* Latin name: *Berberis aquifolium* Pursh; part used: root bark, fruit; uses: antimicrobial, antiinflammatory, antiplatelet, decreases ventricular tachyarrhythmias, topical skin treatment; precautions: causes spontaneous abortion, avoid during pregnancy, cardiac damage, nephritis. Also called *berberry, jaundice berry, pepperridge bush, pipperidge, sour-spine, sowberry, trailing mahonia,* or *wood sour.*

barberry, Indian, *n* Latin name: *Berberis aristata*; parts used: roots, stem, fruits; uses: in Ayurveda balances kapha and vata doshas (bitter, astringent, light, rough), hepatoprotective, antiinflammatory, antibacterial, tonic, cholagogue, stomachic,

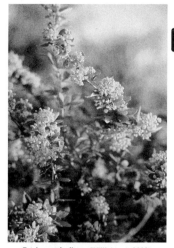

Barberry, Indian. (Williamson, 2002)

fever, diarrhea, hepatitis, splenitis, jaundice, eye infections, precautions: none known. Also called *daruhaldi* or *daru haridra.*

bardo (ba'r·dō), *n* from the *Bardo Thodol* (i.e., the *Tibetan Book of the Dead*), refers to the space between death and rebirth and by extension to the space between any cessation and becoming.

barium enema, *n* a procedure in which barium sulfate is introduced into the intestine through the rectum. Allows medical professionals to image intestinal tumors, obstructions, ulcerative colitis, and the like with x-rays. Also called *contrast enema.*

B

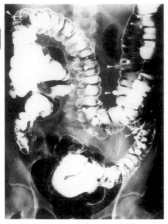

Barium enema. (Heuman, Mills, and McGuire, 1997)

baroreceptor (ba'·rə·ri·sep'·ter), *n* receptor cell in the bloodstream that relays information about blood pressure to the medulla oblongata.

Barosma betulina, *n* See buchu.

Barosma crenulata, *n* See buchu.

Barosma serratifoliata, *n* See buchu.

barrida (bär·rē'·də), *n* in Curanderismo, the Mexican healing system, the ritual of cleansing or sweeping, in which a person is swept from head to toe with an object (e.g., egg, lemon, garlic, broom, or crucifix, depending on the nature of the ailment) that is thought to have the power to give positive energy or remove bad vibrations. Also called *limpia.*

barrier, anatomic, *n* anatomic, structural limitations to motion; any limitation to passive motion.

barrier, elastic, *n* the range between the anatomic, passive motion barrier and the physiologic, active motion barrier.

barrier, pathologic (pa'·thə·lô·jik ber'·rē·er), *n* any permanent limitation to motion created by pathologic transformations of tissues.

barrier phenomenon, *n* a limitation on the ability of chemicals to move across a membrane or into a tissue as a result of pathology, anatomy, or physiology.

barrier, physiologic, *n* the limitation to active motion.

barrier, superficial, *n* the chemical, mechanical, and pathogenic protections offered by the skin, mucous membranes, respiratory and excretory systems. These defenses must be breached to trigger an inflammatory response.

Barthel index, *n.pr* standard, well-validated assessment that measures functional outcomes, including independence in mobility and self-care. Commonly used in rehabilitation medicine.

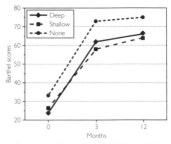

Barthel index. (Samuel Shiflett, PhD, Kessler Medical Rehabilitation Research and Education Corporation, West Orange, NJ)

basal body temperature, *n* temperature of the body determined in the morning, after sleeping and before any activity.

basal metabolic rate, *n* the rate of metabolism at rest.

basal metabolism, *n* the minimum amount of energy that the body requires to carry out normal functions such as respiration, temperature, peristalsis, circulation, and muscle tone.

base, *n* **1.** a compound that can react with an acid in aqueous solutions to form salts. **2.** in aromatherapy, an ingredient specifically prepared to represent a particular natural fragrance source, a blend of natural sources of fragrance sources, or an abstract fragrance concept.

base note, *n* aromatic components of essential perfumes and oils, such as sandalwood and vetivert, that do not readily evaporate and are used as fixatives to provide permanence. See also note.

baseline, *n* the horizontal axis on a graph drawn by the pen recorder.

basic induction, *n* initial phase of hypnosis during which patients are gradually encouraged to relax while being given information about the ensuing hypnosis session.

basic science evidence, *n* objective findings from laboratory experiments that serve to further or confirm conclusions from clinical research or determine mechanisms.

basil (bā´·zəl), *n* Latin names:*Ocimum basilicum, Ocimum sanctum*; parts used: leaves; uses: antiseptic, antidiabetic, immune system stimulant, antiinflammatory, ulcers, arthritis, anxiety, flatulence, coughs; precautions: pregnancy, lactation, infants, diabetes, extended usage; do not use with insulin or antidiabetic medications. Also called *common basil, sweet basil,* or *St. Josephwort.*

basil, holy, *n* Latin name: *Ocimum sanctum;* parts used: leaves, seeds, root; uses: in Ayurveda, pacifies kapha and vata doshas (pungent, bitter, light, dry), immunomodulation, antistress, antimicrobial, antiasthmatic, anticarcinogen, radioprotective, bronchitis, cold, fever, cough, laxative, stimulant, cardiotonic, indigestion, appetite stimulant; precautions: constipation. Also called *sacred basil, surasa, tulsi,* or *vrinda.*

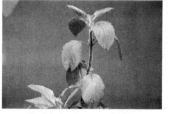

Basil, holy. (Williamson, 2002)

basophil, *n* white blood cell with cytoplasmic granules and histamines used to direct other WBCs to inflamed areas.

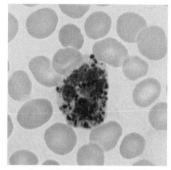

Basophils. (Carr and Rodak, 1999)

bay, *n* Latin name: *Laurus nobilis;* parts used: berries, leaves, oil; uses: antidiabetic, antiulcerogenic, rubefacient, rheumatism, colic, antispasmodic, cirrhosis; oil: antibacterial, antifungal; precautions: pregnancy, lactation, children, asthma, insulin, antidiabetic medications. Also called *bay laurel, bay leaf, bay tree, laurel, sweet bay,* or *Roman laurel.*

bayberry (bā´·ber·ē), *n* Latin name: *Myrica cerifera*; parts used: dried root bark, flowers; uses: diarrhea, jaundice, emetic, skin conditions, promotes healing of wounds; precautions: pregnancy, lactation, children, hepatotoxicity. Also called *candleberry, myrica, wax myrtle, spicebush, sweet oak, tallow shrub, vegetable tallow, waxberry,* or *wax myrtle.*

BBT, *n* See technique, Buteyko breathing.

BCAAs, *n.pl* See acids, branched-chain amino.

BCG, *n.pr* See bacille Calmette-Guérin.

bearberry (ber·ber·ē), *n* Latin names: *Arctostaphylos uvaursi, Arctostaphylos coactylis, Arctostaphylos adenotricha;* parts used: dried leaves; uses: antimicrobial, antiinflammatory, antiseptic, astringent, diuretic, urinary infections; precautions: pregnancy, lactation, children, diuretic medications, NSAIDs, mutagenic, carcinogenic, hepatotoxicity; not recommended for long-term use. Also called *arctostaphylos, bear's grape, crowberry, foxberry, hogberry, kinnikinnick, manzanita, mountain box,* or *rockberry.*

bearwood, *n* See chittem bark.

beating, *n* massage technique that uses the ulnar side of the fist. The technique consists of rapid, heavy percussive tapotement. See also tapotement.

bechic (bā´·shik), *n* a cough suppressant.

bee pollen, *n* mixture of flower pollen, honeybee digestive juices, and nectar. Has been used therapeutically for asthma, allergic conditions, impotence, bleeding stomach ulcers, altitude sickness, as a dietary supplement has been used for cancer, high cholesterol, and cardiac conditions. Should not be used if allergic to pollen or by diabetic patients who are using insulin or hypoglycemic medications.

bee venom, *n* poison extracted from bees. Has been used in the treatment of rheumatic diseases, especially multiple sclerosis and arthritis; can be applied directly or by intramuscular injection.

behavioral kinesiology (BK), *n* a combination of applied kinesiology and psychoanalytical concepts that treats psychological and functional problems with the meridian points used in acupuncture and muscle testing.

behavioral rasayanas (bə·hā´·və·rəl rä´·sä·yä´·nəz), *n.pl* in Maharishi Ayurveda, behaviors such as love, moderation, and respect, which release in the brain beneficial chemicals that boost an individual's immunity. See rasayana.

beimu (pā·mōō), *n* Latin name: *Fritillaria cirrhosa;* part used: bulb; uses: cough aid, mucolytic, expectorant, respiratory tract inflammation; precautions: none known.

Bell's palsy, *n.pr* paralysis of the seventh cranial nerve; affects one side of the face. Can be caused by nerve compression, tumor, nerve trauma, infection, or stress.

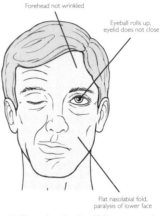

Forehead not wrinkled

Eyeball rolls up, eyelid does not close

Flat nasolabial fold, paralysis of lower face

Bell's palsy. (Lewis, Heitkemper, and Dirksen, 2000)

Bellis perennis, *n* See daisy.

belly bowl, *n* a small device that holds burning moxa directly above a bodily region, usually the navel. See also moxibustion.

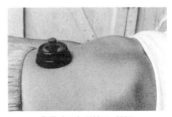

Belly bowl. (Abbate, 2001)

Bence Jones protein, *n.pr* protein commonly found in patients suffering from multiple myeloma.

beneficence (bə·ne´·fi·səns), *n* a principle of medical ethics according to which a person should do good to others, especially when one has a professional duty to do so.

benefit, *n* the condition of promoting improvement or enhancing a sense of well-being.

benevolent spirits (bə·ne'·və·lənt spir'·its), *n.pl* according to the Pima Indian healing system, spirits believed to be responsible for recruiting and training shamans, who diagnose illness and direct the clients to other practitioners for treatment.

benign, *adj* noncancerous; descriptive term for tumors, moles, and growths.

benign prostatic hyperplasia (bi·nīn' prô·sta'·tik hī·per·plā'·zhə), *n* condition marked by enlargement of the prostate gland that exerts pressure on the urethra thereby obstructing the flow of urine.

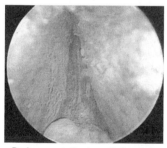

Benign prostatic hyperplasia. (Greig and Garden, 1996)

Benjamin gum, *n* See gum benzoin.

benzene ring, *n* See aromatic ring.

benzoin (ben'·zə·wən), *n* Latin name: *Styrax benzoin, Styrax paralleloneurus, Styrax tonkinesis*; parts used: resin; uses: antiseptic, wound healing, expectorant, bronchial conditions; precautions: may cause rash, allergic reactions, contact dermatitis, gastrointestinal hemorrhage upon ingestion. Also called *Benjamin tree, benzoe, benzoin tree, gum benjamin, Siam benzoin,* or *Sumatra benzoin.*

berberine (bər·bə·rēn'), *n* alkaloid derived from the plants belonging to

the *Berberidaceae* family with long history of medicinal use in both Ayurveda and Chinese medicine; used to treat intestinal parasite infections, ocular trachoma infections, and bacterial diarrhea.

Berberis aquifolium Pursh, *n* See barberry.

Berberis aristata, *n* See barberry, Indian.

berberis bark, *n* See barberry.

beta (bā'·tə), *n* Greek letter represented as β. See Greek letters.

beta-amyloid protein (BAP), *n* a protein found in excess in the brains of Alzheimer's disease sufferers; aggregates into dense plaques on the exterior of brain cells, which in turn destroy the synapses and conduction of nerve impulses.

beta-carotene (bā·tə·ke·rō·tēn), *n* a plant pigment, antioxidant, and biochemical precursor to vitamin A. Large doses may increase the risk of lung cancer and cardiac disease.

beta endorphin, *n* naturally occurring opiate neurotransmitter released when the body is under stress; responsible for pain reduction.

betadine (bā'·tə·dīn), *n* an antiseptic agent used topically to destroy microbes. In comparison to iodine, it is less likely to sensitize or sting the affected area. It is also soluble in water and will not permanently stain clothes. Also called *povidone-iodine.*

beta-sitosterol (bā·tə·sis'·ter·ôl), *n* a mixture of phytochemicals—specifically sitosterolins and phytosterols. Used to treat an enlarged prostate and as an immunomodulator. No known precautions.

beta-thalassemia (bā'·tə·tha·ləs·sē'·mē·ə), *n* type of anemia occurring as a result of reduced synthesis of the beta chains of hemoglobin.

betel palm (bē'·təl pôlm), *n Areca catechu;* parts used: nut, leaves; uses: stimulant, depression, respiratory ailments, coughs, sore throats; precautions: pregnancy, lactation, children, oral cancers, ulcers, kidney conditions, carcinogenic, alcohol, antiglaucoma medications, beta blockers, cardiac glycosides, neuroleptics. Also called *areca nut, betal, chavica betal, hmarg, maag, paan, pan masala, pan parag, pinang,* or *supai.*

beth root, *n* Latin name: *Trillium erectum, Trillium grandiflorum;* parts used: leaves, roots, rhizomes; uses: astringent, antifungal, hemorrhoids, skin ulcers, varicose veins, analgesic, expectorant, skin irritation; precautions: uterine stimulation, pregnancy, lactation, children, cardiotoxicity. Also called *birthroot, cough root, ground lily, Indian balm, Indian shamrock, Jew's harp, purple trillium, rattlesnake root, snake bite, squaw root, stinking benjamin, three-leafed trillium, trillium pendulum,* or *wake-robin.*

betony (be·'tə·nē), *n* Latin name: *Stachys officinalis* L.; parts used: flowers, leaves; uses: seizure disorders, diarrhea, asthma, wounds, high blood pressure, kidney stones, palpitations; precautions: uterine stimulant, pregnancy, lactation, children, patients taking blood pressure medications; may cause hepatotoxicity. Also called *bishops wort* or *wood betony.*

Betula alba, *n* See birch.

Betula lenta, *n* See birch.

Betula pendula, *n* See birch.

Betula pubescens, *n* See birch.

Betula verrucosa, *n* See birch.

between-person cardiac brain synchronization, *n* the aligning of brain and cardiac rhythms of two individuals in close proximity to each other.

bhakti (bhäk·'tē), *n* in Hinduism, devotion and love as a path to salvation.

bhangra (bhäng·'rə), *n* Latin name: *Eclipta alba;* parts used: whole plant, roots, seeds, seed oil; uses: in Ayurveda, balances kapha and vata doshas (pungent, bitter, light, dry), antiinflammatory, hepatoprotection, hypotensive, alopecia, ringworm, liver conditions, catarrh, cough, hemorrhage, indigestion, roots: emetic; purgative; precautions: none known. Also called *babri, bhringaraja,*

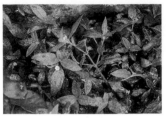

Bhangra. (Williamson, 2002)

false daisy, tekarajah, or *trailing eclipsa.*

bhasma (bhäs·'mə), *n* in Ayurveda, a method of medicine preparation in which purified minerals and animal ingredients (e.g., horn, shell) are macerated and ground with herbal extracts. The resulting mixture is then heated until only the residual ash remains.

bheda (bhā·'də), *n* in Ayurveda, a phase in the progression of a disease characterized by destruction of a tissue or structure within the body, thus leading to changes in other bodily systems and organs. It is difficult to treat a disease at this stage.

bhutagnis (bhōō·täg·'nēs), *n* in Ayurveda, the five enzymes found in the liver that convert partially digested food into a homologous chyle that nourishes the body. See also agnis.

bian zheng (pē·än dzəng), *n* in traditional Chinese medicine, the process of identifying patterns during the diagnosis of illness in order to determine the cause of disease and best course of treatment.

biarticular (bī·'är·tik·'yə·ler), *adj* pertaining to a muscle, which crosses two joints acting on both.

bibliotherapy, *n* use of books, stories, and/or poetry with the intention of affecting therapeutic change, or personal development. See also therapy, poetry.

bidirectionality, *n* in herbalism, the property of tonic herbs that allows them to maintain balance by eliciting a response in opposite directions depending on the needs of the individual taking them. See also adaptogen and tonic herbs.

bigu (bē··gōō), *n* a type of Qi gong practice in which practitioners claim to survive without solid food for a significant length of time, sometimes months or even years. See also Qi gong.

bilberry (bil·ber·ē), *n* Latin name: *Vaccinium myrtillus;* parts used: berries; uses: antioxidant, vasoprotection, glaucoma, cataracts, myopia, diabetic retinopathy, varicose veins, hemorrhoids, venous insufficiency, antidiabetic actions; enhances night vision; prevents macular degeneration; precautions: pregnancy, lactation, children, those taking anticoagulant medications, antiplatelet medications, aspirin, insulin, NSAIDs, antidiabetic medications. Also called *bog bilberries, European blueberries, huckleberries,* or *whortleberries.*

bile (bāl), *n* emulsifying fluid secreted from the gallbladder into the intestines. Bile breaks down fat globules to provide fat-absorbing enzymes with a larger surface area.

bile preparation, *n* remedy derived from raw bile. In Asia, the raw bile of *Ctenopharyngodon idellus* grass carp is thought to promote good health. Use of raw bile derived from sheep is believed to cure diabetes mellitus. Ingestion of raw bile can cause renal toxicity and hepatic failure.

bilirubinemia (bı·le·rōō·bi·nē·mē·ə), *n* the presence of elevated bilirubin in the bloodstream.

bilis (bē·lēs), *n* according to Curanderismo, the Mexican-American healing system, sickness marked by constipation and bitter taste in mouth, believed to be caused by feelings of anger or fear.

bind, *n* a feeling of resistance to motion within a joint or tissue. Also called *resistance.*

binomial (bī·nō·mē·əl), *n* the taxonomic name for plants that always

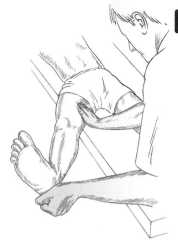

Bind. (Chaitow, 2003)

consists of two parts: the genus, which is the first name and is always capitalized, and the species, which is the second name and is always lowercase. These names should be used instead of common names to avoid confusion in the identification of herbs. Also called *botanical name, Latin name,* or *scientific name.*

bioavailability (bī·ō·ə·vāl·ə·bil·i·tē), *n* the amount of or rate at which a substance or drug is accessible to the body.

biochemical changes (bī·ō·ke·mik·əl chā·ng·gəz), *n* one of the five components of the subluxation model proposed by Dishman and Lantz.

biochemical individuality, *n* the concept that the nutritional and chemical make-up of each person is unique and that dietary needs therefore vary from person to person.

biochemistry, *n* the chemistry of living organisms and vital life processes.

biodiversity prospecting, *n* globally locating medicinally beneficial flora for commercial use.

bioelectrical impedance (bī′·ō·ē· lek′·trik im·pē′·dəns), *n* measurement of tissue conductivity by applying an electric current to the body.

bioelectromagnetics, *n* the study of how changes in electromagnetic fields can alter a person's physical and mental condition.

bioenergetics, *n* **1.** system in which natural healing is enhanced by creating harmony between the patient's body and the natural environment. **2.** therapy created by neo-Reichian physician Alexander Lowen holding that body and mind are functionally identical. Work with the body eases mental tensions and vice-versa, thus creating greater emotional and physical flexibility.

bioenergy, *n* the energy of the body.

biofeedback, *n* **1.** process in which equipment sensors provide measurements of bodily functions (such as heart rate or neural activity) and those signals are displayed to the patient. **2.** a technique used to teach patients to control physiologic events based on feedback provided by various types of equipment. See also biofeedback, electromyographic.

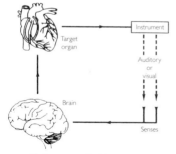

Biofeedback. (Rankin-Box, 2001)

biofeedback training, *n* a technique for learning voluntary control of physiologic functions normally considered autonomic, such as blood pressure and heart rate, to reduce stress, improve overall well-being, and treat functional conditions. Biofeedback uses sensors and computer programs or other devices that measure physiological parameters and give instantaneous feedback to the user so that one may cultivate conscious control of those parameters.

biofeedback-assisted somatic release, *n* the use of myoelectric biofeedback to become aware of and relax habitual muscular tension.

Biofeedback Certification Institute of America, *n.pr* an independent organization founded in 1981 to establish and maintain standards for providing biofeedback services. It also provides certification to practitioners who meet particular requirements. Also called *BCIA.*

biofield, *n* subtle energy fields that permeate the living body. See also therapy, biofield.

biofields (bī′·ō·fēldz), *n.pl* areas of energy that expand past the corporal boundaries of living organisms.

bioflavenoids (bī′·ō·flā′·və·noidz), *n.pl* compounds found in grapes, berries, and other fruits; vegetables; wine; and tea that are claimed to improve endothelial function, reduce LDL-C oxidation, and prevent and treat atherosclerotic vascular disease.

bioinformation, *n* organizational properties of biological systems. Also called *information medicine hypothesis* and *information biology.*

biological response modifiers, *n.pl* substances such as phytochemicals and fibers that modulate mechanisms related to the development of disease, such as hormonal changes, immune function, inflammatory activity, oxidative stress, and homeostasis. Also called *BRMs.*

bioluminescence, *n* light produced by living organisms, such as fireflies, some bacteria, and some deep-sea fish, via chemical reactions. Most cells have low-level bioluminescence.

biomagnetic fields, *n.pl* bodily magnetic fields.

biomagnetics, *n* the scientific study of magnetic fields as applied to living tissue.

B

biomagnetism, *n* the science of examining the properties of living systems that create magnetic fields.

biomedical approach, *n* medical framework that considers illness to be caused by identifiable agents.

biomedicine, *n* the study of diseases of the human body caused by biological, chemical, physical, and psychosocial elements.

biopathography (bī'·ō·pə·thog'·rə·fē), *n* a form of case analysis in which the current malady is contextualized through the patient's biography and case history.

biophoton emission, *n* low-energy endogenous radiation produced by humans and other living organisms and detected as barely visible light.

biophysics, *n* **1.** the principles of physics applied to biological events. **2.** the investigation of physical processes taking place in living organisms, such as electrical or magnetic events.

bioresonance (bī'·ō·re'·zə·nəns), *n* technique in which the practitioner uses a device to analyze the patient's electromagnetic waves and alter them before returning them to the body. Used for treating headaches, skin conditions, pain, and other maladies.

biosynthesis (bī'·ō·sin'·thə·sis), *n* formation of a chemical compound by a living organism. Also called *biogenesis.*

biotin (bī'·ə·tən), *n* a B vitamin synthesized by bacteria within the gut; acts as a cofactor with enzymes; thought useful in the treatment of diabetes and brittle nails. Supplementation is not usually necessary except with pregnancy, inflammatory bowel disease, or antibiotic or anticonvulsant medications. No known precautions.

biphasic activity, *n* **1.** two contrasting stages of activity. **2.** the principle that varying the degree of a stimulus applied on either side of a critical threshold may reverse the results in a living organism. See also hormesis and law, Arndt-Schulz.

bipolar magnets, *n.pl* magnets in which the north and south poles are adjacent. Have been used to relieve pain. See also therapy, magnetic field.

birch, *n* Latin names: *Betula alba, Betula pendula, Betula verrucosa, Betula pubescens, Betula lenta;* parts used: bark, leaves; uses: topical and internal analgesic, antioxidant, diuretic, kidney and bladder stones, gout; precautions: pregnancy, lactation, children, patients with allergic conditions, congestive heart failure, severe kidney conditions. Also called *birch tar oil, birch wood oil, black birch, cherry birch, sweet birch oil,* or *white birch.*

birth trauma, *n* physical injuries experienced by an infant during delivery.

bismuth (biz'·məth), *n* a mineral that is used as an antacid and for removing *Helicobacter pylori.* Several variations of this mineral are found and include bismuth subsalicylate (Pepto-Bismol) and bismuth subcitrate.

bistort (bis'·tōrt), *n* Latin name: *Polygonum bistorta;* parts used: leaves, roots, rhizomes; uses: external—bites, burns, hemorrhoids, snakebites, stings; internal—diarrhea, peptic ulcers, irritable bowel syndrome, ulcerative colitis, possible antiinflammatory and antiviral activities; precautions: pregnancy, lactation, children; may cause hepatotoxicity. Also called *adderwort, common bistort, Easter ledges, Easter mangiant, knotweed, oderwort, osterick, patience dock, snakeroot, snakeweed,* or *twice writhen.*

bitter apple, *n* Latin name: *Citrullus colocynthus;* part used: fruit pulp; uses: only in very small doses as a cathartic; precautions: can be poisonous; can cause severe pain and irritation, bloody discharge, inflammation of bowel. Also called *bitter cucumber* and *colocynth.*

bitter melon, *n* Latin name: *Momordica charantia* L.; parts used: fruit, seeds, seed oil, leaves; uses: antidiabetic, antiinfective, antipyretic, anthelmintic, laxative, possible antifungal, androgenic, antiviral, antimalarial actions; possibly useful for infertility; precautions: pregnancy, lactation, children, patients taking hypoglycemic medications; may cause uterine bleeding or contractions, hepatotoxicity; seeds are toxic to children. Also called *balsam apple, balsam pear, bitter cucumber, bitter pear, carilla cundeamor, fu gwa,* or *karolla.*

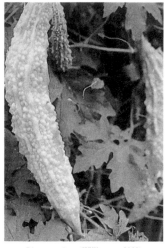

Bitter melon. (Williamson, 2002)

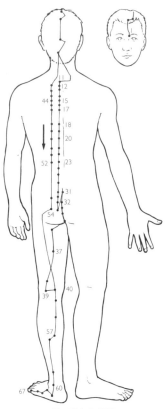

BL. (Chirali, 1999)

bitter orange, *n* an essential oil, expressed from the fruit of the bitter orange *(Citrus aurantium),* useful for treating colds and flu, constipation and flatulence, gum conditions, sluggish digestion, and stress.

bitters, *n* orally administered drugs made from botanical sources. Bitter in taste, they often are used to activate the gastrointestinal tract, to reduce inflammation, and to work as mild sedatives.

BL, *n* bladder channel; an acupuncture channel running from the head to the feet on the back of the body and associated with the kidney (KI) channel. See also KI.

black bryony, *n* Latin name: *Tamus communis;* parts used: roots; uses: homeopathic diuretic, rubefacient, chilblains; precautions: none known.

black cherry, *n* See wild cherry.

black cumin, *n* Latin name: *Nigella sativa;* parts used: seeds; uses: in Ayurveda, pacifies vata and kapha doshas (pungent, bitter, light, dry, sharp), antimicrobial, hepatoprotective, carminitive, stimulant, diuretic, anthelmintic, indigestion, diarrhea, skin disorders, worms, stops vomiting; precautions: none known. Also called *kalajaji, kalajira, kalonji, nigella,* or *small fennel.*

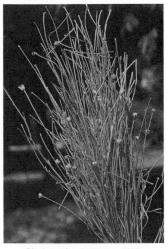

Black cumin. (Williamson, 2002)

black haw (blak˙ hô), *n* Latin names: *Viburnum prunifolium, Viburnum opulus;* parts used: root bark; uses: diuretic, antispasmodic, sedative, relaxes uterine muscles, dysmenorrhea, cardiovascular diseases; precautions: patients with kidney stones, those taking anticoagulant medications. Also called *American sloe, cramp bark, guelder-rose, may rose, nannyberry, sheepberry, shonny, silver bells, sloe, stagbush,* or *sweet haw.*

black hellebore, *n* Latin name: *Helleborus niger;* parts used: dried rhizome, root; uses: anthelmintic, antipsychotic, antianxiety, anticonvulsant, laxative, pregnancy-related hypertension, amenorrhea, meningitis, encephalitis; causes abortion; precautions: pregnancy, lactation, children, considered poisonous, can cause bradycardia, arrhythmias, seizures, respiratory depression, nausea, diarrhea, abdominal cramps, altered vision, coma, and paralysis. Also called *Christe herb, Christmas rose, Easter rose,* or *melampode.*

black mustard, *n* Latin name: *Brassica negra, Brassica alba;* part used: seeds; uses: emetic, diuretic, soothe skin irritation, homeopathic treatment of upper respiratory and gastrointestinal conditions; precautions: individuals with renal disorders, gastrointestinal disorders, skin irritation, contact dermatitis. Also known as *brown mustard, California rape, charlock, Chinese mustard, Indian mustard, white mustard,* and *wild mustard.*

black radish, *n* Latin name: *Raphanus sativus* var. *niger;* part used: leaves, seeds, roots; uses: anthelmintic, inhibition of bacterial and fungal growth, scurvy, prevention or relief of spasms or cramps, contraction of bodily tissues, flatulence, increased flow of bile to intestines, stomachic, diuretic, expectorant, induce bowel evacuation, stimulate appetite, asthma, indigestion, abdominal bloating, relieve acid regurgitation, diarrhea, bronchitis, wound healing; precautions: digestive disorders, can cause miosis, pain, vomiting, slowed respiration, stupor, and albuminuria. Also called *oriental radish.*

black root, *n* Latin names: *Veronicastrum virginicum, Leptandra virginica, Veronica virginica;* parts used: fruit (unripened), oleoresin, roots, rhizome; uses: aromatic, antiperiodic, emetic, diuretic, appetite stimulant, astringent, jaundice, upset digestive system, common cold, seizures, bronchitis, epidermal disorders; precautions: pregnancy, lactation, children, causes headaches, drowsiness, vomiting, stomach cramps, hepatotoxicity (from dried leaves in large doses). Also called *Bowman root, brinton root, Culvert's physic, Culver's root, high veronica, hini, leptandra, physic root, quitel, tall speedwell,* or *Veronica.*

black snakeroot, *n* Latin name: *Cimicifuga racemosa, Actaea racemosa;* part used: root; uses: inflammation, rheumatism, prevention or relief of spasms or cramps, contraction of bodily tissues, induction of perspiration, diuretic, promotion

B

of menstrual flow, expectorant, sleep induction, relaxant, vasodilator, painful menstruation, menopausal symptoms, childbirth, sciatica, chorea, tinnitus, and high blood pressure; precautions: may cause gastrointestinal disturbances. Also called *actee a grappes, American baneberry, amerikansk slangerod, black bugbane, black cohosh, bugbane, cimicaire, cimicifuga, rattle root, sauco, slangenwortel, squaw root, tahta bitiotu,* and *wanzenkraut.*

bleeding, *n* **1.** losing blood, externally or internally. **2.** in traditional Chinese medicine, method used to remove heat from a given location or to drain a channel.

blepharoplasty (ble·'·fa·rō·pla'·stē), *n* plastic surgery procedure by which fat is removed from the upper eyelid.

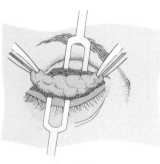

Removal of excess
fat from upper eyelid

Blepharoplasty. (Beare and Myers, 1998)

blind testing, *n* a clinical trial in which participants are unaware of whether they are in the experimental or control group of the study. Also called *masked.*

blinding, *n* within a clinical trial, hiding the knowledge of a particular treatment. The three types of blinding are the following: observer-blind—when the researcher does not know the particular treatment that a patient undergoes; single-blind, when only the patient does not know to which group he or she belongs; and double-blind, when both the patient and the one providing the treatment do not know group identity. These types of blinding ensure—all other factors being identical—that any observed results are not the result of bias of the study participants.

blitz gus (blits' gəs), *n* application of a highly pressurized cold water stream from a specified distance. See also cryotherapy.

blood-brain barrier, *n* barrier formed by epithelial cells in the capillaries that supply the brain and central nervous system. This barrier selectively allows entry of substances such as glucose, some ions, and oxygen, while blocking entry of other substances. Also called *BBB.*

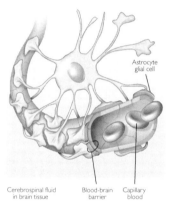

Astrocyte
glial cell

Cerebrospinal fluid   Blood-brain   Capillary
in brain tissue   barrier   blood

Blood-brain barrier. (Mosby's Medical, Nursing & Allied Health Dictionary, ed 6, 2002)

blood circulation system, *n* in Chinese medicine, system that transmits central and local biomolecular elements plus the cellular and biochemical changes stimulated by an acupuncture treatment within the periphery.

blood glucose level, *n* level of glucose in the bloodstream, normally about 70 to 115 mg/dL after fasting overnight. Higher levels may indicate diseases such as diabetes mellitus.

blood group, *n* classification based on the presence of certain antigens on the surface of red blood cells. Types include A, B, AB, O, and Rh+ or Rh–. Used in organ tranplantation, transfusion therapy, genetic studies, and maternal-fetal compatibility testing.

blood pressure, *n* force applied by circulating blood on the walls of the blood vessels and on the chambers of the heart. The pressure in a healthy individual varies but is usually considered below 120 mm Hg during systole and 80 mm Hg during diastole in adults.

Category	Systolic (mm Hg)		Diastolic (mm Hg)
Optimal†	<120		<80
Normal	<130		<85
High normal	130-139		85-89
Hypertension‡			
Stage 1 (mild)	140-159	or	90-99
Stage 2 (moderate)	160-179	or	100-109
Stage 3 (severe)	≥180	or	≥110

Blood pressure. (Potter and Perry, 2001; National High Blood Pressure Education Project, National Heart, Lung & Blood Institute, National Institutes of Health: The sixth report of the Joint National Committee on Detection, Evaluation & Treatment of High Blood Pressure, *Arch Intern Med* 157:2413, 1997)

bloodroot, *n* Latin name: *Sanguinaria canadensis* L.; part used: rhizome; uses: expectorant, antifungal, antiplaque, antiinflammatory, antimicrobial, skin cancer, ear cancer, nose cancer, nasal polyp; precautions: pregnancy, lactation, children, deep wounds, labeled as unsafe by the FDA skin irritations; can cause hypotension, shock, coma, headache, nausea, and anorexia. Also called *coon root, Indian paint, paucon, pausan, red puccoon, redroot, sweet slumber,* or *tetterwort.*

blue, *adj* in Chinese medicine, a facial coloration, often on the nasal bridge, that indicates unresolved emotional shocks. Useful in diagnosis of childhood illnesses.

blue balm (blōō' bälm'), *n* Latin name: *Melissa officinalis* L; parts used: foliage, oil; uses: carminative,

anxiety, insomnia, and menstrual problems, gastrointestinal complaints, sedative, and wound healing; precautions: none known. Also called *lemon balm, sweet balm, garden balm, cure-all,* and *dropsy plant.*

blue flag, *n* Latin name: *Iris versicolor;* part used: rhizomes with root; uses: laxative, diuretic, emetic, antimicrobial, treat sores, bumps, bites; precautions: pregnancy, lactation, children; can cause headache, soreness, and irritation to ear, eyes, nose, and throat, nausea, and death by poison. Also *dagger flower, dragon flower, flag lily, fleur-de-lis, flower-de-luce, liver lily, poison flag, snake lily, water flag,* or *wild iris.*

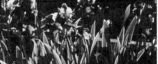

Blue flag. (Scott and Barlow, 2003)

blue food, *n* cool, yin food used to treat headaches and mental and spiritual conditions. Blue foods include grapes, plums, blueberries, asparagus, celery, parsnips, potatoes, and nuts.

blueberry, *n* Latin name: *Vaccinium angustifolium;* part used: fruit; uses: antioxidant, diabetes, cancer prevention; precautions: none known.

blue-gray, *adj* in Chinese medicine, a facial coloration, typically found in infants; indicates indigestion and stomach upset.

BMAS, *n.pr* See British Medical Acupuncture Society.

BMT, *n.pr* See bone marrow transplant.

body armoring (bô·dē-är·mər·ing), *n* a mentalmuscle reflex mechanism in the body, first described by

B

psychologist Wilhelm Reich. It involves tensing of muscle tissue whenever stress or emotion is experienced. To protect itself, the body takes a defensive, tight, and stiff stance. On a tissue level it enters into a muscular holding pattern that resists change and release. Unexpressed emotions such as anger, fear, and grief are common causes of this phenomenon.

body awareness, *n* the felt sense of embodiment; consciousness of our somatic feelings.

body chart, *n* method used by a practitioner to record symptoms experienced by the patient and the affected regions.

body density, *n* a noninvasive, quantitative technique for determining an individual's body fat composition by calculating the specific gravity of the subject. This involves comparing the weight of the body inside and outside of water.

body drop, *n* chiropractic technique in which the practitioner brings his full body weight quickly upon the patient's vertebra to be manipulated.

body mass index, *n* obesity-determining formula according to which an individual's weight in kilograms is divided by the square of the individual's height in meters. A BMI of 27 or more indicates obesity.

body mechanics, *n* in massage, proper and efficient use of the therapist's body during massage to avoid injury to the therapist. Also called *biomechanics.*

body/mind, *n* the interface between physiology and psychology that shows unified function by both.

Body-Mind Centering (BMC), *n* an integrated methodology that uses hands-on repatterning and movement reeducation; based on physiological, anatomical, developmental, and psychophysical principles that use touch, mind, voice, and movement.

body/mind/spirit, *n* in complementary and alternative medicine, the whole person, recognized and treated as a unique living intersection of the physical, mental, emotional, and subtle energies.

body note, *n* aromatic components of essential perfumes and oils, such as lavender and geranium, that provide body to a blend of specific natural sources of fragrance. See middle note.

body unity, *n* an aspect of osteopathic philosophy in which the human body is understood as a dynamically integrated functional whole.

bodywork, *n* **1.** a collection of techniques for restoring health and balance to the entire person by working through the body. **2.** to apply any number and combination of the therapeutic touch paradigms that have been developed.

Boerhaavia diffusa, *n* See punarnava.

bogbean, *n* Latin name: *Menyanthes trifoliata;* part used: leaves; uses: antiinflammatory, upset stomach, anorexia; precautions: pregnancy, lactation, children; can cause nausea, anorexia, and bleeding hemolysis when taken in conjunction with NSAIDs, antiplatelets, or anticoagulants. Also called *buckbean, marsh trifoil,* or *water shamrock.*

bogginess, *n* an abnormal texture of tissues characterized by a feeling of sponginess, usually because of high fluid content.

Boldea boldus, *n* See boldo.

boldine (bōl·dīn´), *n* alkaloid obtained from the plant *Peumus boldus* Molina and used as a diuretic.

boldo, *n* Latin names: *Boldea boldus, Peumus boldus;* part used: leaves; uses: sedative, liver medicine, laxative, flatulence, dysmenorrhea, gout, spastic digestive tract; precautions: pregnancy, lactation, children, patients with lung or neurologic disease, bile duct blockage, liver ailments, and gallstones; can cause paralysis, coma, seizures, death, and the crippling of the respiratory system. Also called *boldea, boldoa, boldine, boldo-do-Chile,* or *boldus.*

bond, *n* the attachment between the atoms in a molecule that is determined by the arrangement of electrons in the outer shell of the atom. See also covalent bond and ionic bonding.

bone densitometry (bōn´ den·si· tô´·me·trē), *n* test that determines bone density according to the radiation absorption rate of the skeletal structure being tested.

bone marrow transplant, *n* transfer of bone marrow tissue from a healthy donor to a recipient to restore the recipient's ability to produce normal blood cells. Usually used to treat hematopoietic or lymphoreticular diseases.

bone matrix, *n* flexible protein matrix in which minerals such as calcium and phosphorus are deposited and form bones.

bone setter, *n* Latin name: *Cissus quadrangularis;* parts used: leaves, stems, roots; uses: in Ayurveda pacifies vata and pitta doshas (sweet, light, dry), alterative, anthelmintic, aphrodisiac, antiasthmatic, bone healing; precautions: skin irritation. Also called *asthisanhari* or *hajora.*

boneset, *n* Latin name: *Eupatorium perfoliatum;* parts used: entire plant, dried leaves, buds; uses: expectorant, sedative, fever, flu, bronchitis; precautions: pregnancy, lactation, patients with liver disease; can cause nausea, anorexia, hepatotoxicity, and diarrhea. Also called *agueweed, crosswort, eupatorium, feverwort, Indian sage, Joe-pye-weed, sweating plant, thoroughwort,* or *vegetable antimony.*

bonesetters, *n.pl* during the Renaissance and Middle Ages, professionals who manipulated the joints or spine to relieve pain or restore range of movement.

Bonnie Prudden myotherapy, *n.pr* manual treatment of trigger points, developed by Bonnie Prudden in 1976. Pressure is applied and is followed by stretching the relaxed muscles to help them return to normal state.

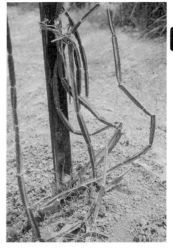

Bone setter. (Williamson, 2002)

borage **(bōr'·əj),** *n* Latin name: *Borage officinalis;* parts used: seeds, stems, leaves; uses: arthritis, hypertension, common cold, bronchitis; precautions: pregnancy, lactation, children. May cause hepatotoxicity. Also called *beebread, common borage, cool tankard, star flower,* and *ox's tongue.*

boron, *n* an element/mineral found in grains, nuts, leafy greens, and (noncitrus) fruits, used in the treatment of osteoarthritis and osteoporosis and in the prevention of prostate cancer. Precaution should be taken by women at risk for hormone-sensitive cancers and for patients who are undergoing hormone replacement therapy for the estrogen-elevating effects.

Boston **Motor** **Inventory,** *n.pr* measures active, isolated range of movement for patients with paralysis or hemiplegia.

boswellia (bôs·wel'·lē·ə), *n* Latin name: *Boswellia serrata;* parts used: resin, bark; uses: in Ayurveda, balances kapha and pitta doshas (astringent, bitter, sweet, light, dry), antiinflammatory, antiarthritic, analgesic, lowering of cholesterol, immunomodulator, antitumor, antifungal, aromatherapy; useful for treating asthma, rheumatoid arthritis, inflammatory bowel disease, malignant glioma; precautions: none known. Also called *Indian olibanum tree, salai,* or *sallaki.*

Boswellia serrata, *n* See boswellia.

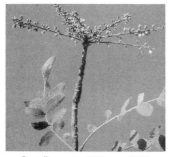

Boswellia serrata. (Williamson, 2002)

botanics, *n.pl* doctors who emerged from the eighteenth century Thomsonian botanical healing movement and expanded the range of herbal practices.

botulism (bô'·chə·li·zəm), *n* fatal form of food poisoning contracted from food or drink that contains the endotoxin produced by the bacillus *Clostridium botulinum.* Double vision, muscle weakness, lassitude, and dysphasia are among the commonly experienced symptoms.

bovine tracheal cartilage (bō'·vīn trā'·kē·əl kär'·tə·lij), *n* an acidic glycosaminoglycan complex, including 20% chondroitin sulfate and smaller amounts of hyaluronic acid, dermatan sulfate, heparan sulfate, and other polysaccharides, derived from the tracheae of cows. Has been used in cancer treatment and arthritis.

bow stance, *n* position assumed by a massage therapist applying continuous pressure to the client's body. The therapist's legs are hip width apart, knees slightly bent, front toes pointing in the direction of movement, and the toes of the back foot facing outward at a 45° angle. Also called *archer stance* or *lunge position.*

bowel nosodes (bou'·wəl nō'·sōdz), *n* homeopathic remedy made from organisms of cultured stool specimen. Used when an appropriate syndrome warrants its use. See also autoisopathy and nosode.

Bowen Moves, *n.pl* the core of the Bowen Technique, Bowen moves are gentle pressures and stretches applied to soft tissue in specific sequences and procedures using the therapist's fingers and thumbs. See also technique, Bowen.

B.P., *n* blood pressure.

B.P., *n.pr* See British pharmacopoeia.

BPD, *n* See disorder, breathing pattern disorder.

brachytherapy (bra'·ki·the'·rə·pē), *n* ionizing radiation applied at a short distance from the body or directly to the surface.

bradycardia (brā·dē·kar'·dē·ə), *n* a heart rate that is less than 60 beats per minute.

bradykinesia (brā·dē·ki·nē'·sē·ə), *n* illness in which an individual moves and speaks in an extraordinarily slow manner; can be caused by extrapyramidal disorders, certain tranquilizers, and Parkinsonism.

Brahman (brä'·mən), *n.pr* according to Vedic tradition, the "soul of the Universe," or the undivided pure consciousness.

brahmi (bräh'·mē), *n* Latin name: *Bacopa monniera;* parts used: dried whole plant, leaves, stems. Uses: in Ayurveda, pacifies kapha and vata doshas (bitter, light, oily), nerve tonic, astringent, cognition, memory, learning ability, anxiolytic, antioxidant, analgesic, and bronchodilator; precautions: none known. Also called *barambhi, nirabarhmi,* or *thyme-leaved gratiola.*

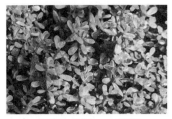

Brahmi. (Williamson, 2002)

brainstem auditory evoked potentials (BSAEPs), *n* neurological test that measures the nervous response of the brainstem and the brain to auditory stimulation. Used to evaluate acoustic neuroma, stroke, multiple sclerosis, and Meniere's disease.

brainwave training, *n* relaxation therapy aimed at learning to identify and control brainwaves, which are the electrical signals generated by brain cells. An individual can produce or change these brainwaves and monitor the same with electroencephalograph instruments. Has been used to treat patients with addiction problems, learning disabilities, seizures, and sleep disorders. See also biofeedback.

Brassica alba, *n* See mustard.

Brassica nigra, *n* See mustard.

breach, *n* action taken by one party in an agreement that serves to convince the other party that the terms of the contract will not be fulfilled. The faithful party may consider the contract canceled at that point.

breach of taboo, *n* violation of values held by a culture. Specifically, in the Native American culture, it refers to the failure to respect a spiritual being, an event, object, person, place, or an animal by committing acts such as visiting a forbidden place of power, offending the spirit of a powerful animal by not addressing the being by its proper name, ignoring the advice of a totem, or sharing guidance provided by totems in waking or sleeping

dreams, which are all believed to result in illness.

breath of fire, *n* a breathing technique used in yoga that incorporates rapid inhalation and exhalation to increase mental and physical energy. Also called *kapalabhati pranayama.*

breathing component, *n* respiration as it relates to meditation and manual therapy, mainly through the techniques of observing, directing, and synchronizing the breath to more fully engage the mind and body connection.

bregma, *n* meeting place on the skull of the anterior sagittal and coronal sutures.

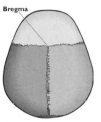

Bregma. (Chaitow, 1999)

Breuss cancer cure, *n.pr* anticancer diet consisting of vegetable juice (up to 1 L daily) and a variety of teas for 42 days.

Brief Symptom Inventory, *n.pr* a short (53-question) test used to assess the patterns of symptoms in those undergoing psychiatric or medical treatment. Useful for initial patient evaluation, clinical situations of patient debilitation, outpatient clinics, and in measuring the progress of treatment.

British Medical Acupuncture Society, *n.pr* the major British professional association for medical doctors who incorporate acupuncture into their practices. It is responsible for professional accreditation of medical acupuncturists.

British pharmacopoeia (bri·'·tish far'·mə·kə·pē'·ə), *n.pr* a list compiled by experts in pharmacology and pharmacy and approved by the government of Great Britain that provides specifications of the characteristics, manufacture, use, and dosage of drugs.

bromelain (brō'·mə·lən), *n* a proteolytic enzyme derived from pineapples that is used as an antiinflammatory and an antiedema agent; to aid digestion; to assist in recovery from surgery and athletic injuries; to treat sinusitis, familial amyloidotic polyneuropathy, ulcerative colitis; and to increase the efficacy of antibiotics. Contraindicated for those taking anticoagulant medications, antiplatelet medications, and sedatives. See also pineapple.

bronchiectasis (brôn·kē·ek'·stə·sis), *n* bronchial tree disorder characterized by the bronchial walls dilating irreversibly resulting in their destruction. Can be congenital but may also be caused by a tumor or by a foreign body that has been accidentally aspirated. Treatment includes expectorants, antibiotics, and (rarely) surgery of the affected part.

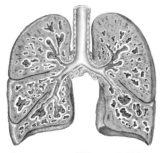

Bronchiectasis. (Wilson and Giddens, 2001)

bronchitis, *n* inflammation of the tracheobronchial tube. May be triggered by viral infections in the upper respiratory system spreading to the bronchi. Symptoms include fever, productive cough, and chest pain.

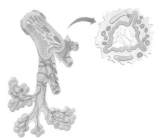

Bronchitis. (Thibodeau and Patton, 1999; Rolin Graphics)

broom, *n* Latin name: *Sarothamnus scoparius;* parts used: branches, buds; uses: emetic, diuretic, antiarrhythmic; precautions: pregnancy, lactation, children; patients with cardiac disease, hypertension, and arrhythmias; labeled unsafe by the FDA can cause headaches, hallucinations (smoking), arrhythmias, nausea, dizziness, tachycardia, shock, and spontaneous abortion through uterine spasms. Also called *bannal, broom top, genista, ginsterkraut, hogweed, Irish broom top, sarothamni herb, Scotch broom,* or *Scotch broom top.*

broom, butcher's, *n* Latin name: *Ruscus aculeatus;* parts used: rhizome (dried), roots (dried); uses: laxative, diuretic, leg edema, varicose veins, hemorrhoids, peripheral vascular disease, arthritis, retinopathy; precautions: pregnancy, lactation, children; patients with hypertension and benign prostate hypertrophy, nausea, anorexia, and gastritis (not often). Also called *box holly, knee holly, pettigree,* or *sweet broom.*

broom, Dyer's (dī'·erz brōōm'), *n* Latin name: *Genista tinctoria;* part used: twigs, leaves, flowering stems, seeds; uses: bowel evacuation, induction of perspiration, diuretic, induction of vomiting, vasoconstrictor, dropsy, rheumatism, gout; precautions: none known. Also called *base-broom, boyaci katirtirnagi, dyer's greenweed, dyer's greenwood, dyer's weed, genista, greenweed, hitotuba-*

enisida, retama de tintoreros, verf-brem, waxen wood, wede-wixen, woodwaxen, woud-wix, and dyer's greenweed.

brown mustard, n See black mustard.

Brucea amarissima (brōō·sā´·ə ä·mä·rēs´·sē·mə), n part used: dried fruit, seeds; uses: antimicrobial, amebic dysentery, malaria; precautions: anaphylaxis. Also called fructus bruceae.

brujos (brōō´·hōs), n in Curanderismo, the Mexican healing system, individuals who practice black magic that causes illness in others.

Bryonia spp., n See bryony root.

bryony root (brī´·ə·nē rōōt´), n Latin name: Bryonia spp.; part used: root; uses: relieves illnesses of the lungs and chest, rheumatism, whooping cough, dizziness, convulsions, dropsy, palsy, leprosy, cramps, kidney stones, cough, shortness of breath; removes freckles; facilitates wound healing; precautions: can cause powerful, watery evacuations of the bowels. Also called kua-lou, ladies' seal, tamus, tetterberry, white bryony, wild bryony, wild hops, wild vine, and wood vine.

buchu (bōō´·chōō), n Latin names: Barosma betulina, Barosma serratifolia, Barosma crenulata; part used: leaves; uses: antiseptic, diuretic, common cold, upset stomachs, urinary tract infections, gout, rheumatism, yeast infections, leukorrhea; precautions: pregnancy, lactation, children, patients with liver or kidney trouble; can cause spontaneous abortion, nephritis, increased menstruation, nausea, anorexia, hepatotoxicity, and diarrhea. Also called Agathosma, betuline, or bucco.

buckthorn, n Latin name: Rhamnus cathartica; parts used: fruit, bark; use: laxative; precautions: pregnancy, lactation, children, elderly; patients with gastrointestinal problems, Crohn's disease, appendicitis, colitis, diabetes; can cause tremors, nausea, diarrhea, stomach cramps, dehydration, and electrolyte imbalance. Also called common buckthorn, hartsthorn, purging buckthorn, or waythorn.

buddhi (bōōd´·dhē), n in Sanskrit, intellect, the faculty responsible for discriminating between good and bad.

bugleweed, n Latin names: Lycopus virginicus, Lycopus europaeus; parts used: buds, leaves, roots, stems; uses: astringent, analgesic, fever, Graves' disease, mastodynia, tachycardia, mild hyperthyroidism; precautions: pregnancy, lactation, children, patients with thyroid growths, hypopituitarism, pituitary adenoma, hypogonadism, heart disease; can cause hypothyroidism. Also called carpenter's herb, common bugle, Egyptian's herb, farasyon maiy, gypsy-weed, gypsy-wort, lycopi herba, menta de lobo, middle comfrey, Paul's betony, sicklewort, su ferasyunu, water bugle, or water horehound.

BUL, n.pr See backward upward laterally.

bulimia, n psychologic eating disorder in individuals of normal weight marked by consumption of excessive amounts of food, followed by self-induced vomiting.

bulking agents, n.pl **1.** fibers, including pectin, psyllium seed, and guar gum, that provide laxative properties, are claimed to maintain the strength of the veins in the body, and decrease the risk of developing varicose veins. These substances reduce the amount of strain produced during defecation by promoting peristalsis and maintaining fecal softness. In general, these fibers produce less irritation than cellulose fiber products such as wheat bran. **2.** supplements thought to assist in adding muscle mass during weight training.

BUM, n.pr See backward upward medially.

bupleurum (bōō·pler´·əm), n Latin name: Bupleurum falcatum L.; part used: roots; uses: antiinflammatory, immunomodulator, hepatoprotective, antitussive, renal disorders, stomach ulcers; precautions: can cause gas, indigestion, slight hepatotoxicity, sedation, nausea. Also called Bupleuri radix, chai hu, hare's ear root, saiko, and siho.

Bupleurum falcatum L., *n* See bupleurum.

burden of proof, *n* in criminal cases, the task of the prosecuting officers to demonstrate the *actus reus* and *mens rea* of the crime; in litigation, to lay out the facts of the case. See also *actus reus* and *mens rea.*

burdock, *n* Latin names: *Arctium lappa, Arctium minus;* parts used: seeds, leaves, roots (dried); uses: (seeds) hypotensive, myodepressant, renotropic; (roots) antiseptic, antitumor, hypoglycemic, toxicopectic; precautions: patients with diabetes or cardiac disorders. Also called *Bardana, beggar's buttons, cuckold, edible burdock, fox's clote, gobo, great bur, great burdock, happy major, hardock, lappa, love leaves, personata, Philanthropium, thorny burr,* or *wild gobo.*

Burkitt's lymphoma, *n.pr* malignant undifferentiated lymphoma usually found in central African children, marked by an enlarged mandible or by a growth in the retroperitoneal area; has been linked to the Epstein-Barr virus.

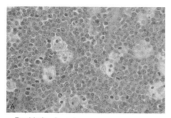

Burkitt's lymphoma. (Cotran, Kumar, and Collins, 1999)

burnout, *n* **I.** a state that occurs when energy is used up faster than it is restored. **2.** psychological and physical fatigue of a caregiver resulting in apathy and depression.

bursae (bur·sā), *n.pl* membrane-lined sacs containing synovial fluid, usually found in and around joints. Bursae provide protective cushioning and lubrication.

bursitis (bur·sī·tis), *n* painful condition in which the connective tissue, or bursa, that surrounds the joints becomes inflamed, often chronically.

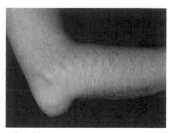

Bursitis. (American College of Rheumatology. Reprinted from the Clinical Slide Collection of the Rheumatic Diseases, 1991, 1995, 1997)

butterbur, *n* Latin names: *Petasites hybridus, Petasites officinalis, Tussilago petasites;* parts used: buds, leaves, roots, stems; uses: sedative, diuretic, pertussis, asthma, cough, arthritis, irritable bowel syndrome; precautions: pregnancy, lactation, children; can cause nausea, vomiting, liver damage, constipation, stomach cramps, discoloration of the epidermis, dyspnea, carcinogenesis from pyrrolizidine alkaloids. Also called *blatterdock, bog rhubarb, bogshorns, European pestroot, flapperdock, langwort, sweet coltsfoot, umbrella leaves,* or *western coltsfoot.*

cacao, *n* Latin name: *Theobroma cacao;* part used: seeds; uses: diuretics, cardiac stimulant, nervous system stimulant (not used by herbalists); precautions: pregnancy, lactation, children, colitis. Also called *cacao, cocoa,* or *cocoa butter.*

cachexia (kə·kek·sē·ə), *n* state of health with

physical atrophy and weakness often found in the last stages of terminal illness.

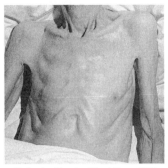

Cachexia. (Kamal and Brockelhurst, 1991)

cactus grandiflora (kak´·təs gran·də·flōr´·ə), *n* **I.** preparation of the night-blooming cereus cactus. As homeopathic, used to alleviate sadness, for physical and emotional pain, weakened heart, and feelings of constriction in the chest. **2.** Latin name: *Selenicereus grandiflorus;* parts used: stem; uses: diuretic, stimulant, heart tonic; precautions: overdose can cause tachycardia, chest constriction, confusion, headaches; caution advised for patients taking cardiac glycosides or other heart medications.

cadmium, *n* a toxic metal that is found in cigarette smoke, industrial waste, paints, and plastics. Exposure has been linked to cancer, hypertension, and lowered activity of specific enzymes.

***cadmium iodatum* (kad´·mē·əm ī·ō·dā´·təm),** *n* a homeopathic preparation of cadmium used to alleviate the symptoms associated with radiation treatments.

***cadmium sulphuricum* (kad´·mē·əm səl·fyur´·i·kəm),** *n* a homeopathic preparation of cadmium used to alleviate facial paralysis, Bell's palsy, nausea, vomiting, and the symptoms associated with chemotherapy.

Caesalpinia bonducella, *n* See fever nut.

caida de mollera (kä·ē´·də dā mō·yā´rə), *n* according to Curanderismo, the Mexican-American healing system, incidence of underdeveloped fontanel in an infant believed to result from the mother's neglect.

cajeput (ka´·jə·pət), *n* Latin name: *Melaleuca leucadendron;* part used: oil extracted from fresh twigs and leaves; uses: flavoring, stimulant, antiseptic, expectorant, anthelmintic; precautions: pregnancy, lactation, persons with hypersensitivity to tea tree plant. May cause hypersensitivity reactions. Also called *cajuput, cajeputol, eucalyptol, swamp tea tree, white tea tree,* and *cineol.*

CAL, *n.pr* See chronic airway limitation.

calcarea carbonica (kal·kar´·ee·uh kar·bō´·ni·kə), *n* a homeopathic preparation of calcium used to treat anxiety, headaches, allergies, constipation, muscle aches and pains, broken bones, asthma, arthritis, teething, and gallstones. Also called *calcium carbonate.*

calcarea fluorica (kal·kar´·ē·ə flōr´·i·kə), *n* a homeopathic preparation of calcium used to treat cataracts, hardened tissues, gout, hemorrhoids, constipation, osteoarthritis, and rheumatism originating from joint injury.

calcarea phosphorica, *n* a homeopathic preparation of calcium used to treat irritability, headaches, stomach conditions, stiff muscles and joints, bone bruises, fractures, carpal tunnel syndrome, osteoarthritis, osteoporosis, teething, and insomnia caused by aches or growing pains.

calcarea sulphurica (kal·kar´·ē·ə sul·fyur´·i·kə), *n* a homeopathic preparation of calcium used to treat acne, boils, burns, and eczema.

calcitonin (kal·si·tō'·nin), *n* hormone originating in the thyroid's parafollicular cells; plays a role in calcium blood level regulation and serves to stimulate bone mineralization.

calcium, *n* an element/mineral that is essential for bone development and maintenance, nerve impulse conduction, and general cellular function. Calcium supplementation is useful for preventing osteoporosis and perhaps colon cancer. It is also used for treating PMS, colon polyps, and may be useful in lowering high blood pressure. Calcium supplements may interfere with the absorption of chromium, magnesium, manganese, iron, and zinc.

calendula (kə·len'·jə·l ə), *n* Latin name: *Calendula officinalis;* parts used: flowers; uses: digestive, antiinflammatory, antiinfective, antitumor, ulcerative skin conditions, varicose veins, stomach conditions; precautions: pregnancy, lactation, children. Also called *garden marigold, pot marigold,* or *poet's marigold.*

Calendula officinalis, *n* See calendula.

California poppy, *n* Latin name: *Eschscholzia californica;* part used: sap, root, plant; uses: relieve pain; prevent or relieve spasms; induce sweating; induce urination; relieve toothache; induce relaxation; suppress milk secretion, incontinence; induce sleep; precautions: none known. Also called *gold poppy, kalifornia hashasi,* and *khishkhash kalifornia.*

calisaya bark (ka·li·sā'·yə bärk'), *n* bark obtained from *Cinchona calisaya,* which is used to extract quinine, an antimalarial.

callings (kä'·lingz), *n.pl* in Native American medicine, the disorders of initiation that should not be treated; the person is believed to suffer through and recover from such conditions to attain a higher level of being.

calmative, *n* a substance that gently induces rest.

caltrops, *n* Latin name: *Tribulus terrestris;* parts used: fruit, root; uses: in Ayurveda, pacifies vata and pitta (sweet, heavy, oily), antiurolithic, nephroprotective, antimicrobial, cardiac stimulant, sexual function, aperient, astringent, antiinflammatory, emmenagogue, stomachic, tonic, diuretic, alterative, hepatitis, rheumatism, skin disorders; precautions: none known. Also called *gokhru* or *gokshura.*

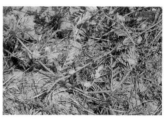

Caltrops. (Williamson, 2002)

calumba, *n* Latin names: *Jateorrhiza calumba, Jateorrhiza palmata;* part used: root; uses: diarrhea, gas; precautions: pregnancy, lactation, children. Also called *Cocculus palmatus* or *columbo root.*

CAM, *n.pr* See medicine, complementary; medicine, alternative and medicine, complementary and alternative.

Camellia sinensis, *n* See green tea.

cancer, *n* any of a diverse group of malignant neoplastic disorders characterized by uncontrolled cell growth in various sites throughout the body. Cancer is the second leading cause of death in the United States, after heart disease.

cancer staging, *n* prognostic tool for cancer treatment where a malignant tumor is charted with respect to its size and location in the patient's body.

cancer-related pain, *n* pain with acute, chronic, and psychological aspects experienced by cancer patients. Associated with the disease process and treatment.

Candida albicans, *n* a pathogenic yeast, which is the causal agent of thrush, vaginal infections, and systemic candidiasis.

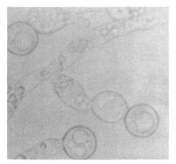

Candida albicans. (Zitelli and Davis, 1997; Dr. Ellen Wald, Children's Hospital of Pittsburgh)

candidiasis (kan·di·dī'·əsis), *n* overgrowth of the microscopic fungal pathogen candida, usually *Candida albicans.*

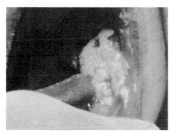

Candidiasis. (Zitelli and Davis, 1997)

cane sugar, *n* sucrose derived from sugarcane *(Saccharum officinarum),* the chemical formula of which is $C_{12} H_{22} O_{11}$. This is used in both solid and syrupy homeopathic medicines.

cantharides (kan·thär'·ə·dēz'), *n* the dried body of *Lytta vesicatoria,* a blister beetle that belongs to genus *Lytta;* active principle in cantharides is cantharidin, used as an aphrodisiac, diuretic, and rubifacient.

cantharidin (kan·thar'·ədən), *n* bitter-tasting, crystalline substance that is the active principle of cantharides and is also found in the bodies of some species of beetles; causes blistering on skin and is lethal to some animals that consume dead bodies of beetles in hay.

canthaxanthin (kan'·thak·san'·thin), *n* an herbal preparation promoted as a tanning agent for the skin. An orange carotenoid approved by the Food and Drug Administration (FDA) only as a color additive for food products. When ingested in excessive doses, it has been shown to produce symptoms of retinopathy and accumulation of yellowish gold–colored deposits around the macula.

caper plant (kā'·per plant'), *n* Latin name: *Capparis spinosa;* part used: bark, buds, leaves; uses: relieves pain; destroys and removes intestinal worms; relieves hemorrhoids; gentle bowel movements; removes obstructions within the body; purifies and cleanses blood; induces urination; stimulates menstrual flow; induces removal of mucus secretion; increases appetite; promotes bowel evacuation; cough, eye infections, stomach pain, vaginal thrush, and gout; precautions: can cause allergic contact dermatitis. Also called *caper, caper bush, kabar,* and *kebre.*

capillaries (kap'·ə·ler·ēz), *n.pl* small, thin-membraned, permeable blood vessels that link arterioles and venules, feeding and removing wastes from the tissues through which they pass.

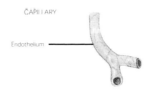

Capillary. (Applegate, 2000)

Capparis spinosa, *n* See caper plant.

capsaicin (kap·sī'·əsin), *n* a major ingredient in hot peppers; eaten to encourage sweating in hot climates and used as a topical pain reliever and to reduce nasal polyps. Capsaicin has also been used in melanoma treatment and may have chemoprotective quali-

C

ties. Toxic effects may include nerve damage and carcinogenesis.

Capsicum annum, *n* See capsaicin and cayenne.

Capsicum frutescens, *n* See capsaicin and cayenne.

capsular patterns (kap'·sə·lər pa'·tərnz), *n.pl* the characteristic ranges of restricted movement exhibited by a joint. Examining this characteristic is common in assessing and treating persons diagnosed with arthritic conditions.

caraway, *n* Latin name: *Carum carvi* parts used: ripe fruit (dried), seeds; uses: spasms in the digestive system, bloating, gas, dyspepsia, common cold, cough, anorexia, colic; precautions: pregnancy, patients with liver disease (oil); can cause diarrhea, burping, and irritation to eyes, oral cavity, and nose. Also called *kummel, kummelol, oleum cari,* or *oleum carvi.*

Carbenia benedicta, *n* See thistle, blessed.

carbon dioxide extraction, *n* in aromatherapy, a method of extracting essential oils using compressed carbon dioxide for a solvent. An expensive method, it uses lower temperature than most methods, thus ensuring that the essential oils are not heat-damaged.

carbonyl group (kär'·bə·nil grōōp'), *n* a functional group in which a carbon atom is joined to an oxygen by a double bond; found in aldehydes and ketones.

carcinogen (kär·sin'·ə·jin), *n* any agent found to be cancer-causing.

carcinoma, *n* a deadly epithelial neoplasm that attacks nearby tissue and tends to metastasize in other areas of the individual's body. A carcinoma is irregular, firm, and nodular with welldefined borders.

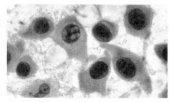

Carcinoma. (McKee, 1997)

cardamon, *n* Latin name: *Elettaria cardamomum;* part used: seeds; uses: dyspepsia, colic, gas, irritable bowel syndrome, gallstones, colds, cough, viruses, congestion, anorexia; precautions: pregnancy, lactation, children; patients with heartburn and gallstones, gallstone colic, and contact dermatitis (not often). Also called *cardamon seeds* or *Malabar cardamom.*

cardiac, *adj* pertaining to or stimulating the heart.

cardiac arrest, *n* condition characterized by the sudden, complete cessation of all cardiac functioning.

cardiac glycosides, *n.pl* steroidal phytochemicals that have a history of use as cardiac medicines, including digitalis and lily of the valley. Not recommended for use without physician guidance. Also called *cardioactive glycosides.* See also therapy, digitalis.

cardiac output, *n* the volume of blood forced out by the ventricles of the heart per beat multiplied by the heart rate. The cardiac output of a normal adult is 4 to 8 L per minute.

cardiac tamponade (kär'·dē·ak tam'·pə·nād'), *n* a condition caused by accumulation of fluid between the heart and the pericardium, thus resulting in excess pressure on the heart. This impairs the heart's ability to pump sufficient blood.

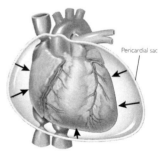

Pericardial sac

Cardiac tamponade. (Mosby's Medical, Nursing & Allied Health Dictionary, ed 6, 2002)

cardiopulmonary resuscitation, *n* life-saving technique for restarting cardiac function and respiration. Includes manual pumping with a rhythmic pressure on the chest and breathing mouth to mouth.

cardiotonic, *adj/n* property of a substance that has an invigorating effect on the heart.

Carduus benedictus, n See thistle, blessed.

Carica papaya, n See papaya.

Carlina acaulis, n See thistle, carline.

carmlnative, *adj/n* ability to provide relief of the expulsion of intestinal gas.

carnitine (kär'·nə·tēn), *n* an amino acid found in meat, dairy sources, avocados, tempeh, and wheat. Claimed to be helpful in endurance and congestive heart failure. Often used by body builders.

carnivora (kär·ni'·və·rə), *n* a phytonutrient derived from the juice of the insectivorous plant, Venus Flytrap *(Dionaea muscipula).* Has been used to treat chronic diseases, including cancer, multiple sclerosis, HIV, and herpes infections.

carotene, *n* an orange- or red-colored pigment found in plants, which is convertible into vitamin A by the body.

carotenoids (kə·rô'·te·noidz), *n.pl* fat-soluble plant pigments whose functions include photosynthesis, providing bright coloration (red, orange, and yellow), and protecting from light and oxygen (antioxidants). In humans, carotenoids are useful as antioxidants (compounds which prevent tissue damage and degeneration). See also beta-carotene, lutein, and lycopene.

carrier gas (kar'·ē·er gas'), *n* a chemically nonreactive gas, such as helium or nitrogen that carries vapor through the column of a gas-liquid chromatograph; known as the mobile phase.

carrier wave, *n* the medium through which signals and energy are delivered from one body to another.

Carthamus tinctorius, n See safflower.

cartilage, *n* tough, fibrous connective tissue without nerves or blood supply that provides protection and support to joints, tubes, ends of long bones,

and facial structures (e.g., ears and nose).

cartilage, elastic, n soft and elastic tissue shaping the outer nose and ears and forming several internal structures, including the auditory tubes, the epiglottis, and the joint linings.

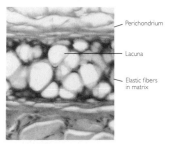

Cartilage, elastic. (Copyright Ed Reschke)

cartilage, hyaline **(hī'·ə·lən kar'·tə·lej),** *n* smooth, pliant tissue that forms most of the skeleton of a fetus. At birth, osseous tissue replaces the hyaline cartilage throughout the body except at the nexus of the ribs and sternum, at the ends of bones, and in parts of the larynx, trachea, and nose. Also called *gristle.*

Carum carvi, n See caraway.

Caryophyllus aromaticus, n See cloves.

CAS, *n.pr* See Chemical Abstracts Service Number.

casanthranol (kəsan'·thrənôl'), *n* a laxative obtained from *Cascara sagrada.*

cascara sagrada (kä·skä'·rə sä'·grə·də), *n* Latin name: *Rhamnus purshiana;* part used: bark (dried, aged); uses: laxative; precautions: pregnancy, lactation, children; patients with stomach bleeding, blockage, pain, nausea, appendicitis, and Crohn's disease; can cause nausea, diarrhea, stomach cramps, urine discoloration, hematuria, albuminuria, osteomalacia, and imbalances in vitamins, minerals, and fluids. Also called *Californian buckthorn, cascara,* or *sacred bark.*

case, *n* **1.** illness episode. **2.** entire account of the historical perspective of the course of a patient's disease and its management. See also anamnesis, biopathography, and case analysis.

case report, *n* a record of a patient's illness, treatment, and recovery.

case taking, *n* the procedure of obtaining and documenting a patient's disease development. See also anamnesis, case analysis, and patient history.

Cassia **spp.,** *n* See senna.

casting, *n* procedure in which a fractured bone is reset and immobilized in bandages impregnated with plaster.

castor, *n* Latin name: *Ricinum communis;* part used: leaves, oil, roots, seeds; uses: birth control, laxative, emetic, stomach antiinflammatory, anthelmintic, leprosy, syphilis, wound healing, boils, tumors, ear infections, migraines, sore throat, facial paralysis, ulcers; precautions: pregnancy, lactation, children; patients with stomach disorders; can cause nausea, stomach cramps, and allergic reactions. Also called *African coffee bean, bofareira, castor bean, castor oil plant, endi, eranda, Mexico seed, Mexico weed, palma Christi, tangantangan oil plant, wonder tree,* or *wunderbaum.*

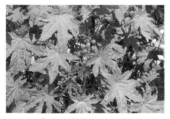

Castor. (Williamson, 2002)

catabolism (kə·ta'·bō·li·zəm), *n* process during metabolism where cells break down complex substances into simple compounds.

catalase (ka'·tə·las), *n* an enzyme that breaks down hydrogen peroxide into water and oxygen.

catalepsy, *n* stiffening of the body or more commonly a specific body part, such as a limb, which can be induced by hypnosis.

cataract, *n* degenerative eye disease marked by the loss of transparency of the lens, resulting in an opaque, milky appearance behind the pupil.

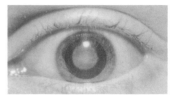

Cataract. (Black, Hawks, and Keene, 2001; Ophthalmic Photography, University of Michigan W.K. Kellogg Eye Center, Ann Arbor, MI)

catatonia (ka·tə·tō'·nē·ə), *n* extreme psychological state characterized by excessively rigid muscles combined with incidental periods of activity; occasionally manifests as impulsive, extreme activity.

catechins (ka'·ti·kinz), *n.pl.* flavonoid phytochemical compounds found principally in green tea. Smaller amounts are contained in grapes, black tea, chocolate, and wine. Considered potent antioxidants, catechins are being studied for their potential to prevent heart disease and cancer.

catecholamines (ka'·tə·kō'·lə·mēnz), *n.pl* a group of substances derived from tyrosine that act as hormones to stimulate cellular activity and carry nerve impulses through the body.

Catha edulis, *n* See khat.

catharsis (kə·thär'·sis), *n* **1.** in medicine, purgation, especially of the digestive system. **2.** a method by which tension and anxiety are relieved by bringing fears and repressed feelings to consciousness, which is often a critical phase of the healing process. See also abreaction.

cathartic, *n* a substance that expels material from or cleanses the gastrointestinal tract.

cation (kat'·ī'·ən), *n* a positively charged atomic or molecular species. See also ion.

catnip, *n* Latin name: *Nepeta cataria;* parts used: leaves (dried), buds; uses: migraines, colic, cold, flu, stomach disorders, arthritis, hemorrhoids; precautions: pregnancy; can cause headaches, nausea, and anorexia. Also called *cataria, catmint, catnep, cat's play, catwort, field balm,* or *nip.*

cat's claw, *n* Latin names: *Uncaria tomentosa, Uncaria guianensis;* parts used: leaves, roots, bark from stems; uses: antiinflammatory, contraceptive, immune system stimulant, colon disease, arthritis, irritable bowel disease, Crohn's disease; precautions: pregnancy, lactation, patients with MS, AIDS, tuberculosis, hemophilia, and organ transplant recipients. Also called *life-giving vine of Peru, samento,* or *una de gato.*

caudad (kô′·dad), *adj* directed toward the rear or tail.

caudal (kô′·dəl), *adj* positioned underneath or toward the bottom. Also called *inferior.*

caulophyllum (kô·lō·fi̇̄′·ləm), *n* a homeopathic preparation of blue cohosh root used to treat dysmenorrhea, weak uterine muscle tone, and difficulty in conceiving. See also cohosh, blue.

Caulophyllum thalictroides, n See cohosh, blue.

causation, *n* the act or agency which produces an effect. See also acausal.

cause of action, *n* the stated circumstances that permit one to bring suit to recover damages.

cause, final, *n* in philosophy, the purpose for, or goal of the existence of a phenomenon. Also called the *telos.*

cavitation, *n* formation of gas bubbles in the synovial fluid caused by a decrease in pressure. This process is responsible for the "cracking" of knuckles and other joints.

cayenne, *n* Latin names: *Capsicum frutescens, Capsicum annuum;* part used: capsaicin extract; uses: analgesia, arthritis, fibromyalgia, neuropathy, indigestion, gastroprotection (particularly that related to NSAID use), heart disease; precautions: patients taking theophylline for asthma. Also called *capsicum, African pepper,* bird pepper, chili, chili pepper, or *hot pepper.*

CBC, *n.pr* complete blood count. Test commonly performed in a clinical laboratory to determine the number of red and white blood cells present in a cubic millimeter of blood.

CCCR, *n.pr* See Consortial Center for Chiropractic Research.

CCP, *n.pr* See common compensatory pattern.

CCP, *n* common compensatory pattern; a common, preferential pattern for rotating the body "left-right-left-right."

CDC, *n.pr* Centers for Disease Control; now called the Centers for Disease Control and Prevention, the U.S. federal agency charged with providing accurate information on managing public health issues and disease outbreaks.

CDSA, *n.pr* See comprehensive digestive stool analysis.

cedarwood, *n* the essential oil from *Cedrus atlantica* used to reduce the effect of sleep induced by barbiturates. See *Cedrus atlantica.*

Cedrus deodar, n See Himalayan cedar.

celandine (se·lan′·dēn), *n* Latin name: *Chelidonium majus;* parts used: buds, leaves, roots; uses: antiinflammatory, digestive aid, spasms in the digestive tract, medicine for the liver and gallbladder; precautions: pregnancy, lactation, children, long-term use, can cause hypotension, dizziness, fatigue, insomnia, nausea, hepatotoxicity, polyuria, and polydipsia. Also called *celandine poppy, common celandine, felonwort, garden celandine, greater celandine, rock poppy, swallow wort, tetter wort,* or *wart wort.*

celery, *n* Latin name: *Apium graveolens;* parts used: seeds, entire plant; uses: (seeds) hypertension, seizures, labor stimulant, (juice) edema, hypertension, anxiety, headaches, aching joints; precautions: pregnancy, lactation, children, patients allergic to mugwort or birch and kidney disease; can cause hampering of the nervous system, uterine stimulant, dermatitis, lesions, anaphylaxis, and angioedema. Also called *apium, celery seed, celery seed oil, marsh parsley, smallage,* or *wild cherry.*

cell cycle, *n* divided into five stages, the resting phase (G$_0$), the first phase of growth and protein synthesis (G$_1$), the DNA synthesis phase (S), a second phase of growth and protein synthesis (G$_2$), and a final phase in which the cell enters mitosis (M).

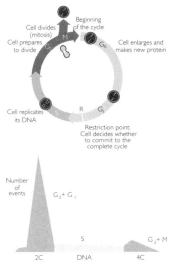

Cell divides (mitosis)
Cell prepares to divide
Beginning of the cycle
Cell enlarges and makes new protein
Cell replicates its DNA
Restriction point: Cell decides whether to commit to the complete cycle

Number of events
G$_0$+ G$_1$
S
G$_2$+ M
2C　　　DNA　　　4C

Cell cycle. (Pizzorno and Murray, 1999)

cellulite, *n* a usually cosmetic defect of the fascia and skin that is indicated by bulging, pitting, and skin deformation. Symptoms include a taut and heavy feeling in the affected regions. When pinched, pressed or strongly massaged, the area becomes quite tender; the areas typically include the thigh and gluteal regions, abdomen, nape of the neck, and upper portions of the arms.

cellulitis (sel·yə·lī'·təs), *n* skin and subcutaneous tissue infection that causes redness, swelling, local heat, and pain; in extreme cases, chills, fever, headache, and malaise.

Antibiotics are the primary course of treatment.

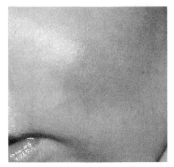

Cellulitis. (Zitelli and Davis, 1997)

cellulose (sel'·yə·lōs), *n* an unbranched 1-4-beta-glucose polymer found in fruits, grains, seeds, and vegetables. A major dietary fiber, cellulose increases fecal size and weight because of its ability to bind water.

cenogenesis (sē·nō·ge'·nə·sis), *n* spontaneously appearing structural developments in a species that occur in response to unique environmental conditions.

Centaurium erythraea, *n* See centaury.

Centaurium minus, *n* See centaury.

Centaurium umbellatum, *n* See centaury.

centaury, *n* Latin names: *Centaurium erythraea, Centaurium umbellatum, Centaurium minus;* parts used: buds, leaves, stems; uses: anthelmintic, antihypertensive, dyspepsia, appetite loss, kidney stones, (infants) anxiety, insomnia, colic, irritable bowel syndrome, ADHD; precautions: pregnancy, lactation, patients with stomach ulcers; can cause anorexia. Also called *bitter clover, bitter herb, bitterbloom, centaurea, common centaury, European centaury, eyebright, feverwort, filwort, lesser centaury,* or *minor centaury.*

centering, *n* **1.** focusing of the attention to relax and become calm. **2.** in therapeutic touch the phase where the practitioner relaxes and brings to bear an internal peace and then a receptiveness to the patient.

centesimal, *n* in homeopathy, a 1/100 part dilution of natural, organic, or mineral substances in alcohol or lactose.

central feature, *n* in homeopathy, the most crucial or essential aspect of an inclusive hierarchy of information gathered to form a diagnosis. The central feature increases the likelihood of a successful prescription.

centrifugation (sen·trif´·yə·gā´·shən), *n* the process by which substances are separated by centrifugal force to increase the rate of filtration or sedimentation of two immiscible liquids or a liquid and a solid.

Cephaelis **spp.,** *n* See ipecacuanha.

cephalad, *adj* headward, directed toward the head.

cephalic (sə·fa´·lik), *adj* **1.** pertaining to the head. *n* **2.** in aromatherapy, a substance that stimulates the mind and clears it.

cerebral palsy (ser´·ə·brəl pôl´·zē), *n* neuromuscular disorder sometimes caused by brain damage in utero or at birth, characterized by loss of coordination and muscle control.

cerebral vascular accident, *n* See stroke.

cerebro (se·rā´·brō), *n* in Curanderismo, the Mexican healing system, the part of the brain found at the posterior base of the skull, which when fully developed is believed to enable a person to become a medium for spirits to communicate with the physical world.

cerebrospinal fluid (sə·rē´·brō·spī´·nəl flōō´·id), *n* colorless, clear fluid that surrounds the central nervous system, that absorbs shocks, delivers nutrients, and removes waste products.

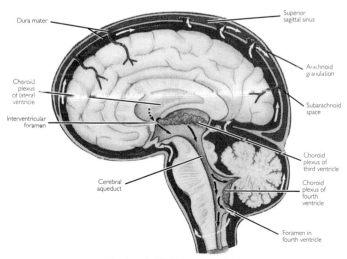

Cerebrospinal fluid. (Applegate, 2000)

cerebrotonia (sə·rē¹·brə·tō¹·nē·ə), *n* one of the three temperaments described by W.H. Sheldon, characterized as introverted, inhibited, controlled, and withdrawn.

ceriod (sē¹·rē·id), *n* age pigment, the levels of which have been shown to increase under conditions of oxidative stress in the absence of adequate antioxidants.

cernilton (ser·nil¹·tən), *n* medicine extracted from flower pollen; used to treat benign prostatic hyperplasia (BPH) and prostatitis. See also benign prostatic hyperplasia.

Certification, Special Proficiency in Osteopathic Manipulative Medicine, *n* a specialized certification that was granted between 1989 and 1999 by the American Osteopathic Association.

certified music therapist (CMT), *n* credential previously awarded (before January 1, 1998) by the American Association For Music Therapy upon completion of required training and education. The National Music Therapy Registry lists music therapists who wish to maintain the designation.

certiorari (sur·shē·ə·rar¹·ē), *n* a legal appeal of a judicial or administrative decision.

cervical (ser¹·və·kəl), *adj* **I.** of or relating to the cervix of the uterus. **2.** of or associated with the neck.

cervical dysplasia (ser¹·vi·kəl dis·plā¹·zhə), *n* abnormal cells in the cervix, with a potential to become cancerous. Typically caused by the human papilloma virus (HPV).

Cetraria islandica, *n* See Iceland moss.

C fibers, *n.pr* unmyelinated fibers that transmit information to the brain about the location of tissue damage and pain.

CFS, *n.pr* See syndrome, chronic fatigue.

chakras (cha¹·krəz), *n.pl* according to Tantric philosophy, the seven centers of energy that constitute our energy system. The chakras act as valves or conduits for energy from consciousness through the endocrine

and nervous systems to different parts of the physical body.

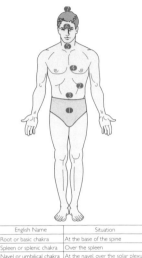

	English Name	Situation
1	Root or basic chakra	At the base of the spine
2	Spleen or splenic chakra	Over the spleen
3	Navel or umbilical chakra	At the navel, over the solar plexus
4	Heart or cardiac chakra	Over the heart
5	Throat or laryngeal chakra	At the front of the throat
6	Brow or frontal chakra	In the space between the eyebrows
7	Crown or coronal chakra	On the top of the head

Chakras. (Fritz, 2004)

chakra connection, *n* healing touch process that uses both manual shadowing and light touch, starting at the feet and working up the body at 60-second intervals until all energy centers (chakras) of the body have been covered.

chakra spread, *n* an approach for treating clients who are undergoing significant emotional, spiritual, and physical stress; practitioner systematically holds each foot, hand, and then moves down the body to open and balance the client's energy centers.

chala (chä¹·lə), *adj* in Ayurveda, "mobile" as a guna, one of the qualities that characterizes all substances. Its complement is sthira. See also gunas and sthira.

chalazion (chə·la¹·zē·ən), *n* nonmalignant swelling in the eyelid area due to an obstruction of or malfunctioning meibomian gland.

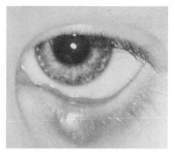

Chalazion. (Zitelli and Davis, 1997)

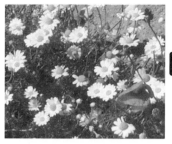

Chamomile. (Scott and Barlow, 2003)

challenge, *n* a stimulating or demanding circumstance. To develop effective problem-solving skills and strategies, it is necessary to perceive such circumstance as inconvenience or burden instead of overwhelming impediments.

Chamaelirium luteum, *n* See false unicorn root.

Chamaemelum nobile, *n* See chamomile.

chamomile, *n* Latin names: *Matricaria chamomilla, Matricaria recutita, Chamaemelum nobile, Anthemis nobile;* part used: buds (dried); uses: antiinflammatory, digestive aid, irritable bowel syndrome, colon disease, Crohn's disease, insomnia, anxiety, spasms, wound healing; precautions: pregnancy, lactation, patients with asthma, hypersensitivity to sunflowers, ragweed, or aster family, can cause burning of the face, eyes, or mucosa, liver disease. Also called *common chamomile, English chamomile, German chamomile, Hungarian chamomile, Roman chamomile, sweet false chamomile, true chamomile,* or *wild chamomile.*

chamomile, Roman (rōˈmən kaˈ·mə·mēl), *n* a colorless to light blue oil that turns yellow upon storage. Commonly used as an antispasmodic; the herb from which it is derived is used to dispel gas and relieve colic. See also *Chamaemelum nobile.*

chamomilla (ka·mə·mēˈ·lə), *n* a homeopathic preparation of chamomile used to treat alcohol withdrawal, asthma, bronchitis, colic, cough, hypersensitivity to pain, diarrhea, dysmenorrhea, ear infections, and teething. See also chamomile.

chancre (shang·ker), *n* extremely contagious symptom of primary syphilis; appears as a lesion at the site of infection, first as a papule and then turns red; is painless and bloodless; has raised edges. Heals without leaving a scar.

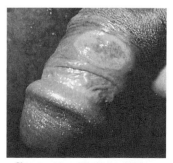

Chancre. (Morse, Moreland, and Holmes, 1996)

ch'ang shan (djäng sän), *n* the root of *Dichroa febrifuga,* used as an antimalarial in Chinese medicine. Has emetic effects. Precaution is advised in the elderly and the infirm.

channels, *n.pl* in acupuncture, a system of pathways running through the body that connect vital organs and carry qi.

channel-structural level, *n* in acupuncture, a disturbance that involves skin, bones, muscles, and fascia.

chaparral, *n* Latin names: *Larrea tridentata, Larrea divaricata;* part used: leaves; uses: fever, bronchitis, cancer, aching joints, diabetes; precautions: pregnancy, lactation, children, patients with liver or kidney disease; can cause liver damage and failure, contact dermatitis. Also called *creosote bush, greasewood,* or *Hediondilla.*

characteristic, *adj* **1.** emblematic or representative. *n* **2.** trait characterizing a person or illness. The most characteristic symptoms are crucial for determining the most efficacious homeopathic remedy. See also pathognomonic.

chassis (cha'·sē), *n* glass plates coated with thin layers of fat over which plant material is spread in layers so that the essential oil is absorbed into the fat. The saturated fat is washed with hexane to dissolve the essential oil and concentrated to yield a purer form. See also enfleurage.

CHD, *n.pr* See disease, coronary heart.

cheilosis (kē·lē·ō'·sis), *n* may indicate riboflavin deficiency in the diet; bilateral fissures and scales appear around the lips and mouth.

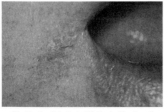

Cheilosis. (Mosby's Medical, Nursing & Allied Health Dictionary, ed 6, 2002)

chelation (kē·lā'·shən), *n* **1.** medical treatment in which heavy metals are flushed from the bloodstream by means of a chelator that binds metal ions; used in cases of mercury or lead poisoning. **2.** the process of ring formation by forming one or more hydrogen bonds.

chelidonium (che·li·dō'·nē·əm), *n* Latin name: *Chelidonium majus* L.; parts used: juice, flowers, leaves, root; uses: choleretic, cholagogic, spasmolytic, antiinflammatory, antiviral, liver and gallbladder conditions, migraines, jaundice, bronchitis, warts, ring-worm, abdominal pains, (uses under research: migraines and psoriasis); precautions: long-term use discouraged; cause nausea; diarrhea, dry mouth, stomach pains. Also called *baiqucai, Chelidonii herba,* and *greater celandine.*

Chelidonium majus, *n* See celandine.

***Chelidonium majus* L.,** *n* See chelidonium.

Chemical Abstracts Service Number, *n.pr* a service based in the United States that provides an abstract of papers and articles in the chemical and scientific literature relating the properties of a substance. By using the code number assigned to a specific compound or substance, one can locate pertinent information.

chemical burn, *n* tissue damage resulting from exposure to a strong alkali or acid.

chemical dependence, *n* reliance on or addiction to mood-altering substances, often to the detriment of the user's life.

chemical property, *n* property shown by a substance when it reacts with a different substance or undergoes a change in composition.

chemical purity, *n* the degree to which a substance is undiluted or unmixed with extraneous material, typically expressed as a percentage (%).

chemical reaction, *n* rearrangement of atoms or ions accompanying energy change. A catalyst, such as heat or an enzyme, may alter the rate of reaction.

chemical symbol, *n* a shorthand interpretation of an element, molecule, or a compound.

Chemicals Hazard Information and Packaging for Supply, *n.pr* an extensive group of policies intended to protect people from hazardous materials. CHIP 2 Regulations 1994 specifically apply to aromatherapy. See also COSHH.

chemotherapy, *n* form of treatment, usually for cancer, in which the drug kills or inhibits diseased cells' viability.

chemotype, *n* plants that are practically indistinguishable from one another in appearance but are nevertheless unique in their composition and therefore are used to treat distinct diseases.

chemovar (kē'·mə·var'), *n* a particular species of plants, the chemical composition of which varies from the average because of different environmental growing conditions.

Chen style (dtsən stīl), *n.pr* the oldest known style of tai chi, derived from Chen family boxing; movements are quick and large. See also tai chi.

Chenopodium ambrosioides, *n* See oil, chenopodium.

cherubism, *n* hereditary condition that causes the mandible to grow excessively; in some cases the eyes are also upturned, increasing the cherubic look on the face.

chest x-ray, *n* an examination of the chest using x-rays. Routinely performed in patients complaining of chest pain to rule out respiratory or heart disease.

Cheyne-Stokes respiration, *n* atypical pattern of breathing where the individual alternates between deep, rapid breathing and apnea.

chhandas (chə·hän'·dəs), *n* in Sanskrit, the acquired knowledge. It is one of the three components of the Vedas, the ancient Hindu scriptures considered sources of pure knowledge. According to Vedic sciences, interactions of chhandas, rishi, and devata give rise to matter. See also veda, rishi, and devata.

chi (dzhē), *n* **1.** in Tibetan medicine, awareness, one of the three functions of the mind, providing the direction for actions. Plays an important role in spiritual development. **2.** in traditional Chinese medicine, qi. See also badahan, schara, and qi.

ch'i, *n* See qi.

chi gong, *n* See qi gong.

chi type (dzhē tīp), *n* in Tibetan medicine, a unique psychosomatic set of characteristics; on a physical level, a chi-type person will have a tall, slender figure; weak muscle tone; slender, elongated neck; narrow, drooping shoulders; slim chest; flat, small abdomen; elongated arms and legs; diminutive, lean feet and hands; rather lengthy toes and fingers; dry, fine nails; dried out skin; noticeable veins; and dull skin tone. A thin layer of soft hair covers an elongated and small-sized head. On a psychological level, he or she may exude nervousness and anxiety. The mind is adaptable and always changing. New ideas, which develop easily with this particular individual, may not be carried out due to an inability to put into action or lack of resolve. The presence of nervous and neurologic conditions is common. This person is often diagnosed with osteoarthritis or rheumatoid arthritis. Typically, a person will have a compilation of all three types—chi, schara, and badahan. One or two of the types may be more prevalent than the other. See also schara type and badahan type.

chickenpox, *n* contagious childhood illness caused by the varicella zoster virus. Symptoms include infectious skin lesions that form crusts before receding, headache, and slight fever. Generally mild in children but may be severe in adults.

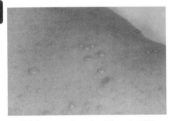

Chickenpox. (Lemmi and Lemmi, 2000)

chickweed, *n* Latin name: *Stellaria media;* parts used: buds, leaves, stems; uses: expectorant, antitussive, demulcent, heartburn, ulcers, sore throat, dyspepsia, wound healing, eczema, psoriasis, rashes, pruritus; precautions: pregnancy, lactation, children; toxic in large doses; can cause headaches, dizziness, paralysis. Also called *mouse-ear, satinflower, star chickweed, starweed, stitchwort, tongue grass, white bird's eye,* or *winterweed.*

chicory, *n* Latin name: *Cichorium intybus;* parts used: leaves, roots; uses: diuretic, laxative, sedative, appetite inducer, cancer; precautions: pregnancy, lactation, children, patients with heart disease or gallstones; can cause contact dermatitis. Also called *blue sailors, garden endive, succory,* or *wild succory.*

chief complaint, *n* the concern that brings a patient to seek therapeutic intervention.

chief ingredient (chēf in·grē´·dē·ənt), *n* one of the four components in a typical Chinese herbal formula, which is responsible for treating the specific illness. See also deputy ingredient, assistant ingredient, and envoy ingredient.

Chimaphila umbellata, n See pipsissewa.

Chinese flower, *n* Latin name: *Paederia foetida;* parts used: whole plant, roots, leaves; uses: in Ayurveda, bal-

ances vata dosha (bitter, heavy), anti-inflammatory, anthelmintic, antispasmodic, arthritis, rheumatic conditions, tonic, leaves: herpes, flatulence; roots: emetic, splenitis; precautions: none known. Also called *gandhaprasarini* or *prasarini.*

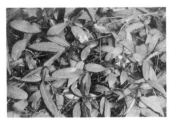

Chinese flower. (Williamson, 2002)

Chinese goldthread, *n* Latin name: *Coptis chinensis;* part used: rhizome; uses: antimicrobial, diarrhea, eye infection, leishmaniasis; precautions: stomach and intestine problems.

Chinese inch, *n* See cun.

Chinese manipulation, *n.pr* See tui na.

Chinese thoroughwax root, *n* Latin name: *Bupleurum chinense;* parts used: roots; uses: rheumatoid arthritis and other inflammatory conditions. In recent times, this medicine has been combined with prescribed drugs like prednisone to enhance the drug's ability to act. Constituents within this type of medicine called saikosaponins promote the release of hormones like cortisone by the adrenal gland and increase the potency of these chemicals. At the same time, it is claimed to prevent the atrophy of the adrenal gland caused by the use of corticosteroids; precautions: dizziness, headache, nausea, vomiting, in TCM associated with liver yang agitation. Also called *bei chai hu, chai hu, Chinese thorowax,* and *hare's ear.*

Chinese time clock, *n.pr* a 24-hour chronological map detailing the precise daily flow of qi throughout the organs and meridians. Knowledge of the zenith and nadir of an organ's energy is useful in diagnosing and treating imbalances and illnesses.

CHIP, *n.pr* See Chemicals Hazard Information and Packaging for supply.

chirality (kī·ral´·i·tē), *n* the "handedness" property of organic compounds (containing an asymmetrical carbon) that gives rise to structures that are mirror images and that cannot be superimposed on each other; the two isomers are called optical isomers, which refers to their ability to rotate plane-polarized light.

chiretta (chē´·re·ta), *n* Latin name: *Swertia chirata;* part used: whole plant; uses: in Ayurveda, balances tridosha (bitter, light, dry), hepatoprotection, antiulcer, CNS depressant, hypoglycemic, antiinflammatory, antimicrobial, appetite stimulant, nausea, tonic, liver conditions, asthma, bronchitis, malaria; precautions: none known. Also called *bhunimba, chirayita, kirat,* or *kirata-tikta.*

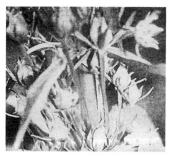

Chiretta. (Williamson, 2002)

chiroenergetics (kī´·rō·en·er·je´·tiks), *n* chiropractic technique that deals with the release of residual muscular tension associated with buried psychological traumas.

chiropractic, *n* a complementary health discipline in which a licensed practitioner corrects vertebral subluxation (improper spinal positioning affecting nervous system functions) by employing manual adjustments to the client's back, neck, and limbs. See also DC (Doctor of Chiropractic).

chiropractic adjustment, *n* any of a variety of physically manipulative techniques used to correct the functions of the spine or joints. May be applied with varying amplitude, velocity, amounts of recoil, and lengths of lever.

chitosan (kī´·tō·san), *n* a fat-binding fiber found in aquatic crustaceans.

chittem bark (chi´·tem bärk´), *n* See cascara sagrada.

chlamydia (kla·mi´·dē·a), *n* an infection caused by the bacterium, *Chlamydia trachomatis* that primarily affects the urethra in males and the cervix in females. Typically, the infection does not present any symptoms, but an atypical discharge from the penis or vagina may appear during urination. If not treated, it can worsen and cause pelvic inflammatory disease in females and epididymitis in males. Worldwide, it is the most common sexually transmitted disease. See also epididymitis; disease, pelvic inflammatory; and providone-iodine.

chlorella (klare´·la), *n* green one-celled algae taken as a food supplement. A rich source of vitamins, proteins, chlorophyll, and nucleic acids.

chlorophyll (klō´·rō·fil), *n* a nontoxic plant pigment used in the treatment of pelvic inflammatory disease, to promote production of erythrocytes and hemoglobin, and to facilitate tissue regeneration. Used by plants to make energy from sunlight.

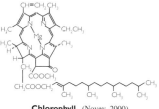

Chlorophyll. (Novey, 2000)

choanae (kō·an´·ā), *n* the large openings over the hard palate through which air leaves the nose.

cholagogic, *n* **I.** a substance that stimulates contraction of the gall bladder to promote the flow of bile. *adj* **2.** having the properties of a cholagogue.

cholagogue (chō'·lə·gôg), *n* a substance that stimulates contraction of the gall bladder, thus promoting secretion of bile.

cholecystitis   (kō·lē·sis·tī'·tis), *n* condition marked by chronic or acute gallbladder inflammation.

cholecystokinin   (kō'·li·sis·tō·kī'·nin), *n* a substance produced in the body that acts as a neurotransmitter, opiate antagonist, and hormonal peptide and that is involved in digestive processes and the experience of satiety.

cholelithiasis   (kō'·lə·li·thē'·ə·səs), *n* gallstones asymptomatically present in the gallbladder. The gallstones form when the relative concentration of bile components is altered.

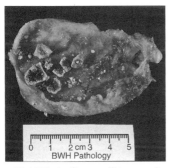

Cholelithiasis. (Kumar, Cotran, and Robbins, 1997)

cholera, *n* bacterial infection of the small intestine caused by the *Vibrio cholerae.* Symptoms include vomiting, diarrhea, dehydration, and electrolyte imbalance. Can be fatal in up to half of cases if left untreated.

choleretic, *n* a substance that stimulates the liver to produce bile.

cholestasis (kō'·lə·stā'·sis), *n* build-up of bile in the liver.

- Estrogen excess or birth control pills
- Pregnancy
- Presence of gallstones
- Alcohol
- Endotoxins
- Hereditary disorders such as Gilbert's syndrome
- Anabolic steroids
- Various chemicals or drugs
- Nutritional deficiencies

Cholestasis. (Pizzorno and Murray, 1999)

cholesterol   (kə·les'·ter·ôl), *n* organic compound produced in the liver and absorbed from food that is essential to the production of metabolic products and hormones.

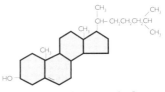

Cholesterol. (Thibodeau and Patton, 1999)

choline, *n* a compound that is used by the body to synthesize acetylcholine (a neurotransmitter), lecithin (phosphatidylcholine), and platelet-activating factor (a blood clotting agent). Choline can be obtained from dietary sources as a supplement and is also synthesized by the body. Has been used for nerve conditions, kidney conditions, liver conditions, headaches, dizziness, and fatigue. Taking regular doses of more than 3.5 g per day can produce a fishy odor, low blood pressure, diarrhea, dizziness, and changes in the ECG. See also lecithin.

cholinergic (kō'·lə·ner'·jik), *adj* pertaining to the parasympathetic part of the autonomic nervous system as well as acetylcholine release and its role as a transmitter agent.

chondroitin (kən·droi'·tin), *n* naturally occurring substance in the body responsible for elasticity of cartilage. Derived from animal cartilage and taken as a dietary supplement. Chemical name: chondroitin sulfate, chondroitin sulfuric acid, chonsurid; part used: bovine tracheal cartilage; uses: antithrombotic, extravasation agent, arthritis, ischemic heart disease, hyperlipidemia; precautions: pregnancy, lactation, children, patients with bleeding or kidney failure; can cause headaches, agitation, euphoria, nausea, bleeding. Also called *CAS, chondroitin sulfate,* or *chondroitin C.*

Chondrus crispus, *n* See Irish moss.

Chow Integrated Healing System and Qi gong, *n.pr* Chinese healing approach developed recently by Effie Chow that integrates the free flow of Qi, harmony of spirit, mind, and body with nature, yin and yang, the five elements, (fire, water, earth, metal, and wood), and elements taken from Western medicine to attain health and maintain youthfulness and vigor. Patients are empowered to take an active role in their recovery through breathing techniques, exercise, relaxation, and nutrition. See also Qi, Qi gong, and yin-yang.

Christian Science, *n* a Christian denomination that teaches that the healing powers of Christ are available to all because the divine mind is the source of all health. Disease is illusory and is based upon wrong perceptions of divine mind. A radical reliance on this mind instead of on medicine is what is needed to heal in cases of illness. Also called *Church of Christ Scientist.*

chromatography (krō'·mə·tä'··grə·fē), *n* analytical technique by which the components of a chemical mixture are separated and identified based on differences in absorption on a stationary phase, such as silica gel or cellulose. See also adsorption.

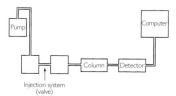

Chromatography. (Tiran, 2000)

chromium, *n* an essential mineral that is associated with glucose tolerance, high cholesterol, blocked arteries, glaucoma, obesity, diabetes, and hypoglycemia. Not for use by children or pregnant or nursing women. Also called *chromium picolinate, chromium polynicotinate,* or *chromium chloride.*

chromoblastomycosis (krō'·mō·bla'·stō·mī'·kō'·sis), *n* fungal infection often appearing along the lymphatic drainage path, characterized by large, wart-like lesions that are small initially but grow over the course of a few weeks to months. Also called *chromomycosis* and *verrucous dermatitis.*

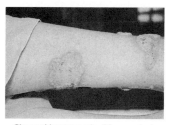

Chromoblastomycosis. (Murray et al, 1998)

chromotherapy (krō'·mə·the'·rə·pē), *n* in Ayurveda and other systems, the use of colors to promote harmony and healing based on the belief that certain colors are infused with healing energies (e.g., red is energizing; blue is calming). Also called *color therapy.*

chronic, *adj* characterized by recurrence or slow development over time, tending to last over a prolonged period.

chronic airway obstruction, *n* a persistent or recurring condition that impedes normal breathing. See also disease, chronic obstructive airways.

chronic candidiasis (krô'·nik kan'·də·dī'··ə·sis), *n* a complex syndrome with multiple symptoms caused by the yeast *Candida albicans* in the gastrointestinal tract and thought to negatively affect the majority of the body's systems. Also called the *yeast syndrome.*

chronic cough, *n* health condition characterized by either a lingering cough or a recurring cough lasting more than a month.

chronic somatic dysfunction, *n* impairment or alteration in function, often for long duration, of interrelated parts of the musculoskeletal system.

chronobiology, *n* the study of effects of time and cycles in biological systems.

Chrysanthemum parthenium, *n* See feverfew.

Chrysanthemum vulgare, *n* See common tansy.

churna (chōōr'·nə), *n* in Ayurveda, medicinal powders that are derived from plants and minerals.

cicatrisiant (si'·kə·trī'·sē·ənt), *n* a substance used to aid in wound healing and scar formation. Also called *cicatrizant* or *cicatriziant.*

cicatrizant (si'·kə·tri·zənt), *n* a substance that enhances the formation of scar tissue.

Cichorium intybus, *n* See chicory.

Cimicifuga racemosa, *n* See cohosh, black; black snakeroot.

Cinchona succirubra, *n* See quinine.

cinchona (kin·chō'·nə), *n* Peruvian shrub, the bark of which is the source of quinine. Samuel Hahnemann repeatedly dosed himself with cinchona to examine its effects and realized that his symptoms paralleled those of malarial patients. This led to his development of the similia principle: "let likes be cured by likes." Also called *quinine, china bark,* or *china.* See also quinine.

cingulate cortex (sing'·gyə·lāt kōr'·teks), *n* a component of the limbic system of the brain, responsible for producing emotional responses to physical sensations of pain.

Cinnamomum spp., *n* See cinnamon.

cinnamon, *n* Latin name: *Cinnamomum* spp.; parts used: bark, leaves; uses: antifungal, aromatic, analgesic, diarrhea, colds, stomach pain, appetite loss, hypertension, bronchitis, internal bleeding; precautions: pregnancy, lactation, children; can cause elevated heartbeat, stomatitis, glossitis, gingivitis, anorexia, labored breathing. Also called *Cassia, Cassia lignea, ceylon cinnamon, Chinese cinnamon, cinnamomom, false cinnamon, Panang cinnamon, Padang cassia, Saigon cassia,* or *Saigon cinnamon.*

circadian reassurance, *n* concept of nature-based therapy, which holds that nature provides dependable rhythms and patterns—for example, through sunrise and sunset, the phases of the moon, and the seasons—that can provide continuity and a sense of hope in the lives of people experiencing the uncertainty of illness.

circadian rhythm, *n* person's biological patterns within a 24-hour cycle, circa a day. See also chronobiology.

circumduction (sir'·kəm·duk'·shən), *n* cone-shaped movement of a limb that includes flexion, abduction, extension, and adduction.

cirrhosis (sə·rō'·sis), *n* chronic liver condition where the lobules are filled with fat, the parenchyma deteriorates, and the lobes become fibrous. Most commonly caused by alcohol abuse.

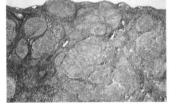

Cirrhosis. (Kumar, Cotran, and Robbins, 1997)

cis, *pref* Latin preposition meaning "on this side." In stereochemistry, it refers to the position of carbon chains extending from a molecule.

cisplatin (sis·pla'·tən), *n* a potent anticancer agent used to treat ovarian, prostatic, testicular, and other tumors.

Cissus quadrangularis, *n* See bone setter.

Citrullus colocynthis, *n* See colocynth fruit.

Citrus spp., *n* See extract, citrus seed.

civil action, *n* proceedings presented in civil courts.

CLA, *n.pr* See acid, conjugated linoleic.

clary, *n* Latin names: *Salvia sclarea, Euphrasia officinalis;* part used: oil from leaves and buds; uses: antiinflammatory, antispasmodic, sedative, astringent, menopause, premenstrual syndrome, exhaustion, adrenal stimulant, sore throat; precautions: pregnancy, lactation, children; patients with uterine, breast, or ovarian cancers, breast tumors, uterine fibroids; can cause sleepiness, headaches, increased menstruation. Also called *clary oil, clary sage, clear eye, eyebright, muscatel sage, orvale, see-bright,* or *toute-bonne.*

classical conditioning, *n* behavioral response resulting from pairing an unrelated (conditioned) stimulus with a related (unconditioned) stimulus before a particular response is elicited. Used in diagnosis and treatment of disease by conditioning the responses of a patient to external stimuli.

clathrate (kla·thrāt′), *n* a lattice at the molecular level. The phenomenon of having the molecules interwoven within the lattice of another component may explain the method of passing on the active aspects of the source material during potentization for a homeopathic remedy.

Claviceps purpurea, *n* See ergot.

cleaning, *v* to expunge all residue of prior materials. Heat or steam is required to remove any hint of previous remedies from the receptacles and tools used in the creation of homeopathic or herbal preparations.

clearing, *n* in therapeutic touch the phase where the practitioner's hands hover (3 to 5 inches above) over the patient's whole body and even out the patient's energy.

clematis, *n* Latin name: *Clematis virginiana* L.; part used: leaves (fresh); uses: migraines, epidermal maladies, hypertension; is used rarely; precautions: pregnancy, lactation, children, patients with vasculitis; can cause mucous irritation, upset stomach, colic, diarrhea, dizziness, seizures,

disorientation, death (rare). Also called *Devil's darning needle, old man's beard, traveler's joy, vine bower,* and *woodbine.*

Clematis virginiana, *n* See clematis.

clinical, *adj* **1.** relating to the examination and healing of patients. **2.** relating to people in a clinic.

clinical aromatherapist (kli′·ni·kəl ə·rō′·mə·the′·rə·pist), *n* a person who is trained and professionally certified in the use of essential oils for therapeutic purposes.

clinical auditing, *n* large-scale measurement and evaluation of patients using questionnaires to gather information on the outcomes of treatments.

clinical ecology (kli′·ni·kəl i·kô′·lə·jē), *n* study of the toxicity levels present in the environment and in foods along with the impact these levels have on human health.

clinical experimental evidence, *n* the results obtained from randomized, blind testing on humans. Also called *RCT evidence.* See also randomization and blind testing.

clinical nutrition, *n* the use of diet and supplements as a therapeutic and preventive approach.

clinical pattern, *n* the association of signs and symptoms presented in a visit to a healthcare professional.

clinical picture, *n* a sketch of symptoms and all facets of the patient's ailment that encompasses the specific, general, and mental features. See also symptom picture, drug picture, disease picture, and clinical.

clinical research, *n* research involving human subjects in a context in which the researcher interacts directly with the subjects.

clinical significance, *n* a level of efficacy that is considered sufficient to adopt the practice.

clinical trial, *n* a clinical study.

clinically standardized meditation, *n* a form of meditation in which participants choose one of 16 standard sounds or create their own and then silently repeat the sounds for a period of 2 to 30 minutes a day. This is a less structured form of meditation used to create a relaxed state.

CLL, *n.pr* See leukemia, chronic lymphocytic.

clonus (klō'·nəs), *n* abnormal neuromuscular activity marked by the involuntary relaxation and contractions of the skeletal muscles.

closed focus, *n* meditation technique where attention is focused on a singular thought, word, or sound.

cloves, *n.pl* Latin names: *Syzygium aromaticum, Eugenia caryophyllata, Caryophyllus aromaticus;* part used: buds (dried); uses: essential oil, antiseptic, antibacterial, antiinflammatory, anesthetic, toothaches; precautions: pregnancy, lactation, children; can cause tissue irritation in eyes, ears, nose, and throat, epidermal irritation, bronchospasms, pulmonary edema. Also called *oil of cloves* and *oleum caryophylli.*

cluster headache, *n* headache characterized by constant pain on one side of the head, around the eye. May be accompanied by constricted pupils, facial swelling, flushed appearance, nasal blockage, runny nose, and/or lacrimation.

Cnicus benedictus, n See thistle, blessed.

CNS, *n* central nervous system; portion of the nervous system comprising the spinal cord and brain, responsible for coordinating the activities of the entire nervous system.

CO₂, *n* carbon dioxide; a heavy, colorless, and odorless gas formed during respiration. It is lethal to humans in large to moderate concentrations.

coaching, *v* to provide assistance, by a therapist, to clients, as they learn new skills, apply themselves in rehabilitation sessions, and keep a positive outlook to help them reach their goals.

COAD, *n.pr* See disease, chronic obstructive airway.

cobalamin, *n* See vitamin B_{12}.

COBRA, *n.pr* See Consolidated Omnibus Budget Reconciliation Act.

coca, *n* Latin name: *Erythroxylum* spp.; part used: leaves; uses: quicken activity of the physiologic process, astringent, anesthetic, relieve hunger, fatigue, nausea, vomiting, stomach pains; stimulate central nervous system; stimulate muscular activity; relieve neurasthenia, dilate pupils; paralyze sensory nerve fibers; precautions: addictive, hallucinations and delusions, can cause restlessness, tremors; convulsions, emaciation, memory loss, sleeplessness, severe agitation, tachycardia, perspiration, elevated blood pressure. Also called *cuca* and *cocaine.*

coccygeal (kôk·si·jē'·əl), *n* caudal spine including the coccyx.

coenzyme, *n* an essential nonprotein component (such as a vitamin or a mineral) of an enzyme.

coenzyme Q₁₀, *n* an enzyme along the electron transport chain. Scientific name: 2,3 dimethoxy-5 methyl-6-decaprenyl benzoquinone; uses: heart disease—including ischemic heart disease, dysrhythmias, congestive heart failure, hypertension, angina pectoris, mitral valve prolapse—diabetes, infertility, Bell's palsy, periodontal disease; precautions: pregnancy, lactation, children; can cause nausea, diarrhea, epigastric pain. Also called *Co-Q10, mito-quinone, ubidecarenone,* and *ubiquinone.*

Coffea spp., n See coffee.

coffee, *n* Latin name: *Coffea* spp.; part used: seeds; uses: digestive aid, appetite stimulant; increase alertness; increase circulation; increase bronchodilation; precautions: pregnancy, lactation, children, patients with heart disease; can cause palpitations, elevated blood pressure, restlessness, headaches, insomnia, dizziness, depression, nausea, heartburn, peptic ulcers, tremors. Also called *bean juice, café, espresso,* and *java.*

cognitive-behavioral stress management (CBSM), *n* the combination of meditation with a variety of cognitive-behavorial strategies, such as problem solving and interpersonal communication, to recognize and alter responses to negative thoughts, often done in a group setting.

cognitive rehabilitation, *n* therapy that connects memory failure with a person's relationship, anxiety, and self-concept issues. Has been used for traumatic brain injury.

cognitive restructuring, *n* any behavior therapy that results in notable shifts in an individual's perception and thought processes.

coherent vibrations, *n.pl.* the vibrations of all molecules in a body that are collective properties of an organism and are radiated into the environment.

cohobation, *n* the process of repeatedly using the water present during distillation to minimize loss of water soluble components from a plant material.

cohosh, black (blak´ kō´·häsh), *n* Latin names: *Actaea racemosa, Cimicifuga racemosa*; parts used: rhizome, roots; uses: relaxes smooth muscles, antispasmodic, antitussive, astringent, diuretic, antidiarrheal, antiarthritic, antiabortion, dysmenorrhea, menopausal complaints, antiasthmatic in children, possible prevention of osteoporosis; precautions: pregnancy except during first trimester to reduce uterine spasms and for antiabortion effects, lactation, patients who have had breast cancer, children except with qualified supervision, those taking blood pressure medications, hormone replacement therapies. Also called *black snakeroot, bugbane, bugwort, cimicifuga, fairy candles, rattleroot, rattleweed,* or *squaw root.*

cohosh, blue, *n* Latin name: *Caulophyllum thalictroides;* parts used: roots, rhizomes, aerial parts; uses: antispasmodic, anticonvulsant, rheumatism; jump start labor; increase menstruation; precautions: pregnancy, lactation, children, patients with cardiac disorders; can cause hypertension, chest pain, hyperglycemia, stomach cramps, diarrhea, and irritation to the mucous membrane; is embryotoxic. Also called *blue ginseng, papoose root, squaw root,* or *yellow ginseng.*

cohosh, white (whīt´ kō´·häsh), *n* Latin name: *Actaea alba*; parts used: rhizomes; uses: menstrual complaints, childbirth, coughs, colds, urinary tract conditions; precautions: pregnancy, lactation, children, toxic (especially roots and fruits); may cause circulatory failure; do not ingest other than homeopathic doses. Also called *baneberry, snakeberry, coralberry,* or *doll's eye.*

Cola acuminata, *n* See tree, cola.

Cola nitida, *n* See tree, cola.

colchicine (käl´·chə·sēn), *n* an alkaloid derived from the toxic plant *Colchicum autumnale* and used to treat the pain and inflammation of gout. Contraindicated for pregnant and lactating women; children; geriatric patients; and those taking antineoplastics, antithyroid medications, azathioprine, chloramphenicol, cyclophosphamide, flucytosine, gancyclovir, interferon, mercaptopurine, methotrexate, phenylbutazone, plicamycin, or zidovudine.

Colchicum autumnale, *n* See meadow saffron.

cold expression, *n* commonly used for citrus fruits, a method of extracting essential oils from their botanical source; either the whole fruit or the peel alone is crushed, and the oils are separated from the pulp by centrifugation. Cold-expressed oils typically have a short shelf life.

coleus (kō´·lē·əs), *n* Latin name: *Coleus forskohli;* part used: root; uses: allergic rhinitis, dysmenorrhea, eczema, hypertension, psoriasis, asthma, angina; precautions: none known.

colitis (kə·lī´·tis), *n* inflammation of the colon and rectum; can result in intestinal ulcerations and bleeding, diarrhea, and weight loss.

collagen, *n* protein that is the major constituent of cartilage and other connective tissue; comprises the amino acids hydroxyproline, proline, glycine, and hydroxylysine.

collateral circulation effect, *n* **1.** the opening up of normally closed blood vessels that connect arteries, thus providing a path for blood to flow around occlusions, such as occur in stroke or myocardial ischemia. **2.** one of the physiologic doctrines used in hydrotherapy to modify blood circulation in an area of the body that has a single artery supplying blood to the deep as well as the superficial areas. A cold application causes a decrease in blood flow to the superficial areas and a simultaneous increase to the deeper areas and a hot application has the opposite effect.

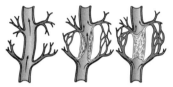

Collateral circulation effect. (Lewis, Heitkemper, and Dirksen, 2000)

colloid, *n* submicroscopic particles suspended in either a gaseous, liquid, or solid medium that does not separate. When homeopathic remedies are created from source materials, a colloidal phase may occur after trituration with lactose.

colocynth fruit (kô'·lə·sinth frŏŏt'), *n* Latin Name: *Citrullus colocynthis;* part used: pulp; uses: cathartic; precautions: can stimulate bowel movements with violent gripping pain plus occasional bloody discharge and dangerous inflammation of the bowels; can cause colitis and death. Also called *colocynth pulp, bitter cucumber,* and *apple (bitter).*

colocynthin (kō'·lə·sin'·thin), *n* glycoside found in *Citrullus colocynthus* used as a laxative. Precautions include violent griping pain plus occasional bloody discharge and dangerous inflammation of the bowels; can cause colitis and death.

colon hydrotherapy (kō'·lən hī'·drō·the'·rə·pē), *n* washing of the rectosigmoid area, usually with an instrument, claimed to cleanse, restore intestinal flora balance, improve muscle tone, and enhance absorption of nutrients. See also *hydrotherapy.*

colonic (kə·lô'·nik), *adj* pertaining to the colon.

colonic (kə·lô'·nik), *n* irrigation of colon for cleansing by injecting large amounts of fluid.

colonic irrigation (kə·lôn'·ik ir·rə·gā'·shən), *n* method that employs colon flushing to cleanse the body of toxins as well as treat gastrointestinal conditions, including diarrhea and constipation. Possible side effects include infection, torn tissue, electrolyte disparity, intestinal perforation, and sometimes death.

colorpuncture (kul'·er·punk'·cher), *n* therapeutic use of small colorzone lamps focused on acupuncture points and other parts of the body.

colostomy (kə·lô'·stə·mē), *n* incision made in the abdominal wall, intended to draw the intestine out and create an artificial anus. Often done after cancer surgery.

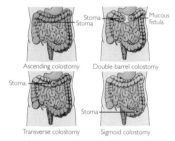

Colostomy. (Beare and Myers, 1998)

colostrum (kə·lä'·strəm), *n* **1.** bovine prelactation secretion that contains antibodies and other immune system–activating substances. Claimed to treat infections, autoimmune diseases, lyme disease, and inflammatory bowel disease. No known precautions, although the possibility of prior contamination exists in bovine products. **2.** human mammary secretion that contains living immune cells, immune factors, and antibodies. Produced in the first few days of lactation.

coltsfoot, *n* Latin name: *Tussilago farfara;* parts used: buds (dried), leaves, roots; uses: asthma, coughs, bronchitis, inflammation of the oral cavity; precautions: pregnancy, lactation, children, patients with liver disorders; those hypersensitive to ragweed, chamomile, or the composite family; do not use for longer than 6 weeks; can cause hypertension, nausea, diarrhea, jaundice, hepatotoxicity (not often), upper respiratory infections. Also called *British tobacco, bullsfoot, butterbur, coughwort, donnhove, farfara, fieldhove, filius ante patrem, flower velure, foal's-foot, foalswort, hallfoot, horsefoot, horse-hoof, kuandong hua,* and *pas díane.*

column, *n* component of gas-liquid chromatography apparatus that contains the stationary phase through which the carrier gas transports the vaporized sample to be separated.

combination essences, *n.pl* mixture of therapeutic plant and/or gem essences in one bottle.

combined movements, *n.pl* the combination of two separate motions to examine a joint and the spine.

comfrey, *n* Latin name: *Symphytum officinale;* parts used: leaves, roots; uses: wound healing, antiinflammatory for bruises and sprains; precautions: pregnancy, lactation, children; external use only; do not use for more than 6 weeks a year; can cause hepatotoxicity, nausea, liver adenoma. Also called *black root, blackwort, boneset, bruisewort, consound, gum plant, healing herb, knitback, knitbone, salsify, slippery root,* and *wallwort.*

comminution (kô·mə nōō·shən), *n* the grinding of a hard material (e.g., wood, seeds) into powder to release the essential oils.

Commiphora molmol, *n* See myrrh.

Commiphora mukul, *n* See guggul.

commitment, *n* in behavioral medicine, one of the three attitudes associated with stress hardiness. Characterized by feelings of fidelity and integrity and recognition that one's actions are important and valuable. See also stress hardiness.

common tansy (kô·mən tan·zē), *n* Latin names: *Tanacetum vulgare,*

Tanacetum aubiderti, Chrysanthemum vulgare, Chrysanthemum tanacetum; parts used: leaves, flowers, seeds; uses: anthelmintic, menstrual irregularities, antispasmodic, carminative, kidney disorders, hysteria, stomach problems, febrifuge, inflammatory skin disease, used to kill lice, fleas, scabies; precautions: may cause the premature expulsion of a premature fetus, may be toxic in large quantities. Also called *bachelor's buttons, bitter buttons, boerenwormkruid, buttons, ginger plant, gold-buttons, ponso, solucanotu, tanaceto, tansy,* and *yomogi-giku.*

community-based systems, *n.pl* healthcare organizations centered in and around a particular community.

comorbidity (kō·mōr·bi·də·tē), *n* presence of additional conditions with the initially diagnosed illness.

comparative clinical trial evidence, *n* a clinical research tool used to measure the efficacy of a given treatment by comparing the test results of two groups (i.e., when group one is administered only the test treatment, while group two is administered the standard treatment or no treatment). May or may not be randomized and/or blinded.

comparative effectiveness, *n* the assessment of the relative merits of two active therapeutic approaches by direct comparison.

compassion, *n* a profound awareness of another's suffering coupled with a desire to alleviate that suffering.

compassion fatigue, *n* emotional drain experienced by caregivers usually after caring for another with a progressive illness.

compassionate nonattachment (kəm·pa·shən·ət nän·ə·tach·mənt), *n* the desire to alleviate another's suffering without being attached to either the recipient or the outcome.

compatible, *adj* 1. congruent. 2. capable of blending with.

competence, *n* the state or condition of being sufficiently qualified to perform a particular action. To achieve this condition, one must possess the proper knowledge, skills, training, and professionalism.

complaint, *n* a patient-described symptom, problem, or malady. See also illness and disease.

complement fixation, *n* an immune reaction in which an antigen-antibody complex inactivates or fixes the complement of the antibody. Complement fixation tests are used to determine antibodies for infectious diseases, such as syphilis and certain viral infections.

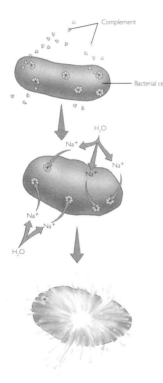

Complement fixation. (Thibodeau and Patton, 1999 [modified])

complementarity (kam´·plə·men·tar´·ə·tē), *n* a concept in quantum physics, proposed by Neils Bohr, in which total information about a subject or system cannot be obtained because the information is located in at least two complementary qualities. Measuring one quality precludes measurement of the other.

complex carbohydrates, *n.pl* polysaccharides; nutritional compounds composed of multiple monosaccharide (simple sugar) building blocks. Complex carbohydrates include starches, glycogen, and cellulose.

complex prescribing, *n* the homeopathic practice, popular in France and Germany, of prescribing a combined remedy of dilutions at different potencies in one container to treat a specific disease state.

complexism (kəm·pleks´·izm), *n* a form of homeopathy that simultaneously uses multiple remedies of highly diluted plant or mineral substances.

compliance, *n* **1.** in physiological terms, the degree of suppleness of a form. **2.** in terms of medical practice, the extent to which a patient implements the prescribed remedy. The term *concordance* has recently been suggested to replace *compliance,* which has the connotation of forcing the patient to follow the regime.

compound, *n* **1.** in chemistry, a distinct substance produced by chemical combination of two or more elements, the atoms of which are held together by chemical bonds. **2.** in herbal medicine, a mixture of two or more herbs that act synergistically. See also element and molecule.

compound muscle action potential (CMAP), *n* a group of almost simultaneous action potentials from several muscle fibers in the same area usually evoked by stimulation of the supplying motor nerve and are recorded as one multipeaked summated action potential.

comprehensive approach, *n* medical philosophy that considers multidimensional factors in disease and emphasizes quality of life or wellness by addressing the emotional, psychosocial, and spiritual aspects of a patient.

comprehensive digestive stool analysis, *n* a diagnostic procedure used to identify gastrointestinal disorders involving detailed stool examination for indications of digestive disorders, malabsorption, and microbiological imbalances.

compress, *n* a method of medicine preparation in which a large cloth is soaked in a hot infusion or decoction; the excess liquid wrung out; and the cloth applied to the affected part of the body.

compress, **cold,** *n* a cloth or pad soaked in cold water or ice (sometimes containing herbs or specific solutes) and applied on a part of the body. In hydrotherapy, used as a single compress to reduce blood flow and as a double compress to increase blood flow.

compress, **hot,** *n* a cloth or pad moistened in warm to hot water and applied to a part of the body. In hydrotherapy, used to ease pain locally, increase blood flow, and relax muscles.

compression, *n* **1.** squeezing or applying pressure, often to remove liquids. **2.** a type of somatic dysfunction in which two different structures or tissues are pressed together.

compression broadening, *n* massage technique designed to encourage full muscular contraction by applying of gliding pressure across the muscle fiber.

compression component, *n* a method of deliberately directing energy through a client's body by working the muscles and limbs through manual techniques such as pushing and pressing, squeezing and pinching, and twisting and wringing.

compression with manipulation, *n* neuromuscular technique in which the practitioner picks up the tissue and then rolls or twists it between the thumb and fingers. The practitioner applies this technique after the tenderness in the tissue has been lessened by static compression and gliding strokes.

compression, **SBS,** *n* condition in which the basilar part of the sphenoid

is tightly held together with the basilar part of the occiput, thus limiting motion of the sphenobasilar synchondrosis. Also called *sphenobasilar synchondrosis (symphysis) compression.*

computed axial tomography (kəm·pyu·tid ak·sē·əl tə·mô'·grə·fē), *n* See computerized tomography.

computed tomography, *n* radiographic imaging technique used to record a cross-section of tissue.

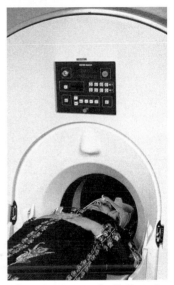

Computed tomography (Perkin et al. 1986)

concentration, *n* the amount of a solute (substance) dissolved in a specific amount of solvent. This number may be represented as a percentage (%), grams per liter, or as a mole fraction.

concentric (kən·sen'·trik), *adj* **1.** referring to a muscle contraction that involves reduction in a muscle's length. **2.** referring to muscles or other tissues that are structured as circles or rings.

conchae (kông'·kə), *n* the three bony plates which curve along the outer wall of the nose, creating turbulence and increasing the inner surface area.

conclusion, *n* result or outcome of an event, action, or process.

concomitants (kən·kä'·mə·tənts), *n.pl* concurrent or consecutive symptoms that emerge during the course of the illness. See also symptom, accessory.

concordances, *n.pl* **1.** items that are in harmony. **2.** homeopathic medicines with affinity to one another and therefore can be used serially during the sequence of treating an illness. This interaction was initially noted by Boenninghausen. See also remedies, alternating; compatible; remedy, complementary; remedy, following; or remedies, relationship of.

concrete (käng'·krēt'), *n* solid or semi-solid plant extract obtained by washing with an organic solvent, such as hexane. It has a fatty or waxy consistency and comprises pigments, wax, and essential oils.

concurrent validity, *n* the degree to which results from one test agree with results from other, different tests.

condensation (kôn'·den·sā'·shən), *n* **1.** change in phase of a substance from a gas or vapor phase to a liquid or solid phase. **2.** the process of combining two different molecules by eliminating a simple molecule like water.

condensed food, *n* **1.** a concentration of food stuffs, usually involving the removal of water. **2.** in Tibetan medicine, mineral and herbal formulations used to treat specific diseases. Based on traditions carried throughout the Badmaev family lineage for more than 100 years, each formula is given a numerical designation and comprises a multitude of mineral and/or herbal components.

condenser (kən·den'·ser), *n* a component of distillation apparatus that cools the vapor produced by heating a substance and returns it to liquid.

condition, *n* **1.** the current health situation of a patient. **2.** the detail of a legal agreement or contract.

condurangin (kôn'·də·ran'·jin), *n* glycoside derived from the bark of

Marsedenia condurango that is poisonous in large quantities but is used in small quantities for homeopathic treatments.

condurango, *n* Latin name: *Marsedenia condurango;* part used: bark (dried); uses: astringent, antisyphlitic, anorexia, (under research: cancer); precautions: pregnancy, lactation, children, those allergic to the milkweed family, patients with liver disease or chronic seizures, can cause seizures, nausea, hepatotoxicity. Also called *condor-vine bark, condurango bark, condurango blanco, eagle vine, gonolobus,* and *condurango triana.*

confabulation (kən·fa'·byə·lā'·shən), *n* fabrication of information that often occurs during hypnosis, when the unconscious encounters a memory gap and fills it with incorrect information.

confession, *n* in spiritual and psychological practice, a process of acknowledging, repenting, and seeking forgiveness for mistakes.

confusion induction, *n* during hypnosis, a technique best used with very reserved, skeptical subjects to bring about a state of trance. Patients are bombarded with numerous vague and disturbing topics until they eventually stop trying to decipher the intent and subside into a relaxed state conducive to hypnosis.

congenital scoliosis (kən·gen'·i·təl skō·lē·ō'·sis), *n* spine abnormality present at birth in which anomalies in certain ribs and vertebrae cause the spine to curve.

congenital sternal foramina (kən·je'·nə·təl stur'·nəl fə·ram'·ə·nə), *n* small perforations present in different regions of the sternum. This condition is considered a potential complication of an acupuncture treatment in which the practitioner uses incorrect insertion technique.

congestive heart failure, *n* inability of the heart to sustain sufficient blood circulation in the lungs and tissues; condition characterized by shortness of breath, weakness, and edema.

Stage	Symptoms
Stage I	Patient is symptom-free at rest and with treatment
Stage II	Patient experiences impaired heart function with moderate physical effort. Shortness of breath with exertion is common. There are no symptoms at rest
Stage III	Even minor physical exertion results in shortness of breath and fatigue. There are no symptoms at rest
Stage IV	Symptoms such as shortness of breath and signs such as lower extremity edema are present when the patient is at rest

Congestive heart failure. (Pizzorno and Murray, 1999)

conjunct rotation (kän'·jənkt rō·tā'·shən), *n* small amount of rotation that occurs at a joint during flexion or extension; caused by the ligaments surrounding a joint and the shape of the joint surfaces.

conjunctiva (kən·jənk·ti'·və), *n* the inner lining and mucous membranes of the eyelids and the front of the sclera.

conjunctivitis (kən·jənk·ti·vī'·tis), *n* condition, typically contagious, in which the conjunctiva, the tissue surrounding the eye, is inflamed. Also called *pink eye*.

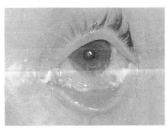

Conjunctivitis. (Newell, 1996)

connective tissue, *n* structural tissue composed of fibrous materials and a substrate that contains a variety of cells. Bone, cartilage, hair, nails, and fibrous tissue between cells and around muscles are all considered types of connective tissue.

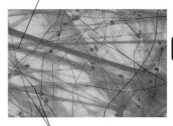

Bundle of collagenous fibers

Elastic fibers

Connective tissue. (Copyright Ed Reschke)

connective tissue consciousness, *n* a form of consciousness, contrasted to neurological consciousness (i.e., ordinary consciousness), in which the entire connective matrix of the body acts as the basis and the medium for responsiveness to environmental stimuli. See also matrix theory.

connective tissue physiology, *n* the biological study of mesodermal tissue that forms tendons and supports organs by filling in the spaces between them; also forms ligaments.

conscious breathing, *n* a relaxation technique in which the practitioners shift the focus of their attention from the stream of mental chatter to the natural rhythms of their breath. Many meditation techniques, including Vipassana and mantra, employ variations of conscious breathing. See also mantra, meditation, relaxation, relaxation response, Transcendental Meditation, and Vipassana.

consegrity (kôn·sā'·gri·tē), *n* a therapeutic modality in which energetic blockages, whether physical, mental, or spiritual in origin, are removed from the cells and connective tissues so that they can return to their innate ability to withstand tension and stress.

consideration, *n* a valued commodity exchanged between two parties in a legal agreement with one another, such as money, services, and so forth.

Consolidated Omnibus Budget Reconciliation Act, *n.pr* law that

C

allows individuals to carry over health coverage from a previous job for a limited time at their own expense.

Consortial Center for Chiropractic Research, *n.pr* an interdisciplinary association of researchers and practitioners who conduct and support scientific studies on chiropractic.

constipation, *n* health condition characterized by hard, dry feces that is difficult to pass, often indicating another health concern. In children, constipation is also characterized by the child not defecating on a daily basis. Can often be remedied through dietary modifications, increasing the fiber in the diet, improving digestion, alleviating stress, and usually as a last resort—using a laxative.

constitution, *n* **1.** the fundamental components that form a human being or thing. **2.** the total configuration of traits, physical and mental, that categorize a person. This compendium will consider both the effects of nature and nurture on that person. See also homeopathic medicine, constitutional; constitutional prescribing, constitution, carbonic; constitution, epidemic; constitution, fluoric; constitution, phosphoric; sensitive type; constitution, sulphuric; susceptibility; and typology.

constitution, carbonic, n one of the three body types developed by Nebel; consists of squat, stout, often obese people with joint hypolaxity. The homeopathic remedy is calcarea carbonica. Also called *brevilinear constitution.* See constitution, fluoric and constitution, phosphoric.

constitution, epidemic, n inherent qualities of people that make them sensitive to epidemic diseases.

constitution, fluoric, n the connection between thin undernourished people (ectomorphic body build) with slack ligaments and hyperextensible joints, and the properties of the homeopathic remedy, calcarea fluorica. See

also constitution, carbonic; constitution; morphology; constitution, phosphoric; constitution, sulphuric; and typology.

constitution, phosphoric, n category of body typified by being tall, lanky, and flexible and associated with the calcarea phosphorica homeopathic remedies. See also constitution, carbonic; constitution; constitution, fluoric; morphology; and constitution, sulphuric.

constitution, sulphuric, n category of body typified by being balanced and average. Also called *normolinear constitution.* See also carbonic constitution, fluoric constitution, phosphoric constitution, and morphology.

constitutional case-taking, *n* in homeopathy, the initial interview between the patient and the practitioner to obtain the totality of symptoms. Based upon such detailed information as the patient's health history, constitution, personality, occupation, habits, relationships, age, and gender/sexuality as well as the symptoms they present, this interview is indepth and may take several hours.

constitutional prescribing, *n* selection of homeopathic remedy centered on the complete makeup of the patient instead of parts of the symptoms alone. See also clinical picture; constitution; medicine, constitutional; morphology; simillimum; and typology.

constitutional types, *n.pl* categorization of individuals by type to predict their vulnerability to certain illnesses.

construct validity, *n* the degree to which an experimentally-determined definition matches the theoretical definition.

constructive knowledge, *n* information and understanding derived from circumstances.

contact dermatitis, *n* skin rash or inflammation following exposure to a primary irritant.

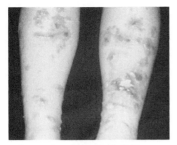

Contact dermatitis. (Lewis, Heitkemper, and Dirksen, 2000)

contact sensitization, *n* irritation of skin exposed to certain oils and other substances after initial application.

containment, *n* psychiatric mode of treatment for patients with conditions with which further deterioration is inevitable. In these cases, the primary goal of therapy is relief from symptoms and prevention of the progression of the illness.

content validity, *n* the degree to which an experiment or measurement actually reflects the variable it has been designed to measure.

contextual thinking, *n* a method of diagnosis in which the practitioner evaluates a patient's symptoms as an individual segment in a complex continuum rather than an effect of a specific cause or influence.

continued treatment in the face of adverse effects, *n* the continuation of a therapeutic approach despite unfavorable effects or outcomes. A risk of incompetent judgment or training.

continuous positive airways pressure, *n* the preferred therapy used to treat obstructive sleep apnea in which a nasal mask is used to facilitate regular sleep patterns by applying sufficient force to keep the upper airways open. See also OSA.

continuum consciousness, *n* See connective tissue consciousness.

Continuum Movement, *n* founded by Emily Conrad, a somatic education approach that develops self awareness

in an individual, which facilitates faster recovery from an illness or injury. See also somatic education.

continuum pathway, *n* the physiologic pathway for the transmission of information and energy; includes both the nervous system and a parallel somatic, energetic transfer via connective tissues.

contraction, *n* shortening or tensing of a muscle.

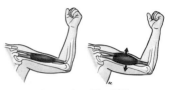

Contraction. (Fritz, 2004)

contraction, concentric, *n* movement accompanied by a shortening of the muscle as in the lifting phase of a biceps curl.

contraction, concentric isotonic, *n* therapeutic technique involving contraction by a client of a target muscle against pressure applied by the therapist. See also contraction, isotonic.

contraction, eccentric, *n* a muscle contraction involving an external force which lengthens the muscle. Used to increase muscle strength and mass but repeated contractions may result in muscle damage.

contraction, eccentric isotonic, *n* therapeutic technique involving the lengthening of a muscle against pressure provided by the therapist. See also contraction, isotonic.

contraction, isolytic, *n* a muscle contraction that occurs against resistance while lengthening the muscle.

contraction, isometric (ī'·sə·me'·trik kən·trak'·shən), *n* a muscle contraction in which the muscle tension increases without moving the points of muscle origin and insertion because a counterforce equal to that of the contraction is being exerted.

contraction, isotonic (ī'·sə·tôn'·ik kən·trak'·shən), *n* a muscle contraction in which the muscle length (shortening or lengthening) changes against a counterforce less than that of the contraction thus resulting in movement.

contractions, multiple isotonic, *n.pl* the muscle contractions that occur as the client moves a joint and accompanying muscles through the complete motion against moderate resistance.

contracture (kən·trak'·chər), *n* a frozen joint in flexion.

contractured muscle, *n* a muscle in which muscle tissue has been replaced by noncontractile tissues, so that the muscle is structurally prevented from relaxing to its normal length.

contradictory modality, *n* antagonistic approach to curing local symptoms in a patient, as in alleviating symptoms by cold applications in a patient who cannot tolerate cold.

contraindication, *n* any reason that a drug should not be taken, including harmful interactions with other drugs and the individual's personal sensitivity and condition.

control group, *n* in a clinical trial, the group of subjects that does not receive the active treatment. Having a control group allows comparisons by factoring out confounding variables so that any remaining differences may be attributed to the variable (i.e., the active treatment).

Control of Substances Hazardous to Health, *n.pr* a set of United States regulations intended to protect people from hazardous materials.

control, *n* **I.** power to direct the outcome of events that occur throughout life. To develop effective problem-solving skills and strategies, one must specifically differentiate between the circumstances that can and cannot be personally managed. For instance, one can direct the events associated with a work but not the outcome of a surgery. In behavioral medicine, it is one of the three unique attitudes associated with stress hardiness. **2.** comparison standard as part of comparative test design. **3.** the group selected for comparison to a test group in order to assess a hypothesis. See also stress hardiness.

Convallaria majalis, *n* See lily of the valley.

convergent strabismus (kôn'ver'·jənt strə·biz'·məs), *n* condition in which the eyes turn inward toward the nose; cross-eyed.

convergent view, *n* a school of thought that states the human body manifests emotions, beliefs, and past experiences within its posture and range of motion.

Convulvus scammonia, *n* See Mexican scammony.

copper, *n* an element and essential mineral that may be useful in the treatment of osteoporosis. Excessive consumption of zinc, use of oral contraceptives, or the drug AZT can lead to copper deficiency, but otherwise deficiency is rare. There are no known precautions for copper supplementation at nutritional doses, but mega-doses may lead to nausea and vomiting.

Coptis spp. **(kôp'·tis),** *n* part used: rhizome; uses: antiinflammatory, vasodilator, antipyretic, cholagogic, hepatitis, gallstones, cirrhosis, jaundice, venereal diseases, conjunctivitis, abscesses, hemorrhage, oral ulcers, scabies, leukemia, cancer, tuberculosis, typhoid fever; relieve heat conditions associated with insomnia, anxiety and nervousness; precautions: can increase risk of jaundice; can injure the stomach. Also called *Rhizoma coptidis, Coptis chinensis,* and *huang lian.*

Cordyceps sinensis **(kōr'·di·seps si·nen'·sis),** *n* part used: fruiting bodies; uses: asthma, chronic bronchitis, antiaging, weakness, lung and kidney functioning; precautions: none known.

core link, *n* the dura mater covering the brain and the spine, internally connecting the occiput to the sacrum and coordinating the synchronized motions of these structures. Also called *craniosacral membrane* and *dural membrane.*

coriander, *n* Latin names: *Coriandrum sativum, Coriandrum sativum* var. *vulgare, Coriandrum sativum* var. *microcarpum;* part used: fruit (dried);

uses: anthelmintic, appetite stimulant, arthritis, dyspepsia; precautions: pregnancy, lactation, children; can cause nausea, fatty liver tumors. Also called *Chinese parsley* and *cilantro*.

Coriandrum sativum, *n* See coriander.

Coriandrum sativum var. microcarpum, *n* See coriander.

Coriandrum sativum var. vulgare, *n* See coriander.

corkwood, *n* Latin name: *Duboisia myoporoides;* parts used: leaves, stems, roots; uses: motion sickness, gastrointestinal spasms; precautions: pregnancy, lactation, children, patients with glaucoma, myasthenia gravis, stomach or genital blockage, congestive heart failure, enlarged prostates, hypertension, dysrhythmias, and stomach ulcers; can cause palpitations, tachycardia, confusion, restlessness, headaches, blurred sight, nausea, dry mouth, constipation, upset stomach. Also called *pituri*.

Cornell Medical Index, *n.pr* a self-report screening instrument used to obtain a large amount of relevant medical and psychiatric information. Specifically, the subject is expected to respond to inquiries regarding his or her health habits, symptoms, and family history. Also called *CMI*.

coronal plane postural decompensation, *n* nonoptimal distribution of body mass in the frontal plane resulting in scoliotic changes in the posture.

coronal suture, *n* meeting place on the skull, of the frontal bone and the anterior parietal bones.

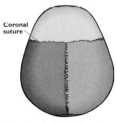

Coronal suture. (Chaitow, 1999)

coronary occlusion, *n* obstruction in the heart's blood-supplying arteries.

corrientes espirituales (kōr·rē·en'· tās e·spē'·rē·tōō·ä'·läs), *n.pl* in Curanderismo, the Mexican healing system, the spiritual currents that can be tapped for information and healing.

corticotropin-releasing factor (kor'· ti·kō·trō'·pin·rē·lē'·sing fak'·ter), *n* substance secreted by the hypothalamus that triggers the pituitary-adrenal axis. The increased release of this substance plays a significant role in immunosuppression and has other secondary effects. Also called *CRF*.

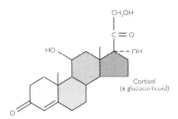

Cortisol (a glucocorticoid)

Corticotropin-releasing factor. (Thibodeau and Patton, 1996 [modified])

cortisol (kōr'·tə·sōl), *n* an adrenal hormone produced in response to stress.

coryza (kə·rī'·zə), *n* nasal discharge often accompanying the common cold and other conditions.

COSHH, *n.pr* See Control of Substances Hazardous to Health.

cotton, *n* Latin name: *Gossypium herbaceum;* parts used: bark, seeds, leaves, flowers, root bark; uses: in Ayurveda, pacifies vata dosha (sweet, astringent, light, oily), antifertility, antibacterial, antiviral, antimutagen, antitumor, emmenagogue, expectorant, amenorrhea, dysentery, (seeds) rheumatism, (leaves) diuretic; precautions: none known. Also called *kapas* or *tundakesi*.

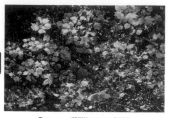

Cotton. (Williamson, 2002)

couchgrass, *n* Latin names: *Agropyron repens, Elymus repens, Graminis rhizomo, Triticum repens* L.; part used: rhizomes; uses: irrigant, demulcent, antimicrobial, cystitis, urethritis, prostatitis, urinary tract infections, renal gravel, upper respiratory disorders, gout, rheumatism, cough, cirrhosis, tumors, cancer; not used today; precautions: patients with edema caused by heart or kidney conditions. Also called *cutch, dog grass, durfa grass, quack grass, quitch grass, Scotch quelch, triticum, twitch-grass,* and *witch grass.*

cough, *n* the expulsion of air forcefully and audibly from the lungs. A cough works to loosen and clear foreign matter and irritants from the air passages and is often a symptom of infection.

coumarin, *n* C_9H_6O, derived from a variety of sources, including tonka bean and sweet clover; may also be artificially manufactured.

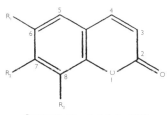

Coumarin. (Beresford-Cooke, 2003)

Council for Homeopathic Education (kôwn´·sil fōr hō´·mē·ō·pa´· thik e·djōō·kā´·shən), *n.pr* an organization founded in 1982 that

accredits homeopathic training programs in the United States and Canada. Also called *CHE.*

Council on Naturopathic Medicine Education, *n.pr* an agency founded in 1978 that accredits naturopathic education. It certifies postdoctoral programs in naturopathic medicine, including naturopathic residencies that provide licensed naturopathic physicians with the opportunity to obtain postgraduate training in naturopathic health care. The agency is recognized by four-year naturopathic colleges and programs within Canada and the United States, the Canadian and American national naturopathic professional associations, and the North American Board of Naturopathic Examiners. See also Examination, Naturopathic Physicians Licensing.

counseling, *n* wisdom and advice offered by a counselor to the patient as a regular part of the healthcare process.

counseling skills, *n* the acquired verbal and nonverbal skills that enhance communication by helping a medical professional to establish a good rapport with a patient or client.

counteraction, *n* instinctive response of the life force to the implementation of the homeopathic remedy. Also called *after action* and *back action.* See also secondary drug action.

counterirritation, *n* technique that relieves irritation in one part of the body by producing superficial irritation in another part.

counternutation, *n* posterior movement of the sacrum around a transverse axis relative to the hip bones.

counterpressure, *n* pressure applied by the therapist against the client's effort, corresponding partially (isotonic contraction) or fully (isometric contraction). See also contraction, isotonic and contraction, isometric.

coupled motion (ku´·pəld mō´· shən), *n* consistent association of one type of motion with an another.

covalent bond (kō·vā´·lənt bônd), *n* chemical bond that involves sharing of electrons between atoms of the same element to give a molecule of that element (e.g., nitrogen) or atoms of two or more elements to give a molecule of a compound (e.g., carbon dioxide); the predominant type of bonding in organic chemistry.

cowhage, *n* Latin name: *Mucuna pruriens;* parts used: seeds, roots, legumes; uses: in Ayurveda, considered a rasayana (sweet, bitter, heavy, oily), anthelmintic, aphrodisiac, seeds: nervine, abortifacient, root: diuretic, kidney stones, coughs, Parkinson's disease; precautions: irritant, inflammation, use as vermifuge is dangerous. Also called *atmagupta, cowitch, kavach,* or *vanari.*

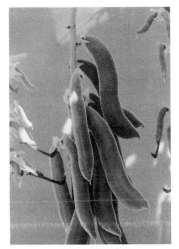

Cowhage. (Williamson, 2002)

cowslip, *n* Latin name: *Primula veris;* part used: buds; uses: insomnia, anxiety; precautions: pregnancy, lactation, children, patients with liver disease and gastrointestinal disorders; can cause nausea, diarrhea, gastritis, hepatotoxicity, contact dermatitis. Also called *artetyke, arthritica, buckles, crewel, drelip, fairy cup, herb Peter, key of heaven, key flower, may blob, mayflower, our lady's keys,* *paigle, palsywort, password, peagle, petty mulleins,* and *plumrocks.*

coxal (käk′·səl), *adj* pertaining to the hip area.

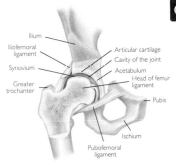

Coxal. (Thompson et al, 1997)

cox/flexion-distraction (kôks′/flek′· shən-dis·trak′·shən), *n* chiropractic technique that treats intervertebral disc pathosis using traction-mobilization.

CP, *n* cerebral palsy; a disorder thought to result from brain damage that occurs before, during, or immediately after birth. The primary indications include disturbances in speech and a noticeable lack of muscle coordination.

CPAP, *n.pr* See continuous positive airways pressure.

CPR, *n.pr* See cardiopulmonary resuscitation.

CR, *n* contract relax; a proprioceptive neuromuscular facilitation (PNF) technique that involves stretching and relaxing taut muscles. It is particularly used for larger muscles of the body. See also PNF.

CRAC, *n* contract-relax, antagonist contract; a proprioceptive neuromuscular facilitation (PNF) technique that uses antagonist and agonist muscles to stretch and relax taut muscles. See also PNF.

cramp bark (kramp′ bärk′), *n* Latin names: *Viburnum opulus;* part used: dried bark; uses: antispasmodic, uterine sedative, prevent or treat scurvy; precautions: none known.

Also called *high bush cranberry, snowball bush, guelder rose,* and *stagbush.*

cranberry, *n* Latin names: *Vaccinium macrocarpon, Vaccinium oxycoccus, Vaccinium erythrocarpum;* part used: berries; uses: kidney stones, prevention of urinary tract infections; precautions: patients with oliguria or anuria. Also called *bog cranberry, isokarpalo, marsh apple, mountain cranberry,* and *pikkukarpalo.*

cranial (krā'·nē·əl), *adj* positioned over or toward the cranium. Also called *superior* or *cephalic.*

cranial concept, *n* in osteopathic medicine, a diagnostic and therapeutic approach associated with the application of osteopathic medicine principles to the skull or cranium; based on the structural studies and clinical observations conducted by William Garner Sutherland, D.O. Dr. Sutherland claimed that a palpable motion within the human body takes place in concurrence with the movement of the bones called the Primary Respiratory Mechanism, or PRM, within the head. The cranial concept is considered an extension of osteopathic philosophy.

cranial electrostimulation (krā'·nē·əl i·lek'·trō·stim·yə·lā'·shən), *n* treatment that applies low-level electrical impulses to the mastoid process and eyelids. Has been used for insomnia and anxiety. Also called *electrosleep.*

cranial osteopathy, *n* an approach to treatment and healing that considers the whole patient, especially in regard to the motion, tissues, and fluids of the skull area. This is practiced by osteopathic physicians.

cranial rhythmic impulse, *n* the concept that a cadence of fluids and tissue in the body is detectable by palpation of the head. Change in speed or strength indicates a correctable problem. See also primary respiratory impulse and Sutherland wave.

cranial suture, *n* structure within the skull that houses layers of ligaments, tissue bundles, and nerve fibers.

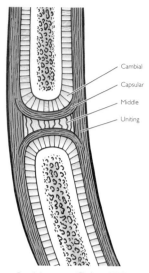

Cambial

Capsular

Middle

Uniting

Cranial suture. (Chaitow, 1999)

craniectomy (krā·nē·ek'·tə·mē), *n* removal of a section of the skull by surgical means.

craniopathy (krā'·nē·ō·pə·thē), *n* area of medicine concerned with the bones that encase the brain.

craniosacral mechanism, *n* a term used by osteopath William G. Sutherland; the dura mater linkage between the sacrum and the occiput. See also core link.

craniosacral outflow (krā'·nē·ō·sā'·krəl aut'·flō), *n* the flow of energy postulated to move between the head and sacrum in cranial osteopathy.

craniosacral system (krā'·nē·ō·sā'·kəl sis'·təm), *n* physiologic system of cerebrospinal fluid and the dura mater membrane as well as attached bones, sutures, and vessels.

craniostenosis (krā'·nē·ō·ste·nō'·sis), *n* birth defect in which the sutures between the cranial bones close prematurely.

craniotomy (krā·nē·ô'·tə·mē), *n* opening of the skull during surgery.

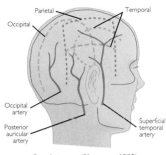

Craniotomy. (Youmans, 1982)

cricoid pressure (krī'·koid pre'·sher), *n* technique used during general anesthesia to lessen the possibility of stomach content aspiration. The practitioner squeezes the cricoid cartilage against the sixth cervical vertebra to stop passive regurgitation. Does not work with active vomiting, however. Also called *Sellick's maneuver.*

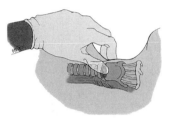

Cricoid pressure. (Sanders et al, 2000)

***Crataegus* spp.,** *n* See hawthorn.

Crataeva nurvala, *n* See varuna.

C-reactive protein, *n* protein usually not present in normal serum but detected with necrosis and a large number of inflammatory conditions, such as bacterial infection, rheumatic fever, and some neoplastic diseases.

creams, *n.pl* emulsions of oil and water containing a substance and used externally for a variety of cosmetic or medicinal purposes.

creatine (krē'·ə·tīn), *n* an amino acid that is created in the body in the kidneys, liver, and pancreas. Used as a supplement by athletes to aid in performance. Not for use by pregnant or nursing women, children, or patients with kidney or heart disease.

creativity, *n* the ability to imagine and create through innovation and synthesis.

crema de belleza (krā'·mə dā·be·yā'·zə), *n* a preparation originating from Mexico; used to cleanse the skin and prevent acne; causes mercury poisoning.

creosote (krē'·ə sōt), *n* a colorless to yellowish, oily liquid obtained by distilling wood tar, particularly *Fagus sylvatica;* used as wood preservative; harmful to animals because they may develop skin irritation by chewing on wood treated with creosote.

crinnion depuration protocol (krin'·nyən dē'·pyŏŏ'·rā·shən prō'·tə·kôl), *n* in environmental medicine, a method of removing xenobiotics from the body by using exercise, heat, hydrotherapy, colonic irrigation, homeopathy, therapeutic manipulation, and counseling. This protocol is followed on a daily basis for 4 to 8 weeks.

Crocus sativus, *n* See saffron stigma.

cross-directional stretching, *n* technique that uses counterdirectional stretching of connective tissue to increase pliability.

cross-sensitization, *n* a phenomenon in which a person becomes sensitized to substances different from the substance to which the person is already sensitized.

Croton tiglium, *n* See oil, croton.

croup (krōōp), *n* viral respiratory ailment that afflicts children ages 3 months to 3 years old; symptoms include but are not limited to fever, dry barking cough, dyspnea, and tachypnea. Also called *angina trachealis, exudative angina,* or *laryngostasis.*

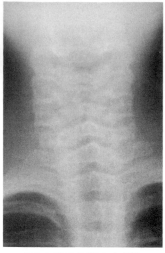

Croup. (Stone and Gorbach, 2000)

CRP, *n.pr* See C-reactive protein.

crural (krur'·əl), *adj* pertaining to upper and lower leg.

cryokinetics (krī'·ō·ki·ne'·tiks), *n* therapeutic process that includes application of external cold therapy to an area and is followed with full passive range of movement.

cryosurgery (krī'·ō·ser'·jə·rē), *n* surgical operation in which a metal probe (chilled to at least −160°C) is therapeutically applied to destroyed tissue.

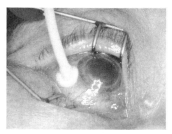

Cryosurgery. (Jaffe, 1996)

cryotherapy, *n* the use of cold applications, such as ice packs, to reduce edema and inflammation, relieve pain, and encourage vasoconstriction. See also vapocoolant sprays.

crystal, *n* distinctive form of molecule created when an element or chemical compound is frozen or slowly solidified. Each element or compound has a unique structure often used in gem healing and in amulets of pendulum.

CSCT, *n.pr* See therapy, Cell Specific Cancer.

CSF, *n.pr* cerebrospinal fluid.

C-SPOMM, *n* See Certification, Special Proficiency in Osteopathic Manipulative Medicine.

CT, *n* cervicothoracic; the region of spine locatced between the C7 and T3 vertebrae. It is one of the locations in which fascial tensions can be indicated.

cubital (kyōō'·bi·təl), *adj* pertaining to the inner fold of the arm at the elbow.

cucumber, *n* Latin name: *Cucumis sativus;* parts used: fruit, seeds; uses: diuretic, anthelmintic, hypertension, hypotension, skin irritations; precautions: pregnancy, lactation, children; can cause heartburn. Also called *wild cucumber.*

cucumber, Chinese, *n.pr* Latin name: *Trichosanthes kirilowii;* parts used: fruit, rind, seeds; uses: antiinflammatory, expectorant (seeds), sedative, demulcent, AIDS (fruit), cancer, ulcers, diabetes; precautions: pregnancy, lactation, children, patients with convulsions or diarrhea; can cause fever, seizures, abortion, damage to heart, death. Also called *Chinese snake gourd, gua-lou,* or *tia-hua-fen.*

cucumber, squirting (skwer'·ting kyōō'·kəm·ber), *n* Latin name: *Ecballium elaterium;* part used: fruits, plant, roots; uses: pain reliever, rheumatism, induce bowel evacuation, kidney disorder, heart condition, paralysis, shingles, sinusitis; precautions: may cause skin irritation, gastroenteritis, and toxicity in large doses. Also called *cohombrillo amargo, esekhiyari,* and *wild cucumber.*

Cucumis sativus, *n* See cucumber.

Cucurbita maxima, *n* See pumpkin.

Cucurbita moschata, *n* See pumpkin.

Cucurbita pepo, *n* See pumpkin.

cultivar, *n* a plant not found in nature; the form used to cultivate in order to propogate desired characteristics.

cultivated, *n* in herbal medicine, used to describe plants that are commercially farmed rather than collected from the wild.

cultural relativity, *n* technique for understanding the various ways in which people explain their behavior.

culture, *n* **1.** language, values, customs, and aesthetics of an individual or a group of people; culture influences attitudes about health and health care. **2.** growth of bacteria, fungi, or viruses on or in nutritive media in the laboratory.

cumbi-resin, *n* Latin name: *Gardenia gummifera;* part used: resin; uses: in Ayurveda, pacifes kapha dosha (bitter, pungent, light, dry, sharp), antiseptic, anthelmintic, insecticide, digestive, stimulant, fevers, teething, gum disease, wound dressing; precautions: none known. Also called *dikamali* or *nadi-hingu.*

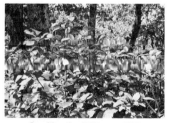

Cumbi-resin. (Williamson, 2002)

cumulative effect, *n* the exaggerated, often adverse, effects of herbs and/or medications taken in conjunction with other herbs or medications that function in physiologically similar ways. See also synergy.

cun (tsōōn), *n* in acupuncture, a variable unit of measure used to determine the location of acupuncture points.

The cun is calculated for each individual based on measurements taken on the thumb or index finger. Also called *Chinese inch.*

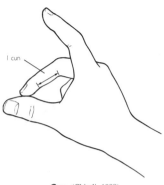

Cun. (Chirali, 1999)

cupping, *n* in traditional Chinese medicine, technique in which rounded glass cups are warmed and applied to an individual's bare skin to treat local qi problems or blood stagnation. Once the cup is warmed, the oxygen in the cup is eliminated so that a vacuum is created; this holds the cup to the skin, and encourages the flow of blood and qi to the area beneath the cup. Recommended only when performed by licensed practitioners, due to nonpermanent marking and bruising. Chosen by some as an alternative to acupuncture. Can cause bruising, bleeding, and burns if not properly applied. See also qi.

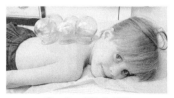

Cupping. (Chirali, 1999)

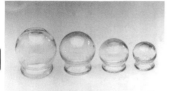

Cupping glass. (Chirali, 1999)

cuprea bark (kōō′·prē·ə bärk′), *n* bark obtained from *Remijia peduncu-lata*, which contains cupreine; used as an antimalarial.

cupreine (kōō′·prē·īn), *n* alkaloid derived from bark of the cuprea tree; used as an antimalarial.

curanderas/curanderos (kōō·rän·de·räs/kōō·rän·de·rōs), *n.pl* folk healers (female and male, respectively) in the medical traditions of Latin America. They treat mental and spiritual maladies in addition to physical illness.

Curanderismo (kōō′·rän·de·rēz′·mō), *n* Mexican-American healing tradition with roots in Moorish, Greek, Judeo-Christian, and Native American practices and beliefs. The Curandero (or healer) is consulted by the people in his community for help and spiritual assistance to resolve health, relational, and financial problems. Continues to be practiced in various forms throughout Mexican-American, Puerto Rican, and Cuban American communities today.

Curcuma longa, *n* See turmeric.

Curcuma santhorrhiza, *n* See temu lawak.

curcumin (kur·kyōō·min), *n* an extract obtained from turmeric. Used as an antioxidant, chemoprotective, and antiinflammatory and in the treatment of dyspepsia and hyperlipidemia. See also turmeric.

cure, *n/v* **1.** to eliminate illness or disease, to return to a healthy state. **2.** elimination or end of symptoms or syndrome. See also direction of cure and healing.

curettage (kyur·ə·täzh′), *n* the scraping, suction, or clearing of cells from an area of concern (i.e., a cavity or infection) with a sharp or blunt curet to improve examination or for removal.

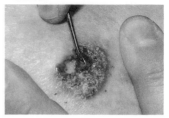

Curettage. (Habif, 1996)

curing, *n* the process of eliminating a particular disease.

curious meridians, *n.pl* in acupuncture, pathways that create links among the principal acupuncture channels and function as an energy storehouse during extreme periods of fullness or emptiness.

cutting, *n* the process of weakening or diluting a substance; in aromatherapy, organic solvents or carrier oils are added to essential oils to increase the volume. Dipropyl glycol (DPG), diethyl phthalate (DEP), and phenylethyl alcohol are common cutting agents.

CV, *n* the conception vessel, an acupuncture channel running from the perineum to the chin along the front of the body.

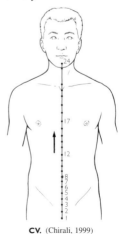

CV. (Chirali, 1999)

CV-4, *n.pr* compression of the fourth ventricle, in osteopathic shorthand.

CXR, *n* chest x-ray; an image of the thoracic cavity, produced by an irradiation scan of the upper torso. Routinely performed to rule out respiratory or heart disease for patients complaining of dyspnea or chest pain.

Cyamopsis tetragonolobus, *n* See guar gum.

cyanocobalamin (sī'·ə·nō'·kō·ba'·lə·mən), *n* See vitamin B₁₂.

cyclic (sik'·lik), *n* a molecule with atoms arranged in one or more rings, such as cyclohexane or benzene.

cyclooxygenases (sī'·klō·ôk'·sə·je·nā'·səs), *n.pl* enzymes that are rate-limiting in the production of thromboxanes and prostaglandins from arachidonic acid. The constitutive form of these proteins is essential for maintaining homeostasis while the inducible form is expressed in leukocytes in response to an inflammatory stimulus, resulting in production of prostanoids. The activity of cyclooxygenases is inhibited by antiinflammatory drugs, such as aspirin, and corticosteroids interfere with gene expression of the inducible form of the enzyme.

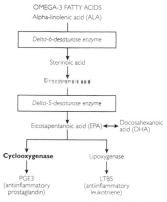

OMEGA-3 FATTY ACIDS
Alpha-linolenic acid (ALA)

Delta-6-desaturase enzyme

Sterinoic acid

Eicosatrienoic acid

Delta-5-desaturase enzyme

Eicosapentanoic acid (EPA) ←→ Docosahexanoic acid (DHA)

Cyclooxygenase   Lipoxygenase

PGE3   LTB5
(antiinflammatory   (antiinflammatory
prostaglandin)   leukotriene)

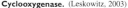

Cyclooxygenase. (Leskowitz, 2003)

Cydonia oblonga, *n* See quince.
Cymbopogon citrates, *n* See lemongrass.
Cynara scolymus, *n* See artichoke.
Cyperus rotundus, *n* See nutgrass.

Cypripedium calceolus, *n* See yellow lady's slipper.

Cypripedium pubescens, *n* See yellow lady's slipper.

cystadenoma (sist'·a'·də·nō'·mə), *n* **1.** cystic glandular tumor related to a glandular tumor. **2.** a glandular tumor that contains multiple cysts.

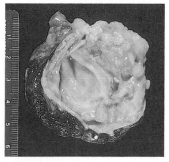

Cystadenoma. (Kumar, Cotran, and Robbins, 1997)

cystic fibrosis, *n* an inherited disorder that causes the exocrine glands to excrete very thick mucus; weakens lung capacity and resistance to infections; changes saliva chemistry, increases electrolyte levels in perspiration; and dysregulates the autonomic nervous system. Also called *mucoviscidosis* and *fibrocystic disease of the pancreas.*

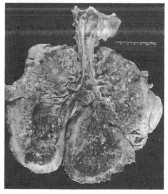

Cystic fibrosis. (Cotran, Kumar, and Collins, 1999; Dr. Eduardo Unis, Children's Hospital of Pittsburgh)

cystic lymphangioma (sis'·tik lim'·fan·gē·ō'·mə), *n* congenital condition in which the lymph vessels form a cystic growth; usually occurs in the groin, neck, or axilla. Also called *cystic hygroma* and *lymphangioma cysticum.*

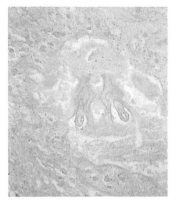

Cysticercosis. (Farrar, 1993)

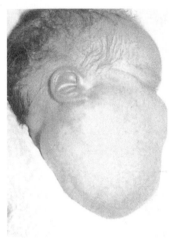

Cystic lymphangioma. (Greig and Garden, 1996)

cystic mastitis, *n* mammary dysplasia accompanied by nodular cysts and inflammation in breast tissue.

cysticercosis (sis'·tə·sər·kō'·sis), *n* food-borne illness caused by the beef or pork tapeworm, usually from eating undercooked beef that contains, *Taenia saginata* or by eating pork that contains *Taenia solium.* When the eggs of either tapeworm are ingested, they will develop inside the intestine and eventually invade the entire body, causing fever, muscle pain, eosinophilia, and malaise. Long-term effects include calcification of infested areas, brain seizures, and personality changes.

cystinuria (sis·tə·nur'·ē·ə), *n* elevation of cystine in urine.

cystitis (sis·tī'·təs), *n* inflammatory condition that occurs in the ureter and urinary bladder with symptoms such as hematuria, pain, frequent urination and persistent urge to urinate.

Cytochrome P-450 enzymes (sī'·tə·krōm' pē'-fōr' fif'·tē en'·zīmz), *n.pl* oxygenating catalysts responsible for the reactions used by the body, especially the liver, to detoxify drugs and other substances.

cytokines (sī'·tō·kīnz), *n.pl* regulatory proteins, such as lymphokines and interleukins that are produced by immune system cells and act as intercellular mediators in the modulation of immune response. Cytokines produced by recombinant DNA technology are administered to people to affect immune status.

cytomegalovirus (sī'·tō·me'·gə·lō· vī'·rəs), *n* species-specific, herpes-type virus capable of causing life-threatening illness in HIV patients, transplant recipients, and newborns; typically causes gastrointestinal or retinal infections.

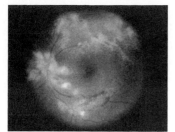

Cytomegalovirus. (Seidel et al, 1999; Douglas A. Jabs, MD, The Wilmer Ophthalmological Institute, The Johns Hopkins University and Hospital, Baltimore, MD)

cytoprophylactic (sī´·tō·prō´·fə·lak´·tik), *n* a substance used to promote new cell growth.

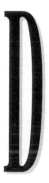

***d*-isomer,** *n* a stereo-isomer whose asymmetric carbon atom rotates plane-polarized light clockwise. See also asymmetric carbon atom.

dacryocystitis (dā´·krō·sis·tī´·tis), *n* an infection in the lacrimal sac that results from nasolacrimal duct obstruction. Responds to antibiotics; in extreme cases surgery may be required.

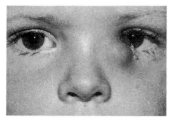

Dacryocystitis. (Zitelli and Davis, 1997)

daffodil, *n* Latin name: *Narcissus pseudonarcissus;* parts used: bulbs,

buds, leaves; uses: emetic, congestion, arthritis, burns, wounds; precautions: pregnancy, lactation, children; eating bulbs or flowers can be fatal; can cause heart collapse, nausea, contact dermatitis, daffodil itch, lung collapse. Also called *daffydown-dilly, fleur de coucou, Lent lily, narcissus,* and *porillon.*

D

daisy, *n* Latin name: *Bellis perennis;* parts used: buds, leaves; uses: antifungal, blood cleanser, pain reliever, diarrhea, cough, stomach spasms, arthritis; precautions: pregnancy, lactation, children. Also called *bairnwort, bruisewort, common daisy, day's eye,* and *wild daisy.*

damages, *n* monetary award from a court as compensation for a legally proven loss.

damiana (dä´·mē·ä·nə), *n* Latin name: *Turnera diffusa;* part used: leaves; uses: aphrodisiac, diuretic, antidepressant; precautions: pregnancy, lactation, children, patients with liver disease; can cause hallucinations, nausea, hepatotoxicity, irritation of the urethra. Also called *herba de la pastora, old woman's broom,* and *rosemary.*

dan tian (dän´ tē·än´), *n* refers to the region in the lower abdomen beneath the navel; also considered the place where qi is cultivated and stored. See also qi.

dan zhong (tän dzông), *n* in traditional Chinese medicine, acupuncture point found in the center of the chest.

dandelion, *n* Latin names: *Taraxacum officinale, Taraxacum laevigatum;* parts used: buds, leaves, roots; uses: laxative, antihypertensive, diuretic, (under research: antitumor, immunogenic, colon disease, urolithiasis); precautions: pregnancy, lactation, those allergic to chamomile or yarrow root, patients with diabetes, irritable bowel syndrome, stomach disorders, bile duct blockage, intestinal blockage, latex allergy; can cause nausea, cholelithiasis, gallbladder infection, contact dermatitis. Also called *blowball, cankerwort, lion's tooth, priest's crown, puffball, swine snout, white endive,* and *wild endive.*

dang gui (täng kwē), *n* Latin name: *Angelica polymorpha* var. *sinensis;* part used: roots; uses: menopause, PMS, menorrhagia, dysmenorrhea, neuralgia, headache, malaria, herpes infection, anemia, vitiligo; precautions: pregnancy, lactation, children, dang gui hypersensitivity, photosensitivity, bleeding disorders, acute illness, heavy menstrual flow. Also called *Chinese angelica, dong quai, dry kuei, tang-kuei, toki,* and *women's ginseng.*

daoyin (dōw·yēn), *n* an ancient Chinese mind-body exercise that combines the principles of meditation techniques and breathing to promote self-development and increase spirituality.

darshanam (där·shä´·nəm), *n* in Ayurveda, observation; the book that provides a fundamental basis for the eight classical methods—urine, pulse, tongue, feces, voice and speech, assessment of the eyes, evaluation by touch, and general physical assessment used throughout the examination. In Ayurvedic medicine, it is thought that each patient resembles a book that lives and breathes. To understand this book, a practitioner must hone his or her abilities in the application of the eight clinical markers listed here to perceive and announce the correct diagnosis. See also sparshanam and prashnam.

datura, *n* See jimsonweed.

Datura stramonium, *n* See jimsonweed.

Daucus carota, *n* See Queen Anne's lace.

DAy, *n* doctor of Ayurvedic medicine.

DC, *n* doctor of chiropractic.

de qui (dequi) (dā kē´), *n* the sensation experienced by a person undergoing acupuncture treatment when the needle is inserted correctly into an acupuncture point.

dearterialization (dē´·ar·ti´·rē·ul·ī´·zā·shən), *n* **1.** the process of turning arterial blood (which is oxygenated) into venous blood. **2.** disruption of the arterial blood supply to an organ.

death rehearsal, *n* a hypnotic technique used to give patients added insight regarding the dying process to relieve fear or anxiety. Patients are directed to project to the time of their death and examine the associated feelings and circumstances and then aided to positively reinterpret them.

deceleration, *n* in osteopathy, the process of decreasing speed or velocity of a manipulative technique.

decimal medicines, *n.pl* homeopathic medicines diluted at a 1:10 ratio and labeled with an X or a D (the latter commonly in Europe).

declarative learning, *n* learning that evolves from procedural learning after language development. Characterized by analytical, language-based, memory-dependent approach to acquiring and retaining knowledge. See also procedural learning.

decoction (dē·käk´·shən), *n* a method of medicine preparation in which herbal roots and stems are boiled in water for several minutes. This increases the efficiency of extraction of medicinal constituents from large, fibrous chunks of herbal material.

decompensation (dē·kôm´·pen·sā´·shən), *n* **1.** a persistent (yet reversible, in some cases) pattern of dysfunction, in which homeostatic mechanisms are overwhelmed, either in part or completely. **2.** postural pattern in which the musculoskeletal system indicates dysfunctional adjustments as a result of a physical anomaly, such as shortened leg.

decongestant, *n* a substance that reduces the production of mucus, thus relieving sinus congestion.

deep, *adj* positioned internally at or toward the center. Also called *central.*

deep breathing, *n* a quick relaxation technique in which attention is focused on breathing: deep inhalation and holding the breath for a few seconds before exhalation.

deep cause, *n* the sociocultural consideration of a person's illness as opposed to the epidemiological causes.

deep fascia (dēp´ fā´·shē·ə), *n* the connective tissue that resides throughout the human body, giving support and form, and connecting all the organs and tissues.

deep intratemporal fossa (dēp′ in′·trə·tem′·pə·rəl fô′·sə), *n* an acupuncture treatment area located at the junction of the zygomatic arch and the mandible, beneath the masseter muscle; useful for treating trigeminal neuralgia. See also acupuncture treatment area.

deep longitudinal stripping, *n* massage technique that uses very slow, intense pressure to decrease hypertonicity. Also called *deep tissue*.

defacilitation, *n* a state of deep calm in which a slower, underlying cranial rhythmic impulse or wave can be detected. See also cranial rhythmic impulse.

defect, *n* **1.** congenital anomaly in structure or function that may or may not be life-threatening. **2.** failure of a product to meet a reasonable expectation of performance and safety to the consumer.

deha prakriti (de′·hə prə·kri·tē), *n* in Ayurveda, the prevalent dosha or body composition of an individual. See also dosha.

dehydroepiandrosterone, *n* See DHEA.

delayed hypersensitivity, *n* sensitivity regulated by T lymphocytes that may take anywhere from 24–72 hours to develop.

Delphinium consolida, *n* See forking larkspur.

delta, *n* a Greek letter symbolized by upper case Δ or lower case δ. See also Greek letters.

delta rhythm, *n* the brain wave pattern connected with deep, dreamless sleep, characterized by a frequency of 1/2–4 Hz.

delta-6 desaturase enzyme (del′·tə-siks′ dē·sa′·chu·ras en′·zīm), *n* the rate-limiting step for converting

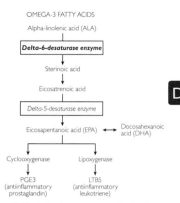

OMEGA-3 FATTY ACIDS

Alpha-linolenic acid (ALA)

Delta-6-desaturase enzyme

Sterinoic acid

Eicosatrenoic acid

Delta-5-desaturase enzyme

Eicosapentanoic acid (EPA) ⟷ Docosahexanoic acid (DHA)

Cyclooxygenase   Lipoxygenase

PGE3   LTB5
(antiinflammatory   (antiinflammatory
prostaglandin)   leukotriene)

Delta-6-desaturase enzyme. (Leskowitz, 2003)

linolenic acid or linoleic acid into longer essential fatty acid metabolites, (eicosapentaenoic acid and gamma linolenic acid).

dementia, *n* general term for a variety of organic brain disorders characterized by a decline in mental acuity, personality deterioration, memory loss, disorientation, and stupor. Certain types of dementia may be partially or completely reversible.

democratization of the arts (də·môk′·rə·tə·zā′·shən əv thə ärts′), *n* concept which states that every individual can engage in arts and that all are free to express the creativity within them, not simply those who are trained or otherwise skilled.

demulcents, *n.pl* remedies that relieve irritation and have soothing properties.

demyelination, *n* breakdown of the myelin sheaths covering nerves and nerve fibers.

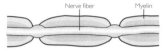
Nerve fiber   Myelin

Normal axon

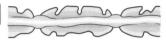
Disintegration of myelin

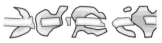
Disruption of axon function

Demyelination. (Phipps, Sands, and Marek, 1999)

denervation hypersensitivity (dē·ner·vā´·shən hī´·per·sen´·si·ti´·vi·tē), *n* interruption of automatic innervation to an organ, following which the degradative enzymes at the site are lost; as a result, the synaptic receptor becomes extremely sensitive to the neurohumoral agent because of loss of the degradative mechanism.

dengue fever (deng´·gē fē´·vər), *n* Flavivirus infection from the bite of the *Aedes aegypti* mosquito that presents symptoms including rash, fever, and acute back, head, and muscle pain. Also called *Aden fever, bouquet fever, breakbone fever, dandy fever, dengue,* and *solar fever.*

dentistry, *n* the medical science concerned with the teeth, gums, and general oral health care.

dentistry, biocompatible **(bī´·ō·kəm´·pa·tə·bəl den´·tis·trē),** *n* See dentistry, biologic.

dentistry, biologic, *n* a profession that treats conditions of the oral cavity. See also dentistry, biocompatible; dentistry, holistic; and dentistry, environmental.

dentistry, environmental, *n* a philosophy of dentistry that considers the biological and environmental impact of dental practice. Often incorporates complementary and alternative approaches. Also called *biologic, biocompatible,* or *holistic dentistry.*

dentistry, holistic, *n* dentistry that emphasizes the relationship of whole body health to the health of the oral cavity, teeth, and jaws. May involve herbal medicine, homeopathy, or other complementary and alternative methods. Also called *integrative dentistry.*

deodorant, *n* a substance that masks or eradicates odors.

depression, *n* a condition identified by loss of energy and ability or desire to function, poor sleep or appetite, and/or exaggerated feelings of hopelessness and discouragement.

depuration (dē´·pyŏŏ´·rā·shən), *n* in environmental medicine, the cleansing of impurities from the body.

depurative, *adj/n* ability of a substance to decontaminate or purify.

deputy ingredient (de´·pyŏŏ·tē in·grē´·dē·ənt), *n* one of the four components in a typical Chinese herbal formula used to help the chief ingredient in the treatment of the primary condition or a coexisting condition. See also chief ingredient, assistant ingredient, and envoy ingredient.

derivative effect, *n* one of the physiologic doctrines used in hydrotherapy to modify blood circulation. The application of heat increases the blood flow to an area while a cold application decreases the blood flow.

dermal toxicity, *n* an adverse skin reaction to the application of essential oils and other substances; includes irritation, (inflammation, itching) sensitization (reactions occurring after initial contact), and phototoxicity, (increased vulnerability to sun).

dermatitis, *n* inflammatory skin condition. Severity, duration, and treatment depend on the type (i.e., contact dermatitis and actinic dermatitis).

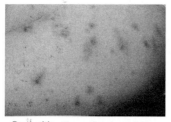

Dermatitis. (Cotran, Kumar, and Collins, 1999)

dermatome, *n* an area of skin innervated by a single spinal nerve and its branches. Dermatomes may overlap.

desarollo (de·sä·rṓ·yō), *n* in Curanderismo, the Mexican healing system, the training period that Curanderos (healers) must undergo in order to work on the spiritual level.

desensitization, *n* removing or neutralizing the allergenic propensity by introducing the patient to serially increasing doses of the offensive material. This allows the immune system to endure the allergen without an allergic response. Used in conventional medicine, and a parallel procedure is used in some homeopathic therapies, such as isopathy. See also isopathy.

designer music, *n* music made specifically to affect the listener on a physiologic or psychologic level, or both.

D

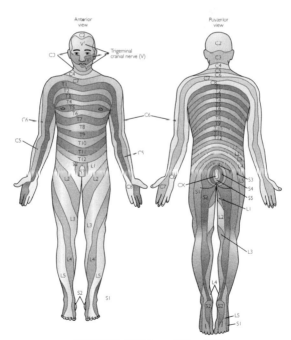

Dermatome. (Thibodeau and Patton, 1997)

desquamation (des·kwə·mā´·shən), *n* sloughing off of the cornified epidermal layer. Also called *exfoliation*.

detector, *n* a device used in analytical instruments that reacts to variations, such as temperature, pressure, humidity, or electrical conductivity charges, and measures the degree of response. This signal from the device is then amplified and plotted by a recorder.

determinism, *n* the notion that events may be predicted and anticipated by knowing the initial conditions and scientific law.

detoxification (dē·tôk´·sə·fə·kā´· shən), *n* cleansing of accumulated harmful substances, such as industrial chemicals and byproducts of metabolism.

devata (dā·vä´·tə), *n* in Sanskrit, the process of gaining knowledge. It is one of the three components of the Vedas, the ancient Hindu scriptures considered sources of pure knowledge. According to Vedic sciences, interactions of devata, rishi, and chhandas give rise to matter. See also veda, rishi, and chhandas.

devil's claw, *n* Latin name: *Harpagophytum procumbens;* parts used: roots, tubers; uses: appetite stimulant, arthritis, allergies, headaches, heartburn, dysmenorrhea, upset stomach, malaria, gout; precautions: pregnancy, lactation, children, patients with chronic peptic and duodenal ulcers and cholecystitis; can cause nausea. Also called *grapple plant* and *wood spider.*

DEXA, *n.pr* See dual-energy x-ray absorptiometry.

dextrorotatory (dek´·strə·rō´·tə· tôr´·ē), *n* a molecule or material capable of rotating plane-polarized light in a clockwise direction. See also enantiomers.

DGLA, *n.pr* See acid, dihomogammalinolenic.

DHA, *n.pr* See acid, docosahexaenoic.

DHANP, *n.pr* See Diplomate of the Homeopathic Association of Naturopathic.

dharana (dhä·rä´·nə), *n* mental concentration, one of the eight limbs or paths of Patanjali's yoga aimed at self-realization and self-knowledge. Con-

centration is here defined as calming the mind by focusing its attention on an object. See also yama, niyama, asana, pranayama, pratyahara, dhyana, and samadhi.

dhatus (dhä·tōōs), *n.pl* in Ayurveda, the seven fundamental principles that support the basic structure of the body. See also rasa, rakta, mamsa, meda, asthi, majja, and shukra.

DHEA, *n* dehydroepiandrosterone, a hormone precursor, exists naturally in yams. Claimed to enhance immunity, memory, and neural functioning; hamper osteoporosis; combat atherosclerosis, hyperglycemia, and cancer. Currently being researched as a treatment for depression, arthritis, asthma, lupus erythematosus, and fraility in the elderly. Not for pregnant or nursing women, children, or patients with breast, uterine, prostate, or ovarian cancers or prostate enlargement; can cause irregular heartbeats, insomnia, anxiety, acne.

DHom, *n* doctor of homeopathic medicine.

dhyana (jyä´·nə), *n* meditation, one of the eight limbs or paths of Patanjalis yoga, aimed at self-realization and self-knowledge. When the mind is no longer distracted from the object of concentration, then dhyana is realized as distinct from dharana. See also yama, niyama, asana, pranayama, pratyahara, dharana, and samadhi.

diabetes, *n* illness often identified by increased urination. Can be characterized by hyperglycemia (as in diabetes mellitus) or by a deficiency of antidiuretic hormone (as in diabetes insipidus).

Features	Type 1	Type 2
Age at onset	Usually under 40	Usually over 40
Percentage of all diabetics	Less than 10%	Greater than 90%
Seasonal trend	Fall and winter	None
Family history	Uncommon	Common
Appearance of symptoms	Rapid	Slow
Obesity at onset	Uncommon	Common
Insulin levels	Decreased	Variable
Insulin resistance	Occasional	Often
Treatment with insulin	Always	Not required
Beta-cells	Decreased	Variable
Ketoacidosis	Frequent	Rare
Complications	Frequent	Frequent

Diabetes. (Pizzorno and Murray, 1999)

diabetes, gestational, *n* a condition characterized by the development of high glucose levels during pregnancy; may be treated through diet, regular exercise, and insulin injections. If untreated, this condition may have ill effects on the health of the mother and the baby.

diabetes, non–insulin-dependent diabetes mellitus, *n* chronic disease marked by elevated levels of insulin and decreased tissue sensitivity to insulin. The condition may be asymptomatic, but an increase in thirst, appetite, and urination as well as fatigue, blurred vision, and weight loss are common.

diabetes, Type 1, *n* disease marked by an inability to use carbohydrates because of an absolute deficiency of insulin. Occurs in adults and children; symptoms include excessive thirst, frequent urination, weight loss, increased appetite, and irritability. Individuals with Type 1 diabetes depend completely on insulin.

diabetes, Type 2, *n* a form of diabetes not necessarily dependent on insulin but exhibits hyperglycemia and insulin resistance. Often linked to obesity, onset is usually after 40 years of age.

diadote (dī·ə·dōt'), *n* substance that blocks the assimilation of homeopathic remedies.

diagnosis, *n* the identification of an illness or condition through evaluation and examination. Diagnostic methods may include clinical examination, blood tests, palpitation, or pulse examination, depending upon the medical system in which the diagnosis is being made.

diagnosis, clinical, *n* the act of identifying a disease by analyzing the symptoms without considering the biological causes.

diagnosis, differential, *n* the act of listing a disease or diseases through comparative analysis of the symptoms.

diagnosis, electrodermal (ē·lek'·trō·der'·məl dī'·əg·nō'·sis), *n* method used to detect disease or an imbalance in energy along the body's acupuncture meridians by measurement of the electrical resistance at acupuncture points.

diagnosis, energy, *n* in energy medicine, use of intuition and trained subtle senses to discern the flow of energies in the body as well as blockages and disruptions of these energies.

diagnosis, hara (hä·rä dī·əg·nō'·sis), *n* a naturopathic method for locating imbalances that originate in the abdominal region. The therapist uses gentle, pressing movements and deeper palpations to identify the affected organs and the severity of the problem.

diagnosis, homeopathic, *n* analysis of a patient's illness according to homeopathic theory and method.

diagnosis, intuitive, *n* an assessment of a person's health performed by attending to subtle cues such as color, smell, and touch, through the use of intuition or via some form of remote sensing. See also anomalous cognition.

diagnosis, iris (ī'·ris dī·əg·nō'·sis), *n* the study of the iris for indications of disease.

diagnosis, Korean constitutional, *n* method based on herbal therapeutic system that uses the four yin and yang divisions to identify illness.

diagnosis, meridian, *n* a whole-body diagnostic method used by shiatsu practitioners to determine the location of energetic distortion in the meridians. It is usually used to supplement hara diagnosis or to treat structural complaints. See also diagnosis, hara, and Shiatsu.

diagnosis, orthodox, *n* diagnostic method that uses conventional Western approaches and models.

diagnosis, segmental, *n* last stage of an osteopathic spinal examination in which the nature of the disorder is described at the level of the spinal segments.

diagnosis, tongue (tung' dī'·ə g·nō'·sis), *n* method of identifying signs of disease by examining the color and moistness of or markings and coating on a patient's tongue.

D

Diagnostic and Statistical Manual IV, *n* comprehensive listing of recognized diseases and conditions, updated and published annually. Also called *DSM-IV.*

diahuang (dä·hwäng), *n* Latin name: *Rehmannia glutinosa;* part used: roots; uses: fever reduction, rheumatism, diuretic; precautions: none known. Also called *rehmannia* and *Chinese foxglove.*

diapedesis (dī'·ə·pə·dē'·sis), *n* disorder in which red and white blood cells pass through the blood vessel walls that house them without injuring the vessels.

diaphoresis (dī'·ə·fə·rē'·sis), *n* excessive sweating; may be associated with exercise or with emotional, physical, and mental stress.

diaphoretic, *adj/n* a substance that produces or encourages perspiration.

diarrhea, *n* frequent loosened, watery stools, often accompanied by abdominal cramping and strong urge to move bowels.

diathermy (dī'·ə·thər·mē), *n* a treatment that uses pulsations of electrical energy to generate heat and enhances local recovery. The high energy pulsations of electrical energy are applied for shortened periods of time. See also disease, pelvic inflammatory.

diathesis (dī·a'·thə·sis), *n* **1.** genetic propensity toward a certain disease. **2.** configuration of a syndrome typical of a fundamental illness. See also constitution, psoric miasm, sycotic miasm, syphilitic miasm, terrain, and tubercular diathesis.

Dictamnus dasycarpus (dik'·tam·nəs dä'·sē·kär'·pəs), *n* part used: root bark; uses: digestive disorders, urogenital conditions, promotion of hair growth, impetigo, eczema, antipyretic, antiarthritic, skin inflammation, scabies, hepatitis, of menstrual disorders, uterine hemorrhage, thread fungus, relaxant, general health, diuretic, antispasmodic, hysteria, epilepsy, vermifugal, prevent pregnancy; precautions: can cause liver damage. Also called *bai xian pi* and *dense-fruit dittany.*

diet, ADA, *n* a regimented plan of eating and drinking recommended by the American Dietetic Association and American Diabetes Association. It is based on an exchange system for foods, which currently recognizes the following six groups of food: milk, fruits, vegetables, meats, breads, and fats. It emphasizes maintenance of an ideal weight while restricting the intake of calories.

diet, ama-reducing (ä·mə rē·dōō·sing dī'·et), *n* in Ayurveda, a light, easily digestible diet that allows the digestive system to function more efficiently and to burn off accumulated ama. See also ama.

diet, anthroposophic (an'·thrō·pə·sô'·fik dī'·ət), *n* a health diet popular in Europe that includes lactovegetarianism, sour milk products such as yogurt, and unrefined carbohydrates.

diet, Atkins, *n.pr* a dietary system developed by Robert Atkins, MD, that recommends eating high-protein foods that are dense in nutrients. Consuming certain nutritional supplements and refined or processed carbohydrates is discouraged.

diet, blood type–based, *n* a dietary system which recommends a diet based on the genotype of a person's blood type. The system comprises four dietary regimens and four programs of exercise based on the four ABO blood groups.

diet, Bristol, *n* anticancer diet that comprises soy and other beans, peas, and raw and partially cooked vegetables.

diet, Bristol Cancer Help Center, *n* anticancer diet of soy protein, raw, and partially-cooked vegetables eaten to enhance attitude and quality of life.

diet, Budwig's oil-protein, *n.pr* anticancer diet that comprises fruit and fruit juices with a mixture of flaxseed oil and curd cheese.

diet, caveman, *n* a food plan in which only natural, unprocessed foods— such as fruits, legumes, nuts, poultry, seafood, seeds, vegetables, and wild game—are eaten for five days to eliminate allergens and toxins from the body. Used to attain a neutral situation at which point suspected food allergens can be introduced and tested.

diet, diversified rotation, *n* a food plan in which only foods on an arranged, scheduled chart are eaten. Foods are arranged by their botanical classifications and are rotated to test suspected food allergens.

diet, elimination, *n* a food plan in which suspected food allergens are avoided for at least five days and then reintroduced individually and tested.

diet, Gerson, *n.pr* See therapy, Gerson.

diet, high-carbohydrate, high-fiber (HCF), *n.pr* a high-carbohydrate, high plant-fiber, nutritional plan that recommends root vegetables, legumes, and cereals and restricts consumption of simple sugars and fat.

diet, Kelley, *n.pr* anticancer therapy that includes a special diet and supplements, including enzymes and internal (enemas, irrigation) and external (sitz baths) cleansing.

diet, Kousmine, *n* anticancer diet comprising the "vital energy" foods, such as raw vegetables and wheat.

diet, living foods, *n* a dietary system that recommends fermented and fresh vegetables, wheatgrass juice, sprouted seeds, and fruits. Raw cheese or milk is permitted occasionally. Advocates also produce their own "seed cheese" or "seed milk" by grinding soaked nuts or rice. The reasoning primarily originates from the thought that cooking destroys several enzymes that are necessary for assimilation of nutrients and proper digestion. The system was developed by Ann Wigmore of the Hippocrates Institute in Boston.

diet, macrobiotic (ma'·krō·bī·ô'·tik dī'·ət), *n* designed to bring yin/yang energies into balance, the macrobiotic diet developed by Michio Kushi is part of a larger philosophy and whole-body regimen.

diet, McDougall, *n.pr* a dietary system developed by John McDougall that emphasizes low-fat, vegetarian whole foods. See also new four food

groups diet, reversal diet, and block integrative nutritional therapy.

diet, Mediterranean, *n* diet that comprises carbohydrates (50%–60%), fats (30%), and proteins (10%); derived from the eating habits of Mediterranean people and thought to lower rates of cardiovascular disease.

diet, modified high-carbohydrate, high-fiber (MHCF), *n.pr* a modification of the HCF diet with substitution of natural and unprocessed foods. Although the plan recommends avoiding foods with toxic effects and higher consumption of legumes, processed grains are limited, and fruit juices, skim milk, margarine, and fruits with low-fiber content are eliminated. See also diet, HCF.

diet, Moerman, *n.pr* anticancer lactovegetarian diet supplemented with eight essential substances: iodine; sulfur; iron; citric acid; and the vitamins A, B, C, and E.

diet, natural hygiene (na'·chə·rəl hī'·jēn dī'·et), *n* a dietary regimen that recommends a particular combination of foods thought to maximize efficiency of the digestive process. Specifically, vegetables and fruits are never consumed together. Foods rich in starch and proteins are also never eaten together. Sylvester Graham initially developed the diet in the early 1800s, but Harvey and Marilyn Diamond, authors of *Fit for Life*, have increased its popularity.

diet, new four food groups, *n* a dietary regimen that recommends foods derived from plants, specifically vegetables, grains, legumes, and fruits eliminating meat and dairy products. The system was proposed by the Physicians Committee for Responsible Medicine or PCRM.

diet, oligoantigenic (ä'·li·gō·an·ti·gen'·ik), *n* See diet, elimination.

diet, Ornish, *n* high fiber, low-fat diet combined with relaxation, exercise, and yoga. The Ornish diet has been shown to reverse heart disease and reduce diabetic insulin dependence.

diet, Oslo, *n* diet of reduced fat and increased fish intake. Has been used

D

to produce a decrease in insulin resistance.

diet, Pritikin, *n* primarily vegetarian, low-fat, high-fiber diet in conjunction with aerobic exercise that has shown positive results in the treatment of diabetes and heart disease.

diet, reversal, *n* a dietary regimen recommended by Dean Ornish in which fat and protein intake is very low while the intake of unprocessed carbohydrates is high. Adherents are recommended to consume nonfat yogurt, skim milk, and egg white as supplemental sources of protein. Along with other lifestyle changes, this system reverses the development of coronary heart disease and atherosclerosis within the body.

diet, rotation, *n* a food plan in which only foods on an arranged, scheduled chart are eaten. Foods are arranged by family classes and rotated to avoid suspected allergens or to allow the body to recover from known allergic reactions.

diet, Swank, *n.pr* a nutritional plan that recommends foods with low amounts of saturated fat; claimed to slow the progression of multiple sclerosis and lessen the number of recurrences. The plan recommends eating less than 10 grams of saturated fat per day, consuming 40–50 grams of polyunsaturated oils and eating fish at least three times a week. Practitioners are also advised to consume 1 teaspoon daily of cod liver oil and normal amounts of protein. See also multiple sclerosis.

diet, very-low-calorie, *n* high protein diet of 400 to 600 kcal/day. This diet, combined with behavior therapy, has been used to lower blood glucose levels and reduce hypoglycemia in patients with diabetes.

diet, waianae (wī'·ə·nī' dī'·ət), *n* a dietary regimen that recommends low fat and protein and high carbohydrate intake. Adherents are recommended to consume foods that are traditional to the Hawaiian culture, such as seaweed, fish, fruit, bread, and yams. Food is served either steamed or raw. Terry Shintani developed the system as a reaction to the increased rate of chronic medical conditions occurring among Westernized native Hawaiians.

diet, zone, *n* a dietary system that recommends consuming a diet that comprises 40% carbohydrates, 30% protein, and 30% fat. Foods with high levels of carbohydrates and fats, such as starches, grains and pastas, are restricted. Vegetables and fruits are emphasized as a source of carbohydrates. The amount of protein is limited to foods that have low levels of fat and are not thicker and bigger than the palm of a hand. Consumption of canola oil, olive oil, macadamia nuts, almonds, and avocados that are sources of monounsaturated fats is advised. The system was developed by Barry Sears. See also diet, Atkins.

dietary fiber, *n* nonnutritive residue and constituent of plant cell walls. Health benefits include enhanced digestion, eased stool passage, energy, anticancer effects, and enhanced colon function.

DIF, *n* deep inframtemporal fossa; an acupuncture treatment area located at a specific point along the mandible; used to treat trigeminal neuralgia.

diffuse noxious inhibitory control (DNIC), *n* one of several explanations for acupuncture's analgesic abilities. Inhibiting pain by using a counterirritant that stimulates an intricate network of impulses and responses within the nervous system.

diffusion (di·fyōō'·zhən), *n* the tendency of molecules to move as a gas or liquid to move from an area of higher concentration to one with lower concentration. The rate of movement depends on the size and weight of the molecules involved.

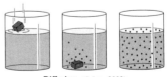

Diffusion. (Salvo, 2003)

digestive, *n* a substance that contributes to the process of digestion.

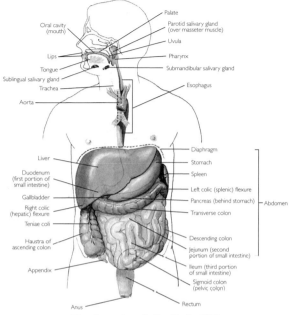

Digestive system. (LaFleur Brooks, 1994)

digestive enzymes (di·jes'·tiv en'·zīmz), *n.pl* proteins that catalyze reactions between other chemicals by reducing the energy required for the reactions.

dilation, *n* widening or opening of any orifice in the body.

dill, *n* Latin name: *Anethum graveolens,* parts used: buds, fruit, seeds; uses: antispasmodic, colic, gas; precautions: pregnancy, lactation, children, patients with fluid imbalances; can cause photodermatitis, alteration in sodium balance. Also called *dill seed, dillweed, garden dill,* and *dilly.*

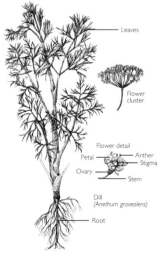

Dill. (Skidmore-Roth, 2004)

D

diluent (di·lōō'·wənt), *n* inert substance added to source material to thin it to the potency desired. Some common diluents are glycerin, isotonic sodium chloride, lactose, purified water, and ethanol.

dilute juice fast, *n* a food plan in which only juices diluted in mineral water or distilled water are ingested for several days to eliminate allergens and toxins. Used to attain a nonreactive state into which suspected food allergens can be introduced and tested.

dilution (di·lōō'·shən), *n* decreasing the concentration; for essential oils used in aromatherapy, the dilution range is between 1% and 5%.

dilutions, ultra-high, *n.pl* in homeopathy, solutions of substances that have been repeatedly agitated and diluted.

dimethyl sulfoxide (dī·me''·thəl səl·fôks'·īd), *n* an industrial solvent used as a treatment for interstitial cystitis; also used as an analgesic and antiinflammatory for muscle aches and arthritic conditions. Caution should be used in selecting high-quality dimethyl sulfoxide because any contaminants and toxins present in it are transported directly into the bloodstream.

dimethylaminoethanol (dī'·meth'·əl·ə·mē'·nō·e'·thə·nôl), *n* pharmacologic supplement, a precursor to acetylcholine, taken to stimulate the central nervous system. Contraindicated in patients with seizure conditions.

dincharya (dēn·chär''·yə), *n* in Ayurveda, time of the day. An important factor in determining an appropriate diet aimed at preventing formation and accumulation of ama. See also ama.

Dioscorea villosa, *n* See wild yam.

diosmin (dī'·ōs·mən), *n* a flavonoid pigment derived from citrus fruits or rosemary, used in combination with hesperidin (in a 9:1 ratio) to improve the tone of veins; normalize the permeability of capillaries; and treat vascular conditions such as hemorrhoids, chronic venous insufficiency,

and fragile capillaries. No precautions known. See also flavonoids and hesperidin.

diphtheria, *n* communicable disease caused by the bacterium *Cornyebacterium diphtheriae,* which releases an extremely damaging toxin to the central nervous system and heart. It also produces an adherent pseudomembrane lining to the throat that may interfere with eating and drinking. Treated by administration of diphtheria antitoxin, antibiotics, rest, and fluids.

Diplomate in Homeotherapeutics (dip'·lə·māt' in hō'·mē·ō·the'·rə·pyōō'·tiks), *n.pr* a designation granted to medical and osteopathic doctors who practice homeopathy by the American Board of Homeotherapeutics. To receive this certification, a homeopathic physician must present proof of clinical and didactic training, complete three years of practice in a clinical setting, and pass oral and written exams testing homeopathic knowledge. Also called *DHt.*

Diplomate of the Homeopathic Association of Naturopathic Physicians (dip'·lə·māt' əv thə hō'·mē·ō·pa''·thik ə·sō'·sē·ā'·shən əv na'·chə·rō·pa''·thik fə·zi''·shə nz), *n.pr* a designation awarded to naturopathic physicians who have received certification from the Homeopathic Association of Naturopathic Physicians. Those who receive this designation have become members of the Homeopathic Association of Naturopathic Physicians by completing training and passing written and oral exams that demonstrate their skill and aptitude in homeopathy. See Homeopathic Association of Naturopathic Physicians.

Dipteryx odorata, *n* See tonka bean.

direct adverse effects, *n.pl* unfavorable outcomes as a direct result of treatment. Includes toxic effects and side effects of various duration.

direct inhalation, *n* the targeting of an aromatherapy treatment to the nose of one patient.

direct mental interaction of living systems (DMILS), *n* **I.** the concept that two individuals can influence each other without direct contact or apparent communication. **2.** an experimental framework from parapsychology in which the interaction between two isolated subjects are investigated.

direct MFR, *n* an osteopathic technique for myofascial release in which a constant force is applied to a restrictive barrier until the tension is released.

direct suggestion, *n* a type of instruction phrased as a firm request that is used by therapists in hypnosis sessions.

directing, *n* a breathing technique in which the practitioner coaches various inhalation and exhalation exercises and patterns to the client.

direction of cure, *n* the cure for a disease proceeds in the opposite direction as that of the disease. Symptoms diminish from above downward, from major to minor organs, from psychological to corporeal, from the newest symptom to the oldest. Also called *Hering's law of cure.* See also law of cure, Hering's.

directions, *n.pl* in the Alexander technique, four specific reminders to keep in mind so one can develop and encourage one's own innate expansiveness and sense of poise. See also Alexander technique.

dirgha (dēr′·ghə), *n* See three-part yogic breath.

disability, *n* according to the World Health Organization (WHO) rehabilitation guidelines, impairment of an individual as it affects his or her role in life, such as an inability to work because of a health condition.

discretion (dis·kre′·shən), *n* in Native American medicine, avoiding the act of bragging or revealing a dream helper's identity. This is one way of circumventing a breach of taboo. See breach of taboo.

disease, *n* abnormal functioning within an organism often expressed by specific bodily symptoms. This term is more concrete than *illness,* which includes mental aspects as well.

disease affinity, *n* a homeopathic remedy's association with a certain illness or symptom.

disease entities, *n.pl* term used for illnesses to emphasize the concept that sickness is separate from the person suffering from it.

disease picture, *n* depiction of all disease-related symptoms in an individual.

disease process, *n* progression of the illness, both mental and physical symptoms involved.

disease(s), autoimmune **(ô·tō′·im·yōōn′ də·zēz′),** *n.pl* conditions caused by immune system dysfunction that results in cells and antibodies attacking one's own tissue.

disease, Adams-Stokes, *n.pr* disease marked by symptoms such as unanticipated and repeated black-out periods, and occasionally seizures due to an incomplete heart block.

disease, Addison's, *n.pr* condition in which the adrenal glands are compromised because of infection, autoimmunity, hemorrhage, or neoplasm. Symptoms include anorexia, skin bronzing, dehydration, and gastrointestinal disturbances, among others. Life-threatening form requires meticulous medical and self care.

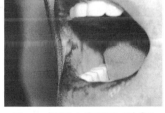

Disease, Addison's (Lawrence and Cox, 1993)

disease, Akureyi, *n.pr* condition marked by extreme and incapacitating fatigue, the cause of which is unknown. Accompanying symptoms can include pain as well as loss of sleep, concentration, and memory.

disease, Albers-Schonberg, *n.pr* osteopetrosis form in which bones display calcification that resemble marbles.

disease, Alexander's, *n.pr* variant of leukodystrophy characterized by an abnormal increase in brain size.

disease, Alzheimer's, *n.pr* brain disease in which the individual gradually loses mental acuity and may become helpless. Characterized by protein deposits and abnormal tissue growth in the cerebral cortex.

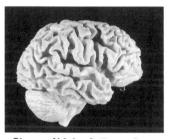

Disease, Alzheimer's (Kumar, Cotran, and Robbins, 1997)

disease, Anderson's, *n.pr* rare, fatal disease characterized by abnormal glycogen deposits in tissues caused by deficiency of the branching enzyme (alpha-1:4, alpha1:6 transglucosidase). Not detectable at birth, infants eventually develop liver cirrhosis or heart failure.

disease, celiac (sē'·lē·ak də·zēz'), *n* metabolic disorder present at birth marked by the inability to hydrolyze the peptides found in gluten. Dietary changes can ensure full recovery. Also called *celiac sprue, gluten-induced enteropathy,* and *nontropical sprue.*

disease, chronic obstructive airway, *n* a progressive lung disorder, caused by blockage of the airways, which inhibits the breathing process;

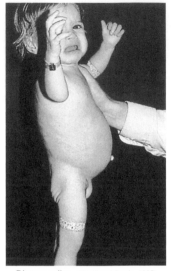

Disease, celiac. (Zitelli and Davis, 1997)

includes chronic bronchitis, chronic obstructive bronchitis, or emphysema, or combinations of these conditions.

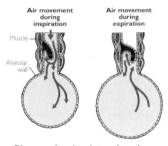

Disease, chronic obstructive airway. (Huether and McCance, 2000)

disease, coronary heart, *n* a condition resulting from poor blood supply to the heart attributable to narrowing of the coronary arteries caused by accumulation of plaque, which ultimately leads to deterioration of heart function. Also called *coronary artery disease.*

disease, Crohn's, *n* colon disease of unknown origin causing chronic inflammation, discomfort, frequent diarrhea, fever, nausea, abdominal pain, and weight loss. Also called *regional enteritis.*

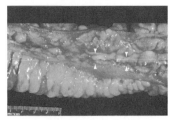

Disease, Crohn's. (Kumar, Cotran, and Robbins, 1997)

disease, Crouzon's, *n* hereditary illness characterized by malformed skull as well as ocular problems including divergent squint, exophthalmos, and optic atrophy.

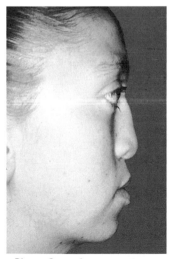

Disease, Crouzon's. (Carlson, 1999; A.R. Burdi, Ann Arbor, MI)

disease, degenerative joint, *n* a medical condition that mostly affects the elderly and is marked by erosion of the joints, cartilage loss, and changes in the subchondral bone. Symptoms include tenderness, swelling, stiffness, worsening pain after use of a particular joint and the decreased functionality of a joint. Several nutritional supplements, vitamins, drugs, botanical medicines, balanced diet, and exercise are used to lessen the symptoms. Also called *osteoarthritis* or *OA.*

disease, drug, *n* **1.** condition caused by the lengthy use of a medication. **2.** collection of symptoms experienced following a homeopathic treatment.

disease, fibrocystic breast (FBD) (fī'·brō·sis'·tik brest' di·zēz'), *n* common condition in premenopausal women characterized by the development of cysts of varying sizes in both breasts and the appearance of a nodular texture in the breasts. Symptoms include cydical tenderness and pain in the breast. Also called *cystic mastitis.*

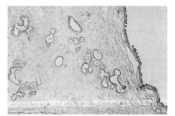

Disease, fibrocystic breast. (Kumar, Cotran, and Robbins, 1997; Dr. Kyle Molberg, Department of Pathology, University of Texas Southwestern Medical Center, Dallas, TX))

disease, gastroesophageal reflux (gas'·trō·ə·sä·fə·jē'·əl rē'·fləks di·zēz'), *n* condition in which the acidic contents of the stomach reflux up into the esophagus. Symptoms include heartburn, regurgitation, and pulmonary irregularities. May cause damage to the esophageal tissues. Causes may include hiatal hernia, alcohol, overeating, smoking, fatty foods, and caffeine. Also called *acid reflux, reflux,* or *reflux esophagitis.*

disease, heart, n any disorder that affects the heart's function.

disease, iatrogenic, n disorders caused by medical intervention or through exposure to healthcare facilities.

disease, Lou Gehrig's, n See amyotrophic lateral sclerosis.

disease, mixed connective tissue, n a systemic disease distinguished by a combination of symptoms that are present in a variety of rheumatic diseases like polymyositis, systemic lupus erythematosus, and scleroderma. Presence of antinuclear antibodies, muscle inflammation, swollen hands, nondeforming arthritis, and arthralgia are some indications. Corticosteroids are commonly prescribed for treatment.

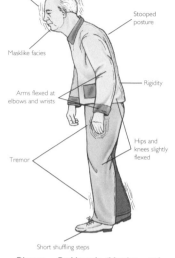

Tremor
Stooped posture
Masklike facies
Rigidity
Arms flexed at elbows and wrists
Hips and knees slightly flexed
Tremor
Short shuffling steps

Disease, Parkinson's. (Monahan and Neighbors, 1998)

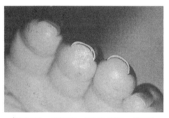

Disease, mixed connective tissue. (White, 1994)

disease, Parkinson's, n.pr neurological disorder characterized by progressive degeneration of neurons producing dopamine. Symptoms include tremors, movement difficulties, speech impediment and often dementia.

disease, pelvic inflammatory, n inflammation and infections affecting the pelvic region. Pain in the lower abdomen, tenderness in the adnexal region to palpitation and sensitivity to touch in the cervical region after movement are common symptoms.

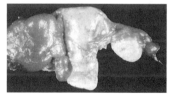

Disease, pelvic inflammatory (PID). (Kumar, Cotran, and Robbins, 1997)

disease, peptic ulcer, n ailment in which a sharply defined area or areas in the gastrointestinal mucous membranes deteriorate. Occurs most commonly in the stomach and duodenum.

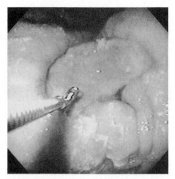

Disease, peptic ulcer. (Wilcox, 1995)

disease, periodontal, *n* inflammatory condition affecting the periodontium or gingival regions, progressing from gingivitis to periodontitis. It can be a manifestation of an underlying medical condition including leukemia, diabetes mellitus, vitamin deficiency, or anemia.

disease, psychosomatic, *n* any condition in which detrimental physiological changes are facilitated by psychological and affective stressors.

disease, somatopsychic (sō·ma'·tə·sī'·kik di·zēz'), *n* any condition in which detrimental psychological changes are facilitated by physical and physiological stressors.

dislocation, *n* forced separation and misalignment of bones in a joint cavity.

disorder, *n* an atypical physical or mental condition.

disorder, attention deficit/hyperactivity, *n* childhood disorder of the brain, marked by lack of intellectual and emotional focus and physical self-control. Generally diagnosed by age 7.

disorder, attention deficit, *n* syndrome characterized by short attention span, difficulty concentrating, and possibly hyperactivity. Affects children and adults; males affected 10 times more often than females. May be caused by various factors, such as genetic predisposition, injury, disease, excessive stimulation, and diet.

disorder, badahan (bä·dä·hän dis·ōr'·der), *n* in Tibetan medicine, a medical condition exhibited by the appearance of eyes that are hollow and a facial expression without emotion. During a careful interview, the mind may be revealed to be blunt and wandering. Feelings of prejudice, persecution, greediness, and self-pity may exist. The patient may feel that he or she does not have a purpose or direction in life. On a physical level, the patient may note fatigue and stiffness of joints. Speech patterns might be slurred and slow. Bodily movements and reactions may be subdued. Body odor may be rancid; breath may smell like tooth decay or periodontal disease.

disorder, bipolar, *n* mental illness marked by episodes of depression, mania, or a combination of the two.

disorder, breathing pattern, *n* a recurring or continuous irregularity in the breathing cycle.

disorder, chi (dzhē dis·ōr'·der), *n* in Tibetan medicine, a medical condition characterized by the appearance of eyes that are fearful, worried, and examining. During careful interview, a patient may describe sentimentalism, premonitions, telekinesis, and telepathy. On a physical level, the patient may report fatigue, uneasiness, and giddiness. Hyperactivity, disorganized speech patterns, and poor coordination may occur. Body odor may smell like acid; breath is sharp with a scent like rust. The tongue may turn dark brown or red, become rough, and form irregularly shaped cracks.

disorder, generalized anxiety, *n* psychologic disorder marked by vague anxiety symptoms such as sweating, irritability, tension, quivering, dizziness; considered a functional disorder.

disorder, obsessive-compulsive, *n* an anxiety condition distinguished by recurring and persisting thoughts, ideas and obsessive or compulsive feelings and/or behaviors. Also called *OCD*.

disorder, post–traumatic stress, *n* a condition in response to trauma or lasting stress. Identified by somatization of feelings and memories, flashbacks, sleep disturbances, depression, and anxiety.

disorder, rLung (lōōng dis·ōr'·der), *n* in Tibetan medicine, a blockage in the flow of vital energy resulting in emotional, mental, and physical illness.

disorder, schara (schä·rä dis·ōr'·der), *n* in Tibetan medicine, a medical condition exhibited by tense and aggressive behaviors. During a careful interview, the patient may reveal a contemptuous and arrogant mind, continually scheming and plotting activities. Perfectionist and workaholic tendencies may be indicated. On the physical level, the patient be warm or have excessive perspiration, increased thirst, a frequent need to urinate, nausea, and purging. Body language might reveal impatience with rushed speech patterns. Body odor may be pungent, and breath may smell putrid or similar to stomach acid. A yellow-green or yellow coat covers the tongue.

disorder, seasonal affective, n a chronic disorder in which symptoms fluctuate with the level of light exposure. In particular, persons affected are normal during the summer months while having feelings of depression during the winter months. Melatonin and light therapy are two common alternative treatments often prescribed. Also called *SAD*.

disorder, upper limb, n collective term for various conditions characterized by pain, stiffness, or immobility of the arms, hands, and/or shoulders.

disorders, autonomic dysregulation (ô'·tō·nô'·mik dis'·re·gyə·lā'·shən dis·ōr'·derz), *n.pl* in medical acupuncture, a loose categorization for medical conditions that are in a premorbid state. Indicated by bowel dysfunction, sleep disturbances, and anxiety.

disorders, immune dysregulation (i·myōōn' dis'·re·gyə·lā'·shən dis·ōr'·derz), *n.pl* in medical acupuncture, a loose categorization for medical conditions that are in a premorbid state. Indicated by recurring inflammatory and infectious conditions that do not have any specific immunodeficiency. Recurrent pharyngitis, sinusitis, gastroenteritis, bronchitis, and viral illnesses are examples.

disorders, pelvic floor, *n.pl* problems originating in the muscles of the pelvic floor, including but not limited to urinary incontinence, pain, constipation, pain during intercourse, muscle tension-related fecal incontinence, and so on; sometimes can be treated with biofeedback.

disorders, Type M (musculoskeletal) (mus'·kyə·lō·ske'·lə·təl), *n.pl* chiropractic classification for musculoskeletal ailments such as sacroiliac joint dysfunction, tension headache, facet syndrome, strain, and sprain injuries.

disorders, Type N (neurogenic) (ne·rō'je·nik), *n.pl* chiropractic classification for ailments with neurological origins, such as Bell's Palsy, migraine, nystagmus, and Tourette's syndrome.

disorders, Type O (organic, stress-related), *n.pl* chiropractic classification for ailments that result from stress and organic causes, such as bladder and bowel dysfunction, hypertension, infantile colic, headache, angina, asthma, and gastritis.

disper (dis'·per), *n* an emulsifier based on lecithin used to hold essential oils in a stable dispersion.

disposition, *n* inherent propensity to a particular condition. See also trait, terrain, and constitution.

distal (dis'·təl), *adj* pertaining to an area relatively farther from the center.

distancing, *n* in goal-directed visualization, a method of pulling back from a situation to gain an objective view.

distillation, *n* process of separating a liquid from a solid by vaporizing it; followed by condensation of the vapor; essential oils are isolated by successively evaporating and condensing the water that contains the plant material.

distillation, portable (pōr'·tə·bəl dis'·tə·lā'·shən), *n* distillation of essential oils using transportable equipment designed for producing small batches.

distinct meridians, *n.pl* in acupuncture, energy channels that travel directly from the body's surface to the organs. These channels serve as a conduit for the energy and nourishment produced by the organs to flow through the body.

distress, *n* harmful stress that tends to disturb the balance of body and mind and promotes ill health.

diterpenes (dī'·ter'·pēnz), *n.pl* naturally occurring organic compounds that comprise two monoterpene molecules; found in some essential oils; have antibacterial, antiviral, antifungal, and expectorant properties. See also monoterpene.

diterpenols (dī'·ter'·pə·nälz), *n.pl* chemical compounds found in some essential oils. Said to effect functions of the endocrine system because of their structural similarity to steroid compounds. See also terpenic alcohols.

diuresis, *n* increase in urine production and passage from the body occurring in conditions such as diabetes mellitus and diabetes insipidus.

diuretic (dī'·yə·re'·tik), *n* a substance that promotes urination.

diversified (di·ver'·sə·fīd), *n* commonly used chiropractic technique in which thrusts are applied to one or more vertebra after the patient's mobility is analyzed and a palpatory exam is performed.

diverticulosis, *n* colon disorder in which small, saclike herniations appear mainly in the sigmoid colon. Occurs in people over the age 50 and is linked to low-fiber diets; can lead to diverticulitis.

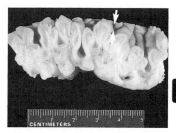

Diverticulosis. (Kumar, Cotran, and Robbins, 1997)

diverticulum, *n* sac-like herniation occurring in a muscular organ wall, such as the small intestine, stomach, or colon.

divine breath (di·vīn' breth'), *n* in Native American Medicine, the manifestation of the divine spirit in all living beings. Also called *life breath, ni,* and *nilch'i.*

DMILS, *n.pr* See direct mental interaction in living systems.

DMSO, *n.pr* See dimethyl sulfoxide.

DNCB, *n* dinitrochlorobenzene, a chemical used to develop color photographs; in alternative medicine, used to treat HIV by topical application.

DNIC, *n* See diffuse noxious inhibitory control.

D.O., *n* See Doctor of Osteopathy (or Osteopathic Medicine).

docere (dō'·se·rā), *n* "doctor as teacher." One of the three guiding principles of functional and natural medicine.

doctor, *n* professional title; used in the medical field if the individual holds an M.D. or D.O. degree.

Doctor of Medicine in Ayurveda, *n.pr* in India, M.D. degree awarded to an individual after completion of a graduate program in Ayurveda. To earn this degree, an individual must successfully complete a Bachelor of Ayurvedic Medicine and Surgery program, perform research, write a thesis based on the research subject, and pass a series of exams. In general, it takes nine or ten years after primary school for a practitioner to earn this degree. See Master of Ayurvedic Science.

Doctor of Osteopathy (or Osteopathic Medicine), *n* degree accredited by the American Osteopathic Association to physicians specially trained to perform osteopathic medicine including manipulations aimed at restoring normal nerve and blood supply thereby enabling self-healing.

doctor-patient relationship, *n* interaction between a physician and a patient.

doctrine of signatures, *n* a principle that assigns healing properties to plants on the basis of the association between their physical characteristics and those of the disease or the affected part of the body.

dog button, *n* Latin name: *Strychnos nux-vomica;* part used: dried seeds; uses: tonic, central nervous system stimulant, veterinary medicine; precautions: pregnancy, lactation, toxic in all but homeopathic doses. Also called *quaker button, poison nut,* and *semen strychnos.*

dong quai (dông kwī), *n* Latin name: *Angelica polymorphia* var. *sinesis;* part used: roots; uses: PMS, dysmenorrhea, menorrhagia, headaches, neuralgia, herpes, malaria, vitiligo, anemia; precautions: pregnancy, lactation, children; patients with breast, uterine, or ovarian cancer, bleeding conditions, inordinate periods, or acute illness, can cause nausea, bleeding, photosensitivity. Also called *Chinese angelica, dang gui, drykuei, tanggwi, tang-kuei, toki,* and *women's ginseng.* See also angelica.

dopamine (dō′·pə·mēn), *n* a neurochemical that supports fine motor activity, blood pressure, focus, inspiration, intuition, enthusiasm, and joy, among other functions.

dorsal (dōr′·səl), *adj* pertaining to the back of the body or the top of the foot.

dorsal respiratory group (dōr′·səl res′·pi·rə·tōr′·ē grōōp′), *n* the group of neurons located in the medulla oblongata, which generates the basic rhythm of breathing.

dosage (dō′·sij), *n* the frequency and quantity of remedy administered to a patient.

dose, *n* 1. a specific quantity of a therapeutic substance. 2. a specific amount of radiation received by an organism.

dose equivalent, *n* number used in radiation safety that is the product of the radiation dose absorbed by a tissue multiplied by a given quality factor specific to the type of radiation used. Expressed in sieverts or rems, dose equivalent is used to determine potential physical injury to the patient.

dose, carbohydrate challenge, *n* a measured quantity of lactulose or glucose taken as part of a breath test used to detect bacterial overgrowth in the small intestine. Bacteria are detected by increased hydrogen and methane in the breath resulting from fermentation of the carbohydrate administered.

dose, effective, *n* dose that produces sufficient or the best results.

dose, infinitesimal, *n* homeopathic remedy, the source material of which is diluted past the Avogadro's number and therefore is not likely to have the original remaining constituent. See also ultrahigh dilution.

dose, lethal, *n* in animal-based product testing, the amount of test product required for 50% of the test subjects to die.

dose, material, *n* a dosage with an assessable quantity of source material in it. Also called *ponderal dose* and *substantial dose.* See also concentration, dilution, infinitesimal dose, ultrahigh dilution, and ultramolecular dilution.

dose, maximum permissible, *n* according to the guidelines for radiation protection for persons working with x-rays or radioactive materials, the maximum ionizing radiation that can be received by a person. Also called *effective dose equivalent unit* or *MPD*.

dose, median effective, n in animal-based product testing, a determined dosage results in 50% of tested animals manifesting the intended effects.

dose, median lethal, n the amount of a substance that, when administered to a group of experimental animals, is expected to kill 50% of the population within a given time.

dose, median toxic, n the amount of a substance that is expected to produce toxic effects in 50% of the patients to whom it is administered.

dose, minimum, n in homeopathy, the highest dilution of a remedy that has curative properties without undesirable side effects elicited at higher concentrations.

dose, minimum lethal, n in relation to the body weight, the smallest amount of a substance that will kill an experimental animal. Also called *minimum fatal dose* or *MLD*.

dose, no-effect, n the largest amount of a substance that induces no effects in cells or organisms.

dose, safe, n the maximum dose of a medicinal substance that can be administered without producing deleterious side effects.

dose, single, n the theory of giving only one dosage at a time. Depending on the type of homeopathy, the dose could be later repeated, or different remedies could be given. Unicist homeopathy is founded on this concept. See also homeopathy, complex and homeopathy, pluralist.

dose, therapeutic, n the dose of a medicinal substance necessary to produce the desired ameliorative effects.

doses, ultra-low, n.pl amounts of medicinal substances that are a fraction of their normal concentration.

dose response curve, n the relationship between the dose level to an external stimulus or a drug and the response of an organism, often depicted graphically. See also law, Arndt-Schulz; dose-dependent reverse effect; and hormesis.

dose-dependent reverse effect, n the situation where one dosage of a remedy produces one effect and another dosage (usually lower) produces the opposite effect. See also antitaxic drug action; law, Arndt-Schulz; biphasic activity; hormesis; primary drug action; and secondary drug action.

doshas (dō′·shäs), n.pl in Ayurveda, the three fundamental principles formed by combination of two elements (mahabhutas) each and that form the basis of homeostasis. See also mahabhutas and tridosha.

Kapha season: Spring early summer (approx. March–June)
Kapha time: Approx. 6 a.m. (sunrise) to 10 a.m. and 6 p.m. to 10 p.m.
Kapha period in life cycle: Childhood

Pitta season: Midsummer–early autumn (approx. July–October)
Pitta time: Approx. 10 a.m. to 2 p.m. and 10 p.m. to 2 a.m.
Pitta period in life cycle: Adulthood

Vata season: Late autumn–winter (approx. October–February)
Vata time: Approx. 2 a.m. to 6 a.m. (sunrise) and 2 p.m. to 6 p.m.
Vata period in life cycle: Old age

Doshas. (Sharma and Clarke, 1998)

dosification (dō′·si·fə·kā′·shən), n in acupuncture, the use of varying quantities of stimulation, preferring low stimulation for treatment unless stronger stimulation is necessary. See also acupuncture, minimalist.

double-bind, n a hypnotic technique in which conflicting messages are communicated to the patient at the same time.

double-blind study, n experimental technique in clinical research in which neither the researcher nor the patient knows whether the treatment administered is considered inactive (placebo) or active (medicinal).

double bond, *n* a covalent bond in which two valence (outer) electrons are contributed by each participating atom. See also covalent bond.

double crush phenomenon, *n* according to which, an individual suffering from a nerve injury is at a higher risk for a second injury to the same nerve.

douches, *n.pl* water-based solutions intended for use on the skin or in a body cavity, sometimes containing herbal decoctions.

DPA, *n.pr* See acid, docosapentaenoic.

D-phenylalanine (dē-fē·nə·la'·lə· nēn), *n* the isomeric form of the amino acid phenylalanine, sometimes used to treat depression. Contraindicated in large doses for those taking antipsychotic medications or those with PKU. Also called *DL-phenylalanine.*

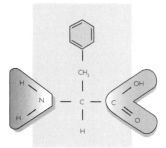

D-phenylalanine. (Mosby's Medical, Nursing & Allied Health Dictionary, 2002)

DPM, *n* **1.** doctor of podiatric medicine. **2.** diploma of psychological medicine.

drag, *n* tension between the stretch or pull of tissue and the tissue's resistance.

Dragon's Mouth, *n.pr* a Shiatsu technique in which the practitioner uses the same hand to simultaneously stabilize the limb being worked on and to apply pressure with the first knuckle of the index finger.

draping, *n* in massage, technique of

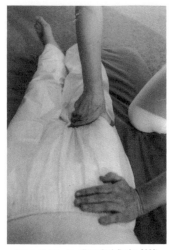

Dragon's Mouth. (Beresford-Cooke, 2003)

securely covering and uncovering parts of the body and moving the client.

drava (drä'·və), *adj* in Ayurveda, liquid as a guna, one of the qualities characterizing all substances. Its complement is sandra. See also gunas and sandra.

Drimia maritima, *n* See squill.

drug, *n* nonfood physical material that alters an organism's normal functioning by affecting physiologic processes. Preferred homeopathic terminology is *medicine* or *remedy* rather than *drug.*

drug abuse, *n* use of a drug, whether over the counter or prescription, for purposes other than those prescribed on the product label, often for recreational reasons.

drug action, *n* in homeopathy, consequence of the application of a homeopathic remedy in a living organism that is different from its potency at a biochemical level. See also autoregulation.

drug interactions, *n.pl* negative (occasionally positive) health consequences arising from the ways in which drugs, herbs, medications, and nutritional supplements interact with each other when taken concurrently. Such interactions arguably represent the largest risk when taking multiple medications and/or supplements.

drug picture, *n* a description of the symptoms resulting from a homeopathic remedy. These pictures can be found in the materia medica and result from provings when the remedy was given to healthy people. Also called *remedy picture.*

drug, nonsteroidal antiinflammatory (nôn'·ste'·roi·dəl an'·tī·in·fla'·mə·tōr·ē drug'), *n* a family of medications that reduce symptoms associated with inflammation, such as pain, swelling, and stiffness. It can also be used to treat other painful conditions like gout, tendonitis, bursitis, sprains, or menstrual cramps. Also called *NSAID.*

drugs, antiviral (an'·tē·vī'·rəl drugs'), *n.pl* a class of drugs used to combat illnesses, such as HIV, that are caused by viruses.

drugs, standardization of, *n* **1.** in pharmacology, the establishment of consistent parameters for a given drug's synthesis, composition, action, and toxicity. **2.** in homeopathy, the requirement that homeopathic remedy preparation be consistent with respect to content and manner of preparation.

drum circle, *n* a spiritual, communal, or therapeutic music experience in which participants join together in a circle with drums, move, dance using various percussion instruments, voices, and other devices. These circles are used to reduce stress, anxiety and blood pressure, to increase immune system function, and to create a sense of community.

Dryopteris filix-mas, *n* See male fern.

DSM-IV, *n.pr* See *Diagnostic and Statistical Manual IV.*

dual-energy x-ray absorptiometry, *n* diagnostic test used to determine bone density and to diagnose and monitor osteoporosis.

dual nervous system, *n* a communication system in the body that comprises the traditional nerve network and the older perineural network. It is postulated that the perineural system

plays a major role in wound healing and is activated by therapies, such as acupuncture.

Duboisia myoporoides, *n* See corkwood.

Duchenne's muscular dystrophy, *n* an X-linked recessive condition present at birth in which the muscles of the pelvis and legs waste away in a symmetric fashion. Appears in children between three to five years of age, with death occurring 10 to 15 years after the onset of symtoms. Also called *pseudohypertrophic muscular dystrophy.*

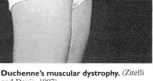

Duchenne's muscular dystrophy. (Zitelli and Davis, 1997)

Duke-UNC Health Profile, *n.pr* a validated questionnaire with 63 items that evaluates the health status of an adult with respect to general health. The four dimensions investigated are physical, emotional, and social functioning and symptom status.

Dupuytren contracture, *n.pr* a pathologic condition of the hand in which the fascia of the palm are shortened and thickened, thus resulting in fibrosis and deformities of the fingers.

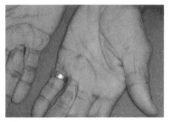

Dupuytren contracture. (Lemmi and Lemmi, 2000)

dural tube, *n* membrane that surrounds the spinal cord. The space between the dural tube and the spinal cord is filled with cerebrospinal fluid (CSF). See also cerebrospinal fluid.

duty of care, *n* the extent to which a healthcare provider must reasonably ensure that no harm comes to a patient under the provider's care.

dyers woad (dī'·erz wōd), *n* Latin name: *Isatis tinctoria* L.; parts used: leaves; uses: antiinflammatory, febrifuge, digestive, antiviral, skin inflammation, jaundice, dysentery, mumps, sore throat, laryngitis, scarlet fever; precautions: feeble patients. Also called *ban lang gen, bei ban lan gen, dyers weed, pan lan ken, pannamgeun,* or *woaddye plant.*

dynamical energy system, *n* the ordering of electromagnetic pulses according to their relative velocities.

dynamis (dī'·nə·mis), *n* word coined by Hahnemann to describe an organism's life force (i.e., prana, ch'i, etc.) See also bioenergetics, dynamisation, life force, potency, potency energy, vital force, and Wesen.

dynamisation (dī'·nə·mi·zā'·shən), *n* the way in which a homeopathic remedy becomes potent. The method may be either forceable trituration or serial dilution and succussion. Also called *potentization.* See also attenuation, plussing, and succussion.

dysaesthesia (dī'·as·thēs'·ē·ä), *n* a disagreeable, atypical sensation; maybe spontaneous or induced.

dysautonomia (dis'·ô'·tə·nə·mē'·ə), *n* in the three-dimensional chiropractic assessment model, dysfunction in the autonomic and sensory nervous systems resulting from incomplete development of the neurons. It is evaluated by taking skin temperature readings.

dysbiosis (dis·bē·ō'·sis), *n* an imbalance in the intestinal bacteria that precipitates changes in the normal activities of the gastrointestinal tract or vagina, possibly resulting in health problems. Also called *dys-symbiosis.*

dysentery, *n* intestinal inflammation, particularly in the colon caused by bacteria, chemical irritants, parasites, or protozoa. Symptoms include abdominal pain; tenesmus; and bloody, frequent stools.

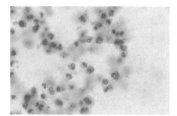

Dysentery. (Auerbach, 1995)

dysesthesia (dis'·es·the'·zhē·ə), *n* symptom of a neurologic disorder in which the patient experiences unusual sensations without any stimulation.

dyskinesia (dis·ki·nē'·zhē·ə), *n* difficulty of movement due to vertebral subluxation; one of the diagnostic components of the three-dimensional chiropractic assessment model. See also subluxation, vertebral.

dyslexia, *n* learning disability in which individuals with normal vision and intelligence have difficulty reading written language and spelling and writing words. Occurs more commonly in males; exact cause is unknown.

dysmenorrhea (dis·′men·ō·rē′·ə), *n* a female condition of painful, disabling menstrual cycles that interfere with daily activities; usually treated with oral medication.

dysostosis (dis·ə·stō′·sis), *n* condition marked by defective ossification, particularly the abnormal ossification of fetal cartilages.

dyspepsia, *n* digestive disturbance characterized by burping, heartburn, and gas.

dysphagia (dis·fā′·jē·ə), *n* inability to swallow. May be caused by physical obstruction or disease or psychological illness.

dysplasia (dis·plā′·zhə), *n* abnormal cell growth or growth patterns in tissues or organs.

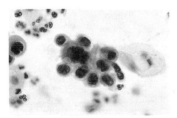

Dysplasia. (Damjanov and Linder, 1996)

dyspnea (disp′·nē·ə), *n* labored breathing may be due to vigorous exercise, anxiety, or heart and lung conditions.

dysponesis (dis′·pə·nē′·sis), *n* condition named by chiropractors to describe misdirected physical reactions to various stimuli (i.e., emotions, bodily sensations, environmental events, and thoughts) and the effects of these reactions throughout the body.

dysthymia (dis·thī′·mē·ə), *n* a chronic form of a depressive disorder, symptoms of which are not as severe as other types of depressive disorders. An individual must present with feelings of depression on a daily basis for a period of at least two years to be diagnosed with this condition. At least three of the following symptoms must also be indicated over the same period of time: fatigue, low self-esteem, pessimistic attitude, a noninterest in typical activities, decreased concentration, irritability, decreased productivity, and excessive guilt. A full criteria for diagnosis is available in the *Diagnostic and Statistical Manual of Mental Disorders* or *DSM-IV*. Counseling, lifestyle changes, nutritional supplements, and botanical medicines may lessen symptoms associated with this condition.

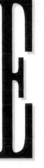

ear infections, *n.pl* infections of the ear usually triggered by bacteria or viruses, often occurring with infections of the throat or respiratory system. There are three types of ear infection: otitis externa (ear canal inflammation), otitis media (middle ear inflammation—the most common type), and otitis interna (inner ear inflammation rare). Serious complications that can arise from ear infections include loss of hearing, a burst eardrum, and mastoiditis, a rare infection of the mastoid process.

eardrops, *n.pl* oil-, water-, or alcohol-based treatment that is placed in the ear. Used to treat inflammation and infections of the ear canal.

early detection, *n* in complementary, conventional, and natural medicine, the act of discovering a disorder or disease before it has fully developed.

earth, *n* one of the five phases, or elements, in Chinese cosmological and medical theory, whose characteristic

E

manifestations include caring, nourishment, stability, support, and familial loyalty.

ease, *n* the feeling of freedom of motion within a joint or tissue. Also called *compliance* or *resilience.*

easing factors, *n.pl* movements or postures that ease the symptoms of a patient used to establish the nature, severity, and irritability of the condition.

EAV, *n.pr* See electroacupuncture according to Voll.

Ecabalium elaterium, *n* See cucumber, squirting.

eccentric (ek·sen'·trik), *n* muscle contraction that involves an increase in the length of the muscle.

eccyhmosis (eh·kē·mō'·sis), *n* evidence of broken blood vessels or capillaries that appear just under the surface of the skin. May appear as irregular blue spots or patches at the site of the injury.

up-hat, comb flower, coneflower, hedgehog, Indian head, Kansas snakeroot, Missouri snakeroot, purple coneflower, red sunflower, rudbeckia, Sampson root, scurvy root, or *snakeroot.*

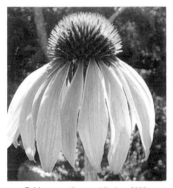

Echinacea. (Scott and Barlow, 2003)

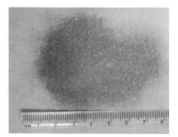

Eccyhmosis. (Lemmi and Lemmi, 2000)

ECG, *n.pr* See electrocardiography.

echinacea (e'·ki·nā'·shə), *n* Latin names: *Echinacea angustifolia, Echinacea pallida, Echinacea purpurea;* parts used: rhizome, roots, flowers, leaves; uses: stimulates immune system; promotes healing; treats bruises, burns, antiinfective; precautions: children, pregnancy, lactation; patients with autoimmune disorders. Also called *American cone flower, black sampson, black susans, cock-*

echo pattern, *n* a pattern of recurring illness resulting from unresolved imbalances in the patient's diet, energy, and stress levels.

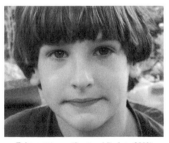

Echo pattern. (Scott and Barlow, 2003)

echocardiography (eh'·kō·kar'·dē·ô'·grə·fē), *n* diagnostic heart examination that utilizes sound wave technology to noninvasively determine the condition of the organ.

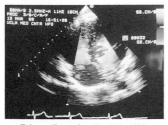

Echocardiography. (Canobbio, 1990)

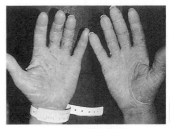

Eczema. (Hill, 1994)

E

often an indication of other health problems.

eclecticism (i·klek'·tə·si'·zəm), *n* the use of multiple approaches in alternative medicine selected and applied according to patient need.

Eclipta alba, *n* See bhangra.

ecology of mind, *n* a phrase coined by anthropologist Gregory Bateson to describe culture as a mutually inter-dependent world wherein individual relationships shape socially shared meanings while these collective meanings simultaneously inform the individuals' understandings of their actions.

ectomorph, *n* one of the three somatotypes described by W.H. Sheldon, characterized by a linear, thin, delicate body with small bone and muscle structure and mass. See also somatotype.

ectomorphy, *n* according to the Heath-Carter model of somatotypology, this body type is characterized by relative thinness and linearity. See also Heath-Carter somatotype.

ectopic (ek·tä'·pik), *n* located in an atypical or unusual place, usually outside its normal location.

eczema, *n* a skin condition character-ized by irritated, dry, and itchy skin. Although usually triggered by an external agent, internal conditions such as poor nutrition, digestion, and circulation; excessive mucus; food allergies; stress; and environmental toxins contribute to eczema.

edema, *n* abnormally high fluid accu-mulation in the interstitial tissues;

Edema. (Christiansen and Grzybowski, 1993)

edetate (e'·də·tāt), *n* Scientific name $C_{10}H_{14}N_2Na_2O_8 \cdot 2H_2O$ of EDTA; uses: treats cardiovascular disease, hypercalcemia, pathologic calcifica-tion; precautions: can cause renal tubular necrosis, acute renal failure, acute hypocalcemia, tetany, cardiac arrhythmias, bone marrow depres-sion, vasculitis, and exfoliative der-matitis. Also called *disodium edetate.*

EDR, *n* electrodermal response; a skin conductance measurement indi-cating the general level of automatic —or involuntary—arousal. See also biofeedback.

EFAs, *n.pl* See essential fatty acids.

effleurage (ef·fler'·aj), *n* a mild massage technique; consists of super-ficial manual movements moving away from the heart to encourage relaxation as well as deep manual movements toward the heart to aid circulation.

effusion, *n* flow of fluid (i.e., blood) into a body cavity; can be an indication of congestive heart disease.

EIA, *n* exercise-induced asthma; a breathing disorder characterized by fits of heavy or irregular breathing, wheezing, coughing, and gasping, which is brought on by physical exertion.

Eighty Percent Rule, *n.pr* the principle that asserts that in an optimal clinical environment, positive outcomes will be generally produced in 70% to 90% of the individuals undergoing any particular treatment.

e jiao (ə jē·ōw), *n* Latin names: *Gelatinum corii asini, Colla corii asini;* part used: gelatin; uses: tonify and enrich the blood; dizziness, palpitation, sallow complexion, myoatrophy, insomnia, myasthenia, stop bleeding, hematemesis, hemoptysis, apostaxis, hemafecia, hematuria, metrostaxis, metrorrhagia, flushed tongue, rapid and thready pulse, chronic cough due to irritant cough or pulmonary tuberculosis, moisten lungs; precautions: weak digestion associated with poor appetite, diarrhea, and vomiting. Also called *donkey hide glue* and *ass hide glue.*

EKG, *n* See electrocardiography.

el don (el dōn'), *n* in Curanderismo, the Mexican healing system, a gift of healing, the inherent ability of a healer to practice his or her work, particularly in the supernatural realm.

elastic deformation, *n* reversible deformation of tissue.

elasticity, *n* the ability of a tissue that has been strained or otherwise deformed to return to its original shape.

elder healers, *n* according to Native American culture, a healing source found in natural elements, such as water, earth, sun, and mountains. Patients who find harmony with these natural elements are said to undergo spontaneous healing or discover insightful resolutions to problems in their lives.

elderberry, *n* Latin names: *Sambucus nigra, Sambucus canadensis;* parts used: buds, fruit; uses: common cold, toothaches, headaches, diaphoresis, hay fever, sinus infections, epidermal irritations, lacerations, liver disorders, inflammation; precautions: pregnancy, lactation; bark and leaves are poisonous; can cause nausea, cyanide poisoning. Also called *black elder, boretree, bountry, common elder, ellhorn, European elder,* and *sweet elder.*

elecampane, *n* Latin name: *Inula helenium;* parts used: rhizomes (dried, fresh), roots; uses: antimicrobial, relaxant, expectorant, antiseptic, anthelmintic, appetite stimulant, digestive aid, diuretic, coughs, pertussis, colds, bronchitis, asthma; precautions: pregnancy, lactation, children younger than age 12; can cause paralysis (large amounts), mucous membrane irritation, nausea, diarrhea, stomach spasms, contact dermatitis. Also called *aunee, elfdock, horseheal, horse-elder, scabwort, velvet dock,* and *wild sunflower.*

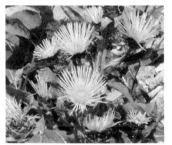

Elecampane. (Scott and Barlow, 2003)

elective affinity, *n* part of the body where a homeopathic remedy is most effective. See also disease affinity, organ affinity, and tissue affinity.

electroacupuncture (EA), *n* process in which acupuncture needles charged with electrical currents are inserted into specific meridian points to stimulate the sites and facilitate healing. See also acupuncture.

electroacupuncture by Voll, *n.pr* method of diagnosis and therapy developed by Dr. Reinhold Voll in which the conductance of electricity across acupuncture points is used to diagnose the clinical and energetic condition of internal organs. Also called *EAV*.

electrobiology, *n* the study of an organism's electrical phenomena.

electrocardiogram (ə·lek'·trō·kär'·dē·ə·gram'), *n* recording of the electrical activity of the heart. Often used to identify heart problems; routinely performed in patients complaining of chest pain to rule out heart disease. Also called *EKG*.

electrocardiography (eh·lek'·trō·kar'·dē·ô'·grə·fē), *n* the recording and graphing of the heart's electrical activity.

electrochemical treatment (ə·lek·trō·ke·mi·kəl trēt·mənt), *n* cancer treatment involving insertion of platinum electrodes directly into tumors and providing a constant low voltage for up to several hours at a time.

electrodermal augmentation (EDA), *n* skin resistance measurements used experimentally to determine the validity of direct mental interaction with living systems (DMILS). See also direct mental interaction in living systems.

electrodermal response (i·lek'·trō·der'·məl rə·spôns'), *n* technique by which sensors monitor the skin's electrical resistance to treat anxiety disorders, chronic pain, hyperhidrosis, and stress. Also called *electrodermal activity therapy*.

electrodermal response biofeedback, *n* process of biofeedback where sensors monitor and feedback skin conductance in order to treat anxiety disorders, chronic pain, hyperhidrosis, and stress. Also called *electrodermal activity therapy*.

electroencephalographic normalization (ə·lek'·trō·en·se'·fə·lō·gra'·fik nōr'·mə·lī·zā'·shən), *n* the normalization of electroencephalogram (EEG) readings through internal (self-induced) or external entrainment. Has been used to treat depression and anxiety.

electroencephalography (ə·lek'·trō·en·se'·fə·lô'·grə·fē), *n* technique used to record the distinct patterns of electrical impulses emitted by brain cells through use of electrodes placed on the scalp. Useful in diagnosis of epilepsy, tumors, and infections.

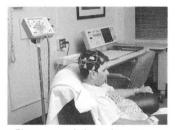

Electroencephalography. (Chipps, Clanin, and Campbell, 1992)

electrolysis (i·lek·trô'·lə·sis), *n* means by which electrical energy is conducted through electrodes into a substance (molten or in solution), thus causing a chemical change in the substance.

electrolytes (ē·lek'·trō·līts'), *n.pl* the ionized salts present in body fluids that play an important role in functioning of the human body. Electrolyte levels in blood plasma and urine are often used as diagnostic tools.

Normal electrolyte content of body fluids*

	Extracellular		
Electrolytes (anions and cations)	Intravascular (mEq/L)	Interstitial (mEq/L)	Intracellular (mEq/L)
Sodium (Na$^+$)	142	146	15
Potassium (K$^+$)	5	5	150
Calcium (Ca^{++})	5	3	2
Magnesium (Mg^{++})	2	1	27
Chloride (Cl$^-$)	102	114	1
Bicarbonate (HCO$_3^-$)	27	30	10
Protein (Prot$^-$)	16	1	63
Phosphate (HPO$_4^=$)	2	2	100
Sulfate (SO$_4^=$)	1	1	20
Organic acids	5	8	0

From Phipps WJ, Sands JK, Marek JF: *Medical-surgical nursing: concepts and clinical practice*, ed 6, St. Louis, 1999, Mosby.
*Note that the electrolyte level of the intravascular and interstitial fluids (extracellular) is approximately the same and that sodium and chloride contents are markedly higher in these fluids, whereas potassium, phosphate, and protein contents are markedly higher in intracellular fluid.

Electrolytes. (Phipps, Sands, and Marek, 1999)

electromagnetic bioinformation system (i·lek'·trō·mag·ne'·tik bī'·ō·in·fer·mā'·shən), *n* system that encompasses perineural and fascial conduction throughout a person's body plus static electricity on the surface. It also includes ionic migration in the interstitial fluid between the acupuncture needles and as currents of injury at the insertion site of the acupuncture needles.

electromagnetic field (EMF), *n* three-dimensional areas that represent the mutual interaction of magnetic and electric forces.

electromagnetic pollution, *n* electromagnetic radiation which has a negative effect on the health of living organisms.

electromagnetic spectrum (ə·lek'·trō·mag·ne'·tik spek'·trəm), *n* the entire range of electromagnetic radiation that extends from the longest (radio waves) to the shortest (gamma radiation) wavelengths.

electromagnetism (i·lek'·trō·mag'·nə·ti·zəm), *n* one of nature's four forces; the electromagnetic force is pervasive, effectual at subatomic distances (the arena where weak and strong nuclear forces are of exceptionally short range) and at astronomical distances (the arena where gravitational forces are significant).

electromotive force, *n* the ability of electrical energy to perform work, measured in volts or joules per coulomb.

electromyographic biofeedback (i·lek'·trō·mī'·ō·gra'·fik bī'·ō·fēd'·bak), *n* therapy in which sensors are placed on the skin in order to detect tension-related electrical activity. A biofeedback instrument translates the electrical activity levels into a description of the varying degrees of muscle tension. Often used to treat tension headaches.

electromyography (ə·lek'·trō·mī'·ô'·grə·fē), *n* a technique used to measure and record the electrical activity in muscles. Used to diagnose neuromuscular disorders and in biofeedback. Also called *EMG*.

electron (i·lek'·trôn), *n* the negatively charged particle that orbits around the nucleus of an atom.

electronic configuration (i·lek·trôn'·ik kən·fig'·yə·rā'·shən), *n* arrangement of electrons within an atom.

electroosmosis (i·lek'·trō·ôz·mō'·sis), *n* process by which a conducting liquid moves through a porous membrane because of a difference in potential between the two electrodes on opposite sides of the membrane.

electrophoresis (i·lek'·trō·fə·rē'·sis), *n* method used to separate particles, such as DNA or proteins, in which an electric current is passed through the medium and the separation of the molecules depends on the rate at which they travel towards the electrode based on their electrical charge.

electropollution, *n* electromagnetic radiation that might contribute to health problems.

electroporation (i·lek'·trō·pə·rā'·shən), *n* technique by which cell membranes are made permeable by rapid pulses of high-voltage current. Has been used to treat cancers.

electrovalency (i·lek'·trō·vā'·lən·sē), *n* the numerical value used for determining the combining power of an atom that equals the number of electrons an atom could lose or gain when forming ions or bonds.

element, *n* any substance that cannot be reduced into a less complex substance, all atoms of which are defined as having the same number of protons.

elemental mercury vapor, *n* a form of mercury released from dental fillings and absorbed through the lungs into tissues.

Elettaria cardamomum, n See cardamom.

eleuthereo, *n* See ginseng, Siberian.

Eleutherococcus, n See ginseng, Siberian.

Eleutherococcus senticosus, n See ginseng, Siberian.

ELISA, *n.pr* See enzyme-linked immunosorbent assay.

ELISA/ACT, *n.pr* a diagnostic test for identifying reactive substances that provoke delayed hypersensitivity of the immune system. A one-step method that uses both lymphocyte blastogenesis and enzyme amplification.

elm bark, *n* See slippery elm.

Elymus repens, n See couchgrass.

EM microcurrent device (ē·em mī'·krō·ker'·ent di·vīs'), *n* machine used to apply electromagnetic cur-

rents to the body in order to target disease. Used for osteoarthritis, bone repair, wound healing, and nerve stimulation. Used in acupuncture by applying currents to acupuncture points.

embedded suggestion, *n* during hypnosis, a more casual type of instruction couched in vague, flexible terms consistent with the patient's natural personality and inclinations, which nonetheless encourage the patient to act on the issue at hand.

Embelia ribes, n See viranga.

embolism, *n* condition in which a foreign object, such as gas, tissue, blood clots, air, small tumor, etc., becomes wedged in a blood vessel.

embrocations, *n.pl* alcohol-based treatments rubbed into the skin for purposes of analgesia or as a rubefacient.

embrujada (em·brōō·hä'·də), *n* according to Curanderismo, the Mexican folk healing system, sorcery involving participation of demonic spirits to inflict sickness on an individual.

embrujados (em·brōō·hä'·dōs), *n.pl* in Curanderismo, the Mexican healing system, individuals often believed to be hexed or bewitched.

embryo, *n* the fertilized ovum, while in its primary developmental stage, two to eight weeks after implantation in the mother's womb.

embryological approach (em'·brē·ə·lô'·ji·kəl ə·prōch'), *n* in osteopathic medicine, an approach compiled by James Jealous, DO, that is based upon the later writings of WG Sutherland, DO, the founder of cranial osteopathy. As part of this approach, the natural healing strength of the breath of life is emphasized. The functions of the body are thought to be structured in a relationship to this vital force of organization. The use of this approach has practical implications for the methods by which diagnostic and therapeutic approaches are performed.

emergency, *n* life-threatening situation requiring immediate medical attention.

EMF, *n* See electromotive force.

EMG, *n* electromyography; test that measures the response of a muscle to nervous stimulation.

-emia, -aemia, *suf* suffix that means *blood condition.*

emmenagogic, *adj* encouraging menstrual flow.

emmenagogue (i·men'·ə·gôg'), *n* a substance that promotes the flow of menstrual blood.

emotional body, *n* See emotional field.

emotional field, *n* in energy medicine, one of the ethereal layers associated with conceptualization, thought, rationalization, and event interpretation. Because the physical and emotional fields are interconnected, emotions influence physical well-being. See also physical level.

emotional level, *n* See emotional field.

emotional strength, *n* emotional stability and resiliency, characterized by assertiveness, caring, coping, and stress-management skills.

empacho (em·pä'·chō), *n* an ethnomedical condition common to Latin America in which the bowel or stomach is thought to be blocked by saliva, soft food such as chewing gum, or hard-to-digest foods like popcorn hulls. Cures consist of massage, popping the back, purgative herbal teas, and occasionally dangerous treatments with heavy metals such as lead or mercury. Also called *tripida.*

empiric soul (em·pir'·ik sōl'), *n* concept in Tibetan medicine; comprises the attributes of the mind, including memory, ego, intellect, emotions, and the five senses. The mind is the most essential element because it is responsible for processing the information provided by the sense organs that leads to understanding. It is believed that a properly functioning empiric soul is important for spiritual development.

empirical formula (em·pi'·rə·kəl fōr'·myōō·lə), *n* the simplest whole-number formula used to express the composition of a chemical compound.

empiricism, *n* philosophical school in which theories must be based upon repeatable observations. Modern science has empiricism as its philosophical foundation.

emulsify, *v* to distribute and suspend small globules of fat in water.

enantiomers (i·nan'·tē·ə·merz), *n.pl* molecules that are nonsuperimposable mirror images of one another resulting from the chirality exhibited by organic compounds (containing an asymmetrical carbon); enantiomers differ in their ability to rotate plane-polarized light. Also called *enantiomorphs.* See also chirality.

encircling (en·ser'·kə·ling), *n* a term used to describe the "loose-tight" interrelationship between some body structures that may be the cause of or affected by breathing dysfunction. Alternatively referred to as *crossover, spiral,* or *wrap-around.*

endangerment site, *n* any part of the body—including the kidney area where veins, arteries, and/or nerves are close to the surface of the skin—unprotected by connective skeletal tissue or muscle.

endemic, *n* the occurrence of certain diseases as they relate to a population or geographic area.

end-feel, *n* the restricted motion felt upon approaching an anatomic or physiologic barrier. See also barrier, anatomic and barrier, physiologic.

end-gaining, *n* in the Alexander technique, the quick expenditure of energy to achieve an end, rather than focusing on the means to achieve the end, which is called the "means whereby." See also technique, Alexander.

endocrine glands (en'·dō·krin glandz'), *n.pl* ductless glands of the endocrine system that secrete hormones directly into the bloodstream.

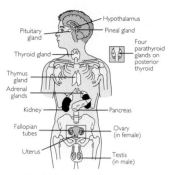

Endocrine glands. (Salvo, 2003)

endocrine system, *n* the group of tissues, organs, and glands within the human body that produce hormones to regulate body functions and processes. Includes small areas of cells in the heart, stomach, kidneys, and small intestines; the hypothalamus, pancreas, ovaries, and testes; and the pituitary, thyroid, parathyroid, adrenal, pineal, and thymus glands.

endogenous **(en·dô′·jə·nəs),** *adj* produced internally; made by the body.

endogenous fields, *n.pl* electromagnetic radiation that is emitted from the human body.

endometrial, *n* relating to the endometrium or cavity of the uterus.

endomorph, *n* one of the three somatotypes described by WH Sheldon, characterized by a round, smoothly contoured, soft body with the body mass concentrated in the abdomen and chest. See also somatotype.

endomorphy, *n* according to the Heath-Carter model of somatotypology, this body type is characterized by relative fatness. See also Heath-Carter somatotype.

endorphin-dependent system (en·dôr′·fin-də·pen′·dənt sis′·təm), *n* in acupuncture, one model system of activating the body's endogenous opioid peptide system and influencing the body's system of regulating pain by using low-frequency (2–4 Hz)/high-intensity electrical stimulation of needles. The onset of the analgesic response is often slow, generalized through the body, and it increases on succeeding stimulations.

endorphins, *n.pl* polypeptides produced in the body that bind the neuroreceptors in brain and act on the central and peripheral nervous system to alleviate pain.

endoscope, *n* an illuminated instrument that is used to investigate the interior of the intestinal lining via the mouth.

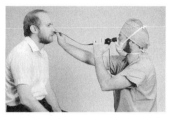

Endoscope. (Bingham, Hawke, and Kwok, 1992)

endotoxin, *n* toxin present in the cell walls of bacteria that is released after the bacteria has died. May cause chills, fever, leukopenia, and shock depending on the bacterial species and the health of the infected person.

end-tidal CO$_2$, *n* the level of carbon dioxide in the air exhaled from the body, the normal values of which are 4% to 6%; that is equivalent to 35 to 45 mm Hg.

endurance strategy, *n* an exercise method that uses extended periods of muscle activity with little or no resistance resulting in extended ability to work.

enduring improvement (in·dur′·ing im·prōōv·mənt), *n* in acupuncture, the desired objective of cumulative therapy sessions in which the patient is able to attain a higher level of function, such as regressed symptoms, reduced medications, or improved function. Typically, the full level of response can be estimated after six or eight visits. However, to attain enduring improvement, a full schedule of 12 sessions is often necessary.

energetic component, *n* encompasses six energy systems in and around the body, including acoustic, thermal, elastic, electromagnetic, photonic, and gravitational; practitioners employ avenues of intuition, balancing, and sensing to harness these elements and bring the body toward homeostasis.

energetic view, *n* paradigm that works on assumption that human beings exist in an interdependent relationship with energy forces in and around the universe. Therapies focus on maintaining an unimpeded flow between the client and universal energies to sustain equilibrium.

energizing, *adj* giving energy to; revitalizing; rejuvenating.

energy, *n* the capability to do work or produce an effect.

energy exchange, *n* in energy medicine, the relation between two human (usually practitioner and patient) fields of energy. Also called *transfer.*

energy field, *n* any force that can do work or produce an effect at a distance.

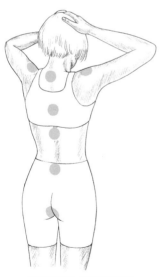

Energy field. (Chaitow, 2003)

energy psychology, *n* a treatment approach that combines a wide range of behavioral psychology theory with concepts informed by bioenergy research and perspectives.

energy psychotherapy, *n* discipline which holds that the causes of negative emotions can be traced to disruptions in the energy system of the human body.

energy scanning, *n* in traditional Chinese Medicine and energy medicine, a diagnostic tool in which the practitioner passes his or her hands over the client's body in order to scan, see, and interpret the patient's aura.

energy shielding, *n* creation of a safe haven in which one's inner peace and energies—psychic and emotional— are protected using focused breathing and visualization.

energy, cold, *n* an energetic style characterized by low metabolism, passive behavior, pale complexion, dislike of cold weather, and finicky eating.

energy, healing, *n* energy that has a beneficial effect on the health of an organism.

energy, hot, *n* an energetic style characterized by high metabolism, active behavior, red complexion, large appetite and thirst, dislike of hot weather, restlessness, light sleep, heavy sweating, and irritability.

energy, muscle, *n* an osteopathic treatment in which the patient's muscular force is used in cooperation with the motions performed by the physician.

energy, orgone (ōr·gōn en´·er·gē), *n* an intelligent, primordial energy that permeates all living things and the biosphere, as described by psychiatrist Wilhelm Reich.

energy, pulsed muscle, *n* therapeutic technique that uses tiny, rapid resisted contractions at the movement barrier. Effects include mechanical pumping, postisometric relaxation (PIR), and reciprocal inhibition (RI). See also postisometric relaxation and reciprocal inhibition.

energy, state of, *n* the quality of a patient's vitality as indicated through various signs.

energy, subtle, n the modern term for *vital energy* or the substance which permeates the environment and all living things.

energy, vibrating (**vī′·brā·ting en′· er·jē**), n oscillating unseen system of power or energy believed to be derived from sources inside and outside the human body. In many healing models, it is believed that these waves of power can be altered or manipulated to bring about healing. See also absent healing, laying-on-hands healing, and SHEN therapy.

energy, vital, n in homeopathy, the energy that imbues the body and mind, which is the ultimate focus of homeopathic treatment. Also called *vital spirit.*

energy cyst release, n a hands-on craniosacral therapy technique used to remove obstructive or disruptive energy from the body. See also therapy, craniosacral.

energy work, n techniques originating from ancient traditions and recent discoveries that are used to manipulate the bioenergy of the patient with the goal of restoring harmony or removing blockages from within the body. See also qi gong, reiki, qi, and prana.

energy-functional level, n in acupuncture, a disturbance that involves the equilibrium between the metabolic and energetic activities of an organ and the bodily region it influences. This especially includes the psychoemotional correlations with an organ.

enfleurage (**ôn′·flə·räj**), n a labor-intensive method for extracting essential oils from plant material in which glass plates coated with thin layers of fat are used over which plant material is spread in layers so that the essential oil is absorbed into the fat. The saturated fat is washed with hexane to dissolve the essential oil.

enkephalins, n.pl either of the two pentapeptides produced in the body that bind neuroreceptors in brain to alleviate pain.

entelechy (**en·te′·lə·kē**), n the fulfillment of all possible capabilities in a biological system. Homeopathic remedies are believed to encourage entelechy in human beings.

enteric-coated (**en·ter′·ik-kō′·ted**), adj covered with a protective layer (as in pills or tablets) so as to pass through the stomach unaltered until it reaches the intestinal tract.

enteritis, n small intestine inflammation affecting the mucosal lining; may stem from viral, bacterial, inflammatory, and functional causes.

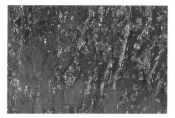

Enteritis. (Damjanov, 2000)

enthesitis (**en·thə·si′·tis**), n condition characterized by recurring, concentrated stress at points of muscle insertion that leads to inflammation and possible calcification and fibrosis.

entrainment (**en·trān′·mənt**), n rhythmic synchronization of two or more beats.

entrapment, n pathologic constriction on a vessel or nerve by swollen or hypertonic soft tissue and/or bone.

entropy (**en′·trə·pē**), n the propensity of matter and energy in a closed system to degrade into an equilibrium of uniform inertness and disorder. The apparent suspension of entropy in animate systems is used to support the philosophy of vitalism.

enuresis, n inability to hold one's urine.

envidia (**ān·vē·dē′·ə**), n according to Curanderismo, the Mexican-American healing system, sickness believed to be caused by jealousy.

environmental contingencies (**en· vī′·rən·men′·təl kən·tin′·jən·sēz**), n.pl in behavioral medicine, associations that exist between a particular behavior and a consequence. These associations can be adapted to encourage or discourage certain behaviors.

environmental poisons (en·vī'·rən·men'·təl poi'·zənz), *n* disease-causing toxins in water, air, and food.

environmentally triggered illnesses, *n.pl* illnesses resulting from exposure to external stressors that compromise biologic functions. Exposure may be low-grade and cumulative or severe and acute; includes multiple factors. Also called *ETI*.

envoy ingredient (ôn'·voi in·grē'·dē·ənt), *n* one of the four components in a typical Chinese herbal formula; used to harmonize all the other ingredients and to convey them to the specific body parts that they are to treat. See also chief ingredient, deputy ingredient, and assistant ingredient.

enzyme (en'·zīm), *n* protein that acts as a catalyst during chemical reactions.

enzyme-linked immunosorbent assay (en'·zīm-linkd' im'·myun·ō·sor'·bənt a'·say), *n* technique used to identify particular antibodies or antigens using enzyme-labeled immunoreactants. Reaction products are recorded by photometry or fluorometry. Commonly used to diagnose HIV infections.

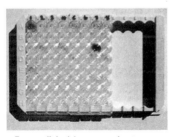

Enzyme-linked immunosorbent assay. (Hart and Broadhead, 1992)

eosinophils (ē'·ō·si·nə·filz'), *n.pl* white blood cells of the granulocyte type that have rough, round granules of cytoplasm that stain with eosin.

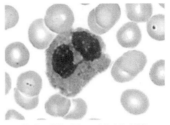

Eosinophils. (Carr and Rodak, 1999)

EPA, *n.pr* See acid, eicosapentaenoic.

ephedra, *n* Latin names: *Ephedra sinica, Ephedra nevadensis, Ephedra trifurca, Ephedra equisetina, Ephedra distachya;* parts used: leaves, seeds; uses: asthma, bronchitis, headaches, congestion, arthritis, weight loss; precautions: pregnancy, lactation, children younger than age 12; patients with sympathomimetics, glaucoma, seizures, hyperthyroidism, diabetes, arrhythmias, heart blockage, hypertension, prostatic hypertrophy, tachycardia, angina pectoris, and psychological disorders; considered unsafe by the FDA; can cause palpitations, tachycardia, hypertension, arrhythmias, stroke, heart attacks, heart failure, insomnia, anxiety, hallucinations, tremors, seizures, nausea, constipation, diarrhea, dysuria, urinary retention, dermatitis, dyspnea, contractions of the uterus. Also called *Brigham tea, cao ma huang, desert tea, epitonin, herba ephedrae, herbal, joint fir, ma huang, mahuanggen, Mexican tea, Mormon tea, muzei mu huang, natural ecstasy, popotillo, sea grape, squaw tea, teamster's tea, yellow astringent, yellow horse,* and *zhong ma huang.* See also ma huang.

Ephedra distachya, *n* See ephedra.

Ephedra equisetina, *n* See ephedra.

Ephedra nevadensis, *n* See ephedra.

Ephedra sinica, *n* See ephedra.

Ephedra trifurca, *n* See ephedra.

ephedrine hydrochloride, *n* chemical employed for treating allergy and asthma caused by its decongestant and bronchodilator properties; administered through the mouth, nose, or by injection.

ephedrine sulfate, *n* chemical employed for treating allergy and asthma for its decongestant and bron-chodilator properties; administered through the mouth or nose or by injection.

ephedrine tannate, *n* chemical employed for its decongestant and bronchodilator properties and administered orally.

epicritic sensitivity, *n* the finely discriminating, interpreted sensations that return to injured parts of the body after a more general sensitivity has been reestablished. See also protopathic sensitivity.

epidemic, *n* disease outbreak that affects more individuals than expected in a population.

epidemiology (e'·pə·dē·mē·ô'·lə·jē), *n* the study of the causes and spread of disease within a population. Commonly, the findings are reported for the benefit of public health.

epididymytis (e'·pə·di'·də·mī'·tis), *n* an inflammatory condition of the epididymis in the scrotum. Common symptoms include pain and tenderness in the affected area. Chills, fever, groin pain, and leukocytosis are also characteristics of the condition.

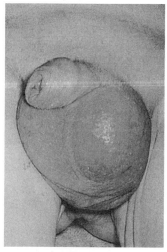

Epididymytis. (Lloyd-Davies, Gow, and Davies, 1994)

epilepsy (e'·pə·lep'·sē), *n* medical condition characterized by repeated episodes of erratic brain electrical discharge. They may be convulsive or nonconvulsive. Epilepsy may be caused by degenerative brain diseases; injuries incurred at birth; infections affecting the brain and central nervous system, head traumas, strokes, drugs, or unknown causes. Also called *falling sickness.*

epinephrine (eh·pi·ne'·frin), *n* neurochemical produced by the adrenal glands that arouses the sympathetic response. Also called *adrenaline.*

epistasis, *n* gene interaction where a gene at a particular locus supercedes or obscures the expression of another gene at a different locus.

epistaxis (e·pə·stak'·sis), *n* nosebleed; caused most commonly by picking but can occur as a result of vigorous sneezing, trauma, irritated mucous membranes, leukemia, vitamin K deficiency, hypertension, and other conditions.

epistemology (ə·pis'·tə·mä'·lə·jē), *n* that branch of philosophy that scrutinizes the nature, foundations, and limits of knowledge.

Epstein-Barr virus, *n.pr* a herpes virus responsible for mononucleosis that is linked to some types of chronic fatigue syndrome and Burkitt's lymphoma.

equilibrial triad (ē'·kwə·li'·brē·əl trī'·ad), *n* a means of maintaining balance. Consists of the visual system, or what the person perceives as reference points; the vestibular system, or internal gyroscope that informs the body of its position as it rotates or accelerates in space; and the proprioceptive system, which provides the person with feedback based upon the position of every joint and contracted muscle in the body.

Equisetum arvense, *n* See horsetail.

erethism, *n* any atypical irritation or sensitivity in human tissue or organs.

ergonomics (er·gə·nô'·miks), *n* applied study of psychology, anatomy, and physiology relating to people and work environments; includes intro-

duction of biomechanically supportive equipment.

ergot (ur'·gət), *n* Latin name: *Claviceps purpurea;* part used: sclerotium;
uses: muscle stimulant, induce uterine
contraction, stop uterine hemorrhage,
relaxant, relieve *delirium tremens,*
spinal congestion, asthma, hysteria,
relieve menstrual disorders, galactogogic, night sweats of phthisis; precautions: pulmonary hemorrhage;
cerebral hemorrhage; can elevate
blood pressure; can cause gangrene.
Also called *argot.*

Ericksonian hypnotists, *n.pl* practitioners of a school of hypnotherapy,
Ericksonian hypnotists follow the
teachings of psychiatrist Milton H.
Erickson (1901–1980).

ERS, *n.pr* See extended rotated side-
bent.

eructation (i·rək·tā'·shən), *n* belch-
ing; the release of air drawn from the
stomach and expelled with a distinctive sound through the mouth.

erythema (er·ə·thē'·mə), *n* mild
redness caused by congested or
dilated capillaries close to the surface
of the skin as in mild sunburns and
blushing due to embarrassment.

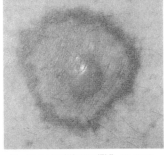

Erythema multiforme (EM). (Goldstein,
1997; Department of Dermatology, University of North Carolina at Chapel Hill)

**erythrocyte sedimentation rate
(ē'·ri'·thrō·sīt se'·di·men·tā'·shən
rāt'),** *n* a measure of erythrocytes
settling in a tube of blood within
1 hour. Used to diagnose infectious
and inflammatory diseases as well as
tumors, arthritis, heart conditions, and
other disorders.

erythrocytes (ē·rith'·rō·sīts), *n.pl*
red blood cells. They circulate oxygen
through the body and remove carbon
dioxide.

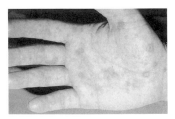

Erythema. (Lemmi and Lemmi, 2000)

**erythema multiforme (EM) (er'·ə·
thē'·mə mul'·tē·fōrm),** *n* a skin
condition marked by vesicular or
papular lesions and discoloration or
reddening of the affected area, caused
by hypersensitivity reaction to a
variety of drugs or viruses.

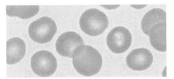

Erythrocytes. (Carr and Rodak, 1999)

erythropoiesis (i·rith·rō·poi'·ē·sis),
n red blood cell production that occurs
in bone marrow and involves matura-
tion of nucleated precursors into
erythrocytes regulated by the hormone
erythropoietin produced in the
kidneys.

***Erythroxylum* spp.,** *n* See coca.

Eschscholtzia californica, *n* See
California poppy.

escin (e'·sin), *n* compound derived
from the seeds of horse chestnut or
Aesculus hippocastanum that reduces

cellulite, inflammation, and edema; decreases the number and size of the small pores located in the capillary walls, thereby reducing capillary permeability. It is also used for thrombophlebitis and varicose veins.

esotericia (eh'·sō·tə·rē'·sē·ə), n a category of health care in which practitioners utilize a personal source of skill or power (or a personal connection to a source of skill and power), through divining techniques, faith, Healing Touch, prayer, or psychic abilities, to diagnose and/or heal.

espiritista (ā·spē·rē·tēs'·tə), n in Curanderismo, the Mexican-American healing system, a healer who serves as a medium for exorcisms and is adept at facilitating the help of benevolent spirits and removing malevolent spirits that surround the client.

espiritos malos (eh·spē'·rē·tōs mä'·lōs), n.pl in Curanderismo, the Mexican healing system, evil spirits believed to cause illness.

espiritualistas (es·pir·ē·tōō·äh·lē'·stäs), n spiritualists, folk healers in Latin American healing systems whose specialty is spiritual maladies.

ESR, n.pr See erythrocyte sedimentation rate.

essence, n defining characteristics of a homeopathic remedy found in materia medica. Also called *genius of the remedy.*

essiac (es·sē·ak), n herbal formula comprising burdock root, sheep sorrel, slippery elm, and turkey rhubarb, discovered by a Canadian nurse Rene Caisse for treating cancer patients; clinical evidence to prove its effectiveness is lacking.

esters (es'·terz), n.pl organic compounds synthesized from acids and alcohols, typically possessing fruity aromas. They have been shown to have antiinflammatory, antispasmodic, calming, and sedative properties.

estriol (es'·trē·ôl), n a form of estrogen synthesized within the liver, used to relieve menopausal complaints. It may increase the risk of endometrial and breast cancers. Also called *E3.*

estrogen (es'·trə·jin), n hormone that maintains secondary female sex characteristics.

ET CO₂, n See end-tidal CO₂.

ether (ē'·thər), n organic compound with molecule containing oxygen atom bonded to two hydrocarbon chains; insoluble in water but soluble in organic solvents such as ether and alcohol. Used as an early anaesthetic.

etheric layers (i·ther'·ik), n.pl in energy medicine, the divisions of energy fields that wrap around the body three-dimensionally; there are believed to be between four and seven etheric layers.

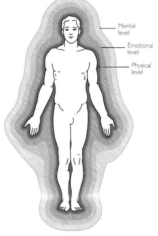

Etheric layers. (Micozzi, 2001)

ethics (e'·thiks), n the standards of conduct that direct a group or individual. In particular, it relates to the appropriate use of the power held by a group or individual.

ethmoid (eth'·moid), n the very thin bone structure of the nose, through which the ethmoid sinuses and other neural structures pass.

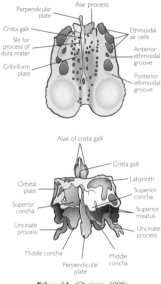

Ethmoid. (Chaitow, 1998)

ethmoid sinus, *n* one of the facial cavities, located beneath the nasal bridge, through which air flows.

ethnobotanical evidence (eth'·nō·bə·ta'·ni·kəl e'·və·dens), *n* data collected by botanists, anthropologists, and others who study the plant medicines of different cultures.

ethnobotany (eth'·nō·bô'·tə·nē), *n* study of how societies perceive and categorize plants and use them for food, medicine, and ritual.

ethnographic studies, *n.pl* methods of qualitative research developed by anthropologists, in which the researcher attends to and interprets communication while participating in the research context.

ethnomedicine (eth'·nō·me'·di·sin), *n* the comparative study of native or indigenous systems of medicine. The topics of this study generally include etiology of disease, practitioners and their role in health care, and types of treatment administered.

ethnopharmacology, *n* study of the medicinal use of plants by different cultures.

etiological prescribing, *n* homeopathic remedy selected by considering the causes of disease. See also etiotropism, isopathy, nosode, and precipitating factor.

etiology (ē'·tē·ô'·lə·jē), *n* the comprehensive study of disease development, including the causative agent, its route of entry into the body, and factors relating to the patient's susceptibility to the disease.

etiotropism, *n* relationship between a remedy and the causes of a disease. See also etiological prescribing.

eubiotic, *adj/n* supportive of life.

eucalyptus, *n* Latin name: *Eucalyptus globulus*; parts used: branch tips, leaves, essential oil; uses: in Ayurveda, pacifies kapha and vata doshas (pungent, bitter, light, oily), decongestant, antioxidant, antibacterial, antispasmodic used to treat IBS, gallstones, kidney stones, cystitis, CNS stimulant, aromatherapy; precautions: avoid mucous membranes; patients with severe renal, hepatic or gastric conditions; patients taking amphetamines, barbiturates, insulin, antidiabetics. Also called *blue gum, fever tree, gum, nilgiri, red gum, stringy bark tree, tailparna,* or *Tasmanian blue gum.*

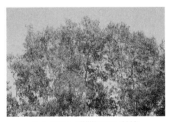

Eucalyptus. (Williamson, 2002)

Eugenia caryophyllata, *n* See cloves.
Euonymus atropurpureus, *n* See wahoo.
Euonymus eurapaeus, *n* See tree, European spindle.

Eupatorium perfoliatum, *n* See boneset.

Eupatorium rugosum, *n* See white snakeroot.

eupeptic, *adj/n* having traits that encourage healthy, functioning digestion.

Euphorbia capitata, *n* See pill-bearing spurge.

Euphorbia hirta, *n* See snakeweed.

Euphorbia piliulifera, *n* See pill-bearing spurge.

Euphrasia officinalis, *n* See eyebright.

European vervain (ye¹·rə·pē¹·ən ver·vān¹), *n* Latin name: *Verbena officinalis;* part used: leaves, flowering stems; uses: pain relief, bacteriostatic, antispasmodic, blood clots, antitumor, bodily tissue contraction, childbirth, purification and cleansing, induction of perspiration, diuretic, menstrual irregularities, milk secretion, wound healing, dysentery, headaches, febrifuge, nervous exhaustion, depression, gall bladder dysfunction, minor injuries, eczema, neuralgia, gum disease; precautions: may cause allergic contact dermatitis, infertility. Also called *ayauhxochitl, bunj, gogerchin otu, herb of the cross, holywort, ijzerhard, kuma-tuzura, ma pien ts'ao, minecicegi, rejil al hamam, texas vervain, verbena, verbena ofici-nal,* and *vervain.*

eustress, *n* beneficial stress; positive emotions.

euthanasia (yōō·thə·nā¹·zhə), *n* the act of facilitating death in a terminally ill patient, whether by deliberate activity, such as the administration of drugs that hasten death (known as *active euthanasia*), or passive, as in the withholding of life-extending treatment *(passive euthanasia).*

euthenics (yōō·the¹·niks), *n* branch of science that seeks to improve the human species by controlling environmental factors, such as prevention of disease, malnutrition, drug abuse, and combating pollution.

evaluation, *n* **1.** in clinical medicine, assessment of the patient for the purposes of forming a diagnosis and plan of treatment. **2.** in research, assessment of a treatment or diagnos-

tic test through experiment and measurement.

evaporation (ē·va¹·pə·rā¹·shən), *n* change of a liquid or a solid to a vapor or gaseous phase; does not form new substances, but the properties of the new phase may be different.

event-related potentials, *n.pl* See somatosensory event-related potentials (SERP).

ex gratia (eks¹ grā¹·shē·ə), *n* a monetary payment to an aggrieved party from the accused party without an admission of wrongdoing.

examination, *n* **1.** general medical procedure for assessing health. **2.** test used to assess skill or understanding.

examination, cun kou **(kōōn kō·ōō eg·zam¹·in·ā·shən),** *n* in a pulse examination, a diagnostic method using only the cun kou (wrist pulse). This pulse is divided into six components or pulse positions, three per hand. See also examination, pulse.

Examination, Naturopathic Physicians Licensing **(na¹·chə·rō·pa¹· thik fə·zl¹·shənz li··sen·sing eg¹· zam·ə·nā¹·shən),** *n.pr* a standard examination used by all licensing jurisdictions in North America for naturopathic physicians. The test evaluates physiology, anatomy, biochemistry, pathology, immunology, and microbiology and is taken after students complete their second year of naturopathic medical school. The test includes physical and clinical diagnosis, diagnostic imaging and laboratory diagnosis, pharmacology, botanical medicine, physical medicine, nutrition, minor surgery, homeopathy, lifestyle counseling, psychology, and emergency medicine and is taken after graduation from the student's fourth year of medical school. Also called *NPLEx.*

examination, osteopathic postural, *n* the component of musculoskeletal examination that concentrates on the body's responses to gravity while in an erect posture.

examination, osteopathic structural, *n* an osteopathic examination protocol that focuses on the neuromusculoskeletal system using palpation and tests on the range of motion of all body parts.

examination, pulse, *n* diagnostic technique in which the pulse of the patient, usually at the radial artery, is palpated with the physician's fingers.

excipient (ik·si'·pē·ənt), *n* ingredient, such as alcohol, which is used as a dilutent or as a vehicle for a drug. Excipients are generally inert, but may cause adverse effects in some individuals.

excipients, *n.pl* all the constituents of a remedy that lack medicinal properties. See also adjuvant, auxiliary substance, and vehicle.

excitatory cause, *n* the direct cause of an illness, such as a trauma or pathogen.

excoriation (ek·skōr'·ē·ā'·shən), *n* any surface injury to the skin; may be caused by scratches, chemical or thermal burns, and abrasions.

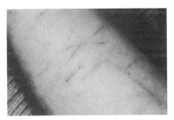

Excoriation. (Lemmi and Lemmi, 2000)

exercise-induced asthma, *n* a breathing disorder characterized by fits of heavy or irregular breathing, wheezing, coughing, and gasping brought on by physical exertion.

exhalation rib, *n* condition characterized by free exhalation and restricted inhalation motions, caused by a rib being caught in an exhalation position. Also called *caught in exhalation, depressed rib, exhalation strain,* or *inhalation restriction of rib.*

exocrine (ek'·sə·krin), *adj* relating to the outward glandular secretion of a substance onto the surface of an organ via a duct.

exoenzyme, *n* any enzyme that works outside the cells in which it is synthesized.

exogenous fields (ek·sô'·gen·əs fēldz), *n.pl* electromagnetic radiation that is emitted from outside the human body and may have either harmful or beneficial effects on human health.

Exogonium purga, *n* See jalap resin.

exopthalmia (eks·ôp·thal'·mē·ə), *n* condition marked by bulging eyeballs; may be caused by a wide array of anomalies, such as edema, tumor, injury to the extraocular muscles, Graves' disease, and other endocrine disorders. Also called *protusio bulbi.*

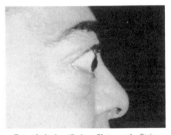

Exopthalmia. (Stein, Slatt, and Stein, 1994)

expansion component, *n* a manual therapy element which advocates manipulating the body and its energies with hands-on techniques including pulling, lifting, and rolling to encourage opening and separation of constricted body parts.

expectorant, *n* a substance that reduces the production of mucus in the lungs and promotes the dislodging of mucus from the bronchioles.

expert witness, *n* a person sufficiently trained in a given area of expertise who can give testimony relevant to a case in court.

expressed juice, *n* fluid extracted from fresh plants used to create a mother tincture.

expression (ek·spre'·shən), *n* the mechanical method used to extract essential oils from plant material by crushing and applying pressure. Commonly used for extracting fluids from citrus fruits like lemons and oranges.

expressivity, *n* variance in the inheritance patterns of genes in people with a common genotype—for instance, polydactyly being expressed as extra fingers in one generation and extra toes in the next.

extension, *n* movement of a limb to increase the angle of the joint. Some joints (at the wrist, in the neck) are able to hyperextend.

extension, bilateral sacral, *n* condition in which the sacrum has rotated around a central transverse axis so that the sacral base moves posterior relative to the bones of the pelvis. Also called *sacral base posterior.*

extension, craniosacral, *n* the movement of the cranial rhythmic impulse, characterized by anterior motion of the sphenobasilar symphysis and posterior motion of the sacrum.

extension, regional, *n* straightening of spinal region in the sagittal plane. Also called *Fryette regional extension.*

extension, sacral, *n* posterior movement of the sacral base relative to the hip bones.

extension, SBS, *n* rotation of the occipital and sphenoid bones in opposing directions about parallel transverse axes, thus resulting in inferior positioning of the basilar portions of both bones and a decrease in the posterior convexity between them. Also called *sphenobasilar synchondrosis (symphysis) extension.*

extension, unilateral sacral, *n* condition involving a one-sided superior sacral shear that results in a shallow sulcus and an ipsilateral upward-forward inferolateral sacral angle.

extracellular matrix (eks'·trə·sel'·yə·ler mā'·triks), *n* substance produced by cells and secreted into the environment in which the cells are embedded; contains collagen, proteoglycans, glycosaminoglycans, and fluid; can influence the behavior of the cells. Also called *ECM.* See also connective tissue.

extract, *n* liquid herbal concentrate obtained by processing crude herbs in alcohol, water, or other solvents.

extract, citrus seed, *n* Latin name: *Citrus* spp; part used: seeds; uses: antiseptic, antibacterial, antifungal, bowel flora conditions, antibacterial mouthwash; precautions: can cause dehydration (overuse). Also called *grapefruit seed extract* and *GSE.*

extract, fluid, *n* in herbal medicine, a substance derived by mixing an herb with a solvent (usually a mixture of water and alcohol).

extract, grapefruit seed, *n* Latin name: *Citrus paradisii;* parts used: seeds, pulp; uses: disinfectant, diarrhea, flu, colds, gingivitis, dental plaques, candidiasis, ulcers, skin conditions; precautions: should be diluted, can cause skin irritation. Also called *GSE.*

extract, grass pollen, *n* a mixture of pollen extracts derived from rye (92%), timothy (5%), and corn (3%) plants; processed to remove any proteins that may trigger allergic reactions. Used to treat benign prostate inflammation and may also be useful in treating prostatitis, prostate cancer, and high cholesterol. Precautions for grass pollen extract include hypersensitivity or allergy.

extract, oyster, *n* a dietary supplement made of oyster extract, taurine, ginseng, and zinc. Its use has been associated with the development of edema.

extract, thymus, *n* a concentrate of bovine or porcine thymus gland. Used to treat asthma, food allergies, respiratory infections, thyroid deficiencies, and viral hepatitis. Precaution urged for patients taking immunosuppressant medications. Caution should be used with bovine glandular extracts because of virus or prior contamination. Also called *thymus gland, calf thymus extract, thymic extract,* or *thymomodulin.*

extracts, adrenal, *n.pl* orally administered extracts of the adrenal gland used to enhance adrenal activity and aid the body's response to stress and fatigue.

extracts, liver, *n.pl* orally administered extracts of liver tissue used to treat hepatic disease and enhance the functions of the liver, including the use of fat and tissue regeneration.

extracts, native, *n.pl* in natural medicine, potent extracts that are concentrated by removing solvent under low pressure and temperature.

extracts, pancreatic, *n.pl* orally administered extracts of the pancreas used to enhance the functions of the pancreas and to treat autoimmune diseases, cancer, cystic fibrosis, infections, and inflammatory diseases.

extracts, plant, *n.pl* products, including absolutes, resinoids, concretes, hydrosols, pomades, and tinctures, that are derived from aromatic plant material by extraction processes such as distillation (steam or water), hydrodiffusion, expression, solvent extraction, carbon dioxide extraction, enfleurage or maceration.

extracts, spleen, *n.pl* orally administered extracts of the spleen. Claimed to enhance the functions of the spleen, aid in white blood cell production, and treat infections and conditions connected to splenectomy.

extracts, standardized, *n* herbal products in which a consistent level of the active chemical ingredient has been established.

extracts, thyroid, *n.pl* preparations made from bovine and porcine thyroid glands available by prescription or over the counter; used to treat hypothyroidism.

extraction (ek·strak'·shən), *n* method used to isolate essential oils and other products, such as absolutes, floral waters, resinoids, and tinctures, from plant material. Distillation, hydrodiffusion, expression, solvent extraction, carbon dioxide extraction, enfleurage, and maceration are commonly used extraction methods. See also distillation, hydrodiffusion, expression, enfleurage, and maceration.

extrasensory perception, *n* perception in which a person gains awareness of events without using the normal senses. Includes experiences such as clairvoyance, precognition,

and telepathy. Also called *ESP* or *psi.*

extravasation (ek·stra·və·sā'·shən), *n* **1.** seeping of blood, lymph, or serum into tissues. **2.** seeping of chemotherapeutic drugs into a tissue.

extrinsic corrective forces, *n.pl* forces used in treatment whose sources are outside the patient (e.g., from a body worker, gravity, etc.).

extubation (ek·stə·bā'·shən), *n* removal of a tube from either a natural body orifice or from a body cavity.

exudation (ek·sōō'·dā'·shən), *n* the steady, slow movement of cells or fluid, from a cell membrane's pores or from small leaks in the membrane.

eye movement desensitization and reprocessing, *n* psychophysiologic treatment that proposes to remove painful memories by providing a moving object for the eye to track while the therapist and patient use deconditioning therapy. Also called *EMDR.*

eye movement integration, *n* therapy in which the practitioner directs a client to recall a traumatic event, while leading the individual to move the eyes in a particular set of patterns to bring about healing and release from the trauma.

eye-fixation induction, *n* in hypnosis, a method whereby patients are directed to focus their eyes on an object until they close; recognized in popular culture as the swinging pendulum technique used to bring about a trance.

eye-roll sign, *n* a biological marker believed to be an indicator of a patient's susceptibility to hypnosis as determined by assessing the white of the patient's eye when it is rolled upward.

eyebaths, *n.pl* water-based solutions, which may contain herbal decoctions, for use in irrigating the eyes. The solutions should always be sterile to avoid infection.

eyebright, *n* Latin name: *Euphrasia officinalis;* part used: blooming plant; uses: eye irritations, nasal catarrh; uses under research: jaundice, lung infections, impaired memory; not recommended because of cytotoxic effects; precautions: can cause disorientation, headaches, fatigue, congestion, photophobia, altered vision, and sneezing. Also called *meadow eyebright* and *red eyebright*.

Eysenck Personality Inventory, *n.pr* questionnaire in a self-report format that measures the personality aspect of extraversion-introversion and neuroticism-stability and includes a lie scale.

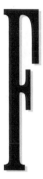

FAAO, *n.pr* See Fellow of the American Academy of Osteopathy.

face validity (fās´ və·li´·di·tē), *n* the degree to which a questionnaire or other measurement appears to reflect the variable it has been designed to measure.

facet asymmetry, *n* condition in which the facet joints of vertebrae are not oriented properly, thereby affecting the mobility of the spine.

facet symmetry, *n* proper orientation of the facet joints of vertebrae. See also facet asymmetry.

facet tropism (fa´·sit trō´·pizm), *n* dissimilar facing and/or size of a vertebra's zygapophyseal joints.

facial, *adj* pertaining to the face.

facilitated positional release, *n* an indirect myofascial release treatment method where the point of dysfunction is gradually moved until a neutral position is realized on all planes; an activating influence (either torsion or compression) is then applied in order to release joint restriction and remove tension from the tissue. Also called *FPR.*

facilitation (fə·si´·lə·tā´·shən), *n* an automatic, impulsive stimulation of a particular muscle to contract.

factual causation, *n* the proven link between a deliberate failure to perform duty of care and the resulting negative impact.

failure to diagnose, *n* a failure to assess a patient's condition. Harm may be inflicted by the failure to administer treatment to a potentially treatable condition.

false unicorn root, *n* Latin name: *Chamaelirium luteum;* part used: roots; uses: diuretic, tonic for the uterus and liver, emetic, genital and urinary system stimulant, abnormal menstruation, morning sickness; precautions: pregnancy, lactation, children. Also called *blazing star, devil's bit, drooping starwort, fairywart, helonias root, rattlesnake,* and *starwort.*

family practice, *n* medical specialization that treats individuals and families by integrating behavioral, biomedical, and clinical sciences and providing comprehensive primary care.

family systems, *n.pl* the social interactions, patterns, and interdependence that exist between members of families, especially as they pertain to the impact of one member's illness on the others in the family.

FAO, *n* See Food and Agriculture Organization.

fascia, *n* elastic connective tissue found throughout the body that surrounds and supports various muscles and organs.

fascial compensation (fa·shē·ül kôm´·pen·sā´·shən), *n* postural pattern in which the musculoskeletal system indicates beneficial functional adjustments as a result of a physical anomaly, such as shortened leg.

fascial unwinding, *n* a manipulative osteopathic technique in which the physician passively moves some part of the patient's body, with constant feedback as to the sensations of motion being given by the patient.

fasciculation (fə·si´·kyu·lā´·shən), *n* localized twitching of a muscle group. Most often idiopathic and benign but also occurs during administration of anesthesia; may be symptomatic of dietary deficiency, fever, cerebral palsy, polio, heart disease, uremia, and several other disorders.

fasting, *v* to abstain from food and any beverages other than water. Used to treat a variety of disorders, including allergies, arthritis, autoimmune disease, diabetes, heart disease, gastrointestinal disease, and obesity.

fat soluble vitamins, *n.pl* a variety of organic substances essential to human health and nutrition that dissolve in fat. Require fat for absorption and is metabolized with fat in the body. High doses of fat soluble vitamins are potentially toxic and should be avoided. Includes vitamins A, D, E, and others.

FDA, *n.pr* See Food and Drug Administration.

febrifuge, *n* temperature-reducing aid. See also antipyretic.

febrile (fe·brīl'), *adj* with a fever.

Federal Emergency Management Agency, *n.pr* a government organization based in the United States that provides assistance, planning, and other services related to disaster management.

Federation of State Medical Boards, *n.pr* an association comprising the medical boards of the United States, the District of Columbia, the Virgin Islands, Guam, Puerto Rico, and 13 state boards associated with osteopathic medicine. The organization strives to enhance the safety, quality, and integrity of health care by promoting elevated standards for medical practice and physician licensure. With regards to complementary and alternative medicine, the Federation advises practitioners to ask patients about their use of complementary and alternative medicine and provide increased education about the scientific basis of such approaches and the risks involved with ceasing conventional treatment.

Feeling Good Thermometer, *n.pr* an illustrated scale that ranges from one to ten used to measure feelings, negative feelings being low on the scale and positive feelings being high.

Feingold hypothesis, *n.pr* hypothesis that states that hyperactivity in children may be caused by food additives such as artificial colors, artificial flavorings, and preservatives.

Fellow of the American Academy of Osteopathy, *n.pr* a designation awarded by the American Academy of Osteopathy to select osteopathic physicians who are certified in both osteopathic manipulative medicine and neuromusculoskeletal medicine.

FEMA, *n.pr* See Federal Emergency Management Agency.

fenestration (fe·nə·strā'·shən), *n* **1.** surgery that accesses a cavity within a bone or organ. **2.** an orifice created in an organ or a bone by surgery.

feng shui (fung shwā), *n* Chinese art of placing objects in accordance with the concepts of yin and yang—the passive (female) and active (male) principles, respectively—in Chinese cosmology, and the flow of qi which may have beneficial or harmful effects on one's health and life. See also qi.

fennel, *n* Latin name: *Foeniculum vulgare;* part used: seeds; uses: abnormal menstruation, hampered lactation, low sex drive; precautions: pregnancy, lactation; essential oil: children; patients with liver disease or stomach ulcers; not for long-term use; can cause convulsions, nausea, contact dermatitis, photosensitivity, lung edemas, and some cancers. Also called *aneth fenouil, carosella, fenchel, funcho, garden fennel, hinojo, large fennel, sweet fennel,* and *wild fennel.*

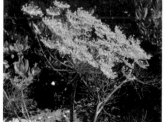

Fennel. (Scott and Barlow, 2003)

fenugreek (fen'·yə·grēk'), *n* Latin name: *Trigonella foenum-graecum;* part used: seeds; uses: dyspepsia, constipation, gastritis. Topically, used to treat cellulitis, leg ulcers, wound healing; precautions: hypersensitivity reactions, pregnancy, children, lactation; causes bruising, bleeding, petechiae; interferes with absorption of other medications, anticoagulants, and antidiabetics. Also called *Bird's foot, Greek hayseed,* and *trigonella.*

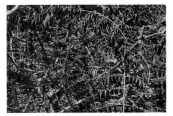

Fever nut. (Williamson, 2002)

Fenugreek. (Williamson, 2002)

ferromagnets, *n.pl* iron-based magnets that generally produce relatively weak fields.

Ferrula assa-foetida, *n* See asafetida.

FEV1, *n.pr* See forced expiratory volume in one second.

fever, *n* condition characterized by a rise in body temperature. Most fevers are mild and can be treated at home, but if they last more than two days, if the temperature rises to over 102.2° F, or if body temperature suddenly rises to 102.2° F within four hours, it is considered dangerous, and professional treatment should be sought immediately.

fever nut, *n* Latin name: *Caesalpinia bonducella;* parts used: seeds, roots, bark, leaves; uses: in Ayurveda, pacifics tridosha (bitter, astringent, light, dry, sharp), antimalarial, antiviral, antiestrogenic, antifilarial, hypoglycemic, hypolipidemic, uterine stimulant, antiinflammatory, febrifuge, tonic, anthelmintic, fever, worms, tumors, smallpox, liver conditions;

precautions: none known. Also called *bonduc nut, kankarej, kuberakshi,* or *katikaranja.*

feverfew, *n* Latin names: *Chrysanthemum parthenium, Tanacetum parthenium;* part used: leaves; uses: abortifacient, abnormal menstruation, inflamed joints, fever; uses under research: migraines; precautions: pregnancy, lactation, children; can cause oral ulcers, nausea, and inflammation in muscles and joints. Also called *altamisa, bachelor's button, chamomile grande, featherfew, featherfoil, midsummer daisy, mutterkraut, nosebleed, Santa Maria, wild chamomile,* and *wild quinine.*

FI, *n.pr* See functional integration.

fiber, *n* threadlike structure found in various plant and animal tissues.

fiber, small myelinated, *n* See A delta fiber.

fiber, soluble, *n* one of three types of fiber; soluble fibers are pectin, gum mucilage, and glucomannan and are found in pears, apples, vegetables, and wheat bran.

fiber, sweeping cross, *n* massage technique that closely resembles gliding or effleurage. Distinguished by the addition of light cross-fiber strokes (direction of movement is perpendicular to the pattern of muscle fibers) that penetrate deeper tissues. See also effleurage.

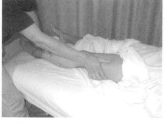

Fiber, sweeping cross. (Lowe, 2003)

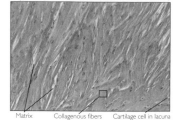

Matrix   Collagenous fibers   Cartilage cell in lacuna

Fibrocartilage. (Thibodeau, 1999; Rob Callantine and James M. Kron)

fiber, unmyelinated (un'·mī'·ə·lə·nā'·tid fī'·ber), *n* a neuron that is not surrounded by a myelin sheath.

fibrillation (fī·brə·lā'·shən), *n* rapid localized contraction of a nerve fiber bundle or a solitary muscle fiber.

fibrin (fī'·brin), *n* white, insoluble protein that makes up a blood clot by forming a network in which red blood cells and platelets are trapped; formed by the action of thrombin on fibrinogen.

fibrinolytic activity (fī·bri·nō·li'·tik ak·ti'·vi·tē), *n* the ability of some proteolytic enzymes to dissolve the fibrin in blood clots facilitating wound healing. See also fibrin.

fibroblast (fī'·brō·blast'), *n* an undifferentiated connective tissue cell that develops into a number of precursor cells, such as collagenoblasts, osteoblasts, and chondroblasts, and then becomes supporting tissue. Also called *fibrocyte* or *desmocyte*.

fibrocartilage (fī'·brō·kar'·tə·lej), *n* very strong, relatively inflexible cartilage found in the meniscus (in the knee joint), intervertebral discs, and pubic symphysis.

fibromuscular dysplasia (fi'·brō·mu'·skyə·ler dis·plā'·zhə), *n* an arterial disease characterized by abnormal development of intraluminal folds of endothelial tissue that are fibrous. Typically affects renal arteries and is related to hypertension.

fibromyalgia (fī·brō·mī·al·jē·ə), *n* a disease primarily indicated by noticeable, extensive pain in muscles, tendons, joints, and soft tissues. The condition can develop as a singular condition or accompanying other conditions such as rheumatoid arthritis or lupus. A successful diagnosis of this condition includes the presence of tenderness and pain in a minimum of 11 tender points on the body. Also called *fibromyositis.* See also FMS and myodysneuria.

fibrositis (fī·brə·sī'·tis), *n* condition marked by inflammation of white fibrous connective tissue, such as muscle sheaths that results in pain and stiffness.

Ficus religiosa, *n* See tree, bo-tree.

field, *n* three-dimensional zone in which an array of forces interact in tangible, recognizable ways.

fierce grace, *n* term coined by spiritual teacher Ram Dass to describe the paradoxical spiritual insight he experienced (growth through suffering) as a result of a stroke.

fight-or-flight response, *n* the psychophysiologic response to a perceived threat that prepares the organism for action.

figwort, *n* Latin name: *Scrophularia nodosa, Scrophularia ningpoensis;* parts used: buds (dried), leaves (dried); uses: antiinflammatory, epidermal maladies, digestive disturbances, cardiac aid; precautions: pregnancy, lactation, children; patients with grave heart disease; can cause low heart rate, cardiac block, asystole, nausea, diarrhea. Also called *carpenter's square, kernelwort, rosenoble, scrofula plant, square stalk, stinking christopher,* and *throatwort.*

filiform needles (fi'·lə·form nē'·dəlz), *n.pl* solid, extremely fine, stainless steel needles commonly used in acupuncture.

Filipendula ulmaria, *n* See meadowsweet.

fire, *n* one of the five phases, or elements, in Chinese cosmological and medical theory, the characteristic manifestations of which include empathy, expressiveness, extreme emotions, extroversion, and sociability.

fire flame bush, *n* Latin name: *Woodfordia fruticosa* ; parts used: flowers; uses: in Ayurveda, pacifies pitta and kapha doshas (astringent, pungent, light); antiinflammatory, antipyretic, antitumor, antiviral, immunomodulator, stimulant, diarrhea, dysentery, hemorrhage, liver conditions, hemorrhoids; used to ferment aristas and aravas; precautions: none known. Also called *dhai, dhanuki,* or *shhan-jitea.* See also arista and arava.

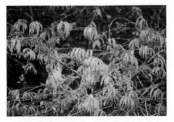

Fire flame bush. (Williamson: Major Herbs of Ayurveda)

fissure, *n* **1.** cracklike groove on an organ's surface. **2.** lesion resembling a crack—for example, anal fissures.

Fissure. (Lemmi and Lemmi, 2000)

five elements, *n.pl* fire, water, earth, wood, and metal; in Chinese medicine, each of these five components is used to organize phenomena for use in clinical applications. Each of the elements corresponds to a specific function (i.e., metal means a decline in function; wood indicates growth; earth is equated with neutrality and balance; water relates to rest and imminent change in direction; and fire is associated with reaching a peak and imminent decline).

five flavors, *n* in the dietary component of Chinese medicine, the five basic tastes into which foods are divided, each of which has different physiologic actions. Sour has astringent effects, retaining and generating fluids; bitter flavored foods are purgative, drying the body; sweet tastes replenish and strengthen, harmonize the stomach and spleen, and are generally tonic; pungent flavors eliminate toxins and alleviate stagnation by supporting movement of qi; and salty tastes soften congestions and tissue masses. The goal of Chinese dietary medicine is to achieve balance among these five tastes. See also qi.

five food groups, *n.pl* a rough guide to good daily nutrition, comprising the following groups: meat/nuts/legumes, breads/cereals, vegetables/fruit, dairy products, and fats.

Five Spirits, *n.pl* five body-mind aspects recognized in Chinese medicine and housed in the yin aspects of the person. They are shen, hun, yi, zhi, and po.

Five Virtues, *n.pl* desirable qualities associated with each of the Five Spirits of Chinese Medicine. They are li, ren, xin, zhi, and bao. See also Five Spirits.

5-HTP, *n* an amino acid that is a precursor to the neurotransmitter serotonin. Supplementation of this amino acid is claimed to be useful in treating depression, fibromyalgia, tension, and migraine headaches; as an anxiolytic; and as an adjunct to weight loss. There are no known side effects. It should not be taken concurrently with SSRI medications, carbidopa, or zolpidem.

5-hydroxytryptophan, *n* See 5-HTP.

five-step nursing process, *n* procedure involving the patient, nurse, and the patient's family or significant other, in which the nurse facilitates a patient-care plan with an application of five stages. The five steps which are assessing, analyzing, planning, implementing, and evaluating.

fixable (fik′·sə·bəl), *adj* a broad category used to refer to patients with curable illnesses.

fixators (fik·sā′·ters), *n.pl* soft-tissue structures that act as synthesizers during movement. Also called *stabilizers.*

flat back posture, *n* posture characterized by the presence of a slight plantar flexion of the ankle joints, an extension of the hip joints, a tilt of the pelvis towards the back, flexion of the upper portion of the thoracic spine, and a slight extension of the cervical spine.

flat compression, *n* a compression technique in which soft tissue is pressed against a bone or muscle lying underneath. See also compression technique.

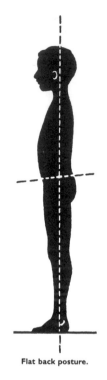

Flat back posture.

flavonoids, *n.pl* common plant pigment compounds that act as antioxidants, enhance the effects of vitamin C, and strengthen connective tissue around capillaries.

flax, *n* Latin name: *Linum usitatissimum;* part used: seeds; uses: inflammatory, laxative, anticholesteremic; uses under research: colon disease, eczema, psoriasis, irritable bowel syndrome, diverticulitis, arthritis, allergies, multiple sclerosis, cancer, lupus, menopause, renal cysts, hypertension, and hyperactivity; precautions: pregnancy, lactation, children; patients with digestive blockage or dehydration, diabetes; unripened seeds are poisonous; can cause nausea, diarrhea, and gas, (overuse: weakness, dyspnea, tachypnea, paralysis, convulsions, and death). Also called *linseed, lint bells, linen flax,* and *linum.*

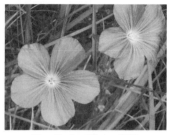

Flax. (Scott and Barlow, 2003)

flexion (flek´·shən), *n* movement of a limb to decrease the angle of a joint.

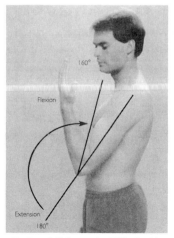

Flexion. (Seidel et al, 1995; Patrick Watson)

flexion, bilateral sacral, *n* condition in which the sacrum has rotated around a central transverse axis so that the sacral base moves forward between the bones of the pelvis. Also called *sacral base anterior.*

flexion, craniosacral, *n* movement characterized by ascending motion of the sphenobasilar symphysis and backward motion of the sacral base.

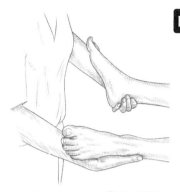

Flexion, craniosacral. (Chaitow, 2003)

flexion, sacral, *n* anterior movement of the sacral base relative to the hip bones.

flexion, SBS, *n* rotation of the occipital and sphenoid bones in opposing directions about parallel transverse axes, thus resulting in superior positioning of the basilar portion of both bones and an increase in the posterior convexity between them. Also called *sphenobasilar synchondrosis (symphysis) flexion.*

Flexner report, *n.pr* a 1910 publication, stemming from the Pure Foods and Drugs Act of 1906; established science is the foundation for medical education and formulation of medicines.

Flexyx neuropathy system (flek´· siks ner·ô´·pə·thē sis´ təm), *n* noninvasive method in which low-intensity light stimulation is used to reset EEG patterns, specifically for individuals suffering from motor paralysis and cognitive and emotional impairment after mechanical or psychologic trauma.

flinch sign, *n* See jump sign.

Flor-Essence (flōr'-es'·səns), *n* a proprietary herbal mixture, marketed as a tea for assisting in cancer and with other health concerns. The herbs have antiinflammatory, antioxidant, anticancer, and immunostimulant properties. Contraindicated for pregnant and lactating women. See also essiac.

flow cytometry (flō' sī·tô'·mə·trē), *n* technique used to determine cell size and granularity by shining a strong, focused beam of light on the cell and then measuring the scattered light.

flower essences, *n.pl* homeopathic dilutions of flowers systematized by Edward Bach, MD; used to address emotional imbalance.

fluid metabolism, *n* the constant maintenance of moisture balance in the body's tissues through intake, absorption, and excretion of water.

fluid retention, *n* condition in which the body fails to flush or otherwise exude excess liquid; often caused by cardiovascular, renal, or metabolic disorders.

fluorescence, *n* the emission of light of a particular wavelength by a substance upon absorption of electromagnetic radiation of a shorter wavelength.

fluorescent microscopy (flə·re'·sənt mī·krō'·skə·pē), *n* a type of microscope examination, usually of microorganisms or tissue stained with a fluorescent dye. Also called *ultraviolet microscopy.*

fluoridation, *n* the technique of infusing public water supply with fluoride to reduce dental decay.

fluoride, *n* a mineral important in bone formation used for the treatment of osteoporosis and prevention of tooth decay. Overdose can produce tooth mottling, joint pain, stomach pain, and nausea.

fluorosis (flə·rō'·sis), *n* problem caused by excessive or protracted ingestion of fluorine. Causes a mottled appearance of the teeth and in extreme

cases, pitting in the deciduous and secondary teeth. May be present in the offspring of females whose fluoride intake was high during pregnancy.

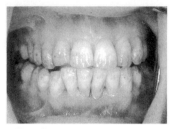

Fluorosis. (Regezi, Sciubba, and Pogrel, 2000)

flux, *n* **1.** an excessive discharge or flow. **2.** undulation or changing course of a condition.

fluxion, *n* a homeopathic process by which a liquid potency is created with injected water, thus producing the potentizing effect in the liquid remedy. Also called *continuous fluxion.*

FMS, *n* fibromyalgia syndrome, a disease primarily indicated by extensive tenderness and pain affecting muscles, tendons, joints, and soft tissues; can develop as a singular condition or concurrently with other conditions like rheumatoid arthritis or lupus.

focusing, *n* **1.** a mental component of manual therapy; helps clients to find areas of pain or tension in their bodies and allows the practitioners to more accurately treat the region. **2.** an introspective psychologic tool developed by philosopher and psychologist Eugene Gendlin, in which the person focusing attends to the subtle physical sensations that underlie grosser emotional experiences and derives understanding of his or her problems from these sensations.

Foeniculum vulgare, *n* See fennel.

folate (fō'·lāt), *n* a B vitamin that is present in leafy green vegetables, dry peas and beans, and fortified breads and cereals. Folate deficiency may increase the risk of certain cancers, Alzheimer's disease, and certain birth defects, such as neural tube defects. Also used by some to enhance the effects of SSRI medications; to maintain cardiovascular health; to prevent tolerance of nitrates during nitrate therapy; and to treat gout, bipolar depression, osteoarthritis, osteoporosis, rheumatism, and vitiligo. Folate supplementation may be contraindicated for patients with seizure disorders and for those taking phenytoin. Also called *folic acid.*

fontanel (fŏn´·tə·nel), *n* the membrane-covered area between an infant's cranial bones before they close. The anterior fontanel usually closes at 14 months of age while the posterior fontanel closes 2 months after birth. There can be a significant bulge in the fontanel during some infections, such as meningitis. Also called *fontanelle* or *fonticulus.*

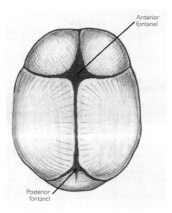

Fontanel. (Potter and Perry, 1995)

Food and Agriculture Organization, *n.pr* a specialized agency of the United Nations that strives to improve agricultural productivity, raise levels of nutrition, and better the living conditions of rural populations. It is also responsible for setting the values associated with the Provisional Tolerable Weekly Intake (PTWI). Also called *FAO.* See also Provisional Tolerable Weekly Intake.

Food and Drug Administration, *n* U.S. agency that oversees the regulation of biotechnology, food, supplements, drug products, and cosmetics.

food challenge, *n* a process of testing for food allergies in which the patient is given, often in double-blind conditions, a sample of a different, potentially allergenic, food once a day and reactions are noted. In some forms the challenge is preceded by a diet from which all common allergens have been eliminated for several weeks, after which foods are introduced as above.

food immune–complex assay, *n* a diagnostic test for identifying reactive substances that cause delayed hypersensitivity of the immune system. Uses a solid-phase radioimmunoassay that detects immune complexes and IgG.

food pyramid, *n* graphic issued by the U.S. Department of Agriculture and Health and Human Services that details recommendations for a balanced diet. Through the illustration of a triangle, it labels daily food choices according to recommended frequency of ingestion. Includes daily serving quantities for bread, rice, and cereal (6–11 servings daily); fruit (2–4 servings daily); vegetables (3–5 servings daily); dairy (2–3 servings daily); meats (2–3 servings daily); and fats, oils, and sweets (use sparingly).

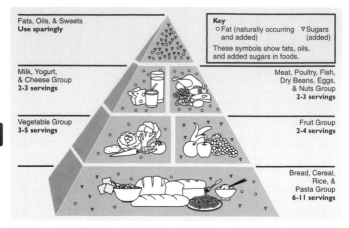

Food pyramid. (US Department of Agriculture: USDA Human Nutrition Information, Pub No 249, Washington DC, 1992, US Government Printing Office)

food supplements, *n.pl* nonfood substances that are used to augment the dietary intake of minerals, vitamins, amino acids, and/or herbs.

foramen (fə·rä´·mən), *n* a naturally occurring opening in human bones or membranous structures that allows the passage of nerves and blood vessels.

force, *n* unseen energy which influences living beings. See also dynamis.

forced expiratory volume in one second (fōrsd´ ek·spī´·rə·tō´·rē vôl´·yōōm in wun´ se´·kənd), *n* an individual test measure used to assess limitations in airflow, which measures the amount of air exhaled in one second.

forced vital capacity, *n* a measure of the maximum rate of exhalation. Deviance from normative patterns based on age, size, and gender may indicate possible dysfunction.

foremilk, *n* thirst-quenching milk with a watery consistency, produced at the beginning of a feeding.

forking larkspur, *n* Latin name: *Delphinium consolida;* part used: plant,
flower, leaves; uses: destroy and remove intestinal worms; induce urination; induce sleep; lower blood pressure; promote bowel evacuation, relax and dilate blood vessels, remove skin parasites, spasmodic asthma, dropsy, hemorrhoids, relieve violent purging, colic; precautions: can cause toxicity in large doses. Also called *doubtful knight's spur, field larkspur, forked larkspur, hezaren, larkspur, royal knight's spur,* and *wilde ridder-spoor.*

forma, *adj/n* minor elements between the members of a botanical species.

formulation (fōr´·myə·lā´·shən), *n* a systematic description of components used in a formula for a variety of products like massage blends or creams.

forward bending, *n* flexion of the spine.

fossa (fä´·sə), *n* dent or visibly lowered area, particularly on the surface of a bone end.

fo-ti, *n* Latin name: *Polygonum multiflorum;* part used: roots; uses: laxative, sleeping aid, autoimmune disorders, diabetes, general aging, diverticular disease, hemorrhoids; precautions: pregnancy, lactation, children; patients with diarrhea, nausea. Also called *Chinese cornbind, Chinese knotweed, flowery knotweed,* and *ho shou wu.*

four examinations, *n* the diagnostic protocol of Chinese traditional medicine; looking, hearing and smelling, questioning, and palpation.

four examinations, hearing and smelling, *n* the second of the four examinations in traditional Chinese medicine, in which the physician scrutinizes the qualities of the patient's voice and body odors.

four examinations, looking, *n* the first of the four examinations in traditional Chinese medicine, in which the physician observes the skin, hair, carriage, and attitude of the patient. Thorough examination of the tongue is also essential at this stage.

four examinations, palpation, *n* the fourth of the four examinations in traditional Chinese medicine, in which the physician gently touches the abdomen looking for tender points, especially those along acupuncture meridians.

four examinations, questioning, *n* the third of the four examinations in traditional Chinese medicine, in which the physician interviews the client to uncover any patterns of disease and discord.

four orders, *n* in Native American medicine, the four degrees awarded to a male or female candidate of the Ojibway tribe being trained in the ways of healing and communing with spiritual powers and energies.

fractional distillation (frak'·shən·əl dis·tə·lā'·shən), *n* the process of separating the portions of a mixture by heating it and condensing the components according to their different boiling points.

fracture, *n* break of bone tissue, usually caused by injury; fractures are classified according to the bone that has been damaged and type of damage produced.

frankincense, *n* See boswellia.

fraudulent, *adj* **1.** relating to actions without proper qualifications. **2.** relating to actions that purposely intend to deceive.

free radicals, *n.pl* compounds with an unpaired electron, which makes them extremely reactive.

freeze-drying, *n* a method for preparing herbs or glandular extracts in which the material is rapidly frozen to between $-40°$ F and $-60°$ F and then dried under vacuum. This method ensures preservation of biologically active molecules in the extracts.

friction, *n* massage technique that uses superficial tissue to engage deeper layers. Friction increases circulation and fibroblast activity.

frontal bone, *n* portion of the skull composed of two parts: the squama, or vertical piece, which forms the forehead, and the horizontal portion, which forms spaces for the eyes and nasal passages.

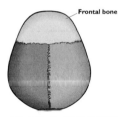

Frontal bone. (Chaitow, 1999)

frontal sinus, *n* the cavity located behind the forehead through which air flows.

F

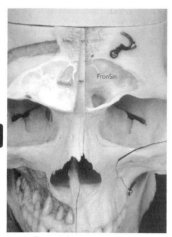

Frontal sinus. (Carreiro, 2003)

frontozygomatic suture, *n* location where the zygomatic bone and the zygomatic process of the frontal bone meet.

frostbite, *n* skin and subcutaneous tissue damage caused by prolonged exposure to extreme cold. Characterized by cessation of blood circulation, frostbite results in a number of signs and symptoms including edema, pain, vesiculation, anoxia, and necrosis.

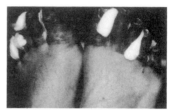

Frostbite. (Auerbach, 1995)

FRS, *n* "flexed rotated side-bent," an osteopathic abbreviation used to describe vertebral position in cases of spinal dysfunction.

fruit, *n* the fully developed seed of a plant, including the surrounding flesh.

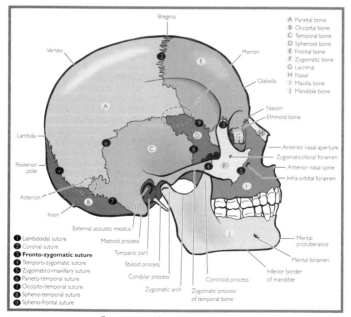

A Parietal bone
B Occipital bone
C Temporal bone
D Sphenoid bone
E Frontal bone
F Zygomatic bone
G Lacrimal
H Nasal
I Maxilla bone
J Mandible bone

❶ Lambdoidal suture
❷ Coronal suture
❸ **Fronto-zygomatic suture**
❹ Temporo-zygomatic suture
❺ Zygomatico-maxillary suture
❻ Parieto-temporal suture
❼ Occipito-temporal suture
❽ Spheno-temporal suture
❾ Spheno-frontal suture

Bregma
Vertex
Pterion
Glabella
Nasion
Ethmoid bone
Anterior nasal aperture
Zygomaticofacial foramen
Anterior nasal spine
Infra-orbital foramen
Lambda
Posterior pole
Asterion
Inion
External acoustic meatus
Mastoid process
Tympanic part
Styloid process
Condylar process
Zygomatic arch
Coronoid process
Zygomatic process of temporal bone
Mental protuberance
Mental foramen
Inferior border of mandible

Frontozygomatic suture. (Chaitow, 1999)

frustration (of contracts), *n* a statutory termination of a legally binding agreement because of unforeseen circumstances.

Fryette's Laws, *n.pr* a set of guiding principles developed by Harrison Fryette, DO, and used by practitioners of osteopathic medicine to discriminate between dysfunctions in the axial skeleton. Three kinds of patterns are classified. The first two solely apply to the lumbar and thoracic spinal regions, and the third applies to the spinal region.

FSR, *n* "flexed side-bent rotated," an osteopathic abbreviation used to describe vertebral position in cases of spinal dysfunction.

fu (fōō), *n* Chinese term for one of two groups into which organs are classified. The gall bladder, small intestine, large intestine, stomach, and bladder belong to the fu group. See also zang.

fu ling (fōō lēng), *n* Latin names: *Poriae cocos, Sclerotium poriae cocos,* part used: fruiting body, outer peel; uses: diuretic, relaxant; decrease blood glucose; improve general health; clear dampness; tonify spleen functions; calm the mind; act as an edema; relieve mucus imbalances; relieve urinary imbalances, diarrhea, palpitations, vertigo, relieve restlessness, anxiety; insomnia; precautions: recurring, profuse urination associated with coldness and deficiency. Also called *Poria, hoelen, poria cocos, fu ling pi,* and *fu shen.*

Fucus vesiculosus, *n* See kelpware.

fugue (fyōōg), *n* dissociative response in which an individual experiences amnesia and physically flees specific circumstances. Person may exhibit normal reactions to the situation but will have no recollection of the event or his response.

Fumaria indica, *n* See pitpapra.
Fumaria officinalis, *n* See fumitory.
fumaric acid esters (fyə·mar´·ik a´·sid es´·terz), *n.pl* Scientific names: *monoethyl fumarate, dimethyl fumarate;* uses: psoriasis; precautions: can cause nephrotoxicity; partially reversible acute renal failure, osteomalacia, gastrointestinal disturbances, flushing, skin reactions, reversible elevated levels of transaminases, eosinophilia, and reversible lymphopenia. Also called *FAE.*

fumitory, *n* Latin name: *Fumaria officinalis;* part used: flowering parts, leaves; uses: laxative, diuretic, epidermal maladies, biliary disease; uses under research: arrhythmias; precautions: pregnancy, lactation, children; patients who suffer from convulsions or elevated internal pressure within the eye; can cause lower pulse and blood pressure, convulsions with overuse, nausea. Also called *earth smoke, hedge fumitory,* and *wax dolls.*

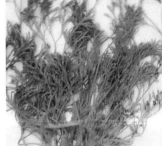

Fumitory. (Williamson, 2002)

functional adequacy, *adj* measure of a particular nutrient to determine marginal deficiency that may require dietary change or supplementation.

functional complaints, *n.pl* interruptions in a patient's health, such as daily aches and pains, sleep disorders, digestive problems, fatigue, and mild depression, that can significantly affect the quality of life but have no organic cause.

functional group (funk'·shən·əl grōōp'), *n* an atom or group of atoms of a molecule that is chemically reactive and imparts the chemical characteristics of a molecule. Alkenes, aldehydes, alcohols, carboxylic acids, ketones, and esters are common functional groups.

functional integration, *n* in the Feldenkrais method, refers to the application of techniques in a one-on-one lesson in which the instructor may use vocal or tactile instruction or a combination of the two.

functional limitation, *n* according to the World Health Organization (WHO), any health problem that prevents a person from completing a range of tasks, whether simple or complex.

functional magnetic resonance imaging (fMRI), *n* a diagnostic tool that uses Magnetic Resonance Imaging (MRI) equipment to study ongoing brain activity. Provides a real time depiction of brain functioning by tracking blood flow in the brain, an indicator of brain activity. Used to study mental illnesses.

functional neuromuscular stimulation (funk'·shə·nəl ner'·ō·mus'·kyə·ler sti'·myə·lā'·shən), *n* rehabilitative therapy for paralysis that involves sequential electrical stimulation of muscles to retrain movement patterns.

functional (neutral) range, *n* a painless range of motion in which maintaining proximal stability and proper form occurs during exercise training.

functional spinal unit (FSU), *n* the smallest possible representation of the spine that can demonstrate the biomechanical characteristics of the spine. Made up of the intervertebral disc, two vertebrae, and the interconnecting ligaments.

functional view, *n* the belief that patterns of movement are learned; treatments that flow from this paradigm focus on the improvement of strength, posture, range, and quality of movement.

fundus (fən·dəs), *n* the part of an organ that is farthest from the opening of the organ, for example, the fundus of the stomach, or uterus.

fungicide (fun'·ji·sīd'), *n* a substance that kills fungi, used to treat fungal infections.

furocoumarins (fyur'·ō·kōō·mar'·inz), *n.pl* chemical substances that sensitize the skin to the effects of the sun, thus leading to irregular pigmentation and increasing the risk of sunburn and phototoxicity.

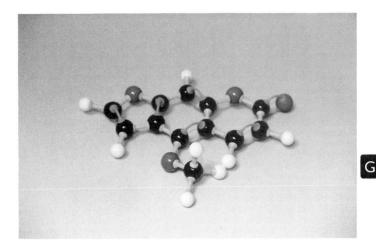

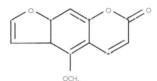

Furocoumarins. (Clarke, 2002)

G

FVC, *n* See forced vital capacity.

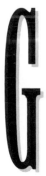

GABA, *n.pr* See acid, gamma-aminobutyric.

L - Glutamic acid ⟶ GABA

Glutamic acid decarboxylase
(B₆ complex dependent)

GABA. (Pizzorno and Murray, 1999)

galactagogic, *adj* inducing lactation. See also lactogenic.

galactagogue (gə·lak'·tə·gôg), *n* a substance that promotes the flow of breast milk.

galanthamine (gə lan' thə mēn), *n* Latin name: *Galanthus nivalis;* part used: bulbs; uses: polio-induced paralysis, myasthenia gravis, Alzheimer's disease; precautions: pregnancy, lactation, children; patients exposed to organophosphate fertilizers; can cause dizziness, confusion, insomnia, nausea, stomach cramps, diarrhea.

Galanthus nivalis, *n* See galanthamine.

Galega officinalis, *n* See goat's rue.

gall, *n* **1.** a bulbous plant structure that is formed in response to an injury or invasion by microorganisms. Often, plant galls contain medicinal phytochemicals. **2.** See also bile.

G

gall bladder, *n* a small pouchlike organ located beneath the liver; responsible for storing bile and secreting it into the small intestine (duodenum).

gall stones, *n.pl* pieces of solid material comprised of numerous inorganic and organic substances, including bile salts, electrolytes, bilirubin, fatty acids, water, and cholesterol that develop within the gallbladder and can potentially obstruct the flow of bile and digestive enzymes. Age, diet, race, gender, obesity, gastrointestinal diseases, and certain drugs can increase the risk of development.

gallows humor, *n* a dark or morbid sense of humor unique to people who deal with suffering and tragedy—for example, patients who are terminally ill joking about their illness or death as a means of coping with the illness.

galvanic skin response, *n* change in electrical conductivity of the skin usually brought on by changes in emotion—for example, fear. Also known as *electrodermal response*. See also biofeedback.

galvanometer (gal'·və·nô'·mə·ter), *n* a device for measuring the electrical conductivity of the skin.

gamma (gya'·mə), *n* Greek letter represented by γ. See also Greek letters.

gamma-hydroxybutyrate (gya'·mə -hī·drôk'·sē·byōō'·tə·rāt), *n* uses: induce sleep; stimulate release of growth hormone; treat narcolepsy; weight control; and use for recreation as a euphoric and hallucinogen; precautions: seizure disorders, bradycardia, cardiovascular disease, Cushing's syndrome, severe hypertension, hyperprolactinemia. Not to be used with benzodiazepines, alcohol, opioids, skeletal muscle relaxants, barbiturates, anticonvulsants, antihistamines, protease inhibitors, major tranquilizers. Can produce hallucinogenic or euphoric states; can cause nausea, depression, vertigo, respiratory distress, lightheadedness, vomiting, abnormal muscle movements, confusion, drowsiness, lack of coordination, loss of bladder control, diarrhea, temporary amnesia, loss of consciousness, seizure-like activity, somnambulism and coma; can become addictive. Also called *cherry meth, liquid X, fantasy, organic quaalude, GBH, salty water, Georgia home boy, scoop, sleep-500, soap, liquid E, somatomaz, liquid ecstasy,* and *vita-G.*

gamma-oryzanol (gya'·mə-ō·rī'· zə·nôl), *n* a nutritional supplement, which is found in grains and isolated from rice bran oil; used to treat menopausal symptoms and to lower blood cholesterol triglyceride levels.

Gandharva Veda (gən'·dhär·və vā'· də), *n.pr* ancient classical music of India used in Ayurveda, the components of which—ragas (melodies) and rhythms—are believed to rectify imbalances in doshas. Listening to a particular raga at the right time brings about harmony between the body and nature while the same raga may have an antagonistic effect at another time. See also doshas.

gangrene, *n* tissue death due to loss of blood circulation and bacterial activity. Usually affects extremities but can occur as a complication from other diseases such as the gall bladder and intestines.

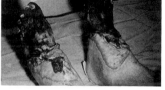

Gangrene. (Auerbach, 1995; Cameron Bangs, MD)

Ganoderma lucidum, *n* See reishi.

ganzfeld (gyanz'·fəld), *n* a technique developed to research mental imagery and anomalous cognition using visual deprivation, in which a subject is situated in a uniform visual field by wearing translucent, monochromatic goggles and in an analogous audio field using white noise playing through headphones.

gap junction, *n* channel between two cells through which communication with neighboring cells occurs.

gap junction complex, *n* areas in the membranes of contiguous cells that permit intercellular communication and transfer.

garbling, *v* in herbal medicine, to separate the useable part of the plant from any irrelevant matter, including dirt or other plant parts.

Garcinia cambogia, n See acid, hydroxycitric.

Gardenia gummifera, n See cumbiresin.

gargles, *n.pl* alcohol- or water-based solutions that are used to treat throat conditions. Typical uses are as demulcents or astringents.

garlic, *n* Latin name: *Allium sativum*; part used: roots (bulbs); uses: antilipidemic, antimicrobial, antiasthmatic, antiinflammatory, antioxidant, antiplatelet, antidiabetic, and potential anticancer; precautions: patients with hyperthyroidism, gastritis; those taking anticoagulants, insulin, antidiabetics, or acidophilus. Also called *ail, allium, camphor of the poor, dasuan, knoblauch, la-suan, nectar of the gods, poor-man's treacle, rustic treacle, or stinking rose.*

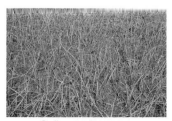

Garlic. (Williamson, 2002)

GAS, *n.pr* See syndrome, general adaptation.

gas-chromatography/mass spectrometry information (gyas'-krō·mə·tô'·grə·fē/mas' spek·trô'·mə·trē in·fər·mā'·shən), *n* details about the relative concentration of components in an essential oil, used as an aid in determining the oil's purity.

gas discharge visualization, *n* the appearance of images of the fluorescence (and, some argue, the biofield or aura) that surrounds living tissue after it has been exposed to a high-intensity field of electricity. The term describes both the technique and the device used. Also called *bioelectography, biological emission and optical radiation stimulated by electromagnetic field amplified by gas discharge with visualization through computer data processing, Kirlianography,* or *Kirlian photography.*

gas-liquid chromatography, *n* technique used to test essential oils and other substances for quality.

gastrectomy (gya·strek'·tə·mē), *n* surgical removal of the stomach, either complete or partial.

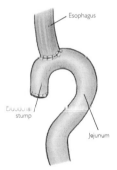

Gastrectomy. (Monahan and Neighbors, 1998)

gastric stapling, *n* surgical procedure in which the stomach is divided with stainless steel staples into two compartments—one large and one small—so food is prevented from entering one compartment. The procedure is used to assist weight loss in cases of morbid obesity. Also called *vertical silastic ringed gastroplasty.*

gastrin, *n* a digestive hormone produced in the antral part of the stomach that stimulates production of hydrochloric acid in the gastric glands.

gastroenteritis, *n* inflamed stomach and intestines, often associated with diarrhea. Also called *enterogastritis.*

gastroesophageal reflux (gas'·trō·eh·sô'·fə·gē·əl rē'·fləks), *n* a condition in which contents of the stomach flow up into the esophagus.

gastrointestinal (gas·trō·in·tes·tə·nəl), *adj* of or pertaining to the stomach and intestines.

gastrotomy (ga·strō'·tə·mē), *n* opening created surgically in the abdominal wall for the purpose of providing access to the stomach to feed an individual who is incapable of normal food intake.

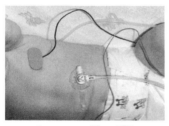

Gastrostomy. (Wong, 1993)

Gaultheria procumbens, *n* See wintergreen.

gay-related immune deficiency, *n* the term adopted in the 1980s in reference to AIDS, when it was considered to affect only homosexual males.

GB, *n* gall bladder channel; an acupuncture channel running from the head to the feet on the sides of the body and associated with the liver (LR) channel. See also LR.

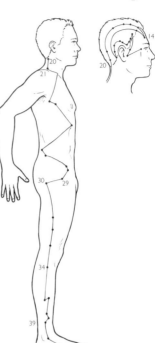

GB. (Chirali, 1999)

GC/GLC, *n.pr* See gas-liquid chromatography.

Gelidium cartilagineum, *n* See agar.

gels, *n.pl* herbal suspensions made from gums, gelatin, or pectin that are used on mucosae and in cases in which long-lasting, slow-acting astringent properties are needed.

Gelsemium sempervirens, *n* See yellow jessamine.

gemmotherapy (je'·mō·the·'rə·pē), *n* the use of plant/glycerin or plant/alcohol macerates mixed according to the French Pharmacopia to treat the tissues and organs for which the mixtures have an affinity.

gene, *n* the unit of heredity that is made of a DNA sequence occupying a specific location on a chromosome and codes for a polypeptide chain.

gene pool, *n* the sum of genes in a given population.

general practitioner, *n* a medical doctor who attends to the everyday medical needs of individuals within a community.

generalized entanglement, *n* in quantum physics, a state wherein what previously seemed to be manifold, discrete phenomena subsequently appear as unitary through time and space.

generals, *n.pl* information gathered by homeopathic doctors about a patient's tendencies. Generals are further divided into the categories of preferences and modalities.

generous, *adj* in Chinese medicine, pertaining to warm, giving behavior. When imbalanced, these traits can transform into heated, aggressive behaviors. This may be a normal aspect of a person's character, or it may indicate an illness or imbalance.

genetics, *n* branch of scientific study concerned with heredity and the causes of variance between related organisms.

Genista tinctoria, *n* See broom, Dyer's.

genistein **(ge´·nə·stīn),** *n* an isoflavone derived from soy that acts as both an antioxidant and a source of phytoestrogen, used to prevent osteoporosis, to reduce cholesterol, to relieve menopausal complaints, and as a chemopreventive.

genotype (jē´·nō·tīp), *n* an organism's genetic makeup.

gentian (jen´·shən), *n* Latin names: *Gentiana lutea* L., *Gentiana acaulis* L.; parts used: roots, rhizomes; uses: appetite stimulant, digestive ailments; precautions: pregnancy, children; patients with chronic upset stomachs, ulcers, or liver disease; can cause headaches and nausea. Also called *bitter root, bitterwort, feltwort,* and *gall weed.*

Gentiana acaulis **L.,** *n* See gentian.

genus, *n* in biology, a group of related species. In the binomial system of nomenclature, the genus is listed first.

geomagnetic field, *n* the magnetic field produced by the earth.

geopathic stress, *n* negative health affects on the body caused by geo-electromagnetic frequencies.

geophagia (gē·ō·fā´·zhē·ə), *n* compulsive drive to eat dirt or clay. A type of pica, believed to be related to a mineral deficiency or imbalance.

Geranium maculatum **L,** *n* See tormentil.

GERD, *n.pr* See disease, gastro-esophageal reflux.

gestation, *n* the period of time between the fertilization of a mammal's egg until the time it is born.

Geum urbannum, *n* See avens.

GH, *n.pr* See growth hormone.

ghasard (ghä·särd´), *n* a traditional preparation originating from India; used to facilitate digestion.

ghrita (ghrē´·tə), *n* in Ayurveda, medicated oils derived from plants or minerals.

ginger, *n* Latin name: *Zingiber officinale*; parts used: roots; uses: stimulates digestion, colic, flatulence, nausea, indigestion, expectorant; precautions: none known, but long-term use of large doses can aggravate heat sensitivities.

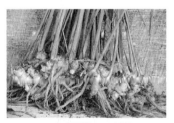

Ginger. (Williamson, 2002)

gingivitis, *n* an inflammatory periodontal disease that affects the area within the oral cavity called the gingiva. Inflamed tissue in the gingival region, bleeding, and changes in contour are common symptoms. See also disease, periodontal.

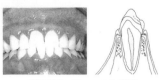

Gingivitis. (Murray et al, 1994)

gingko, *n* Latin name: *Gingko biloba;* parts used: leaves; uses: vascular insufficiency, antioxidant, circulation, cognitive enhancement, depression, headaches, tinnitus, altitude sickness, intermittent claudication; precautions: patients with bleeding disorders; those taking anticoagulants, MAOIs, platelet inhibitors. Also called *maidenhair tree, rokan, sophium, tanakan, tebofortan,* or *tebonin.*

Gingko biloba, *n* See gingko.

ginseng, *n* Latin names: *Panax ginseng, Panax quinquefolius;* part used: uses: adaptogen, immunostimulant, endurance, fatigue and stress, concentration, tonic, diabetes; occasionally used for hyperlipidemia, cancer, rheumatism, male infertility and sexual dysfunction; precautions: high blood pressure, cardiac conditions; patients taking anticoagulants, insulin, MAOIs, antidiabetics, stimulants, or ephedra. Also called *American ginseng, Asian ginseng, Asiatic ginseng, Chinese ginseng, five-fingers, Japanese ginseng, jintsam, Korean ginseng, ninjin, Oriental ginseng, schinsent, seng and sang, tartar root, true ginseng,* or *Western ginseng.*

ginseng, American, *n.pr* See ginseng.

ginseng, Asian (ā'·zhən jin'·sing), *n* Latin name: *Panax ginseng;* part used: roots; uses: general health, illness protection, antiinflammatory, muscle relaxant, tumor prevention, stimulant; precautions: pregnancy; can cause high blood pressure, diabetes, sleeplessness, diarrhea, painful breasts, mania, vaginal bleeding.

ginseng, eleuthero, *n* See ginseng, Siberian.

ginseng, Siberian (sī·bē'·rē·ən gin'·sing), *n.pr* Latin names: *Acanthopanax senticosus, Eleutherococcus senticosus, Hedera senticosa;* parts used: roots; uses: adaptogen, radiostimulant, anticancer, immunostimulant, immunomodulator, genital herpes, athletic performance, energy, antiinflammatory, insomnia; precautions: pregnancy, lactation, children; do not use over three concurrent months; do not use with antidiabetic medications, immunosuppressive medications, cardiac glycosides, stimulants, ephedra. Also called *devil's shrub, Russian ginseng, shigoka,* or *touch-me-not.*

ginseng, true, *n* See ginseng, Asian.

giveaway ritual and feast (giv'·ə·wā ri'·chə·wəl and fēst'), *n* in Native American culture, a ceremony held to redistribute a person's possessions within the community. The purpose of the rite is to honor significant events including birth, naming ceremony, or healing from a disease. Within a Native American community, a person is given a higher status if he or she gives away more possessions. This selfless attitude is an indication that a person is following the original instructions given to him or her by the great spirit.

giving-up/given-up complex, *n* a psychologic condition in which negative emotional states hinder an individual's capabilities to cope with day-to-day challenges. Often precedes an illness.

G-Jo, *n.pr* a system derived from acupuncture in which pressure is applied to specific points of the body in order to induce a reflex response.

GLA, *n* gamma linoleic acid, an essential fatty acid found in rosehip seed, evening primrose, blackcurrant seed, starflower, borage, and other foods.

gland, *n* an organ with specialized cells that secretes or excretes materials into the body. Classified into exocrine glands that secrete via ducts and endocrine glands that secrete directly into the bloodstream.

glaucoma, *n* a disease of the eye caused by an increase in the fluid pressure within the eyes. Initially, the disease is asymptomatic. However, as it progresses, the field of vision may decrease eventually resulting in blindness. Nutritional supplements such as vitamin C, bioflavonoids, magnesium, chromium, and fish oil may help.

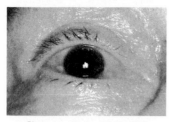

Glaucoma. (Apple and Rabb, 1998)

GLC, *n.pr* See gas-liquid chromatography.

Glechoma hederacea, *n* See ground ivy.

gliding, *n* massage technique that comprises long and smooth strokes toward the heart. Commonly used for preparation and warming. Also called *effleurage*.

global muscles, *n.pl* muscles located toward the front of the external and internal obliques, quadratus lumborum's lateral fibers, erector spinae's lateral segments, and rectus abdominus. These muscles control the ability of the spine to resist bending and impact the alignment of the spine by complying and balancing two imposing forces.

glove anesthesia, *n* a hypnotic technique used to relieve pain. The patient's hand is made to feel numb; the numbness then acts as an anesthetic by transferring the numbness to any other body part that it touches.

glucomannan (glōō·ko·man·nən), *n* Latin name: *Amorphophallus konjac;* part used: tubers; uses: laxative; uses under research: weight loss, antidiabetic, cardiovascular disease; precautions: pregnancy, lactation, children; can cause hypoglycemia, nausea, diarrhea, gas, abdominal cramps, dyspepsia, and stomach

blockage. Also called *konjac* and *konjac mannan.*

glucosamine (glōō·kō'·sə·mēn), *n* 2-amino-2-deoxyglucose in chitin, mucopolysaccharides, and mucoproteins. Used with chondroitin for osteoarthritis. Not for consumption by children, pregnant or nursing women, and people with diabetes. Can cause sleepiness, headaches, nausea, constipation, diarrhea, esophageal reflux, upset stomach, and rashes. Also called *chitosamine* and *GS.* See also chondroitin.

glucose metabolism, *n* the process by which simple sugars found in many foods are processed and used to produce energy in the form of ATP. Once consumed, glucose is absorbed by the intestines and into the blood. Extra glucose is stored in the muscles and liver as glycogen. When needed, it is hydrolyzed to glucose and released into the blood.

glucosinolates (glōō·kō'·sin·ō·lāts), *n.pl* glycoside compounds that are found in broccoli, Brussels sprouts, and cabbage and that contribute to the pungency of mustard and horseradish. They act as irritants and are sometimes used as antiinflammatories, antifungals, and antibacterials. They may have anticarcinogenic effects.

glucosuria (glōō·kō'·sə·rē·ə), *n* atypical occurrence of glucose in urine, may be due to excessive carbohydrate ingestion or a disorder, such as diabetes mellitus.

glucuronidation (gloo·kə·ro·nə·dā'·shən), *n* a phase II detoxification pathway occurring in the liver in which glucuronic acid is conjugated with toxins. Effectively detoxifies the majority of commonly prescribed drugs.

glutamate (glōō'·tə·māt), *n* an excitatory neurotransmitter found in the central nervous system of mammals and used as a flavor enhancer in its sodium salt form, monosodium glutamate (MSG). Controversy surrounds MSG and glutamate because of its role in MSG symptom complex (also known as the *Chinese restaurant syn-*

G

drome) and its deleterious effects as a potential excitotoxin.

glutamine (glōō'·tə·mēn), *n* an amino acid synthesized within the body from glutamic acid. Used in preventing immunosuppression after exercise and as an aid in recovery after a critical illness. Precaution urged for those sensitive to monosodium glutamate, those who suffer from manic conditions, and patients who are taking anticonvulsants. Also called *L-glutamine*.

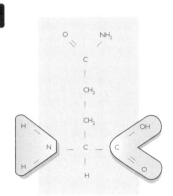

Glutamine. (Mosby's Medical, Nursing & Allied Health Dictionary, ed 6, 2002)

glutathione (glōō'·tə·thī'·ōn), *n* a tripeptide that comprises cysteine, glutamic acid, and glycine. An important antioxidant, instrumental in the glutathione conjugation detoxification pathway. See also glutathione conjugation.

glutathione conjugation, *n* a phase II detoxification reaction in the liver; glutathione combines with toxins and converts them into water-soluble mercaptates. Effectively detoxifies acetaminophen and nicotine.

gluten, *n* a protein, found in wheat and rye. It is a common cause of food allergies.

gluten enteropathy, *n* See disease, celiac.

glycemic index, *n* a measurement of how much particular foods raise blood glucose levels; based on comparing the food to an equal quantity of glucose taken orally.

Food	Glycemic Index
Sugars:	
• Glucose	100
• Honey	75
• Sucrose	60
• Fructose	20
Fruits:	
• Apples	39
• Bananas	62
• Oranges	40
• O.J.	46
• Raisins	64
Vegetables:	
• Beets	64
• Carrot, raw	31
• Carrot, cooked	36
• White potato	98
Grains:	
• Bread, white	69
• Cornflakes	80
• Oatmeal	49
• Pasta	45
• Rice, white	70
• Wheat cereal	67
Legumes:	
• Beans	31
• Lentils	29
• Peas	39
Other Foods:	
• Nuts	13
• Sausages	28

Glycemic index. (Rakel, 2003)

glycine (glī'·sēn), *n* a nonessential amino acid used as an adjunct to therapy for schizophrenia. It may also improve memory; have hepatoprotective, kidney protective, and antitumor effects; and benefit those with 3-phosphoglycerate dehydrogenase deficiency and isovaleric anemia. Precaution is advised for patients taking clozapine.

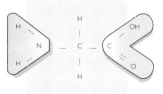

Glycine. (Mosby's Medical, Nursing & Allied Health Dictionary, ed 6, 2002)

Glycine max, *n* See soy.

glycoside, *n* plant-derived compound that breaks down into a sugar and an aglycon when processed with water.

glycosylation (glī·kō'·sə·lā'·shən), *n* process in which a carbohydrate is covalently attached to another molecule.

Glycyrrhiza glabra, *n* See licorice.

goat's rue, *n* Latin name: *Galega officinalis;* parts used: leaves (dried), buds, stalks; uses: diuretic, antidiabetic; precautions: pregnancy, lactation, children; can cause headaches, anxiety, and nausea. Also called *French honeysuckle, French lilac,* and *Italian fitch.*

goiter, *n* distended thyroid gland, usually manifested as a noticeable bulge in the neck.

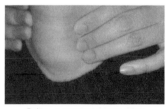

Goiter. (Lemmi and Lemmi, 2000)

gokshura (gŏk·shŏŏ'·rə), *n* Latin name: *Tribulus terrestris;* part used: seed, plant, flower, stem, fruit; uses: improve general health, anthelmintic, sexual desire, carminative, softening of irritated tissues, diuretic, milk production suppression; respiratory disease, infertility, menstrual dysfunction, blood circulation, impotency, nocturnal emissions, gonorrhea, incontinence of urine, painful urination, gout, relieve kidney dysfunction, cancer, leprosy, skin disease, congestion, headache, liver dysfunctions, ophthalmia, stomatitis; precautions: abortifacient. Also called *caltrop, abrojo, burra gokeroo, burra gokhru, burra gookeroo, chi li, chih hsing, goatsheads, gokru kalan, gotub, hasach, ji li, kadava gokharu, kathe nerinnil, khasake kalan, kon jarah,*

nd, pai chi li, puncture vine, sha yuan chi li, tu chi li, and *tzu.*

goldenrod, *n* Latin name: *Solidago virgaurea;* parts used: buds, leaves; uses: antispasmodic, diuretic, abortifacient, antiinflammatory, urinary tract infections, urolithiasis, earaches; precautions: pregnancy, lactation, children; patients with heart or kidney disease; can cause nausea, rashes, difficulty during breathing, hemorrhage in digestive tract, stomach edemas, tachypnea, enlargement of the spleen, and death. Also called *Aaron's rod, blue mountain tea, denrod,* and *woundwort.*

goldenseal, *n* Latin name: *Hydrastis canadensis;* part used: rhizomes (dried); uses: antimicrobial, expectorant, antiinflammatory, gastritis, digestive and oral ulcers, bladder infections, sore throat, epidermal infections, cancer, tuberculosis; precautions: pregnancy, lactation, children; patients with heart conditions or ruptured eardrums; not recommended for more than 6 weeks at one time, can cause bradycardia, asystole, anxiety, convulsions, nausea, diarrhea, stomach cramps, and paralysis (elevated doses). Also called *eye balm, eye root, goldsiegel, ground raspberry, Indian dye, Indian paint, Indian turmeric, jaundice root, orange root, turmeric root, yellow paint, yellow puccoon, yellow root, warnera,* and *wild curcuma.*

gomphosis (gôm'·fō'·sis), *n* a fibrous articulation within the periosteal lining, such as that present in the tooth socket.

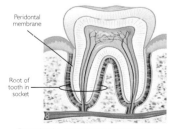

Peridontal membrane

Root of tooth in socket

Gomphosis. (Mosby's Medical, Nursing & Allied Health Dictionary, ed 6, 2002)

Gonstead, *n.pr* chiropractic technique in which thrusts are directed in the direction opposite to that of the complaint area. X-rays assist the chiropractor in pinpointing the area to be treated.

Gonzalez protocol, *n.pr* a therapy for cancer characterized by a regimen of pancreatic enzymes, nutritional supplements (including papaya enzymes, glandular extract, and trace minerals), and coffee enemas.

Gossypium herbaceum, *n* See cotton.

Gossypium hirsutum, *n* See gossypol.

gossypol (gä˙·sə·pōl), *n* Latin name: *Gossypium hirsutum;* parts used: stalks, roots, seeds; uses: contraceptive, dysmenorrhea, labor inducer; precautions: pregnancy, lactation, children; patients with kidney and liver disease; can cause cardiac failure, nausea, diarrhea, muscle weakness, and paralysis. Also called *American upland cotton* and *cotton.*

goti (gō·tē), *n* in Ayurveda, pills that are derived from plants or minerals.

gotu kola (gō˙·tōō kō˙·lə), *n* Latin name: *Centella asiatica;* part used: leaves (dried), aerial parts; uses: stimulant, nerve tonic, antipyretic, leucoderma, hypertension, cancer, liver disease, abdominal maladies, bronchitis, seizure disorders, intestinal cysts, gum disease, lacerations, psoriasis, eczema, leprosy, poor memory; precautions: pregnancy, lactation, children; people allergic to celery; can cause rashes, photosensitivity, pruritus, elevated glucose and cholesterol levels, and sleepiness. Also called *centella, hydrocotyle, Indian pennywort, Indian water navelwort, kula kudi, mandukparni, marsh penny,*

talepetrako, teca, water pennywort, and *white rot.*

gout (gaut), *n* a type of arthritis, which affects primarily males, that is triggered by increased uric acid in serum and joints. The uric acid forms crystals. A common symptom is intense pain and swelling of the metatarsophalangeal joint of the big toe. Also called *rich man's disease.*

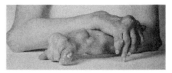

Gout. (American College of Rheumatology. Reprinted from the Clinical Slide Collection of the Rheumatic Diseases, 1991, 1995, 1997)

GP, *n.pr* general practitioner, medical doctor.

Gracilaria confervoides, *n* See agar.

grade V mobilization, *n* See HVT.

grafting, *n* **1.** transplantation of tissue from one side to another, as in skin grafting with burns. **2.** in homeopathy, a controversial method of augmenting the remainder of an existing remedy with a different dosage form or other nonmedicated tablets.

Graminis rhizomo, *n* See couchgrass.

granulation promotion, *n* property of some substances that aids in healing tissue damage and scar formation.

granulocytes (gran˙·yə·lō·sāts), *n.pl* white blood cells with granules of cytoplasm.

granulocytopenia (gran˙·yu·lō·sī˙·tə·pē˙·nē·ə), *n* decreased volume of granulocytes in the blood. Also called *granulopenia* or *neutropenia.*

granuloma (gran·yə·lō˙·mə), *n* persistent, inflamed lesion notable for its abundance of macrophages.

Gotu kola. (Williamson, 2002)

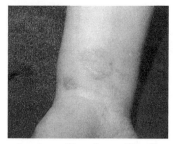

Granuloma. (Weston, Lane, and Morrelli, 1996)

grapeseed, *n* Latin name: *Vitis vinifera;* part used: seeds; uses: antioxidant, cataracts, poor circulation, cancer; precautions: pregnancy, lactation, children; can cause disorientation, nausea, rashes, and hepatotoxicity (possible). Also called *muskat.*

gravitational line, *n* an imaginary line used to visualize the ideal posture, so as to evaluate the anteroposterior curvature of the spine.

grazing, *n* See irregular feeding.

great wing of the sphenoid, *n* portion of an irregularly shaped bone at the cranium's base.

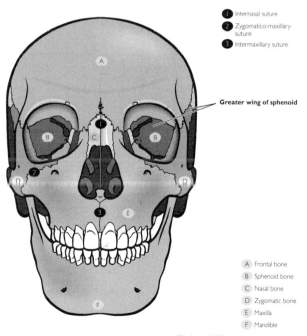

1 Internasal suture
2 Zygomatico-maxillary suture
3 Intermaxillary suture

Greater wing of sphenoid

A Frontal bone
B Sphenoid bone
C Nasal bone
D Zygomatic bone
E Maxilla
F Mandible

Great wing of the sphenoid. (Chaitow, 1999)

Greek cancer cure, *n.pr* a questionable cancer treatment propounded by Athenian microbiologist Dr. Hariton-Tzannis Alivizatos, in which a blood test is said to determine the presence, type, size, and location of cancers after which the patient receives daily injections (including niacin in water) for a period of one to four weeks. Also called *Cellbal* or *METBAL.*

Greek letters, *n.pl* symbols based on the Greek alphabet that are used to represent phenomena and objects in science.

green, *adj* in Chinese medicine, a facial coloration that indicates poor, sluggish digestion, particularly when accompanied by a muddy look in the eyes.

green food, *n* a food mixture that includes avocado, sprouts, wheatgrass, and leafy greens.

green hellebore (grēn´ he·´lə·bōr´), *n* Latin name: *Veratrum viride;* part used: root and rhizome; uses: treat pneumonia, seizure disorders, and nerve pain; precautions: individuals with cardiovascular disorders. May cause nausea, vomiting, abdominal pain, change in vision, coma, paralysis. Also called *false hellebore, Indian poke, itchweed,* and *swamp hellebore.*

green juice, *n* blended drink containing green vegetables and spices.

green tea, *n* Latin name: *Camellia sinensis;* part used: leaves (dried, unfermented); uses: antibacterial, anticancer, antilipidemic, antioxidant, diuretic, gum disease; precautions: patients with sensitivity to caffeine, kidney disease, or heart disease, or who are taking anticoagulant medications. Also called *matsucha.*

greta (grā´·tä)), *n* a traditional preparation originating from Mexico used to relieve empacho, an infection thought to be related to the obstruction of the gastrointestinal tract. There have been reports of lead poisoning from greta. See *Azarcón.*

Grifola frondosa, *n* See maitake.

grinding, *n* pulverizing solid source material together with a liquid, such as lactose to create homeopathic remedies by trituration or herbs to create a powder. See also trituration, ball mill.

groin, *n* area where the abdomen and thigh meet. Also called *inguinal.*

ground ivy, *n* Latin name: *Glechoma hederacea;* parts used: flowers, leaves; uses: sinusitis, allergies, diarrhea, bronchitis; precautions: nausea. Also called *alehoof, cat's foot, creeping Charlie, haymaids,* or *hedgemaids.*

ground system, *n* See connective tissue.

groups, *n.pl* columns of elements within a periodic table. All elements within a group have the same number of electrons in the outer shell.

growth hormone (grōth´ hōr´· mōn), *n* a hormone produced by the pituitary gland; involved in the division of cells and the growth and maintenance of tissues. Also called *GH, HGH, human growth hormone,* or *somatotropin.*

gSowa rigpa (sō-wä rēg-pä), *n* ancient form of Tibetan medicine or the "healing knowledge," believed to be based on the teachings of the Buddha.

GSR, *n.pr* See galvanic skin response.

gua sha (kwä sà), *n* technique used in traditional Chinese medicine; a porcelain soup spoon is scraped across the patient's skin in order to produce a rash—"sha"—that will fade in two or three days. Raising "sha" removes blockages in blood stagnation, thereby promoting normal circulation and metabolic processes.

guan (gwän), *n* in traditional Chinese medicine—in addition to "cun" and "chi"—one of the three divisions of the pulse that is used for diagnosis. Specifically, its position is near the styloid process of the radius. On the left hand, the pulse of guan is associated with the condition of the liver and on the right hand, it is associated with the condition of the spleen.

guar gum (gwär gəm), *n* Latin name: *Cyamopsis tetragonolobus;* part used: endosperm; uses: hyperlipidemia, obesity, diabetes mellitus;

precautions: none known. Also called *guar flour, gucran, Indian cluster bean,* or *jaguar gum.*

guarana (**gwä·rä'·nə**), *n* Latin names: *Paullinia cupana, Paullinia sorbilis;* part used: seeds; uses: antioxidant, stimulant, weight loss; precautions: pregnancy, lactation, patients with sensitivity to caffeine, high blood pressure, kidney disease, and heart disease. Also called *Brazilian cocoa, guarana gum, guarana paste,* or *zoom.*

guarding (**gär'·ding**), *n* **1.** phenomenon in which muscles react to an injury to a joint, bone or ligament by contracting in order to form a protective splint. **2.** a sign detected during physical pain whereby the patient involuntarily contracts muscles second to pain.

guduchi (**gōō·dōō'·chē**), *n* Latin name: *Tinospora cordifolia;* part used: stem; uses: relieve pain, reduce joint inflammation, treat chronic fever; precautions: none known. Also called *cochinnaruha, gulancha, gurach, heartleaved moonseed, k'uan chin t'eng, k'uan chu hsing, moonseed, nirjara,* and *putrawuli.*

guggul (**gōōg'·gəl**), *n* Latin name: *Commiphora mukul;* part used: resin; uses: astringent, antiseptic, antiinflammatory, gum disease, high cholesterol, arthritis, obesity, acne, diabetes; in Ayurveda, pacifies tridosha (pungent, bitter, light, dry, sharp); precautions: pregnancy, lactation. Also called *gugulipid, guggulu, Indian bdellium tree, mukul myrrh tree,* or *myrrh.*

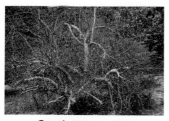
Guggul. (Williamson, 2002)

guided imagery, *n* directed relaxation and visualization to support changes in health.

guided imagery and music, *n* therapy that combines music and deep relaxation states to explore and guide thoughts and feelings.

guiding, *n* gentle assisted movement by an osteopath, of a body part through its normal range of motion.

gum Arabic, *n* Latin name: *Acacia senegal;* part used: gum; uses: lower cholesterol, kidney conditions, gum disease, oral health, sore throat, diarrhea; precautions: none known. Also called *Egyptian thorn* or *senega.*

guru, *adj* **1.** in Ayurveda, "heavy" as a guna, one of the qualities characterizing all substances. Its complement is laghu. **2.** a spiritual teacher, particularly in Tantric traditions. See also gunas and laghu.

gutika (**gōō·tē'·kə**), *n* manual containing specific details for yoga-based meditation, including phrases that the individual is instructed to chant repeatedly during a session.

GV, *n* the governor vessel, an acupuncture channel running from the tailbone to the upper lip along the back of the body.

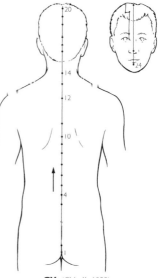
GV. (Chirali, 1999)

G

gymnastik, *n* a somatic education learning approach developed by Elsa Gindler in Germany around 1910 which emphasizes inward focus during external movements, thus resulting in greater self-control.

gymnema (jim·nē´·mə), *n* Latin name: *Gymnema sylvestre;* parts used: leaves, root; uses: in Ayurveda, pacifies kapha and pitta doshas (astringent, bitter, light, dry), antiviral, antioxidant, hepatoprotection, dysentery, diabetes mellitus, tooth decay, uterine tonic; precautions: patients with diabetes who take hypoglycemic medications. Also called gurmar, meshasringi, or *periploca of the wood.*

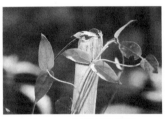

Gymnema. (Williamson, 2002)

Gymnema sylvestre, *n* See gymnema.

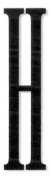

habituation, *n* the process of decreased response to repeated stimulation.

hachimijiogan (a·chē· mē·jē·ō·gän), *n* a medicinal formula that comprises eight herbs developed in Chinese medicine and currently used for the treatment of cataracts. Therapeutic effects include increased antioxidant level within the lens of the eye.

hacking (ha´·king), *n* a massage technique consisting of quick, rhythmic chops, using the blade of the hand. See also tapotement.

Hahnemannism (hô´·nə·ma·nizm), *n.pr* homeopathic force that is believed to allow one remedy to confer its healing ability on other nonmedicated substances. Glass and cork were thought to be a barrier to this force. This notion is not commonly recognized by homeopaths. See also grafting.

half homeopaths, *n* derogatory name coined by Hahnemann for practitioners who blend homeopathy with allopathy. Also called *mongrels.*

halisteresis (ha·lis·te·rē´·sis), *n* a theoretical bone resorption process, in which humoral mechanisms transfer bone salts to body tissue fluids, thereby rendering the bone matrix decalcified.

halitosis, *n* offensive-smelling breath; may be caused by inadequate oral hygiene, fasting, infections, smoking, eating strong-smelling foods, or certain diseases.

hallucination, *n* a phenomenon where-by subjects believe that they see another person or object that is not really present.

hallucinogen, *n* substance which distorts a person's sensory perception, inducing false perceptions such as noises and images that do not really exist.

Hamamelis virginiana, *n* See witch hazel.

hambleceya (hôm·blā·chā·yä), *n* a traditional pipe fast revived by healers of the Cheyenne River Indian Reservation at Eagle Butte as part of an alcohol treatment program.

handedness posture, *n* posture influenced by a person's dominant hand, right or left.

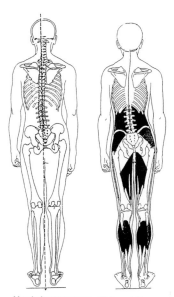

Handedness posture. (Petty and Moore, 2001)

hands-over, *n* technique used in Reiki; the practitioner's hands are held one to two inches above the surface of the client's body to transfer the universal energy rather than laying the hands directly on the person. Used for burn victims or for those who dislike being touched.

hao style (hōw stīl), *n* a traditional form of tai chi developed by the Wu family.

haploid, *adj* possessing just one set of nonhomologous chromosomes. Also called *monoploid* or *monoploidic.*

haptenization (hap·te·nī·zā·shən), *n* the combination of an antigenic compound with a carrier protein molecule, intended to achieve a high enough molecular weight to stimulate an immune response.

hara (hä·rä), *n* a Japanese term that represents the abdomen, where the internal organs are housed.

hard scientists, *n.pl* slang term used primarily to describe laboratory scien-

tists such as molecular biologists and physicists.

hardening (här·də·ning), *n* technique for the cultivation of effective physiologic responsiveness to stress.

hardiness, *n* a cluster of attitudes and behaviors that allow people to maintain health and well-being in situations of stress. These include attitudes of commitment, control and challenge; coping habits; and the creation of social support networks.

harm, *n* the condition of promoting injury or damage. The injury or damage can be described as physical, psychologic, or both.

haronga bark (hə·rông·gə bärk'), *n* Latin name: *Harungana madagascariensis;* part used: bark, leaves; uses: excretory function of the pancreas, gastric juice secretion, choleretic, cholagogic, painful digestion, mild exocrine pancreatic insufficiency; precautions: acute pancreatitis, severe liver function disorders, gallstones, ileus, gall bladder empyema, obstruction of bile ducts; can cause photosensitivity.

Harpagophytum procumbens, *n* See devil's claw.

Harrison biophysics, *n.pr* a subluxation measurement standard that uses a mathematical model of the spine to determine correct alignment; adjustments attempt to bring the spine into uniform agreement with the model.

Harvard Group Scale of Hypnotic Susceptibility, Form A, *n.pr* a standardized test used to measure an individual's ability to be hypnotized. Unlike the Stanford Hypnotic Susceptibility Scale, Form C, the test is used for clinical research purposes. A trained technician working under the supervision of a clinician can administer the assessment to a group of five to ten persons within one hour.

Haungana madagascariensis, *n* See haronga bark.

hawthorn, *n* Latin name: *Crataegus* spp.; parts used: flowers, fruits, leaves; uses: high blood pressure, arrhythmias, arteriosclerosis, Buhrger's disease, congestive heart disease, angina pectoris; precautions: patients taking beta-blockers, cardiac glycosides, CNS depressants, *Adonis vernalis,* or lily of the valley. Also called *Li 132, may, maybush, quickset, thornapple tree,* or *whitethorn.*

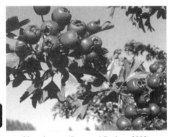

Hawthorn. (Scott and Barlow, 2003)

hay fever, *n* pollen allergy that occurs seasonally that includes sneezing, congestion, and itching of the eyes, ears, nose, and throat due to release of histamines. Antihistamines help control this condition. Also called *pollenosis* or *seasonal allergic rhinitis.*

Hb, *n.pr* See hemoglobin.

HCA, *n.pr* See acid, hydroxycitric.

HCFA, *n.pr* See Health Care Financing Administration.

HCP, *n* healthcare provider, a professional who specializes in treating and managing a person's general or specific health needs.

headache diary, *n* an approach used to monitor the headache progression of a patient throughout the treatment period. This ongoing journal provides a measurement of the intensity and frequency of a patient's headaches.

healee, *n* a person seeking healing; patient, client.

healers (hē·lerz), *n.pl* **1.** one who heals or who is trained in a healing/therapeutic art. **2.** in the traditional culture of the Cherokee, persons who employ prayer, tobacco rituals, and invocation of spirits to restore the health of a person affected by disease. Also called *dida:hnvwi: si(i).*

healing, *n* **1.** the process of recovery, repair, and restoration. **2.** return to wholeness.

healing crisis, *n* in naturopathic medicine, a healing reaction. Symptoms of bodic defense are observable and successful.

healing touch, *n.pr* nontouch therapy that employs an energy-based approach. Also called *HT.*

Healing your Heart, *n* program developed by the Department of Cardiac Rehabilitation at Union Hospital in Lynn, Massachusetts to aid recovery of cardiac patients by incorporating meditation, guided imagery, facilitated group meetings, and yoga along with traditional therapies.

healing, absent, *n* a process of relieving suffering and pain that takes place when the practitioner and patient are not in direct contact with one another. Prayer, meditation, LeShan, and Reiki are common types of practices used. Also called *distant healing.*

healing, crystal, *n* method that employs gems to alter the body's energy to treat certain mental and physical conditions.

healing, distant, *n* healing via a hypothesized form of consciousness that apparently works without recourse to any physical medium or energies.

healing, faith, *n* faith-based processes that restore the psychologic, physical, social, and spiritual aspects of a patient.

healing, lay, *n* the use of gentle techniques aimed at rebalancing either the patient's energy or the energy flow between patient and practitioner.

healing, laying-on-of-hands, *n* technique in which the practitioner places his or her hands in different positions over or on the patient to promote energy flow through them to relieve pain and suffering. Often used in spiritual healing. Also called *apostolic healing.*

healing, mental, *n* mental techniques and processes that restore the psychologic, physical, social, and spiritual aspects of a patient.

healing, miracle, *n* any healing that cannot be accountd for (or one for which the odds against are very high) through medical or psychosomatic means.

healing, paranormal (**pa'·rə·nōr'·məl hē'·ling**), *n* processes which cannot be explained scientifically that restore the psychologic, physical, social, and spiritual aspects of a patient.

healing, psychic (**sī'·kik hē'·ling**), *n* mental or psychic processes that restore the psychologic, physical, social, and spiritual aspects of a patient.

healing, qi, *n* See qi gong.

healing, self, *n* the notion that the body is capable of healing itself, regularly evidenced through the placebo effect. A highly regarded tenet of most alternative healing practices.

healing, spiritual, *n* system of faith or belief, that involves healing through meditation, prayer, or touch, in which the healer serves as a channel through which spiritual energy flows to the client.

healing, supernatural, *n* healing effected through nonmaterial or miraculous means. See also healing, miracle and supernatural mechanism.

healing, Type I, mental-spiritual, *n* practice in which the healer, through a meditative state of consciousness sees himself as completely unified with the patient. The healer does not try to consciously heal the patient but seeks to experience love, oneness, and unity with the person.

healing, Type II, mental-spiritual, *n* practice in which the healer physically touches the patient with the intent to heal, and transmits his energy to the patient.

healing, wound, *n* the natural process of repair in damaged tissues, comprising the inflammation response, the creation of a fibrin framework upon which the scab develops, the defensive action of white blood cells, the epithelial closure of the wound with myofibroblasts, and the creation of a scar.

healing community, *n* in behavioral medicine, a group of individuals

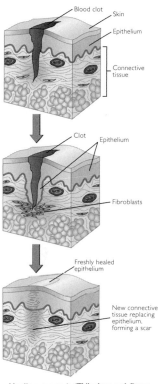

Healing, wound. (Thibodeau and Patton, 1999)

working in tandem to facilitate repair and recovery. Comprises family members, significant others, and healthcare practitioners representing several disciplines, such as primary care physicians, nurses, psychologists, and social workers.

healing energy light process, *n* meridian-based psychotherapy treatment that combines yoga-influenced visualization, HeartMath, psychologic reversal, and neurologic disorganization corrective therapies. See also HeartMath.

H

healing environment, *n* any circumstances that promote recovery from people in the direction of wholeness and healing.

healing reaction, *n* the response of a living organism to heal and defend itself in response to a pathogenic or therapeutic agent.

health, *n* a state of well-being that takes into account an individual's physical, mental, and emotional vitality and desires.

Health Care Financing Administration, *n.pr* department in the U.S. agency of Health and Human Services responsible for the oversight of the Medicaid and Medicare benefit programs, including guidelines, payment, and coverage policies.

health maintenance organization, *n* corporation formed to provide health care, often financed by the employer and employee insurance premium payments. Participating physicians, clinic, and hospital staff provide prevention and treatment to enrolled members and their families.

health professional, *n* one who uses skills and knowledge to treat patients and promote wellness in a clinic environment.

health promotion, *n* cultivation—for both individuals and communities—of habits that promote optimal physical, mental, spiritual, and environmental well-being.

health-promotion practices, *n.pl* activities and habits—including balanced diet, exercise, nutritional education, and public health initiatives that encourage healthy lifestyles.

health psychology, *n* a term used primarily in naturopathy in which counseling is provided to a patient or family.

HeartMath, *n* company that developed tools to enhance overall health; based on the crucial link between emotions, brain function, and heart rhythms. Used in the healing energy light process for correcting psychological problems.

heating pattern, *n* the measure of heat distribution in the human body or model.

heavy metals, *n.pl* metallic compounds, such as aluminum, arsenic, cadmium, lead, mercury, and nickel. Exposure to these metals has been linked to immune, kidney, and neurotic disorders.

Hedeoma pulegioides, *n* American pennyroyal. See pennyroyal.

Hedera senticosa, *n* See ginseng, Siberian.

heiaus (hā·ē·ä·ōōz), *n.pl* in the Hawaiian culture, places of power. It is believed that ancient spiritual beings guard these locations and that violation by offenders results in adversity or disease.

Heidelberg pH capsule system, *n.pr* a diagnostic test in which a miniature transmitter is swallowed and used to measure the acid secretions and pH of the stomach.

Heimlich maneuver, *n.pr* technique designed to assist a person suffering from a windpipe obstruction; the person helping wraps his arms around the person choking, and then with both hands grasped together, employs a quick, upward thrust just under the breastbone.

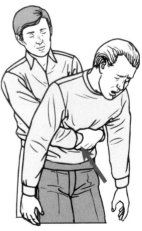

Heimlich maneuver. (Lewis, Heitkemper, and Dirksen, 2000)

Helianthus annuus, *n* See sunflower.

Helicobacter pylori (he·li·kō·bak´·ter pī·lō´·rē), *n* a bacterium implicated as a predisposing factor for most pyloric ulcers.

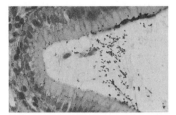

Heliobacter pylori. (Cotran, Kumar, and Collins, 1999)

helicy (hē´·lə·sē), *n* a continuously mixing and rotating property of environmental and human energy fields.

Helleborus niger, *n* See black hellebore.

Hellerwork, *n.pr* See Hellerwork Structural Integration.

Hellerwork Structural Integration, *n.pr* holistic system of bodywork and reeducation developed by Joseph Heller from the work of Dr. Ida Rolf that starts at the surface or sleeve of the body, moves to the deeper core, then unifies and integrates the changes.

helplessness, *n* a perception held by a person because of which he or she feels powerless or unable to act independently. Typically associated with persons diagnosed with chronic disease.

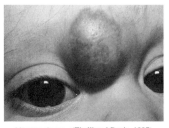

Hemangioma. (Zitelli and Davis, 1997)

hemangioma (hē·man·jē·ō´·mə), *n* a benign tumor that consists of an accumulation of blood vessels.

hematemesis (hem·ə·tə·mē´·sis), *n* the oral expulsion of blood; indicative of peptic ulcer, esophageal varices, or other conditions.

hematocrit (hē·ma´·tə·krit), *n* the number of red blood cells in a sample expressed as a percentage of the total blood volume. The normal hematocrit range is between 43% to 49% in men and 37% to 43% in women.

hematoma (hē´·mə·tō´·mə), *n* an accumulation of clotted blood that develops within an open body space, organ, or tissue as a result of damage to a blood vessel.

H

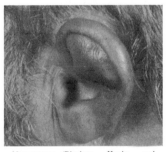

Hematoma. (Bingham, Hawke, and Kwok, 1992)

hemicelluloses, *n.pl* noncellulose polysaccharides of a branched pentose and hexose compound structure. A type of dietary fiber.

hemiplegia (he·mi·plē´·jē·ə), *n* paralysis that affects just one side of the body.

Hemiplegia. (Salvo, 2003)

hemochromatosis (hē'·mə·krō'·mə·tō'·sis), *n* a rare metabolic condition in which excess iron is deposited throughout the body. May lead to skin pigmentation, hepatomegaly, cardiac failure, or diabetes mellitus. Related to sickle-cell anemia and other hemolytic anemias.

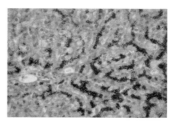

Hemochromatosis. (Kumar, Cotran, and Robbins, 1997)

hemodialysis, *n* mechanical process for removing waste products and impurities from the blood. Blood is drawn out and filtered through a dialysis machine and then reinfused. Often used in patients suffering from renal failure as well as other toxic blood conditions.

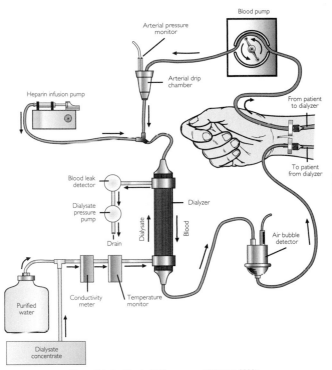

Hemodialysis. (Lewis, Heitkemper, and Dirksen, 2000)

hemoglobin, *n* a protein-iron compound in red blood cells that carries oxygen from the lungs to body cells. The normal hemoglobin levels in the blood are 12 to 16 g/dL in women and 13.5 to 18 g/dL in men.

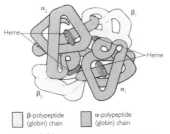

Hemoglobin. (Huether and McCance, 2000)

hemophilia (hē'·mō·fē'·lē·ə), *n* genetically transmitted condition that impairs or prevents blood from clotting.

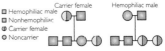

Hemophilia. (Beare and Myers, 1998)

hemorrhoids (he'·mə·roidz), *n.pl* swollen and inflamed veins in the lower portion of the anus or rectum. A common condition that typically develops during the latter months of pregnancy and after childbirth. Contributing factors include straining, low-fiber diet, anal infection, constipation, or sitting for extended periods of time during bowel movements. For some, it may be an indication of another condition such as cirrhosis of the liver. Treatment methods for this condition include eating a diet with a high amount of fiber, regularly taking bulking agents to lessen strain during bowel movements, and consuming preparations of flavonoids to strengthen the blood vessels. Topical treatments, botanical medicines, hydrotherapy, surgical options, and monopolar direct current therapy are also considered beneficial for preventing and treating this condition. See also therapy, monopolar direct current.

hemostatic, *adj/n* ability of a substance to stop the flow of blood.

hepatic (hə·pa ̍ **·tik),** *adj* **1.** pertaining to the liver. *n* **2.** a substance that stimulates healthy liver and gall bladder function.

hepatic function (hə·pa ̍ **·tik funk** ̍ **· shən),** *n* the multifarious role of the liver in the metabolism of carbohydrates, fats, proteins, alcohol, and drugs; storage of vitamins and iron; production of bile; and filtering of potential toxins from the bloodstream.

hepatic pump (hə·pa ̍ **·tik pəmp),** *n* application of rhythmic compression to the body over the liver to increase the flow of hepatic blood, lymph, and bile.

hepatitis (he ̍ **·pə·tī** ̍ **·tis),** *n* a family of infectious viral diseases characterized by inflammation of the liver.

hepatotoxicity (hep ̍ **·ə·tō·tôk** ̍ **·si· sit·ē),** *n* liver toxicity.

herb, *n* naturally occurring plant with nonwoody stems; used for medicinal and wellness purposes.

herb, crude, *n* a fresh medicinal plant, before it has been dried and processed.

herb, marsh, *n* Latin name: *Ledum palustre;* parts used: leaves, flowers; uses: bowel evacuation, diuretic, perspiration, tissue contraction, pain sleep induction, appetite stimulation, asthma, colds, cough, stomach pain, wound healing; precautions: can induce premature expulsion of a fetus; kidney irritation, urinary tract irritation, and gastrointestinal irritation.

Also called *bataklik biberiyesi, labrador tea, marsh labrador-tea, marsh labradortea, marsh tea,* and *wild rosemary.*

herbs, dispersing, *n.pl* herbs used to relieve pressure (whether physical, psychologic, and/or energetic) and as purgatives, sedatives, and for cooling and calming effects. Contraindicated for those with relatively weak constitutions.

herbs, tonic, *n.pl* herbs whose purpose is increasing strength and energy. Contraindicated for those with relatively strong, vigorous constitutions.

herbalism (er ̍ **·bə·li·zəm),** *n* study and practice of using plants to treat illness and promote health.

herbalista (yār·bä·lēs ̍ **·tə),** *n* in Curanderismo, the Mexican-American healing system, a healer who supervises herbal therapies. Also called *medica* and *herbolaria.*

herb-drug interactions, *n.pl* See drug interactions.

herbolaria, *n* See herbalista.

heredity, *n* the passing on from one generation to their offspring of genetic traits or other tendencies. See also constitution, disposition, terrain, and trait.

Hering's law of cure, *n.pr* in homeopathy, principles that govern the process of healing. Healing should occur in the following way: the opposite order that the symptoms appeared—in the vital organs before the nonvital organs, from inside the body to outside, and from the head down to the extremities.

hermeneutic circle (hur ̍ **·mə·nōō** ̍ **· tik ser** ̍ **·kəl),** *n* the interpretation of the underlying insights and understandings embodied in a treatment program, which involves both the practitioner and client as they determine the reason for the unsatisfactory health status of the client and work toward a program for his or her betterment.

hernia, *n* condition in which a part of the peritoneum or an intestine protrudes through weakened muscles, either of the diaphragm or of the abdominal wall. Hernias are typically classified based on their location.

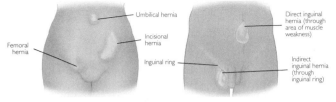

Hernia. (Leonard, 2001)

herniation of the medulla oblongata, *n* dire medical condition in which the medulla oblongata protrudes from the foramen magnum.

herpes simplex, *n* disease caused by the herpes simplex virus characterized by episodic blisters on the mucous membranes and skin.

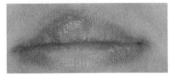

Herpes simplex. (Lemmi and Lemmi, 2000)

herpes zoster (her·'·pēz zôs·'·ter), *n* infection that tends to afflict adults caused by activation of the latent varicella zoster virus along a nerve pathway. Symptoms include painful blisters and red skin eruptions that are responsive to antiviral medications if taken early. Also called *shingles.*

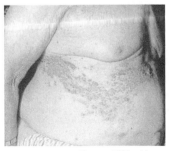

Herpes zoster. (Bryant, 2000; Mary Brahman, Abbott Northwestern Hospital, Minneapolis)

Herxheimer reaction, *n.pr* an increase in the number or degree of symptoms caused by a rapid destruction of antigens, cell particles, and toxins, that occur during treatment.

hesperidin (hes·'·pə·ri·din), *n* a flavonoid pigment derived from citrus fruits, used in combination with diosmin (in a 1:9 ratio) to improve the tone of veins; to normalize the permeability of capillaries; and to treat vascular conditions such as hemorrhoids, chronic venous insufficiency, and fragile capillaries. No precautions known. See also diosmin, flavonoids.

heteropathy, *n* **1.** sensitivity to generally painless touch. Also called *hyperesthesia.* **2.** method of treatment using interventions that counter the disease. Opposite of homeopathy. Also called *allopathy.*

heterostasis (he·'·tə·rō·stā·'·sis), *n* maintenance of physiologic stability in circumstances of change, whether predictable or unpredictable, through adaptation. Also called *allostasis.*

heuristic, *n* self-education built from actual events rather than theory. Also called *empirical.*

hex, *n* a curse; a transcendent force or energy employed for malevolent purposes or a type of imagery shared between two persons via an imaginary, unseen channel that is used to harm instead of heal. In Western tradition, it is considered to be a self-fulfilling prophecy, a prediction of an event due to a strong belief in the outcome.

hierarchy of evidence, *n* the sequence of scientific evidence; a means of judging evidence presented in medical literature. Criteria for judging include how the clinical subjects were selected, the nature of the control group, the means by which the data were collected, and how the statistics were analyzed. See also medicine, evidence-based.

high-dose effect, *n* the biological reaction to elevated dosage. Not the same as high potency in homeopathy. See also law, Arndt-Schulz; biphasic activity; and hormesis.

high-velocity, low-amplitude thrust, *n.pr* a direct method of osteopathic treatment that employs careful patient positioning in concert with the practitioner's short, quick thrusts (high velocity) applied over short distances (low amplitude) across areas of restriction.

Himalayan cedar, *n.pr* Latin name: *Cedrus deodar;* parts used: heartwood, bark, leaves, oil; uses: in Ayurveda, pacifies vata and kapha doshas (bitter, light, oily); antimicrobial, molluscicide, insecticide, skin conditions; precautions: none known. Also called *deodar* or *devadaru.*

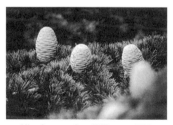

Himalayan cedar. (Williamson, 2002)

hindmilk, *n* thick, nourishing milk that is produced following foremilk during breast-feeding. See also foremilk.

HIO toggle recoil, *n* a chiropractic technique that employs rapid manual thrusts to correct vertebral subluxation complex; does not cause joint cavitation.

hip bone, *n* large bone comprised of the ilium, ischium, and pubis, which in turn is one of the three components

of the pelvis, along with the sacrum and coccyx.

hippocampus (hip·pō̄·kam'·pəs), *n* a part of the brain in the lateral ventricle that is important in learning and memory.

histamine (his'·tə·mēn), *n* a chemical produced during allergic reactions that promotes vasodilation and gastric secretions.

histopathology (his'·tō̄·pə·thä'·lə·jē), *n* the study of diseased tissue, with a focus on changes that are anatomically microscopic.

HIV, *n* human immunodeficiency virus; one of two retrovirus strains, HIV-1, or HIV-2, that attacks the T cells of the immune system with debilitating effects, producing a syndrome called acquired immune deficiency (AIDS).

HMA, *n.pr* See analysis, hair mineral.

HMB, *n.pr* See hydroxymethyl butyrate.

HMO, *n.pr* See health maintenance organization.

holarchy (hō̄·lär'·kē), *n* philosophy that holds that every entity is a holon—that is, an entity unto itself and simultaneously a part of an entity larger than itself.

Holarrhena antidysenterica, n See kutaja.

holding and supporting, *v* involves a practitioner cradling a client's limb and briefly cradling and then alternately carrying it to gauge how the client responds to touch. A kinetic manual therapy component used to establish safety in a therapeutic setting and to encourage client relaxation.

holism (hō̄'·li·zəm), *n* **1.** the characteristic of being whole, complete, interconnected, indivisible, ordered. In medicine the concept is used to address the entire individual and context rather than focusing only on a part or diagnosis. **2.** in biology, the concept according to which the sum of a phenomenon or system cannot be measured, reduced, or observed at the level below that of the entire system.

holistic nursing, *n* philosophy of nursing that seeks to facilitate patient healing by creating a caring, interactive atmosphere; incorporates energy field principles, patient empowerment, scientific knowledge, and personal interaction to assist patients in becoming whole, integrated individuals.

holistic response (hō·lis'·tik rē·spôns'), *n* therapeutic engagement with the patient as a whole, taking into account the patient's physical, emotional, psychologic, social, and spiritual aspects.

Holographic Memory Release, *n* a style of bodywork based on a holographic understanding of mind-body communication. It uses light touch on "touch points" to connect with this psychophysical network and to release energetic and emotional blockages.

Holographic Repatterning, *n* a therapeutic modality in which incoherent patterns in the body-mind energetic fields are identified. Various techniques are used to return the organism to higher orders of coherence.

holon (hō'·lôn), *n* in Greek philosophy, both the individual and the universe. Used in functional medicine to describe the holistic concept of health in which the emotional, mental, physical, and spiritual aspects are all essential for health.

holotropic breathwork (hō'lə·trô'·pik breth'·wurk), *n* a technique developed by Drs. Stanislav and Christina Grof that uses connected breathing, music, and artwork to alter consciousness and explore deep dimensions of the psyche.

homeochord, *n* in homeopathy, a combination of more than one attenuation of the same remedy in a single preparation.

homeodote (hō'·mē·ō·dōt), *n* a second homeopathic remedy used to offset the symptomatic consequences of the first remedy. See also antidote.

homeodynamics, *n* one of the basic concepts of functional medicine in which the body maintains biochemical individuality by constantly undergoing physiologic and metabolic processes.

homeopathic, *adj* relating to the practice of homeopathy, the principle that "like treats like" or referring to the miniscule dilutions used in homeopathic treatments.

Homeopathic Association of Naturopathic Physicians (hō'·mē·ō·pa'·thik ə·sō'·sē·ā'·shən əv na'·chə·rō·pa'·thik fə·zi'·shənz), *n. pr* a specialized group of naturopathy professionals that promotes activities related to the development and improvement of curriculum associated with homeopathic education at naturopathic colleges. A naturopathic physician earning this certification receives the designation of Diplomate of the Homeopathic Association of Naturopathic Physicians or DHANP. On a quarterly basis, it publishes *Simillimum,* a professional homeopathic journal. See also DHANP.

homeopathic drug provings (HDPs), *n.pl* drug experiments in homeopathy that are undertaken to produce symptom pictures for matching with illness.

homeopathic pathogenic trials (HPT), *n.pl* See provings.

homeopathic pathological prescribing, *n* procedure in which single or a combination of medicines are given based on allopathic indications in order to treat symptoms.

Homeopathic Pharmacopoeia Convention of the United States, *n.pr* an independent organization that works closely with the Food and Drug Administration and other homeopathic groups like the American Association of Homeopathic Pharmacists and American Institute of Homeopathy. The organization is responsible for continuously updating and producing the Homeopathic Pharmacopoeia of the United States or HPUS, which provides guidelines for the regulation of homeopathic drugs. It has been continuously published since 1897, but unofficial homeopathic pharmacopoeia, which preceded the publication of HPUS, began in 1841. The FDA officially recognized HPUS in 1938, and the American Institute of Homeopathy published it until Homeopathic Pharmacopoeia Convention of the United States was formed in 1980. Also called *HPCUS.*

homeopathicity (hō'·mē·ō·pə·thi'·si·tē), *n* the state in which congruence exists between the cluster of symptoms for a disease and the medicine.

homeopathy (hō'·mē·ô'·pə·thē), *n* system of medicine using remedies that produce the similar effects in healthy subjects as the illness produces in the patient.

homeopathy, anthroposophic (an'·thr ə·pō·sô'·fik   hō·mē·ô'·pə·thē), *n* a homeopathic approach that identifies the cause of illness and then develops a remedy that shares the "essential nature" of that cause, according to anthroposophic philosophy.

homeopathy, classical, *n* a form of homeopathy in which the remedy consists of highly diluted animal, drug, plant, or mineral substance that most closely matches the essence of the malady and the totality of symptoms.

homeopathy, clinical, *n* homeopathic discipline centered on symptoms that are strong indicators that a specific remedy would be most effective for a disease. The use of clinical homeopathy concentrates on affinities for the disease, organ, or tissue as indicated by the symptoms and the specific remedy. Clinical homeopathy contrasts with classical homeopathy in that the classical viewpoint looks at the totality of symptoms rather than the disease entity. See also clinical.

homeopathy, combination, *n* See complexism.

homeopathy, complex, *n* a system of homeopathic medicine that has more than one remedy combined together in one dosage form.

homeopathy, pluralist, *n* homeopathic theoretical framework that promotes the use of a regime employing multiple medicines simultaneously and/or sequentially to cure illness. Each medicine targets specific symptoms. See also homeopathy, complex; remedies, combination; polypharmacy; and homeopathy, unicist.

homeostasis, *n* the state of balance in the internal environment of the body achieved by various control mechanisms.

homeostatic healing system (hō'·mē·ō·sta'·tik hē'·ling sis'·təm), *n* the physiologic regulatory system in the body that works to correct internal imbalances in order to restore equilibrium.

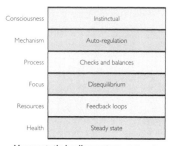

Consciousness	Instinctual
Mechanism	Auto-regulation
Process	Checks and balances
Focus	Disequilibrium
Resources	Feedback loops
Health	Steady state

Homeostatic healing system. (Micozzi, 2001)

homeostatic mechanism, *n* physiologic control system that uses negative feedback to maintain dynamic balance.

homeovitics (hō·mē·ō·vī'·tiks), *n* contemporary homeopathic approach that views toxicity as a cause for all chronic conditions and uses remedies to detoxify and strengthen the body at the cellular level.

homocysteinuria (hō'·mō·sis'·tə·i·nōō'·rē·ə), *n* abnormal metabolic condition in which excessive levels of homocysteine are present in the blood and urine. High homocysteine levels are considered a risk factor for heart disease and stroke.

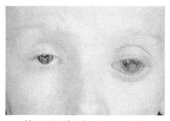

Homocysteinuria. (Newton, 1995)

homolateral (hō'·mə·la'·tə·rəl), *adj* pertaining to the same side or laterality of the body. Also called *ipsilateral.*

homologous series (hə·mô'·lə·gəs sir'·ēz), *n* compounds that have the same general formula and similar properties (physical and chemical) but differ by the number of methylene groups.

homotoxicology (hō'·mō·tôks'·i·kô'·lə·gē), *n* analysis of sickness within the framework of the body's failure to deal with the burden of toxins. Homeopathic remedies often are used as treatment. Developed by Hans Heinrich Reckeweg.

hookup, *n* in the Trager method of therapy, the practitioner enters into a meditative state along with the patient, which allows him or her to work more intuitively and to feel subtle changes in the patient's movement and tissue texture.

hops, *n* Latin name: *Humulus lupulus;* part used: whole fruit; uses: analgesic, anthelmintic, digestive, sedative, possible phytoestrogenic effects; precautions: depression, breast, uterine, or cervical cancer.

horehound, *n* Latin name: *Marrubium vulgare;* parts used: leaves, flowers; uses: diuretic, abortifacient, congestion, coughs, respiratory conditions, diarrhea, laxative; precautions: pregnancy, lactation, children; can cause arrythmias, nausea. Also called *common horehound, hoarhound, hounshane, marvel,* or *white horehound.*

horizontal plane postural decompensation, *n* nonoptimal distribution of body mass in the horizontal plane resulting in rotational changes in the posture.

hormesis, *n* the phenomenon in which low doses of toxins produce stimulating effects.

hormonal, *adj/n* beneficial component in some essential oils that helps to bring hormone secretions to normal levels.

hormone (hōr'·mōn), *n* a chemical transmitter produced by endocrine glands.

horned toad sickness, *n* in the Pima Indian healing model, circulatory disorders, which can lead to fatal heart attacks.

horse chestnut, *n* Latin names: *Aesculus hippocastanum, Aesculus california, Aesculus glabra;* parts used: seeds (extract), bark; uses: varicose veins, chronic venous insufficiency, phlebitis, fever, hemorrhoids, edema, inflammation; precautions: whole seeds are toxic; patients on anticoagulant medications or who have kidney or liver dysfunction. Also called *aescin, buckeye, California buckeye, chestnut, escine, Ohio buckeye,* or *Spanish chestnut.*

horseradish, *n* Latin name: *Armoracia rusticana;* part used: roots; uses: abortifacient, joint inflammation, diuretic, anthelmintic, antibacterial, sinusitis; precautions: pregnancy, lactation, children, toxic (internally in large amounts); patients with thyroid conditions, kidney disease, and ulcers. Also called *great mountain root, pepperrot, great raifort,* or *red cole.*

horsetail, *n* Latin name: *Equisetum arvense;* part used: stems (dried); uses: anticancer, diuretic, gout, kidney stones; strengthens bones, teeth, hair, and nails; precautions: patients with heart disease, kidney disease, nicotine sensitivity, or nicotine toxicity. Also called *bottle brush, corn horsetail, dutch rushes, horse willow, horsetail grass, paddock pipes, pewterwort, scouring rush, shave grass,* or *toadpipe.*

hospice, *n* system for care of a patient during the final phases of a terminal illness, often involving family, emotional support, and professional health care in the patient's home.

hot full immersion bath, *n* soaking of the body in water that is between 100° F and 106° F. Used in hydrotherapy to cleanse the body, relax muscles, treat rheumatoid arthritis, and induce sweating.

Hoxsey herbal treatment (hôk'·sē trēt'·mənt), *n.pr* an herbal treatment used for cancer. Propounded by naturopath Harry Hoxsey and comprising an externally applied paste (containing arsenic sulfide) and an orally administered tonic (containing ingredients such as berberis root,

H

burdock root, buckthorn bark, cascara, licorice, pokeroot, prickly ash bark, red clover, and stillingia root, with proportions varying on a case-by-case basis).

hozhon (hō'·zhôn), *n* Navajo Indian term for beauty, harmony, health, and happiness.

HR, *n* See Holographic Repatterning.

HR, *n* hold-relax; a proprioceptive neuromuscular facilitation (PNF) technique that involves stretching and relaxing taut muscles. See also PNF.

HT, *n.pr* See Healing Touch.

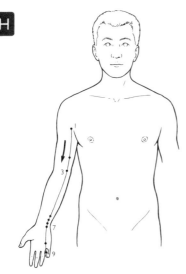

HT. (Chirali, 1999)

huang lian (hwäng lē·en), *n* Latin name: *Coptis chinensis;* part used: root; uses: pain relief, bacteriocidal, poisoning, febrifuge, cramps or spasms, digestion, flow of bile, repair of the intestinal lining, secretion of glycogen and insulin, blood purification, carminative, flow of bile, digestion, nerves, skin conditions, general health, vasodilator, diabetes mellitus, diarrhea, acute enteritis, dysentery, insomnia, fidgetiness, delirium as a result of high fever, leukemia, and

otitis media, wound healing, conjunctivitis, oral ulcers, swollen gums, toothache; precautions: may be toxic.

huang lian e jiao tang (hwäng lē·en ə jyōw täng), *n* in traditional Chinese medicine, a classic herbal formula used to treat high heart fire, a deficiency of yin, characterized by a tongue with a red tip that is covered with a yellow coating and a thin, rapid pulse. The patient will also present symptoms of being mentally overworked and restless. Insomnia will be an indication in addition to frequent dreams, dry mouth, boils within the tongue and mouth, neurasthenia, and forgetfulness. Coptis and e jiao are the two chief ingredients used in the formula. Also called *ass-hide gelatin decoction.* See also chief ingredient, coptis, e jiao.

huang qi (hwäng· chē), *n* root of *Astragalus*; used in traditional Chinese medicine for lowering blood pressure, promoting vasodilation, protecting the liver and regulating blood glucose levels.

Hubbard purification rundown, *n.pr* a method for eliminating xenobiotics from the body. Uses sauna therapy with electrolyte replacement, exercise, and niacin supplements to reduce the levels of polybrominated biphenyls and polychlorinated biphenyls in the body.

huesero (wā·se'·rō), *n* in Curanderismo, the Mexican-American healing system, a bonesetter and healer who works to meet the needs of the community he serves on the material level.

human papillomavirus (hyōō'· mən pa'·pə·lō'·mə·vī'·rəs), *n* any of the group of papoviruses that are sexually transmitted and associated with oral or genital carcinomas.

humanistic health care, *n* approach to medicine that emphasizes the relationship between caregiver and patient. Characterized by collaboration, dignity, empathy, and trust.

humor, *n* **1.** fluid found in the body, particularly lymph or blood. **2.** any amusing, funny, or ludicrous insights that medical personnel and patients can share to laugh and relieve stress, release anger, form relationships, and cope with difficult situations.

humoral immunity, *n* a defense system of the immune system, including antibodies and sensitized white cells that are produced to fight specific pathogens.

Humulus lupulus, n See hops.

hun (hōōn), *n* in Chinese medicine, one of the five spirits. Hun, stored in the liver, is often translated as ethereal soul and is said to complement shen through inspiration, insight, and courage and is further associated with planning and direction, sleep, and dreaming. See also five spirits and shen.

huperzine A (hōō´·pər·zēn), *n* a potent alkaloid obtained from the *Huperzia serrata* club moss; used to improve memory both in healthy individuals and in those suffering from memory loss. Precaution advised for those with high blood pressure, kidney disease, and liver disease. Self-medication is not advised.

HVLA thrust, *n.pr* See high-velocity, low-amplitude thrust.

HVPT, *n.pr* See test, hyperventilation provocation.

HVT, *n* high-velocity/low-amplitude thrusts; a set of techniques used in manipulative therapy for the thorax, spine, and pelvis; distinguishable by quick thrusting impulses by the practitioner. Also called *mobilization with impulse, adjustment,* and *grade V mobilization.*

hybrid plant, *n* the creation of a new plant from natural or artificial fertilization between two species. The letter *x* in the middle of the plant name indicates its hybrid status.

hydergine (hī´·der·jĕn), *n* a chemical derived from ergot mold that grows on the rye grain, said to have antiaging and cognitive enhancement effects.

Hydnocarpus anthelmintica, n See oil, chaulmoogra.

Hydnocarpus wightiana, n See oil, chaulmoogra.

hydrastis root, *n* See goldenseal.

hydrazine sulfate (hī´·drə·zēn sul´·fāt), *n* a monoamine oxidase

inhibitor and drug that has been used for the treatment of cachexia and cancer. Should not be taken with alcohol, tranquilizers, or with foods containing tyrosine.

hydrocarbons (hī´·drō·kär´·bənz), *n.pl* compounds that only contain carbon and hydrogen atoms, such as alkanes, alkenes, alkynes, terpenes, and arenes.

hydrocephalus, *n* abnormal condition in which cerebrospinal fluid collects in the cranium, thus causing the ventricles to dilate. May be present at birth or may manifest in early adulthood. Caused by brain tumors, infection, trauma, or developmental anomalies. Also called *hydrocephaly.*

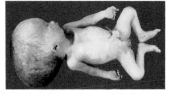

Hydrocephalus. (Carlson, 1999; M. Darr, Ann Arbor, MI)

hydrodiffusion (hī´·drō·di·fyōō´·zhən), *n* a method of extracting essential oils in which steam at atmospheric pressure is passed through the plant material from the top of the extraction chamber, thus resulting in oils that retain the original aroma of the plant; process is less harsh than steam distillations is. See also steam distillation.

hydrogen bond, *n* a weak electrostatic bond between two atoms with opposite charges.

hydrogen peroxide (hī´·drə·jin per·ôk´·sīd), *n* compound (H_2O_2) generally recognized in traditional medicine as an antiseptic and cleansing agent; used externally. Has been used by injection and IV for HIV and other infections.

hydrogenoid, *n* conditions in which excess water is not tolerated.

hydrolat, *n* a French term for the condensed steam used to infuse water with the essence of beneficial plants.

See also water, aromatic; waters, floral; hydrosol; water, essential; and water, prepared.

hydrolysis (hī·drô'·lə·sis), *n* a chemical reaction in which a substance reacts with water.

hydrolytic enzymes (hī·drō·li'·tik en'·zīmz), *n.pl* complex catalytic proteins that use water to break down substrates. See also hydrolysis.

hydropathy (hī·drô'·pə·thē), *n* a system of alternative medicine in which baths are administered to stimulate the patient in order to eliminate disease. Developed in Austria in the 1820s, this system was popularized in the United States in the 1840s but lost its popularity soon after the Civil War. The system was enhanced by a series of changes to regulate lifestyle, such as exercise, diet, dress, and sleep patterns. Also called *water-cure*.

hydropenia (hī·drō·pē'·nē·ə), *n* condition marked by water deficiency in body tissues.

hydrosol, *n* water-based solution that contains tiny particles.

hydrotherapy (hī'·drō·the'·rə·pē), *n* therapeutic modalities that use water, such as whirlpools or Sitz baths.

hydroxyl group (hī·drôk'·səl grōōp'), *n* the functional group (—OH) found in molecules of alcohols and water.

hydroxymethyl butyrate (hī·drōk'·sē·me·thəl byōō·tī·rāt), *n* a compound produced in the body as a byproduct of leucine degradation; used to enhance muscle growth and to protect against muscle damage during weight training. Precaution advised in patients with severe liver or kidney disease. Also called *beta-hydroxy beta-methylbutyric acid.*

hygeiotherapy (hī·gē'·ō·the'·rə·pē), *n* a system of alternative medicine in which the cold baths used in hydropathy are combined with healthy behaviors, such as abstinence from tobacco and alcohol, vegetarian diet, fresh air, exercise, and sexual restraint. See also *hydropathy.*

hygiene, *n* **I.** cleanliness and aseptic practices. **2.** therapy through detoxification.

hygiene hypothesis, *n* the theory that excessive prevention of early childhood exposure to dirt and pathogens can stunt the development of the immune system.

hyperactivity, *n* excessive and often inappropriate activity, often associated with attention-deficit disorder. See also disorder, attention-deficit.

hyperbarism (hī·per·bar'·izm), *n* any of a number of disorders caused by excessive atmospheric pressure, generally occurring after an abrupt increase in pressure.

hyperchloremia, *n* disproportionate levels of chloride in the blood. Causes acidosis.

hypercholesterolemia (hī'·per·kə·les'·ter·ə·lē'·mē·ə), *n* condition marked by excessive amounts of cholesterol in the blood; leads to plaques in the arterial walls, thereby obstructing the blood flow to the heart, brain, and other organs. This increases the risk of cardiovascular disease that can lead to heart attack or stroke.

hyperemia (hī'·pə·rē'·mē·ə), *n* condition of increased circulatory flow, warmth, and flushed appearance in an area. Massage therapists often create hyperemia to warm and soften tissue in preparation for specific or deeper work.

hyperemic, *adj* having a large volume of blood in any given place in the body.

hyperesthesia (hī'·per·es·thē'·zhē·ə), *n* heightened sensitivity to touch, often perceived as painful or irritating; commonly caused by nerve compression, shingles, chronic pain, or stress.

hyperglycemia, *n* a disorder characterized by elevated glucose levels in the blood.

hyperhydrosis, *n* inordinate perspiration.

hypericin (hī·per'·i·sin), *n* an extract from the plant *Hypericum perforatum,* commonly known as St. John's wort; used to treat depression, sleep disorders, and viral infections; the potential to treat HIV is currently under investigation.

Hypericum perforatum, *n* See St. John's wort.

hyperkinesis (hī'·per·ki·nē'·sis), *n* disorder of childhood and adolescence marked by restlessness, short attention span, excessive activity, and impulsive behavior. See also therapy, craniosacral.

hypermenorrhea, *n* extended or excessive menstrual bleeding.

hypermnesia (hī'·perm·nē'·zhē·ə), *n* the ability to remember past events in vivid detail, often enhanced when under hypnosis. See also hypnosis.

hypermobility, *n* condition in which ligaments are loose; a click may be heard when the joint moves through a reasonable range of motion.

hyperpnea (hī·perp'·nē'·ə), *n* rapid and deep respiration that occurs normally after exercise or abnormally when associated with fevers or other disorders.

hypersensitivity reactions, *n.pl* any of several forms of overly responsive actions of the immune system to normally encountered, antigens. Also called *allergic reactions*.

hyperstimulation analgesia (hī'· per·stim'·yə·lā'·shən a'·nəl·jē'· zē·ə), *n* the relief of pain through the stimulation of large-diameter nerves using a variety of techniques, such as acupuncture, acupressure, ice packs, etc. See also counterirritation.

hypertension, *n* high blood pressure; a condition in which an individual's blood pressure regularly exceeds 140/90 mm Hg. Risk factors include family history of hypertension, excessive alcohol intake, high sodium levels, and obesity.

hypertensive (hī'·per·ten'·siv), *n* a substance that increases the blood pressure.

hypertensor, *n* an agent that tends to raise blood pressure.

hyperthermia, *n* See therapy, heat.

hyperthyroidism, *n* the overproduction of triiodothyronine and/or tetraiodothyronine by the thyroid gland. Symptoms include sweating, weakness, nervousness, loss of weight, frequent and loose defecation, increased sensitivity to heat, fatigue, and irritability. Graves' disease, an autoimmune disorder, is the most common cause of hyperthyroidism.

hypertrophy (hī'·per·trō'·fē), *n* increased size of a tissue or cells not attributable to cell division.

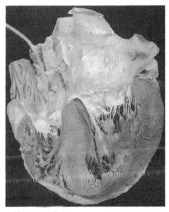

Hypertrophy. (Cotran, Kumar, and Collins, 1999)

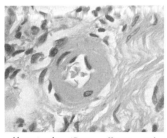

Hypertension. (Cotran, Kumar, and Collins, 1999; Helmut Rennke, MD, Brigham and Women's Hospital, Boston)

hyperventilation (hī'·per·ven'·tə· lā'·shən), *n* condition in which the body exhales carbon dioxide at a rate faster than which it is being produced. May cause dizziness and tingling of toes and fingers and chest pain if continued. Also called *overbreathing*.

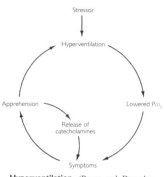

Hyperventilation. (Payne and Donaghy, 2001)

	No	Mild	Moderate	Severe
Crave sweets	0	I	2	3
Irritable if a meal is missed	0	I	2	3
Feel tired or weak if a meal is missed	0	I	2	3
Dizziness when standing suddenly	0	I	2	3
Frequent headaches	0	I	2	3
Poor memory (forgetful) or concentration	0	I	2	3
Feel tired an hour or so after eating	0	I	2	3
Heart palpitations	0	I	2	3
Feel shaky at times	0	I	2	3
Afternoon fatigue	0	I	2	3
Vision blurs on occasion	0	I	2	3
Depression or mood swings	0	I	2	3
Overweight	0	I	2	3
Frequently anxious or nervous	0	I	2	3
Total				

Scoring:
<5, hypoglycemia is not likely a factor
6–15, hypoglycemia is a likely factor
>15, hypoglycemia is extremely likely.

Hypoglycemia. (Pizzorno and Murray, 1999)

H

hypnosis, *n* an altered state of consciousness, usually resembling sleep or trance, which may use relaxation techniques, suggestion, and imagery.

hypnotherapy, *n* the practice of using hypnosis for the treatment of illness. See also hypnosis.

hypnotic induction profile, *n* a set of indicators assessing a person's degree of susceptibility to hypnosis. See also hypnosis.

hypnotic language, *n* language with metaphors, implied meaning, or linguistic matching designed to promote positive effects.

hypnotism, *n* the practice of hypnosis. See also hypnosis.

hypochlorhydria (hī'·pō·klōr·hī'·drē·ə), *n* condition characterized by an abnormally low level of hydrochloric acid in the stomach. Also called *hypohydrochloria.*

hypoglycemia (hī·pō·glī·sē'·mē·ə), *n* a disorder characterized by lower than normal blood glucose levels. May cause lightheadedness, weakness, excessive hunger, anxiety, headaches, visual disturbances, or personality changes.

hypokalemia (hī'·pō·kä·lē'·mē·ə), *n* low potassium in blood; leads to mental depression, weakness, confusion, atypical electrocardiographic readings, and flaccid paralysis. Causes include diuretic therapy, starvation, diabetic acidosis, and adrenal tumor. Also called *kaliopenia.*

hypomobility, *n* condition in which ligaments are tight and movement is restricted.

hypotension, *n* low blood pressure; a condition in which a person's blood pressure is not sufficient for tissue oxygenation or normal perfusion.

hypotensive (hī·pō·ten'·siv), *n* a substance that decreases the blood pressure.

hypothermia, *n* **1.** life-threatening condition usually caused by prolonged exposure to extreme cold; categorized by an oral temperature of below 95° F, or a rectal temperature of below 96° F. **2.** the purposeful lowering of body temperature before performing surgery.

hypothesis, *n* an experimentally testable proposal given as the basis for additional examination.

hypothyroidism, *n* underactivity of hormones. Symptoms include increased sensitivity to cold, depression, recurring infections, weight loss difficulties, problems with menstruation, dry skin, and fatigue are common symptoms. The condition can be caused by a defect in the synthesis of hormones, a decrease in the pituitary gland's rate of stimulation or limited cellular conversion.

hypoventilation (hī'·pō·vēn'·tə·lā'·shən), *n* breathing dysfunction characterized by insufficient respiration, resulting in inadequate oxygenation and build-up of excess carbon dioxide in the body.

hypoxemia (hī·pôk·sē'·mē·ə), *n* condition in which oxygen levels in arterial blood are low. Typical symptoms are apnea, increased blood pressure, tachycardia, restlessness, stupor, coma, Cheyne-Stokes respiration, hypotension due to increased initial cardiac output that has rapidly fallen, ventricular fibrillation, and other conditions.

hypoxia (hī·pôk'·sē·ə), *n* insufficient oxygen supply to tissues in the body; symptoms include hypertension, dizziness, peripheral vasoconstriction, tachycardia, mental confusion, and other manifestations.

hyssop (hi'·səp), *n* Latin name: *Hyssopus officinalis;* part used: extract; uses: antiasthmatic, expectorant, sore throat, possible antiviral; precautions: abortifacient.

Hyssopus officinalis, *n* See hyssop.

hallucinogenic at high doses; used in lower doses to treat addiction, primarily in Europe. In the United States, ibogaine is a schedule I substance (a substance that has a high potential for abuse).

Iceland moss, *n.pr* Latin name: *Cetraria islandica*; parts used: entire plant; uses: cold, respiratory ailments, bacterial infections, HIV; precautions: patients with liver disease; can cause hepatotoxicity. Also called *consumption moss, eryngo-leaved liverwort,* or *Iceland lichen.*

icthyosis (ik'·thē·ō'·sis), *n* any of several hereditary skin conditions characterized by the appearance of dry, hyperkeratotic skin that closely resembles fish scales. The condition develops shortly after birth, but an acquired, uncommon type that accompanies multiple myeloma or lymphoma may develop in adults. In some conditions, lactic acid or bath oils may provide temporary relief from symptoms.

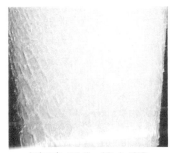

Icthyosis. (Zitelli and Davis, 1997)

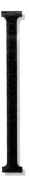

***i*-isomer,** *n* a stereoisomer whose asymmetric carbon atom rotates plane-polarized light counter-clockwise. See also asymmetric carbon atom.

iatrology (ī'·ə·trä'·lə·jē), *n* term used for medical science.

ibogaine (ī'·bō·gyān), *n* stimulant that can be

ida (ē·dä'), *n* according to ancient Indian philosophy, the female or negative energy, one of the two components of prana (life force), the other being pingala. Good health indicate balance between ida and pingala, while an imbalance between the two leads to disease. See also prana and pingala.

ideal, *n* in the treatment of musculoskeletal dysfunction, a clinical classification of a postural pattern in which the minimum adaptive load is shifted to a different area.

ideomotor phenomenon, *n* test for hypnotic susceptibility; relates to involuntary movement induced by an idea.

ideomotor responses (i'·dē·ō·mō'·tər rē·spän'·səz), *n* reflexive motions exhibited by a patient under hypnosis that indicate the thoughts and feelings of the patient. See also hypnosis.

ideomotor signals, *n* the automatic muscle movements, such as a nod, blink, or finger motion, sometimes used in place of verbal responses during hypnosis to indicate that the patient is hearing the therapist. The patient and therapist usually agree upon them in advance. See also hypnosis.

idiopathic (i'·dē·ō·pa'·thik), *adj* relating to the development of a disease from an unknown cause.

idiopathic hypertrophic cardiomyopathy (i'·dē·ō·pa'·thik hī'·per·trō'·fik kar'·dē·ō·mī·ô'·pə·thē), *n* a condition of the cardiac muscle in which the septum between the two ventricles is extraordinarily thick, so that the heart muscle does not relax completely during diastole. This condition often blocks the flow of blood from the heart, resulting in shortness of breath, palpitations, chest pain, fainting, and sudden death.

idiosyncrasy, *n* individualistic reaction to a treatment. See also adverse drug reaction.

idiotype (i'·dē·ō·tīp'), *n* the region of an immunoglobulin molecule responsible for the unique characteristics of the molecule. In most cases, this includes the antigen-binding location.

IFRA, *n.pr* See International Fragrance Association.

IgE, *n* immunoglobin E.

IgG ELISA, *n.pr* a diagnostic test for identifying reactive substances that provoke delayed hypersensitivity of the immune system. A solid-phase immunoassay that uses enzymes to test for IgG subclass reactions.

iha' kicikta (ē·hä' kē·chēk'·tä), *n* Lakota Indian term meaning community mindedness, that is, demonstrating concern for the needs of others in the tribe.

ikce wicasa (ēk·chā' wē·chä'·sä), *n* Lakota Indian term for human being.

Ilex paraguariensis, *n* See yerba maté.

illness, *n* 1. sickness or disorder. 2. malady of either body or mind the symptoms of which may be physically unobservable. Within general medical practice, *disease* is nearly synonomous; however, illness has a more general connotation encompassing the subjective aspects of the patient as a whole rather than just physical or diagnostic symptoms; thus an alternative medical practitioner may prefer to treat illness rather than only the disease. See also disease and complaint.

illness, acute, *n* illness with swift beginning and rapid course.

illness, layers of, *n.pl* in homeopathy, multiple sets of symptoms in chronic disease, where as one set is cured with a specific remedy, the next set is revealed requiring a different remedy. See also symptoms, alternating; metastasis; suppression; and syndrome shift.

illness, level of, *n* the depth of disease manifestation in an individual. The deepest level affects the person's integrity and creativity and major vital organs. See also direction of cure, syndrome shift and symptoms, hierarchy of.

illness, onset of, *n* the pattern of situations and symptoms of the illness that is often crucial for determining the beginning or start of the condition. See also biopathography, etiological factor, causality, occasion, pathogenesis, and precipitating factor.

illnesses, environmental, *n.pl* adverse health effects that result from exposure to chemical toxins found in the environment, such as heavy metals, pesticides, and solvents. Include disorders of the endocrine, immune, and neurological systems.

imageorator (im·ag·ōr·ə·tōr), *n* the art therapist's role in translating the meaning of art that may be painful or disturbing and in evoking the patient's own transformation.

imbalance (im·bal'·əns), *n* **1.** excess supply of one characteristic or energy in unhealthy proportion. **2.** unsteadiness, state of being near falling over.

imedeen (i'·mə·dēn), *n* trade name of a dietary supplement administered orally that is intended to improve the quality of skin and remove wrinkles; comprises proteins derived from the cartilage of a deep-sea fish. Use of the supplement has been associated with edema and generalized skin reaction.

immediate hypersensitivity, *n* a type-1 hypersensitivity reaction in which exposure to an antigen causes an rapid immune response. Immunoglobulin E binds to the antigen, thus causing release of cytokine and histamine. Reactions can include bronchoconstriction, hives, itchy eyes, or more serious responses, such as anaphylaxis or asthmatic attacks.

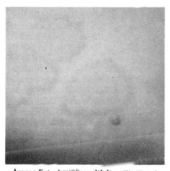

Immediate hypersensitivity. (Zitelli and Davis, 1997; Dr. Donald W. Kress, Children's Hospital of Pittsburgh)

immune complex–mediated hypersensitivity, *n* a type-3 hypersensitivity reaction in which exposure to an antigen causes a delayed response. Antibodies (IgG, IGA, or IgM) combine with antigens to form complexes in tissues, thus causing the release of proinflammatory chemicals and immunologically active cells that

damage those tissues and result in autoimmune disorders (rheumatic fever, rheumatoid arthritis), Arthus reaction, and serum sickness. It may take several hours or days for this response to develop.

immune conditioning, *n* a process by which functions of the immune system are caused to respond to previously unresponsive stimuli (conditioned response).

immune modulators, *n.pl* chemicals that influence the immune system. Also called *cytokines*.

immune system, *n* the group of organs, cells, and chemicals that protect the body from harmful viruses, bacteria, and abnormal cells. It includes bone marrow, proteins, the thymus, the spleen, the lymphocytes, and other white blood cells.

immunization, *n* defense against contagious illnesses acquired either through contact with the contagion or a less virulent form of it as through vaccination. See also immunotherapy and vaccinosis.

immunoglobulin A (IgA) (im'·myə·nō·glô'·byə·lin ā'), *n* protein located in body fluids that guards against infection in mucosal surfaces.

IgA

Immunoglobulin A (IgA). (Thibodeau and Patton, 1999; Rolin Graphics)

immunoglobulin G (IgG) (im'·myə·nō·glô'·byə·lin jē'), *n* protein found in the blood that guards against infection. Also called *gamma globulin.*

IgG

Immunoglobulin G (IgG). (Thibodeau and Patton, 1999; Rolin Graphics)

immunoprophylaxis (im'·myə·nō· prō'·fə·lak'·səs), *n* prevention of illness by the introduction of active immunization by vaccines or passive immunization through antisera.

immunostimulant, *n* a substance that encourages and sustains the immune system and its responses.

immunotherapy, *n* improving the performance of the body's immune system by using immunization and immune factors. See also isopathy.

impairment (im·per'·mənt), *n* any disturbance in the function or structure of an organ.

imperforate (im'·pur'·fə·rāt'), *adj* absence of a typical opening in an organ or passageway of the body, such as the hymen or anus.

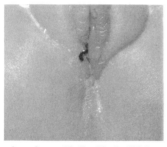

Imperforate. (Zitelli and Davis, 1997; Dr. Christine Williams, New York Medical College)

imponderabilia, *n* homeopathic remedies whose source material is intangible (e.g., magnetism, electricity, and x-rays).

impotence (im'·pə·təns), *n* poor sexual function and reproduction in the male, including erectile dysfunction, in which erection of the penis cannot be achieved or maintained.

impulse, *n* chiropractic technique characterized by a short, quick thrust.

IMS, *n.pr* See intramuscular stimulation.

IMT, *n.pr* See inspiratory muscle training.

in vitro (in vē'·trō), *adj* located outside the organism in a simulated environment.

in vivo (in vē'·vō), *adj* located within the organism.

inanition (i'·nə·ni'·shən), *n* 1. exhaustion due to deficiency of water or food. 2. lethargic state distinguished by a lack of vigor or vitality in all aspects of life, including intellectual, moral, and social aspects.

incensing (in·sen·sing), *n* in Curanderismo, the Mexican-American healing system, purification ritual performed to treat businesses, farms, and homes by praying and walking through building with a pan filled with smoking incense. Every corner of the structure is filled with the incense to bring peace and remove bad luck. Also called *sahumerio*.

INCI, *n.pr* See International Nomenclature of Cosmetic Ingredients.

incontinence (in'·kän'·tə·nəns), *n* inability to control evacuative functions, such as defecation or urination.

Indian apple, *n* Latin name: *Podophyllum peltatum*; parts used: roots, resin; uses: antibilious, cathartic, hydragogue, purgative; precautions: pregnancy, elderly; can cause gastrointestinal inflammation, irritation, overstimulation, nausea, vomiting. Also called *duck's foot, hog apple, mandrake, American mandrake, mandrake root, May apple, podophyllum, racoonberry,* and *wild lemon.*

Indian birthwort, *n* Latin name: *Aristolochia indica*; parts used: roots, rhizomes, leaves; uses: in Ayurveda, balances kapha and vata doshas (bitter, astringent, light, dry), antifertility, antiestrogenic, abortifacient, antitumor, immunomodulator, antiinflammatory, skin conditions, anthelmintic, snake bite, diarrhea, bowel disorders, leprosy; precautions: pregnancy, carcinogenic, nephrotoxic; too poisonous for medical use. Also called *isharmul* or *sunanda*.

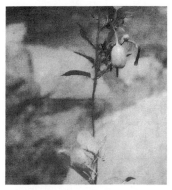

Indian birthwort. (Williamson, 2002)

Indian gooseberry, *n.pr* See amla.

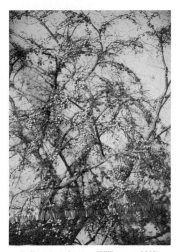

Indian gooseberry. (Williamson, 2002)

Indian licorice, *n* Latin name: *Abrus precatorius;* parts used: roots, leaves, seeds; uses: in Ayurveda, pacifies vata and pitta doshas (bitter, light, dry, sharp); seeds: contraception, antidiarrheal, anthelmintic; roots: antiemetic, anthelmintic; precautions: unprocessed seeds are highly toxic if ingested.

Also called *crab's eye, gunja, jequirity,* or *rati.*

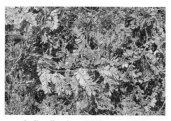

Indian licorice. (Williamson, 2002)

Indian madder, *n* Latin name: *Rubia cordifolia*; parts used: dried roots and stems; uses: in Ayurveda, pacifies kapha and pitta doshas (astringent, bitter, sweet, heavy, dry, hot), antioxidant, antiinflammatory, anticancer, hepatoprotection, tonic, paralysis, jaundice, urinary infections, thoracic inflammations, rheumatism, tuberculosis, allergies; precautions: none known. Also called *chitravalli, dyer's madder, majeeth, manjista,* or *manjit.*

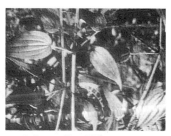

Indian madder. (Williamson, 2002)

Indian tobacco, *n* See lobelia.

indication (in·də·kā´·shən), *n* an appropriate therapeutic treatment for a given condition; will have beneficial effects and promote healing.

indigestion, *n* abdominal discomfort caused by the improper digestion of food. Factors responsible include excessive or deficient acid production, bacterial overgrowth, and pancreatic malfunction.

indigo, *n* Latin name: *Indigofera* spp.; parts used: branches, leaves; uses: liver purification, antiinflammatory, diabetes, mumps; precautions: teratogenic. Also called *qinqdai.*

***Indigofera* spp.,** *n* See indigo.

indirect adverse effects, *n.pl* unfavorable outcomes due to the practitioner's failure to properly perform a diagnostic procedure or administer a therapeutic approach.

indirect inhalation, *n* inhalation of an aroma, of an essential oil not directed at a patient's nose when it is used, for example, in a room.

indirect MFR, *n* indirect myofascial release; an osteopathic technique for myofascial release in which the therapist guides the dysfunctional tissues gently along a path with little resistance until the tension is released.

indirect suggestion, *n* a type of instruction, phrased as an offhand recommendation, used by therapists during hypnosis to encourage patients to follow a desired course of action without actually directing them to do so. See also hypnosis.

indisposition, *n* minor malady curable by altering some facet of behavior.

individualization, *n* the process of tailoring remedies or treatments to cure a set of symptoms in an individual instead of basing treatment on the common features of the disease. See also characteristic, constitution, idiosyncrasy, prescribing strategy, and symptom selection.

induction, *n* the initial phase of the hypnotic process that is used to bring about the state of trance in a patient. See also hypnosis.

inebriant (i·nē'·brē·ənt), *n* an intoxicating substance. Also called *intoxicant.*

inebriated (i·nē'·brē·ā'·təd), *adj* intoxicated.

inert gases (i·nert' ga'·səs), *n.pl* a group of stable elements, such as neon and argon, that do not easily react with other atoms because of their filled outer or valence shell. Also called *noble gases* or *rare gases.*

infantile colic, *n* a health condition encountered in infants and small children; characterized by short, intensely painful intestinal spasms that often wake the distressed child. Can be helped through dietary modifications, warming herbs, essential oils, or abdominal massage.

infarct (in·färkt'), *n* localized tissue death resulting from an interruption of blood supply to that area. Also called *infarction.*

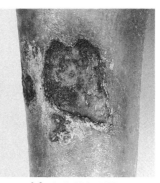

Infarct. (du Vivier, 1993)

infertility, *n* the inability to produce offspring. Causes can be complex and varied, and a wide range of treatment options are used.

inflammation (in·flə·mā'·shən), *n* response of bodily tissues to a chemical or physical injury indicated by heat, redness, swelling, and pain.

inflared innominate, *n* a condition in which the movement of the hipbone is restricted in a sideward direction and unrestricted in a medial direction because the anterior superior iliac spine (ASIS) is positioned medially.

influential points, *n.pl* See great points.

influenza, *n* a viral infection transmitted via airborne droplets; highly contagious, with a sudden onset of symptoms including sore throat, headache, fever, chills, and myalgia. Recovery normally occurs within three to ten days but can be fatal.

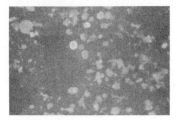

Influenza. (Murray et al, 1990; Richard Thomas, Akron, OH)

information, *n* **I.** coherent, data-bearing pattern that can be separated from its medium of transmission. **2.** concept in meridian based psychotherapy, which posits that information manifests as a function of shape and structure; also believed to be a demonstration of the reality of energy and energy fields.

informed consent, *n* **I.** an aspect of research in which the consent of the subject is obtained and the subject is informed of possible risks and benefits from participating in the research. **2.** consent to medical procedures/treatment given by a patient after the potential risks, hazards, and benefits of the treatment have been explained.

infrared (IR) (in'·fra·red'), *n* electromagnetic radiation of longer wavelength than red light in the range of 730 nanometres (nm) to about 1 millimetre (mm).

infrared spectroscopy (in'·fra·red' spek·trôs'·ka·pē), *n* an instrumental technique used to identify substances —in particular the functional groups present in organic compounds by measuring their absorption of infrared radiation over a range of frequencies. The absorption pattern is then compared to the infrared spectra of known substances for identification.

infusion, *n* a method of medicine preparation in which aromatic herbs are steeped in hot (slightly below boiling) water. This prevents medicinal constituents from being boiled off.

inhalants, *n.pl* **I.** chemical vapors that are inhaled for their mind-altering effects. **2.** in herbology, volatile herbal compounds that are delivered by holding a soaked pad to the nose and mouth, by placing the herbs in steaming water, or by rubbing on ointments that contain the substances.

inhalation (in'·ha·lā'·shan), *n* the entry of vapor into the body by means of the respiratory tract.

inhalation rib, *n* dysfunctional condition characterized by free inhalation and restricted exhalation; caused by a rib being caught in an inhalation position. Also called *anterior rib, caught in inhalation, elevated rib, exhalation restriction of rib,* or *inhalation strain.*

inhibition, manual, *n* **I.** blocking or interfering with a process. **2.** a massage technique in which pressure is applied directly to hypertonic muscles or problematic soft tissues and then released. Also called *ischemic compression* and *trigger point pressure release.*

inimical, *n* a homeopathic remedy whose actions hinder, but do not counteract those of another. Also called *incompatible.*

inipi (ē·nē'·pē), *n* See sweat lodge.

INIT, *n* See technique, integrated neuromuscular inhibition.

injuring movement, *n* the movement responsible for injury; tested when the patient reports temporary symptoms or when symptoms are not observed by other active physiological joint movements.

innate immunity, *n* the ability of the body to protect itself against foreign organisms and toxins. The defense mechanisms of skin, white blood cells, macrophages, stomach acid, and chemicals in the bloodstream are all part of innate immunity.

innate intelligence (in·nāt' in·te'·la·gans), *n* term coined by D.D. Palmer to refer to the force within the body (originating in the spine) that produces healing and proper health unless impaired by spinal subluxation.

innervation (i·nər·vā'·shan), *n* the process of distributing or supplying nerves to a specific region of the body.

innocuous (i·nä'·kyoo̅·əs), *adj* unable to harm or injure.

innominate bone, *n* See hip bone.

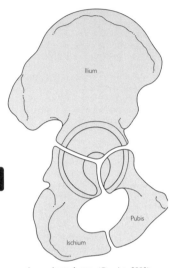

Innominate bone. (Carreiro, 2003)

insertion (in·sir'·shən), *n* the tendinous attachment of a muscle to the bone on which the muscle operates (i.e., the bone moves when the muscle contracts).

insoluble fiber, *n* one of three types of fiber, this group includes cellulose, hemicellulose, and lignins. Insoluble fiber creates a full feeling and helps to ease constipation.

insomnia, *n* sleeplessness; may be short- or long-term; has a variety of causes, including some psychiatric disorders.

inspiratory muscle training (in·spī'·rə·tōr'·ē mus'·əl trā'·ning), *n* a technique used to correct or increase respiratory function by improving the performance of the muscles involved in inhalation.

instinctotherapy (in·stink'·tō·the'·rə·pē), *n* anticancer diet that comprises raw foods (including meat) and no milk products.

insulin (in'·sə·lin), *n* hormone produced by the pancreas that regulates blood glucose levels by stimulating the absorption of sugars into the cells.

inorganic chemistry (in·ōr·ga'·nik ke'·mə·strē), *n* the chemistry of all inorganic compounds (i.e., those that do not contain carbon).

inosine (ī'·nō·sēn), *n* a nucleoside and precursor to adenosine, important biochemical in energy production. It may be useful as an adjunct treatment for cardiovascular conditions and for Tourette's syndrome. High doses may increase the levels of uric acid in the blood.

inositol (ī·nō'·sə·tôl), *n* See vitamin B_8.

inositol hexaniacinate, *n* See vitamin B_3.

inotropic (ī'·nə·trō'·pik), *adj* regarding muscle contraction, particularly the contraction of cardiac muscle.

inquiring, *v* to draw information from a client—whether by verbal questioning or physical examination—to assess the person's state of health.

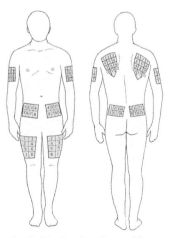

Insulin injection sites. (Potter and Perry, 1997)

integrality (in'·tə·grā'·lə·tē), *n* a principle in energy field work, according to which environmental and human energy fields are open and they constantly pass through each other.

integrated health care, *n* healthcare services combining the best of conventional and complementary health care.

integrator (in'·tə·grā'·ter), *n* a computer that processes results produced by analytical machines such as a gas chromatograph.

integrins (in'·tə·grinz), *n.pl.* proteins that mediate interactions between two cells as well as between a cell and the extracellular matrix.

intending, *v* to apply the impetus, visualization, and course of action taken in goal setting, best when done cooperatively between client and practitioner, so that therapeutic goals are understood, and shared.

intention, *n* 1. consciously committing to act in a definite way. 2. wound healing of approximated edges.

Incision with blood clot   Edges approximated with suture   Fine scar

Primary Intention

Intention. (Lewis, Heitkemper, and Dirksen, 2000)

intention imprinted electrical device, *n* a simple electronic device to which is imparted (by an experienced meditator) the intent to effect a measurable change in some experimental condition. These devices have been used by William Tiller to explore the relationships between consciousness and matter.

intentional immunomodulation (in·ten'·shən·əl im'·myu·nō·mä'·jə·lā'·shən), *n* the conscious suppression or enhancement of immune function through the use of mental techniques such as hypnosis. See also hypnosis.

intentionality (in·ten'·shə·na'·li·tē), *n* the characteristic of any action engaged in intentionally.

interaction, *n* in traditional Chinese medicine, the restricting nature of the five elements (wood, fire, earth, metal, and water), which is considered to be a normal activity.

Interactive guided imagery, *n* therapeutic approach involving visualization drawing from several humanistic psychological theories.

intercalate (in·ter'·kə·lāt'), *v* to place between two adjacent structures or surfaces.

intercession, *n* a prayer in which a request is made on behalf of another person.

intercessors, *n.pl* in spiritual healing, individuals who offer prayer to a higher power on behalf of another person in need of assistance or healing.

interconnectedness (in'·ter·kə·nek'·ted·nes), *n* idea that all objects are connected; therefore a change in the state of one produces change in the rest.

interior-exterior relationship, *n* in traditional Chinese medicine, another term for the yin and yang association between specific pairs of organs, such as the small intestine and the heart or the stomach and the spleen. See also yin and yang.

interleukin (in·tər·lōō'·kin), *n* any of the family of proteins produced by lymphocytes and macrophages in the presence of antigens, responsible for T-cell proliferation.

intermittent claudication, *n* set of symptoms produced by low blood circulation in the lower limbs; characterized by pain, weakness, or tension when in use. Symptoms generally subside completely when the limb is at rest.

International classification of disease codes, *n. pr* a comprehensive system of classification developed and maintained by the World Health Organization (WHO) for the purpose of coding and classifying data related to the causes of mortality. It promotes comparability on an international level regarding the compilation, categorization, processing, and formal presentation of health statistics. It is periodically reviewed and revised to keep abreast with developments in medical science. Also called *ICD-9*.

International Fragrance Association, *n.pr* an organization that represents the interests of the fragrance industry from around the world.

International Nomenclature of Cosmetic Ingredients (in·'·ter·na'·shə·nəl nō'·men·klā'·cher əv kôz·me'·tik in·grē'·dē·entz), *n.pr* an official document that lists the ingredients used in fragrances, including aromatic compositions and perfumes.

International Organization of Standardization, *n.pr* a nongovernmental federation of worldwide bodies that publishes international agreements covering a broad range of services and technologies to promote the use of common standards across the world. For example, one committee of the federation (TC 54) is specifically concerned with procedures relating to the manufacture, sale, and storage of essential oils.

International Society for the Study of Subtle Energies and Energy Medicine, *n.pr* founded in 1989, this is an interdisciplinary research organization whose purpose is the scientific study of subtle energies and their therapeutic applications.

International Society of Hypnosis, *n.pr* an organization of health practitioners who use hypnosis within the context of their practice. The organization works to improve research and clinical practice related to hypnosis, provides informal and formal communication, supports the scientific application of hypnosis, and sponsors the International Congress of Hypnosis on a triennial basis. It establishes codes of ethics defining and limiting persons who are eligible to learn hypnosis. The *International Journal of Clinical and Experimental Hypnosis,* which is published by the Society for Clinical and Experimental Hypnosis, has been adopted as the official

journal of the International Society of Hypnosis. Also called *ISH.*

international units, *n.pl* a unit of measurement that evaluates the potency of a substance. Because it measures potency instead of quantity, there is a different international unit-to-mg conversion ratio for each particular substance.

interpromotion (in'·ter·prə·mō'·shən), *n* in traditional Chinese medicine, the creation or promotion of one element by another in the following sequential order: wood, fire, earth, metal, and water, which is considered to be a normal activity. Wood promotes fire, fire promotes earth, and so forth.

interspersal approach (in·ter·sper'·səl ə·prōch'), *n* method of induction in which suggestions for relaxation are intermingled within a casual discussion on a topic of interest to the patient. See also induction.

interstitial cystitis, *n* a chronic bladder condition resulting in recurring pain in the pelvic area. Possible causes include autoimmune response to bladder infection, bacteria that are not found in the urine, or irritating urine chemistry.

intervention, *n* an intervention designed to improve the health of a patient or change the conditions which have negative impact on the well-being of the patient.

intolerance, *n* undesirable response to a substance (i.e., food, allergen, or remedy) or conditions. See also aggravation, idiosyncrasy, and tolerance.

intra-articular, *adj* administered to or occurring inside of a joint.

intracranial aneurysm (in'·trə·krā'·nē·əl an'·yə·ri'·zəm), *n* localized ballooning of any of the cerebral arteries, symptoms of which include severe headache, nausea, stiff neck, and sometimes loss of consciousness. Rupture of an intracranial aneurysm results in fatality in 50% of the cases.

intradermal, *n* in acupuncture, a fine, short needle that may be left in the skin for up to several days to keep qi moving. See also qi.

intramuscular, *adj* administered to or occurring inside of a muscle.

intramuscular stimulation (in'·trə·mus'·kyə·ler sti'·myə·lā'·shən), *n* a method developed by Dr. Chan Gunn; uses acupuncture to relieve chronic pain of neuropathic origin by releasing muscle shortening, which presses on nerves.

intrinsic corrective forces, *n.pl* forces arising within a patient—voluntary or involuntary—that assist in the therapeutic process of manipulation.

introducer, *n* in acupuncture, a plastic tube used to guide needles for accurate insertion, typically used by beginning acupuncturists. Also called *guide tube.*

intubation (in'·tə·bā'·shən), *n* the insertion of a cannula or a tube into a hollow organ, such as intestines or trachea, to maintain an opening or passageway.

intuiting, *v* to use impression, insight, or premonition to gain information about a client.

Inula helenium, n See elecampane.

investing layer, *n* superficial fascia, lying between the skin and the deeper, tougher fascia.

invitation to treat, *n* an exploratory fact-finding, preliminary step toward entering into a possible agreement with another party, such as a letter asking for more information or an advertisement.

Invocation, *n* a prayer requesting and inviting the presence of God.

involuntary, *adj* an action without conscious control.

iodine (ī'·o·dīn), *n* an element/mineral used in the synthesis of thyroid hormones and whose deficiency is implicated in preventable mental retardation and brain maldevelopment. Iodine is present in kelp and seafood, with the most common supplemental source being iodized table salt.

ion (ī'·ôn), *n* an atom or a molecule that has gained or lost electrons, thus giving rise to a charged particle. See also anion and cation.

ion pump, *n* a complex of proteins located in the cell membrane that is responsible for actively transporting ions across the membrane against a concentration gradient using energy rich ATP molecules. Functions in maintaining osmotic balance in cells and in the conduction of nerve impulses. See also ATP.

ionic bonding (ī·ôn'·ik bôn'·ding), *n* bond between two ions formed from atoms that lose or gain electrons rather than sharing electrons. Also called *electrovalent bonding.*

ionization (ī'·ən·ī·zā'·shən), *n* a process wherein an atom or a molecule loses or gains at least one electron to form an ion (a charged particle).

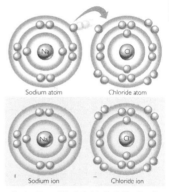

Sodium atom   Chloride atom

Sodium ion   Chloride ion

Ionization. (Mosby's Medical, Nursing & Allied Health Dictionary, ed 6, 2002)

ion pumping cords, *n* copper cords used in variants of electroacupuncture. The cords connect needles placed in different points on the client's body forming polarized (one-way) circuits that conduct the client's own bioelectricity.

ipecac syrup (i'·pi·kak' sir'·əp), *n* over-the-counter remedy made from the root of the *Cephaelis ipecacuanha* plant to induce vomiting.

ipecacuanha (i'·pi·ka'·kyə·wä'·nə), *n* Latin names: *Psychotria ipecacuanha, Cephaelis ipecacuanha;* part used: root; uses: induction of vomiting, perspiration, cough, facilitate digestion, stimulate aperitive, stomach action, intestinal action, liver action, bronchitis, laryngitis, dysentery; precautions: can cause skin irritation; can produce pustules; gastroenteritis, cardiac failure, vasodilator, severe bronchitis, pulmonary inflammation, sneezing, mild inflammation of the nasal mucous membrane, severe myopathy, lethargy, erythema, dysphagia, and cardiotoxicity.

ipriflavone (ī'·prə·flā'·vōn), *n* a synthetic isoflavone used to treat Paget's disease and to protect bones from damage due to osteoporosis, hyperparathyroidism, and corticosteroid therapies. Precaution advised for patients with renal disorders, lymphopenia, immunosuppression, gastrointestinal disorders, or a history of breast or reproductive cancers and those taking theophylline, caffeine, theobromine, phenytoin, warfarin, tolbutamide, NSAIDs, and immunosuppressant medications. Use of ipriflavone has also caused asymptomatic lymphopenia in test subjects, so regular blood cell counts are recommended during supplementation. Also called *7-isopropoxyisoflavone.* See also isoflavones.

iridology, *n* See diagnosis, iris.

iridoscope (i·ri'·də·skōp), *n* specialized microscope used by iridologists to examine the iris of the eye for diagnosis.

Iris versicolor, *n* See blue flag.

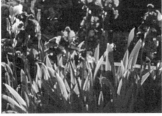

Iris versicolor. (Scott and Barlow, 2003)

Irish moss, *n.pr* Latin name: *Chondrus crispus;* parts used: entire plant; uses: antiinflammatory, diarrhea, gastritis, bronchitis; precautions: patients with ulcers or low blood pressure. Also called *carrageen, carrageenan,* or *chondrus.*

iron, *n* an essential mineral and element (Fe) found in leafy greens, meat, beans, peas, blackstrap molasses, and enriched breads and cereals; used as a supplement to relieve conditions associated with dietary deficiency and to enhance athletic performance. Excessive iron supplementation may also increase risk of cardiovascular conditions.

irregular feeding, *n* feeding behavior in which family members snack continuously throughout the day, instead of taking regular meals that may cause digestive problems or obesity.

irregular pattern, *n* in physical therapy, a classification given to describe symptoms that neither fit into the regular stretch pattern nor regular compression pattern categorizations. Symptoms are typically brought forth by provoking a combination of compressing and stretching movements. See also regular stretch pattern or regular compression pattern.

Isatis tinctoria **L.,** *n* See dyers woad.

Iscador (is'·kə·dōr), *n* a homeopathic preparation of fermented European mistletoe *(Viscum album L.)* and highly diluted metals (copper, mercury, or silver). Has been used in Europe as an adjunct to cancer therapy. Similar mistletoe extract preparations include *Eurixor, Helixor, Isorel, Iscucin, Plenosol,* and *ABNOBA viscum.*

ischemia (is·kē'·mē·ə), *n* a condition characterized by a deficit of oxygen for a tissue.

ischemic reoxygenation (is·kē'·mik rē·ôk'·sə·jə·nā'·shən), *n* the reintroduction of oxygenated blood into a tissue that had previously been oxygen-deficient. Concomitant increase of oxygen free radicals may lead to tissue damage. Also called *hypoxia-reoxygenation,* *ischemic reperfusion,* or *postischemic reoxygenation.*

ischemic reperfusion, *n* the restoration of blood flow to an area that had previously experienced deficient blood flow. Oxidative stresses associated with this situation may cause damage to the affected tissues or organs.

ISO, *n.pr* See International Organization of Standardization.

iso principle (ī'·sō prin'·si·pəl), *n* concept according to which a patient's musical mood can be matched to assist him or her in becoming aware of thoughts and recapture memories.

isodes (ī'·sōdz), *n* in contemporary homeopathy, highly diluted and successed preparations of organic or synthetic substances that are thought to be the cause of disorder or disease. Given as a remedy based on the principle, "the cause is the cure." Also called *detoxodes.*

isoflavones (ī'·sō·flā'·vōnz), *n.pl* phytoestrogenic compounds found in various plants, including red clover and soy. Used in lowering blood cholesterol levels, in relieving menopausal complaints, in protecting against osteoporosis, and as possible preventive against hormone-dependent cancer. Caution in patients with thyroid conditions or with a predisposition to breast cancer, and those taking thyroid medications.

isogenesis (ī'·sō·je'·nə·sis), *n* development from similar processes and having the same origin.

isokinetic exercise, *n* a form of exercise in which the body parts being exercised are moved at a constant speed.

isolate (ī'·sə·lət), *n* the term for a single component, which has been separated from a volatile mixture.

isomerism (ī·sō'·mer·i·zəm), *n* dissimilar arrangement of atoms within the molecules of two chemical compounds that have identical molecular formulae. See also geometric isomerism and optical isomers.

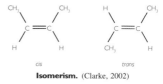

cis trans

Isomerism. (Clarke, 2002)

isomerism, geometric, *n* a form of isomerism in compounds containing at least one double bond where atoms or atomic groups attached to the doubly bound carbon atoms have no free rotation around the axis of the double bond. Geometric isomers with specific atomic groups on opposite sides of the double bond are called trans-isomers, while cis-isomers have those groups on the same side.

isometric (ī'·sō·me'·trik), *n* muscle contraction that does not involve any change in the muscle length.

isometric exercise, *n* exercise in which the muscles contract without the movement of the affected joints. Strengthens bones, builds muscle mass, and increases metabolism. Also called *anaerobic exercise, resistance training,* or *strength training.* See also isometric contraction.

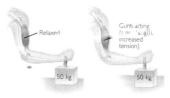

Relaxed

Contracting (non-length, increased tension)

50 kg 50 kg

Isometric exercise. (Thibodeau and Patton, 1999; Rolin Graphics)

isoniazid (ī'·sə·nī'·ə·zid), *n* a drug, $C_6H_7N_3O$ that is used in the treatment of tuberculosis. Also called *INH* or *isonicotinic acid hydrazide*.

isopathy, *n* in homeopathy, treatment involving remedies whose source material is the disease specific antigen or a product of the disease. See also autohemic therapy, autoisopathy, autonosode, nosode, sarcode, and tautopathy.

isoprene (ī'·sō·prēn), *n* the fundamental unit of compounds known as terpenes. It has a molecular formula of C_5H_8 and can be described as aliphatic or acyclic. See also terpenes.

isotherapy (ī·sō·the'·rə·pē), *n* in contemporary homeopathy, the use of isodes as remedies based on the principle "the cause is the cure." See also isodes, isopathy.

isotonic (ī'·sō·tô'·nik), *n* muscle contraction that involves change in the muscle length.

ispaghula seed, *n* See psyllium.

ISSSEEM, *n.pr* See International Society for the Study of Subtle Energies and Energy Medicine.

itch diathesis, *n* a syndrome defined by itching and crusty skin rash, currently associated with a *Sarcoptes scabiei* var. *hominis* infection. Hahnemann considered this to be the main symptom of the psoric miasm. See also psoric miasm.

IU, *n.pr* See international units.

ivy, *n* Latin name: *Hedera helix;* part used: leaves; uses: expectorant, antimicrobial, pain relief, antispasmodic, chronic respiratory problems; precautions: contact dermatitis.

ivy gourd, *n* Latin name: *Coccinia indica;* parts used: leaves; uses: Ayurvedic treatment for diabetes mellitus and improved glucose tolerance; precautions: patients taking antidiabetic medications.

iyus' kiniya (ē·yŏŏs' kī·nī·yä'), *adj* Lakota term for the ability to perform tasks with an upbeat, happy disposition.

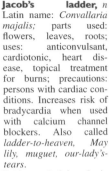

Jacob's ladder, *n* Latin name: *Convallaria majalis;* parts used: flowers, leaves, roots; uses: anticonvulsant, cardiotonic, heart disease, topical treatment for burns; precautions: persons with cardiac conditions. Increases risk of bradycardia when used with calcium channel blockers. Also called *ladder-to-heaven, May lily, muguet, our-lady's-tears.*

jalap resin (ja'·ləp re'·zin), *n* Latin names: *Exogonium purga, Ipomea purga, Convolvulus jalapa, Convolvulus purga;* part used: root; uses: cathartic, colic, pain in the bowels, general intestinal inactivity, vermifugal; precautions: none known. Also called *calapa, jalap bindweed,* and *scammony.*

Jamaican dogwood, *n.pr* Latin name: *Piscidia erythrina;* parts used: bark, roots; uses: insomnia, menstrual conditions, asthma, migraines, analgesia; precautions: toxic, children, pregnancy, lactation, geriatric patients, cardiovascular conditions; not to be used intravenously. Also called *fish poison tree, fishfuddle,* or *West Indian dogwood.*

jambul (jäm·bəl), *n* Latin name: *Syzygium cuminii;* parts used: fruit, seeds, leaves; uses: diarrhea, diabetes mellitus; precautions: none known. Also called *black plum, jamba, jambolana, jambolo, jambool, jambula, jambulon plum,* or *java plum.*

jamun (jä'·mōōn), *n* Latin name: *Syzygium cumini*; parts used: bark, fruit, seeds, leaves; uses: in Ayurveda, pacifies kapha and pitta doshas (astringent, sweet, light, dry), hypoglycemic, diuretic, antiinflammatory, diarrhea, dysentery, diabetes, bark:

gum disorders, oral health; precautions: none known. Also called *Indian blackberry, jambu, jambul,* or *Java plum.*

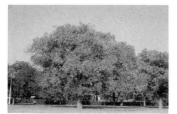

Jamun. (Williamson, 2002)

janma prakriti (jan´·mə prə·kri·tē), *n* in Ayurveda the dosha predominant at birth; determined at conception and based mainly on heredity among other factors. See also dosha.

Jateorrhiza columba, n See calumba.

Jateorrhiza palmata, n See calumba.

jatharagni (jä·thä·räg´·nē), *n* in Ayurveda the enzyme active in the oral cavity and the gastrointestinal tract; catalyst for breaking down food. See also agnis.

Jeffersonia **(je´·fər·sō´·nē·ə),** *n* a genus of the Asian and American herbs of the family Berberidaceae. The root of *Jeffersonia diphylla* is used as a tonic, expectorant, diuretic, and emetic in large doses.

jellies, *n.pl* See gels.

Jenkins activity survey, *n.pr* multiplechoice inventory that assesses type-A behavior patterns, a risk factor in the formation of coronary disease.

Jesuit's bark, *n* See calisaya bark.

jiedu yanggan gao (jē·ä·dōō yäng· gän gä·ō), *n* mixture of herbs used in Chinese medicine to treat chronic hepatitis B.

jimsonweed, *n* Latin name: *Datura stramonium;* parts used: flowers, leaves, roots; uses: asthma, Parkinson's disease, irritable bowel syndrome; precautions: children, pregnancy, lactation, patients with nervous disorders; liver disease, heart conditions, or kidney disease; all parts are highly toxic, especially seeds;

can cause horrifying hallucinations. Also called *angel's trumpet, angel tulip, apple-of-Peru, datura, devil weed, devil's apple, devil's trumpet, Estramonio, green dragon, gypsyweed, inferno, Jamestown weed, loco seeds, locoweed, mad apple, moon weed, stramoine, stechapfel, stinkweed, thorn apple, tolguacha, trumpet lilly,* or *zombie's cucumber.*

jin shin, *n.pr* See jin shin jitsu.

jin shin do (jēn shēn dō), *n* "way of compassionate spirit," a form of acupressure particularly used on hypersensitive acupuncture points.

jin shin jitsu (jin shin jitsōō), *n.pr* a style of bodywork originating in Japan; promotes energetic movement through gentle pressure on multiple acupressure points. This is considered an inner bodywork modality because the techniques release emotional and spiritual—as well as physical— energies.

jing (jēng), *n* Chinese term for acupuncture channels. See also channels.

jing level (jēng´ le´·vəl), *n* the core level of energy located in the kidney and the eight extraordinary meridians that comprises prenatal, encoded materials and can guide development and growth.

jing-luo (jēng lō), *n* according to traditional Chinese medicine, the meridians or channels that form a network of energy pathways that link and balance the various organs. The meridians have four functions: to connect the internal organs with the exterior of the body and the person to the environment and the universe, to harmonize the yin and yang principles within the body's organs and five substances, to distribute qi or the basic life force within the body, and to protect the body against environmental imbalances. When jing-luo are blocked, qi and blood cannot circulate resulting in illness. See also qi.

jin-ye (djēn-yə), *n.pl* body fluids; in traditional Chinese medicine theory, the liquids that nourish, protect, and lubricate the human body. These fluids include tears, sweat, stomach acid, semen, saliva, breast milk, mucus, and other secretions. *Jin* refers to the lighter fluids, which nourish and moisten the muscles and skin; *ye* refers to the denser, darker fluids that feed the internal organs, bones, brain, and body orifices.

jitsu (jē'·tsōō), *n* "full," the active, expressive, energetic component of qi, according to the theory of zen shiatsu. Jitsu is similar to the concept of *yang* in Chinese medical theory. See also ki, kyo, and yang.

jivanti (gē·vän·tē), *n* Latin name: *Leptadenia reticulata;* parts used: leaf, root, whole plant; uses: in Ayurveda, considered a rasayana; balances tridosha (sweet, light, oily), stimulant, restorative, antibacterial, antifungal, lactogenic, skin conditions, wounds, cough, asthma; precautions: none known. Also called *dori, leptadenia,* or *svarnajivanti.*

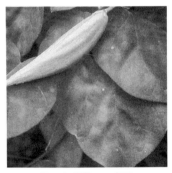

Jivanti. (Williamson, 2002)

johrei (jōh·rā·ē), *n* a healing art from the Japanese tradition. It is a form of energy healing similar to the "laying on of hands" practiced in other cultures.

joint, *n* a point of articulation between bones.

joint capsule, *n* two-layered structure that surrounds, supports, and lubricates synovial joints.

joint centration **(joint' sen·trā'·shən),** *n* a neutral positioning of a joint by which maximum equilibrium exists between the surfaces and the tension or length relationships of antagonist muscles are stabilized.

joint kinesthetic receptors **(joint' ki'·nis·the'·tik rə·sep'·terz),** *n* pressure receptors in the capsules of joints. They are sensitive to the motion, acceleration, and deceleration of the joint.

joint range, *n* the complete range of motion measured with a tape measure or a goniometer. In most cases, a practitioner determines the range by visual examination.

joint, ball-and-socket, *n* joints such as the coxa or glenohumeral that consist of a knoblike ball of bone rotating in a smooth, concavity of bone, thus allowing full range of movement. Also called *triaxial joint.*

joint, sacroiliac **(sa'·krō·i'·lē·ak joint'),** *n* the pelvic joint which connects the sacrum and the ilium. It is supported by the hamstring muscles and can be adversely affected by weaknesses or dysfunction in them.

joints, ellipsoidal **(i'·lip·soi'·dəl joints'),** *n.pl* joints similar to the ball and socket joints; allow flexion, extension, abduction, adduction, and some rotation. Also called *biaxial* or *condyloid joints.*

joints, saddle, *n.pl* joints that permit all movements with limited rotation. Also called *biaxial joints.*

Joint Commission on Accreditation of Healthcare Organizations, *n.pr* the United States body that accredits healthcare organizations.

jojoba (hə·hō'·bə), *n* Latin names: *Simmondsia chinensis, Simmondsia californica;* parts used: seed oil; uses: antioxidant, dry or irritated skin conditions, hair care, hair loss, acne; precautions: none known. Also called *deernut, goatnut,* or *pignut.*

JPRT, *n.pr* See therapy, Jacobson's Progressive Relaxation.

judo, *n* Japanese martial art and sport derived from jujutsu; relies primarily on grappling techniques and a philosophy that emphasizes yielding instead of resistance.

judo revival, *n* a system derived from acupuncture; pressure is applied to specific points of the body to induce a reflex response.

jue yin (jā yin), *n* in Chinese medicine, one of the six principle meridians through which the vital force qi flows; further subdivided into yin division (liver), and yang division (master of the heart). The balance of yin and yang components and the proper flow of qi in an individual indicate sound health. See also qi, tai yang, shao yang, yang ming, tai min, and shao yin.

Juglans regia, n See walnut.

jugular, *adj* relating to the neck or throat regions.

jui (jōō·ē), *n* therapy used to move qi in the body; involves burning dried leaves of the plant *Artemesia vulgaris* close to or directly on the skin. See also qi.

jump sign, *n* an indication of trigger point location in which the patient forcefully pulls away when the trigger point is contacted.

Jungian psychology, *n.pr* psychologic approach based on the ideas and theories developed by Carl Jung (1875–1961). Includes the concepts of the collective unconscious and symbolic archetypes.

juniper, *n* Latin names: *Juniperus communis, Juniperus oxycedrus* L.; part used: berries (dried); uses: diuretic, antiflatulent, antiinflammatory, abortifacient, diabetes mellitus, urinary infections; precautions: pregnancy, lactation, children. Also called *a'ra'r a'di, andie, baical juniper, common juniper, dwarf, gemener, genievre, ground juniper, hackmatack, harvest, horse savin, juniper mistletoe, yoshu-nezu,* or *zimbru.*

Juniperus communis, n See juniper.

Juniperus oxycedrus L., n See juniper.

justice, *n* principle of medical ethics according to which a person treats another person with fairness in both medical and nonmedical settings.

jyotish (jyō·tē'·sh), *n* in Ayurveda, a discipline that involves the comprehensive study of cosmology, astrology, and astronomy. Similar to the ways the moon and sun have significant physical effects upon individuals and the planets, the complete cosmos also possesses certain levels of influences. Specifically, this discipline is claimed to uncover karmic patterns associated with a person's past, present, and future plus his or her strength and potential for affecting future and ongoing events. Also called *jyotisha* or *Vedic astrology.*

kahuna ana'ana (kä·hōō·nə ä·nə·ä·nə), *n* in Hawaiian culture, black magician who can cast spells to bring about death to a person.

kahuna lapa'au (kä·hōō·nə lä·pä·ä·ōō), *n* in Hawaiian culture, healer who employs prayer, herbs, love (aloha), and touch to restore health to an ailing person.

kaliuresis (ka'·lē·yə·rē'·səs), *n* the secretion of potassium, particularly in large amounts, in the urine.

kalka (käl'·kə), *n* in Ayurveda, a method of medicine preparation in which herbs are ground to the consistency of paste.

kalmegh (käl'·məgh), *n* Latin name: *Andrographis paniculata*; parts used: leaves, roots; uses: in Ayurveda, pacifies kapha and pitta doshas (bitter, light, dry), anthelmintic, symptomatic relief and prevention of the common cold, liver disorders, jaundice, diarrhea, malaria, atherosclerosis; precautions: none known. Also called *bhunimba, creat,* or *green chiretta.*

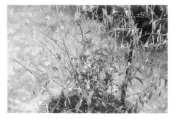

Kalmegh. (Williamson, 2002)

kamalahar (kä·mä·lä'·här), *n* mixture of herbs used in Ayurveda to treat acute viral hepatitis.

kampo (käm·pō), *n* traditional Japanese herbal medicine. By Japanese law, all kampo practitioners must be either Western-trained doctors or pharmacists.

kampo formulations (käm'·pō fōr'·myə·lā'·shənz), *n.pl* Herbal combinations from traditional Japanese medicine.

kampoyaku (käm·pō·yä·kōō), *n* Japanese term used to indicate traditional Chinese herbal medicine. It involves the application of over 210 different types of herbal preparations, including juzen-taiho-to, hochu-ekki-to, and sho-saiko. Also called *juzen-taiho-to, hochu-ekki-to, sho-saiko,* and *kampo.*

kapalabhati pranayama (kä'·pä·lä·bhä'·tē prä·nä·yä'·mə), *n* See breath of fire.

kapha (kä'·fə), *n* in Ayurveda, one of the three organizing principles (doshas) that are responsible for maintaining homeostasis. Formed by a combination of water and earth, kapha is responsible for body stability and cohesion. See also doshas.

kapha, avalambaka **(ə·və·ləm'·bə·kə),** *n* in Ayurveda, a subdivision of the kapha dosha whose influence is evident in the upper torso, heart, and lungs. It promotes upper body strength and cardiac health; when imbalanced, back pain, heart, or respiratory diseases may result. See also doshas.

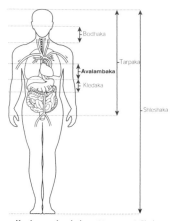

Kapha, avalambaka. (Sharma and Clarke 1998)

kapha, bodhaka **(bō'·dhə·kə),** *n* in Ayurveda, a subdivision of the kapha dosha whose influence is evident in the tongue and throat. It promotes mucus secretion and the sense of taste; imbalance may result in dry mouth, indigestion, and a loss of gustation. See also doshas.

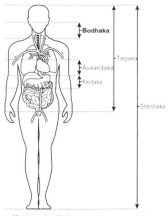

Kapha, bodhaka. (Sharma and Clarke, 1998)

kapha, kledaka (**klā̇·də·kə**), *n* in Ayurveda, a subdivision of the kapha dosha whose influence is evident in the stomach. It promotes the initial stages of food digestion; when imbalanced, digestive disorders may result. See also doshas.

illnesses, and loss of olfaction. See also doshas.

Kaposi's sarcoma, *n.pr* a type of cancer characterized by purplish spots which develop on the feet and spreads from the skin to the lymph nodes and internal organs; commonly seen in patients with compromised immune function, such as AIDS.

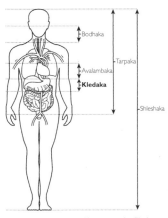

Kapha, kledaka. (Sharma and Clarke, 1998)

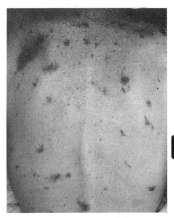

Kaposi's sarcoma (KS). (Callen et al, 1993)

kapha, sama (**sä·mə kä·fə**), *n* in Ayurveda, ama in combination with a kapha imbalance, manifesting in the form of severe mucilaginous conditions. Remedied with pungent and bitter herbs. See also ama and kapha.

kapha, shleshaka (**shlā̇·shä·kə**), *n* in Ayurveda, a subdivision of the kapha dosha whose influence is evident in the joints. It promotes lubrication of the joints and maintenance of connective tissues; imbalance may result in joint diseases such as arthritis. See also doshas.

kapha, tarpaka (**tər·pə·kə**), *n* in Ayurveda, a subdivision of the kapha dosha, the influence of which is evident in the head, sinuses, and cerebrospinal fluid. It promotes healthy moisture levels in the eyes, nose, and throat and also contributes to maintenance of the CSF. Imbalance may result in sinus problems, respiratory

kapu (**kä·pōō**), *n* in the Hawaiian culture, a code of taboos, strictly practiced until the midnineteenth century. Violators of the code were banished or put to death.

karaya gum (**kə·rī·yə gəm**), *n* Latin name; *Sterculia urens;* part used: sap (dried); uses: bulk laxative, demulcent, sore throat; precautions: patients on medication. Also called *Indian tragacanth, kadaya, kadira, katila, kullo, mucara,* or *sterculia gum.*

karma (**kär·mə**), *n* in Sanskrit, action. Karma is understood as the consequence of thought and behavior, thus providing causal continuity from moment to moment and lifetime to lifetime.

karyokinesis (**kar·ē·ō·kə·nē·sis**), *n* the splitting up of the nucleus and equivalent sharing of nuclear material during meiosis and mitosis. Precedes cytokinesis. Also called *karyomitosis.* See also cytokinesis.

kathina (kä·tē'·nə), *adj* in Ayurveda, "hard" as a guna, one of the qualities characterizing all substances. Its complement is mrudu. See also gunas and mrudu.

kava (kä·və), *n* Latin name: *Piper methysticum;* parts used: rhizomes, roots; uses: anxiolytic, antiepileptic, antidepressant, muscle relaxant, analgesia, insomnia, alcohol dependency; precautions: children, pregnancy, lactation; patients with depression, pulmonary hypertension, Parkinson's disease; liver disease, or kidney disease; patients who drink alcohol. Also called *ava, ava pepper, awa, intoxicating pepper, kava-kava, kawa, kew, sakau, tonga,* or *yagona.*

kava kava, *n* See kava.

kayacikitsa (kä·yä·sē·kīt'·sə), *n* the branch of Ayurveda associated with internal medicine.

keiraku chiryo (kä·ē·rä·kōō chē·ryō), *n* Japanese term for meridian therapy.

kelp, *n* Latin names: *Laminaria digitata, Laminaria japonica, Laminaria saccharina, Marcrocystis pyrifera;* part used: fronds; uses: antiobesity, anticancer, antioxidant, antiviral, abortifacient, anticoagulant, high blood pressure, dietary source of iodine; precautions: children, pregnancy, lactation; patients with hyperthyroidism; can cause possible heavy metal toxicity. Also called *brown algae, horsetail, kombu, sea girdles, sea vegetables, seaweed, sugar wrack,* or *tangleweed.*

kelpware, *n* Latin name: *Fucus vesiculosus;* part used: whole plant; uses: obesity, goiter, kidney inflammation, dietary source of iodine; precautions: patients with cardiac conditions, kidney disease, cancer, liver disease, diabetes mellitus, or thyroid disorders other than goiter. Also called *black-tang, bladder focus, bladder-wrack, blasen-tang, quercus marina, sea wrack, sea-oak,* and *seetang.*

keratosis (ke'·rə·tō'·sis), *n* skin condition indicated by the presence of noticeable increased growth and thickening of cornified epithelium. Actinic keratosis, seborrheic keratosis, and keratosis senilis are examples of this skin condition.

Kestenberg movement profile, *n* diagnostic measure in dance/movement therapy.

ketoacidosis (kē'·tō·a·si·dō'·sis), *n* acidosis accompanied by an increase of ketones caused by widespread breakdown of fats as a result of inefficient carbohydrate metabolism. Typically a complication of diabetes mellitus. Characteristics include the presence of a noticeable fruity scent of acetone on a person's breath, dyspnea, mental confusion, nausea, weight loss, and dehydration.

ketoaciduria (kē'·tō·a·sə·dōō'·rē·ə), *n* the presence of a large amount of ketone bodies in a person's urine due to diabetes mellitus, starvation, or a metabolic condition wherein fats are quickly catabolized. Also called *ketonuria.*

ketone, *n* compound that contains a carbonyl group attached to a carbon in a chain. Used as analgesics, antiinflammatories, expectorants, and stimulants.

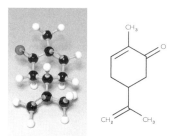

Ketones. (Clarke, 2002; Spring Enterprises Ltd.)

key change, *n* in the Mitchell method, the joint change that the individual finds most beneficial for reducing tension. See also method, Mitchell.

key lesion, *n* a bodily dysfunction that supports a complete pattern of improper anatomic and physiologic functioning.

keynotes, *n.pl* in homeopathy, concise characteristic indications for a remedy.

khara (khə·rə), *adj* in Ayurveda, "rough" as a guna, one of the qualities characterizing all substances. Its complement is slakshna. See also gunas and slakshna.

khat (khät), *n* Latin name: *Catha edulis;* part used: leaves (raw); uses: stimulant, depression, obesity, stomach ulcers; precautions: patients with kidney disease, heart disease, or liver disease; can cause hepatotoxicity; may cause cerebral hemorrhage; is possibly teratogenic. Khat is illegal in the United States and Great Britain. Also called *cat, chat, gad, kaht, kat, miraa,* or *tschut.*

khella (khel'·lə), *n* Latin name: *Ammi visnaga;* parts used: fruit, roots, seeds; uses: angina, cramps, colic, allergies, asthma, diabetes, cholesterol; precautions: pregnancy, lactation, children; patients with liver conditions, severe heart conditions, bleeding disorders, or hypotension. Also called *ammi, bishop's weed, khellin,* or *visnagin*

KHT, *n.pr* See therapy, Koryo hand.

KI, *n* an acupuncture channel running from the feet to the chest, named after the kidney, and associated with the bladder (BL) channel. See also BL.

kidney stones, *n* precipitates of calcium salts, uric acid, or struvite that develop within the upper urinary tract or bladder. The presence of these materials within the body may not initially produce symptoms, but the progression of the condition may result in severe, sporadic pain that radiates from the kidney or flank region.

kieraku chiryo system (kā·ē·rä·kōō chē·ryō sis'·təm), *n* diagnostic system in acupuncture that focuses on problems of repletion and vacuity in the 12 channels. See also acupuncture.

kinaesthetic sense, *n* perception through neuromuscular feedback of a body movement.

kindling (kin'·dling), *n* change in brain function wherein repeated chemical or electrical stimuli induce seizures.

kinesia (ki·nē'·zhə), *n* condition resulting from regular or irregular motions while moving in any combination of directions, such as riding in a car, boat, or an airplane. General discomfort or headaches are characteristic of mild cases, whereas severe cases are marked by nausea and dizziness. Also called *kinetosis* or *motion sickness.*

kinesiology (kə·nē'·zē·ä'·lə·jē), *n* study of the body's structure and processes as they relate to movement.

kinesophobia (ki·nē'·sō·fō'·bē·ə), *n* irrational fear of movement or motion, often following a traumatic injury. Also called *kinetophobia.*

kinesthesia (ki'·nəs·thē'·sē·ə), *n* the sense through which somatic elements such as body position, muscle tension, and weight are perceived.

kinesthetic dystonia (ki'·nəs·the'·tik dis·tō'·nē·ə), *n* concept explored in the Feldenkrais method in which students lie on the floor and when scanning their own bodies, discover disconnections in terms of kinesthetic linking. See also method, Feldenkrais.

kinesthetic identification, *n* movement empathy, a foundational technique of dance/movement therapy in which practitioner and client move in synchrony. Also called *attunement.*

kinetic component, *n* in manual therapy, relating to the interrelationships that exist between body parts and how those connections influence movement.

kinetic energy, *n* a property of a particle that describes the energy of motion and directly correlates with the particle's rate of motion. For example, transfer of gaseous particles is an important factor in the field of aromatherapy.

kinetics, *n* **1.** area of study that examines the effects of outside influences on the movement of material bodies. **2.** the study of the interrelationships that exist between body parts and how those connections influence movement.

Kirlian photography, *n.pr* technique named after Seymon Kirlian, which

K

involves photographing subjects in a high-frequency, low-amperage electrical field, which display bright emanations usually around the fingers or toes.

klapping, *n* using cupped palms to strike the body, with the intent of using the vibrations so produced to loosen material in the hollows and sacs of the body.

kneading, *n* a massage technique in which the whole hand is moved in a circular pattern while the fingers and thumbs squeeze the tissues beneath.

Kneippkur (nē'·pə·kər), *n* a system of natural healing developed by German priest Sebastian Kneipp. The five pillars of Kneippkur are hydrotherapy, movement therapies, herbs, diet, and a consciously ordered lifestyle. Also called *Kneipp cure, Kneipp's cure, Kneippism,* or *Naturheilverfahren.* See also naturopathy.

ko cycle (khô sī'·kəl), *n* in traditional Chinese medicine, one of the two cycles of the five elements, where one element disciplines or controls the next (i.e., metal controls wood, fire controls metal, earth controls water, wood controls earth, and water controls fire.) The ko cycle is compared to the relationship between a father and child in terms of discipline and control. The therapeutic application of the ko cycle involves bringing balance between the elements to restore proper relationship.

koketsu (kō·kāt·sōō), *n.pl* one-hundred-twenty acupuncture points corresponding to underlying, often neurological structures. See also acupuncture.

kombucha (kōm·bōō'·chə), *n* a colony of different species of bacteria and yeast, including *Schizosaccharomyces pombe, Saccharomycodes ludwigii, Bacterium gluconicum, Bacterium xylinum, Bacterium katogenum, Bacterium xylinoides, Pichia fermentans,* and *Torula* spp., kept together by a thin membrane and commonly brewed into a highly acidic tea containing ethyl acetate alcohol,

lactate, and acetic acid. The tea has been promoted as a remedy for insomnia, baldness, arthritis, intestinal disorders, multiple sclerosis, chronic fatigue syndrome, cancer, and AIDS. The tea is claimed to boost the activities of the immune system and reverse the process of aging. Use of kombucha tea has been associated with metabolic acidosis and hepatotoxicity.

koryo sooji chim (kō·ryō sō·ō·jē chēm), *n* Korean system of hand and finger acupuncture in which small filiform needles are inserted and magnets are applied according to a mapping system where the entire body is represented on points on the surface of the hands.

kPA, *n* kilopascal. See pascal.

Krameria triandra, *n* See rhatany root.

kriyas (krē'·yäs), *n.pl* brain exercises taught by Yogi Bhajan; they involve regenerating sound currents, breathing, and finger movements to facilitate a state of meditation and to stimulate the central nervous system.

ksira paka (kshē'·rə pä'·kə), *n* in Ayurveda, a method of medicine preparation in which a paste of fresh herbs is mixed with sugar syrup until it has a gelatinous consistency, at which time it is dusted with a flavoring herbal powder.

kudzu (kud'·zōō), *n* Latin name: *Pueraria lobata;* part used: roots; uses: alcoholism, muscle aches, measles, respiratory conditions; precautions: patients with heart disease. Also called *Japanese arrowroot, kudzu vine, ge gen,* or *mile-a-minute vine.*

kundalini, *n* spiritual energy "coiled" in the root chakra that can be uncoiled and released through special forms of meditation or yoga. See also chakra.

kupipakva rasayana (kōō'·pē·pək·wə rə·sä'·yä·nə), *n* in Ayurveda, a method of medicine preparation in which medicinal substances are heated until they vaporize.

kushta (kōōsh'·tə), *n* a traditional preparation originating from India and Pakistan, used as an aphrodisiac. The preparation contains oxidized metals (zinc, arsenic, mercury, and lead) that are combined with a variety of herbs. Metal poisoning is a risk associated with application and use of kushta.

kutaja (kōō'·tə·jə), *n* Latin name: *Holarrhena antidysenterica;* parts used: stem, root bark, seeds; uses: in Ayurveda, pacifies kapha and pitta doshas (bitter, astringent, light, dry), antibacterial, immunomodulator, vermifuge, laxative, dysentery, bleeding disorders, diabetes, tumors, bronchitis, colic, diarrhea, splenitis; precautions: none known. Also called *conessi, kurchi,* or *tellicherry.*

kutki (kōōt·kē), *n* Latin name: *Picorrhiza kurroa;* parts used: root, rhizome; uses: in Ayurveda, pacifies kapha and pitta doshas (bitter, light, dry), antioxidant, anticholestatic, laxative, antiinflammatory, hepatoprotective, antiasthmatic, liver conditions, jaundice, fever, dysentery, digestive conditions; precautions: laxative, gastric irritation in large doses. Also called *dhanwantary grastya, kutaki, katukarohini,* or *yellow gentian.*

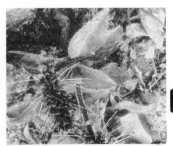

Kutki. (Williamson, 2002)

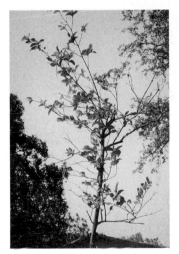

Kutaja. (Williamson, 2002)

kvatha (kwä'·thə), *n* in Ayurveda, a method of medicine preparation in which herbs are decocted in boiling water.

kyo (kyō), *n* "empty," the passive, needful, open component of qi, according to the theory of zen shiatsu. Kyo is similar to the concept of yin in Chinese medical theory. See also jitsu, ki, and yin.

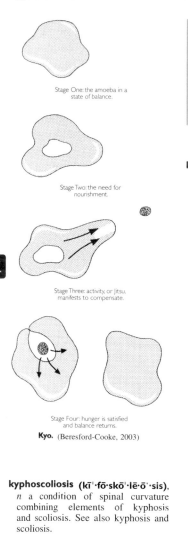

Stage One: the amoeba in a state of balance.

Stage Two: the need for nourishment.

Stage Three: activity, or Jitsu, manifests to compensate.

Stage Four: hunger is satisfied and balance returns.

Kyo. (Beresford-Cooke, 2003)

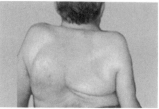

Kyphoscoliosis. (Lemmi and Lemmi, 2000)

kyphosis (kī·fō'·səs), *n* an atypical, exaggerated, backward curve of the thoracic spine caused by tuberculosis of the spine or rickets. Also called *hunchback*.

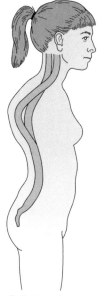

Kyphosis. (Salvo, 2003)

kyphoscoliosis (kī'·fō·skō'·lē·ō'·sis), *n* a condition of spinal curvature combining elements of kyphosis and scoliosis. See also kyphosis and scoliosis.

kyphosis-lordosis posture (kī·fō·səs-lōr·dō´·səs pǎs´·chər), *n* posture characterized by a convex curvature of the thoracic spine and an inwardly curved lower back resulting from the pelvis being tilted forward. See also kyphosis and lordosis.

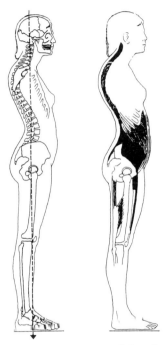

Kyphosis-lordosis posture. (Petty and Moore, 2001)

L, *adj* See lumbar.

LA, *n.pr* See acid, linolenic.

Lactobacillus acidophilus, *n* See acidophilus.

lactogenic, *adj/n* that which promotes milk secretion. See also galactagogue.

lactone (lak´·tōn), *n* a compound with a high molecular mass that comprises an ester linked to a ring structure of carbon atoms. Significant members of this group are coumarin and its derivatives. It is found in expressed oils and some absolutes. It has been used as an anticoagulant, sedative, and antipyretic. Harmful effects include skin allergies and potential toxicity to the nervous system.

lactose, *n* sugar extracted from milk, often used as a diluent in the creation of homeopathic remedies and in non-medicated tablets.

lady's mantle, *n* Latin names: *Alchemilla mollis, Alchemilla vulgaris;* parts used: flowers, roots, leaves; uses: topically controls bleeding, astringent, menstrual cramps, symptoms of menopause, diarrhea; precautions: pregnancy, lactation, children, hepatotoxicity. Also called *bear's foot, dewcup, leontopodium, lion's foot, nine hooks,* or *stellaria.*

laetrile (lā´·ə·tril), *n* anticancer treatment used for centuries that became popular in the 1950s. Ernest Krebs, Jr. coined the trade name *Laetrile.* Controlled clinical studies have failed to confirm the drug's efficacy. See also amygdalin.

laghu (lä´·ghōō), *adj* in Ayurveda, "light" as a guna, one of the qualities characterizing all substances. Its complement is guru. See also gunas and guru.

Lamaze, *n* a philosophy of natural childbirth that recognizes the innate, biological wisdom that women bring to pregnancy and labor. This philosophy attempts to create a supportive birthing atmosphere for mother and child, using such practices as non-supine positions, freedom of movement, a lack of routine interventions, and characteristic breathing exercises for relaxation and pain control.

lambdoidal suture, *n* meeting place of the parietal and occipital bones, which is shaped like the Greek letter lambda.

laparoscopy **(la'·pə·räs'·kə·pē),** *n* an examination of the internal aspects of the body with a thin optical or fiberoptic instrument known as a laprascope. Also called *peritoneoscopy.*

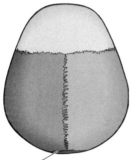

Laparascopy. (Chabner, 2001)

Lamboidal suture. (Chaitow, 1999)

Lambdoidal suture

lamentation, *n* a prayer expressing affliction or sorrow and requesting defense, retribution, or comfort.

Laminaria digitata, *n* See kelp.

Laminaria japonica, *n* See kelp.

Laminaria saccharina, *n* See kelp.

lapacho, *n* See pau d'arco.

laparotomy, *n* any major surgical procedure that involves opening the abdomen.

Larrea divaricata, *n* See chaparral.

Larrea tridentata, *n* See chaparral.

larynx **(lar'·ingks),** *n* the structure between the pharynx and the trachea that contains the vocal cords.

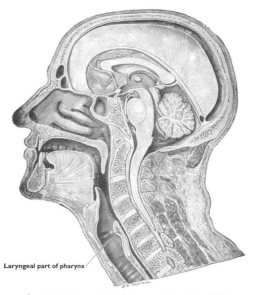

Larynx. (Chaitow et al, 2002; Reproduced from Gray, 1989)

laser, *n* acronym for light amplification by stimulated emission of radiation.

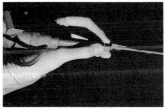

Laser. (Ball, 1995)

lateral flexed, *adj* vertebral position where a point on the anterosuperior aspect of a vertebra moves in the frontal plane around an anteroposterior axis.

lateral masses, *n.pl* the bulkiest, solid parts of the atlas (C1) vertebra, upon which the skull is supported.

laterality, *n* **1.** the side of the body in which the symptoms of disease are manifested. **2.** participation of upper left side and lower right sides of the body and rotation of symptoms from side to side. Some homeopathic remedies are linked to certain laterality, which may help determine the treatment regimen.

laughing spirit listening circles, *n.pl,* form of therapy in which groups of six to 10 people give each person in the circle an opportunity to receive undivided, positive attention while the individual speaks until he or she feels connected to the members within the group. See also therapy, humor.

Laurus nobilis, *n* See bay.

lavage (lə·vazh´), *n* the process of flushing or washing out a hollow organ, particularly the paranasal sinuses, bladder, bowel, or stomach for therapeutic purposes.

Lavandula angustifolia, *n* See lavender.

Lavandula latifolia, *n* See lavender.

Lavandula officinalis, *n* See lavender.

Lavandula stoechas, *n* See lavender.

lavender, *n* Latin names: *Lavandula officinalis, Lavandula latifolia, Lavandula angustifolia, Lavandula stoechas;* part used: flowers; uses: sedative, anxiolytic, insomnia, appetite stimulant, aromatherapy; precautions: CNS depression. Also called *aspic, echter lavendel, English lavender, esplieg, French lavender, garden lavender, lavanda, lavande commun, lavandin, nardo, Spanish lavender, spigo, spike lavender,* or *true lavender.*

law, *n* **I.** any rule within a legal system. **2.** in science, a general principle describing an observed regularity. **3.** a general organizing principle.

law of cure, *n* in homeopathy, the pattern through which healing occurs. Specifically, from within to without, from top to bottom, from more serious to less serious, and in reverse order of development.

law of mother and child, *n* in Chinese medicine, the natural order that dictates the association between the five elements—wood, metal, water, fire, and earth—to ensure harmony. Each element is believed to generate or "give birth" to another element in a cyclical pattern of wood-fire-earth-metal-water-wood. The interaction of these five elements serves as an example for familial behavior.

law of similars, *n* in homeopathy, the principle governing the selection of a remedy. A substance that has been tested and shown to induce particular symptoms in a healthy person is administered to an individual suffering from those same symptoms to enhance the body's recovery mechanisms.

law, Arndt-Schulz, *n.pr* law that describes the link between the potency of a stimulus and its effectiveness on physiologic performance. Weak stimuli promote biologic life functions, moderate stimuli interfere with them, and strong stimuli reduce or annihilate them.

law, common, *n* statutes created through a judge's decisions.

law, Head, *n.pr* according to which a painful stimulus, when applied to an area of low sensitivity which is bounded by an area of higher sensitivity, will be felt at the latter area rather than at the former.

law, Sherrington, *n.pr* **I.** states that specific regions of the skin are innervated by specific posterior spinal nerve roots, although adjacent nerve fibers may also be present. **2.** states that a contraction impulse to a muscle is paired with a relaxation impulse to that muscle's antagonist.

law, statute, *n* ruling established by the governing authority.

laws, access to treatment, *n* legislation that guarantees that patients have the right to obtain a procedure, device, or medication that is intended to be used as a mitigation, cure, therapeutic approach, or preventive measure.

laws, natural living, *n.pl* in naturopathic medicine, general principles that govern a healthy lifestyle, including eating foods that are natural and unrefined, exercising and resting for appropriate period of time, maintaining a moderately paced schedule, maintaining positive and stimulating emotional states, avoiding pollution and toxins, and properly eliminating wastes from the body.

laxative, *n* ability of a substance to promote bowel loosening and movement.

lay herbalist, *n* a person with extensive knowledge of plants useful in healing ailments.

lay homeopath, *n* homeopath without medical training. In the United States and Europe (except the United Kingdom, Ireland, and Norway), it is illegal for a lay homeopath to practice medicine.

LDJ, *n* See lumbodorsal junction.

lead, *n* a toxic metal that can be found in lead-based paints, leaded solder joints, and some fuel substances. Exposure has been linked to poor functioning of central nervous system as well as learning and behavioral difficulties.

lecithin (le'·sə·thən), *n* Scientific name: 1,2,diacyl-sn-glycero-3-phosphatidylcholine. A naturally occurring emulsifier, antioxidant, and dietary supplement used to lower cholesterol, to provide cardiovascular support, to treat kidney and liver conditions, and to aid in the treatment of some central nervous system disorders. See also phosphatidylcholine.

Ledum palustre, *n* See herb, marsh.

lemon balm, *n* Latin name: *Melissa officinalis* L.; parts used: leaves, whole plant; uses: herpes (genital and cold sores), anxiolytic, insomnia, migraines, high blood pressure, bronchial disorders, Graves' disease, ADD; precautions: pregnancy, lactation, infants and children, hyperthyroidism. Also called *balm, balm mint, cure-all, dropsy plant, honey plant, Melissa, sweet balm,* or *sweet Mary.*

lemongrass, *n* Latin name: *Cymbopogon citratus;* part used: leaves; uses: antitussive, antirheumatic, antiseptic, anxiolytic, antibacterial, antifungal, insomnia, vomiting, high blood pressure, fever; precautions: none known. Also called *capimcidrao, Guatemala lemongrass,* or *Madagascar lemongrass.*

lengthening (lengk´·the·ning), *n* the use of various massage or muscle energy techniques to relax and stretch muscle and connective tissue.

lentigo (len´·ta·gō), *n* brown or tan spot on the skin resulting from exposure to sun; usually benign.

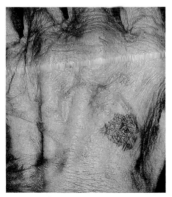

Lentigo. (Habif, 1995)

lentinan (len´·ta·nən), *n* Latin names: *Lentinula edodes, Lentinus edodes;* part used: fruiting body (mushroom); uses: immunomodulator, antibacterial, antiviral, cancer, high blood pressure; precautions: pregnancy and lactation, infants and children. Also called *forest mushroom, hua gu, pasania fungus,* or *snake butter.*

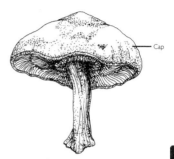

Lentinan. (Skidmore-Roth, 2004)

Lentinula edodes, *n* See lentinan.

Lentinus edodes (len´·ti·nəs ē´·dōdz), *n* part used: fruiting body; uses: tumors, immune system, viral diseases, antibacterial, decrease of blood levels of cholesterol and lipids, hepatitis, HIV; precautions: can cause allergic skin reactions, abdominal bloating; can induce temporary diarrhea. Also called *shiitake, black mushroom, hua gu,* and *mushroom (shiitake).*

Leonurus cardiaca, *n* See motherwort.

leopard's bane (le´·perdz bān´), *n* Latin name: *Arnica montana* L; parts used: flowers, oil; uses: acne, antibacterial, antiinflammatory, antiseptic, joint and muscle sprains or strains, seasickness, wound healing; precautions: children, elderly, pregnancy, breastfeeding, heart conditions, stomach irritant; poisonous when ingested. Also called *arnica, mountain snuff, mountain tobacco, wolf's bane,* and *wolfbane.*

Leptadenia reticulata, *n* See jivanti.

Leptandra virginica, *n* See black root.

LeShan (lə·sän), *n.pr* healing technique developed by Lawrence Le Shan based on the belief that every individual has an innate ability to heal and that a "flow process" takes place once the healer reaches a certain state of consciousness.

letting go and dropping, *v* to release the client's limb after holding or supporting it; as it is let go, the energy flow is broken. A kinetic manual therapy technique, dropping a limb allows the practitioner to see any holding patterns and encourages surrender.

leukemia (lōō·kē´·mē·ə), *n* a group of chronic or acute malignant disorders characterized by an abnormal increase in the number and types of white blood cells; permeation of liver, lymph nodes, and spleen; replacement of bone marrow with proliferating precursors to white blood cells. Lethargy, paleness, loss of weight, and easy bruising are early signs. Fever, extreme weakness, hemorrhages, and pain in the joints or bones may be later indications. An intensive combination of chemotherapy, antibiotics, and blood transfusions or bone marrow transplant is currently the most effective treatment.

leukemia, acute lymphocytic (ə· kyōōt´ lim·fō´·tik lōō·kē´·mē·ə), *n* malignant blood disease, where healthy blood cell numbers are reduced while underdeveloped cells and lymphoblasts proliferate in blood vessels, bone marrow, lymph nodes, and organs. One of the most common malignancies in children.

leukemia, acute myelocytic (ə·kyōōt´ mī´·ə·lō·si·tik   lōō·kē´·mē·ə), *n* bone marrow disease most often occurring in young adults in which undeveloped granular leukocytes multiply in the body. Individuals exposed to high amounts of radiation are at higher risk of developing this disease, as are those with a variety of blood dyscrasias, such as refractory anemia, among others. Also called *acute granulocytic leukemia, acute myelogenous leukemia, acute nonlym-*

phocytic leukemia, myeloid leukemia, splenomedullary leukemia, or *splenomyelogenous leukemia.*

leukemia, chronic lymphocytic, *n* cancer of hematopoeitic tissues common in older men distinguished by proliferation of lymphocytes, especially B cells. Symptoms include malaise, weight loss, fatigue, nighttime sweating, and lymphadenopathy.

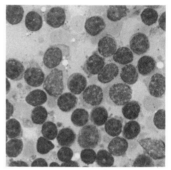

Leukemia, chronic lymphocytic. (Skidmore-Roth, 2004)

leukocytes (lōō·kō·sīts), *n.pl* white blood cells. They protect the body from disease-causing viruses, bacteria, toxins, parasites, and tumor cells.

leukopenia (lōō´·kə·pē´·nē·ə), *n* a condition characterized by the atypical decrease in circulating white blood cells (less than 5000 cells per cubic millimeter). The condition may be related to radiation poisoning, a reaction to a drug, or other pathologic conditions. Also called *leucocytopenia.*

leukoplakia (lōō·kō·pla´·kē·ə), *n* plaque like white lesion that develops in the oral mucosa. Typically a sign of bodily irritation in response to cigarette smoke or tobacco chewing. In 10% of cases, these lesions are considered precancerous.

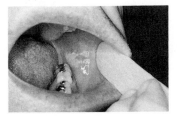

Leukoplakia. (Callen, Greer, and Hood, 1993)

leucopoiesis (lō'·kō·poi·ē'·sis), *n* the process by which white blood cells are produced and developed. Also called *leukocytopoiesis.*

leukotrienes (lōō·kō·trī·ēnz), *n.pl* regulators of inflammatory and allergic reactions. Biologically active leukotrienes are made up of 20-carbon carboxylic acids derived from arachidonic acid.

levant wormseed (lə·vant' werm'· sēd), *n* Latin name: *Artemisia cina;* part used: seeds; uses: anthelmintic, antipyretic, digestive aid; precautions: none known. Also called *centonique, chamomile-leaved artemisi, horasani, santonica,* and *seu wormwood.*

level of manifestation, *n* in acupuncture, a specific region in the body in which an obstruction exists and blocks the flow of blood or energy through the principal meridians, thus resulting in pain.

leverage (le'·və·rij), *n* chiropractic technique in which the thrust is applied with counterstabilization so that the force of the initial thrust is not lost.

Levisticum officinale, n See lovage.

Levisticum radix, n See lovage.

levitation, *n* in psychiatry, a hallucinatory sensation of rising or floating into the air.

levorotatory (lē'·və·rō'·tə·tōr'·ē), *adj* **1.** having the quality of rotating the plane of polarized light in the counterclockwise direction. Applies to many organic compounds. **2.** In aromatherapy, used to describe a characteristic of essential oils. Also known

as *laevorotatory.* Webster's Revised Unabridged Dictionary.

L-fields, *n.pl* See life fields.

li (lē), *n* benevolence and propriety, one of the five virtues in Chinese medicine for which shen is responsible. See also shen.

LI, *n* large intestine channel; an acupuncture channel running from the hand to the face along the radial surface of the arm and associated with the lung (LU) channel. See also LU.

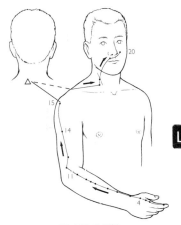

LI. (Chirali, 1999)

lian xian (lē·en zhē·än), *n* Latin name: *Nelumbinis nucifera plumula;* part used: seed embryo; uses: reduce blood pressure, control internal bleeding; precautions: none known. Also called *lotus plumule* and *lian zi xin.*

license, *n* certificate required to practice a professional healing approach.

licensed dietitian, *n* a nutrition specialist who holds a license to practice dietetics and nutrition services. A licensed dietitian facilitates nutrition therapy. Licensure may or may not be required for registered dietitians and requirements are determined on a state-by-state basis Also called *LD.* See also registered dietitian.

licensed health professional, *n* an individual who has successfully completed a prescribed program of study in a variety of health fields and who has obtained a license or certificate indicating his or her competence to practice in that field.

licorice (li·'kə·rish), *n* Latin name: *Glycyrrhiza glabra;* parts used: rhizomes, roots; uses: in Ayurveda, pacifies vata and pitta doshas (sweet, heavy, oily), laxative, asthma, malaria, hepatitis, gastric complaints, chronic fatigue, antiinflammatory, antibacterial, antiviral activities; precautions: patients with hepatic conditions, kidney disease, hypokalemia, hypertension, arrhythmias, congestive heart disease; patients taking antiarrhythmics, antihypertensives, cardiac glycosides, corticosteroids, diuretics, hypokalemia. Also called *Chinese licorice, licorice root, madhuka, mulethi, Persian licorice, Russian licorice, Spanish licorice, sweet root,* or *yashtimadhu.*

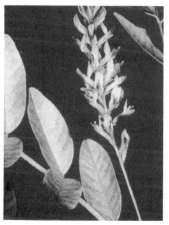

Licorice. (Williamson, 2002)

life fields, *n.pl* the scientifically measured biofields surrounding living beings and inanimate objects. Coined by Yale anatomist Dr. Harold Saxton Burr, Ph.D., in the 1930s.

life force, *n* metaphysical animating force in a system. This term corresponds to qi, prana, ka or ga-ilama, lung, mana, cheim, ruh, akasha, pneuma, apeiron, enormon, Archeus, animal magnetism, etc. See also vital energy, vital force, autoregulation, bioenergy, dynamis, and vitalism.

life scripts, *n.pl* autobiographies that provide maps for psychotherapeutic or hypnotherapeutic work.

lifestyle diary, *n.pr* documentation of physical activity, health, entertainment, leisure, eating, and drinking for evaluation purposes and to monitor changes.

lifting, *v* to raise a client's body or body part above its starting position. Used to facilitate practitioner access to the client's body; helpful in controlling circulation.

ligament, *n* strong connective tissue that binds the bones of the skeleton together at the joints.

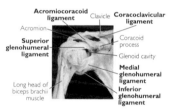

Ligament. (Thibodeau and Patton, 1999)

light-emitting diode (LED), *n* a semiconductor device that produces light when activated with an electrical current.

lignans (lig·'nənz), *n.pl* chemicals derived from flaxseeds, pumpkin seeds, cranberries, tea, and whole grains; have phytoestrogenic properties and are used as chemopreventives, to lower blood cholesterol, and to treat atherosclerosis. Precaution advised for those at risk for developing hormone-dependent cancers.

Likert self-report, *n.pr* a scoring approach for evaluation of attitudes, their dimensionality and strength; uses a wide continuum of numbers from 1 (strongly agree) to 7 (strongly disagree).

lily of the valley, *n* Latin name: *Convallaria majalis;* parts used: flowers, leaves, roots; uses: anticonvulsant, cardiotonic, heart conditions, topically to treat burns; precautions: pregnancy and lactation, infants and children, heart failure, cardiac arrhythmias, labeled unsafe by FDA. Also called *Jacob's ladder, ladder-to-heaven, lily constancy, lily convalle, male lily, May lily, muguet,* or *our-lady's-tears.*

limbic system (lim'·bik sis'·təm), *n* system of nuclei in the brain that modulates the mind's emotional tone, labels events as significant, adjusts motivation, encourages bonding, moderates libido, and filters events that are in the environment through the person's internal state of mind (also termed emotional coloring). Also involved in processing the sense of smell, storing powerful emotional memories, and controlling sleep cycles and appetite.

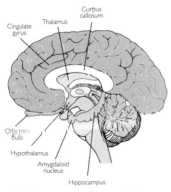

Limbic system. (McKenry and Salerno, 1998)

limpia (lim'·pē·ə), *n* See barrida.

linear causation, *n* unidirectional causality, in which each cause is itself the effect of a prior cause, and where

no effect can precede its cause. Also called *classical causation.* See also acausal and causation.

liniments, *n.pl* oil-based treatments rubbed into the skin for purposes of analgesia or as a rubefacient.

linkage, *n* **1.** in genetics, the location of two genes on the same chromosome such that they are typically transmitted as a cohesive unit during meiosis. **2.** in psychology, the relationship between a response and its stimulus.

linseed, *n* Latin name: *Linum usitatissimum;* part used: seeds; uses: emollient, laxative, anticholesterolemic; topically used as an inflammatory; precautions: persons with bowel obstruction or dehydration. Overdose may cause weakness, seizures, paralysis, and death. Also called *flaxseed, linseed, lint bells, linen flax,* and *linum.*

Linum usitatissimum, *n* See flax.

lipedema (li·pi·dē'·mə), *n* accumulation of fat in the lower extremities of the body indicated by tenderness in the affected region.

lipemia (li'·pə·rnē'·ə), *n* presence of high concentration of lipids in the bloodstream; normally observed after eating.

lipid, *n* fat or a similar greasy substance that dissolves in alcohol and organic solvents but not in water.

lipid profile, *n* a series of tests used to gauge a person's risk for coronary heart conditions. Blood levels examined in a lipid profile include those for total cholesterol, LDL- and HDL-cholesterol, and triglycerides.

lipid-soluble vitamins, *n.pl* See vitamins, fat-soluble.

lipofuscin (lī'·pō·fyōō'·sin), *n* brown-colored pigment characteristic of aging. Found in liposomes and product of peroxidation of unsaturated fatty acids.

lipolytic, *adj/n* the ability to break up fat.

lipophilic, *adj/n* the ability to dissolve or attach to lipids.

liposarcoma (li'·pō·sar·kō'·mə), *n* a malignant tumor that comprises immature fat cells.

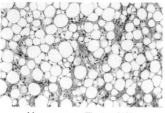

Liposarcoma. (Fletcher, 2000)

liposuction (lī'·pō·suk'·shən), *n* procedure in which fat deposits are removed from beneath the skin using a suction device; mostly performed in the area surrounding the abdomen, breasts, legs, face, and upper arms. Also called *suction lipectomy.*

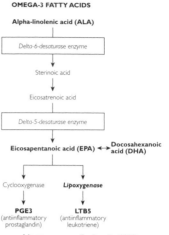

OMEGA-3 FATTY ACIDS

Alpha-linolenic acid (ALA)

Delta-6-desaturase enzyme

Sterinoic acid

Eicosatrenoic acid

Delta-5-desaturase enzyme

Eicosapentanoic acid (EPA) ⟷ **Docosahexanoic acid (DHA)**

Cyclooxygenase **Lipoxygenase**

PGE3 (antiinflammatory prostaglandin) **LTB5** (antiinflammatory leukotriene)

Lipoxygenase. (Leskowitz, 2003)

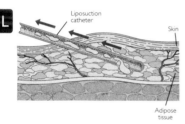

Liposuction. (Beare and Myers, 1998)

lipotropic (lī'·pō·trō'·pik), *adj* the ability to promote the movement of bile and lipids to and from the liver with improved hepatic function.

lipoxygenase (lip'·äk'·sə·jə·nās), *n* catalytic enzyme that facilitates the synthesis of leukotrienes by converting arachidonic acid to hydroxyeicosenoic acid via an oxidative process.

Liquidambar orientalis, *n* See storax.

listening posts, *n.pl* in craniosacral therapy, the places on the body from which the therapist can perceive the flow of cerebrospinal fluid or energy in the patient. The ankles or the occiput (i.e., the base of the skull) are the standard listening posts.

liter (lē'·ter), *n* a metric unit of measure defined as one cubic decimeter or the amount of volume occupied by one kilogram of pure water. It is written as L or dm^3.

lithium, *n* a metal/element (Li) used in the treatment of bipolar disorders and sometimes used in the treatment of herpes.

litholytic, *adj/n* the ability to break up stones.

lithotomy (li·thô'·tə·mē), *n* **1.** the removal of a stone (calculus) from the urinary tract by surgery. **2.** position assumed for rectal or vaginal examination.

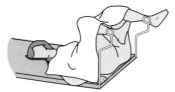

Lithotomy. (Potter and Perry, 2001)

lividity (li·vi'·di·tē), *n* a condition in which tissues appear blue or red due to a congestion in the veins, as caused by a contusion.

living matrix, *n* the collective whole of an organism, including its energies, tissues, cells, systems, and that which connects them.

Livingston-Wheeler regimen, *n.pr* alternative cancer treatment developed by Dr. Virginia Livingston, who asserted that cancer was bacterial in origin, caused by *Progenitor crypto-cides* (later discovered to be a common bacterium in the skin). Her treatment regimen included vaccinations (one vaccine was derived from the urine of the patient), enemas, vegetarianism, digestive enzymes, stress reduction, and visualization.

lobelia (lō·bēl'·yə), *n* Latin name: *Lobelia inflata;* part used: leaves; uses: expectorant, asthma, bronchitis, cough, possible cardiac effects, potential smoking deterrent; precautions: geriatric patients, liver conditions, kidney conditions, cardiovascular conditions, pneumonia, sensitivity to nicotine; patients using nicotine or mayapple, toxic. Also called *asthma weed, bladderpod, cardinal flower, emetic herb, eyebright, gagroot, great lobelia, Indian pink, Indian tobacco, pukeweed, rapuntium inflatum, vomit-root,* or *vomitwort.*

Lobelia inflata, *n* See lobelia.

lobotomy (lə·bä'·tə·mē'), *n* an infrequently performed surgical separation of the nerve fibers that connect the thalamus to the frontal lobes. This procedure is typically used in the treatment of certain mental disorders, such as severe depression. Also called *leukotomy.*

local muscles, *n.pl* muscles located deep within the body that have portions with attachments to the spine. In addition to multifidi, interspinales, intertrasversarii, and transversus abdominus, the central portion of the erector spinae, the medial fibers of quadratus lumborum, and the posterior segment of the internal oblique fit within this classification.

local sidereal time, *n* in astronomy, the right ascension (an equatorial coordinate) of a star on the observer's meridian.

local treatment, *n* application of medicine to a specific location or a specific symptom.

localization, *n* **1.** in manipulative therapies, the positioning of the client and precise application of the forces needed to produce specific, desired therapeutic results. **2.** the referral of sense impression to a specific bodily location.

local-naturalistic mechanisms, *n.pl* explanations for the efficacy of spiritual healing and prayer that include the placebo effect, the psychologic and stress-relieving qualities of prayer and the social support of spiritual communities.

locus of control, *n* the orientation that a person holds as to where control over life events is relative to the self—internal or external meaning self control, or other-controlled.

lodhra (lō'·dhrə), *n* Latin name: *Symplocos racemosa;* parts used: bark, root; uses: in Ayurveda, balances kapha and pitta doshas (astringent, light, dry), antimicrobial, antifibrinolytic, antispasmodic, astringent, diarrhea, dysentery, liver conditions, tonic, conjunctivitis, gum conditions, uterine conditions; precautions: none known. Also called *lodh* or *symplocos.*

L

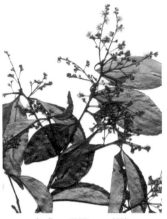

Lodhra. (Williamson, 2002)

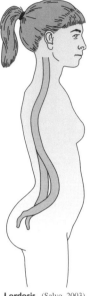

Lordosis. (Salvo, 2003)

Logan basic, *n* chiropractic technique with emphasis on sacrotuberous ligament to relieve sacral dysfunctions.

long tide, *n* a cranial rhythmic impulse or wave deeper and slower than that achieved during defacilitation.

longitudinal luo (lôn¹·jə·tōō¹·də·nəl lōō¹·ō), *n* in traditional Chinese medicine, a channel that serves as a connection between the main and extraordinary channels through which qi flows. See also qi.

Lophophora williamsii, *n* See peyote.

lordosis (lōr·dō¹·sis), *n* exaggerated anterior spinal curvature at the lumbar concavity. Also called *swayback.*

Loschmidt's number, *n.pr* the number of atoms in elements or molecules in compounds that exist in 1 mL of gas at 1 atmosphere of pressure and 0° C which is projected to be approximately 2.687 (10^{19} particles/mL.

lotions, *n.pl* nonoily treatments intended to be applied to the skin for a variety of cosmetic or medicinal purposes.

lovage (lu¹·vij), *n* Latin names: *Levisticum officinale, Levisticum radix;* parts used: roots, seeds; uses: kidney conditions by acting as a diuretic, antilithic, renal antiinflammatory, sedative, stomach disorders, congestion; precautions: pregnancy and lactation, infants and children, kidney irritation, kidney disease. Also called *maggi plant, sea parsley,* or *smellage.*

Lovett brother, *n.pr* the name for a vertebra in the upper or lower spine that moves synchronously with a paired vertebra in the opposite spinal segment to maintain a balanced vertical posture.

low dose effect, *n* the outcome from a small amount of a substance used in homeopathy and hormesis. See also law, Arndt-Schulz; hormesis; biphasic activity; and dose-dependent reverse effect.

lowampi (lō·wäm'·pē), *n* in Lakota Indian medicine, a spirit ceremony during which the spirits instruct the healer about the remedies that would heal the sick person. The ceremony is performed with the support of the sick person's extended family.

low-density lipoprotein cholesterol (lō'-den'·sə·tē li·pō·prō'·tēn kə·les'·ter·ôl), *n* a type of cholesterol that contains lipoproteins with less protein than fat. Low-density lipoproteins contribute to a buildup of fat in the arteries and are a risk factor in atherosclerosis.

lower back pain (LBP), *n* acute and/or chronic discomfort in the lumbar region of the spine caused by a number of factors.

LR, *n* liver channel; an acupuncture channel running from the feet to the chest and associated with the gall bladder (GB) channel. Also called *LV*. See also GB.

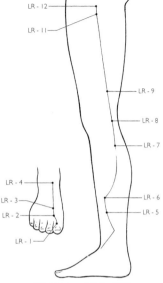

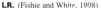

LR. (Fishie and White, 1998)

LS, *adj* lumbosacral; relates to a structure within the lumbar and sacral regions of the body, such as the lumbosacral joint.

LU, *n* lung channel; an acupuncture channel running from the shoulder to the hand along the radial surface of the arm and associated with the large intestine (LI) channel. See also LI.

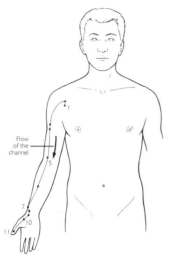

LU. (Chirali, 1999)

Flow of the channel

lucid dreaming, *n* a dream in which the dreamer is aware that he or she is dreaming.

lucid sleep, *n* an early nineteenth-century description for the state of hypnosis which was advanced as an alternative to the magnetism theories of Franz Mesmer. It proposed that no healing magnetic fluid is transmitted by the therapist, and that the patients created the state of trance themselves, which also accounted for differences in patient behavior during treatment. See also hypnosis.

lumbago (ləm·bā′gō), *n* pain in the lower back caused by muscle strain, osteoporosis, arthritis, or scoliosis.

lumbar (lum′·bär), *adj* pertaining to the lower back area between T12 vertebra and the sacrum.

lumbodorsal junction (ləm·bō·dōr′·səl junk′·shən), *n* the area of spine located between the T10 and L2 vertebrae.

lungwort (lung′·wərt), *n* Latin name: *Pulmonaria officinalis;* part used: leaves; disorders: diarrhea, menstrual conditions; precautions: pregnancy, lactation, children, anticoagulant medications. Also called *dage*

of Jerusalem, Jerusalem cowslip, Jerusalem sage, lung moss, lungs of oak, or *spotted comfrey.*

luo (lō), *n* in traditional Chinese medicine, the networks through which qi, or the vital energy, circulates. See also jing luo.

lupus (lōō′·pəs), *n* an inflammatory, autoimmune disorder of connective tissue; occurs mainly in young women. Citation,

lutein (lōō′·tēn), *n* a carotenoid pigment with antioxidant properties that may be useful in preventing cataracts, macular degeneration, and atherosclerosis; no known precautions.

lycopene (lī′·kō·pēn), *n* a carotenoid pigment and an antioxidant that is present in tomatoes (concentrated in processed products like tomato paste and sauce), guavas, watermelons, and grapefruit. May have preventive effects against prostate, lung, colon, and breast cancer; also reduce the risks of cataracts and macular degeneration.

Lycopus europaeus, *n* See wolf's foot.

Lycopus virginicus, *n* See bugleweed.

Lycoris (lī·kōr′·is), *n* a genus of the poisonous plants of the family Amaryllidaceae, whose bulbs contain lycorine, a toxin. The bulbs of *Lycoris radiate* are used as expectorant and emetic in Chinese medicine.

lymph (limf), *n* colorless fluid that is carried by the lymphatic system and that contains leukocytes and cytokines that help fight disease and infection.

lymph nodes, *n.pl* compound structures in the lymphatic circulation system that filter the lymph.

lymph nodes, cervical, *n.pl* chains of lymph nodes found in the neck, behind the chin and below the ear, divided into two levels: superficial and deep.

lymph nodes, occipital, *n.pl* lymph nodes found near the lower back of the skull (i.e., the occiput) that drain into the deep cervical lymph nodes. Palpated to diagnose possible health complaints. See also cervical lymph nodes.

lymph nodes, submaxillary, *n.pl* lymph nodes belonging to the chains of superficial cervical lymph nodes, located on the sides of the mandible, midway between the chin and the corner of the jaw.

lymphadenitis (lim'·fə·də·nī'·tis), *n* an inflammation of the lymph nodes due to infection or any other inflammatory condition.

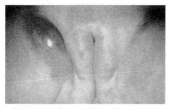

Lymphadenitis. (Zitelli and Davis, 1997)

lymphadenopathy (lim·fə·də·nô·pə ·thē), *n* a condition characterized by an abnormal increase in the size of the lymph nodes or lymph vessels.

lymphangitis (lim'·fan·jī'·tis), *n* an inflammation of at least one lymphatic vessel within the body that is typically caused by an acute streptococcal infection in one of the extremities. Fine red streaks that extend from the area of infection to the groin or axilla, headache, fever, chills, and myalgia are some indications.

lymphatic drainage (lim·fa'·tik drā'·nij), *n* specific type of massage which supports and assists circulation in the lymphatic system.

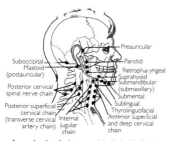

Lymphatic drainage. (Mosby's Medical, Nursing & Allied Health Dictionary, ed 6, 2002)

lymphatic pump, *n* original name given to the thoracic pump technique, used to describe the relationship between changes in intrathoracic pressure and the flow of lymph. See also thoracic pump.

lymphatic system, *n* a widespread network of thin vessels, capillaries, ducts, valves, organs, and nodes that primarily produces, filters, and conveys lymph along with producing various blood cells; maintains the internal fluid environment of the body and transports proteins, fats, and other substances to the bloodstream. The tonsils, thymus, and spleen are other major components of the lymphatic system. Also called *lymph system* or *lymphoid system.*

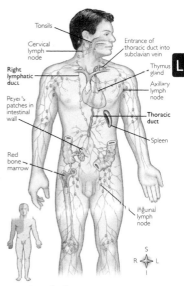

Lymphatic system. (Fritz, 2004)

lymphocyte blastogenesis (lim'·fə· sīt blas'·tō·jen'·ə·sis), *n* multiplication of agranulocytic leukocytes (which normally constitute one quarter of an individual's white blood cell count), whose numbers increase in response to infection.

lymphocytes (lim'·fə·sāts), *n.pl* white blood cells of the agranulocyte type, originally from stem cells, that produce antibodies and attack harmful cells. There are two categories of lymphocytes: B cells and T cells.

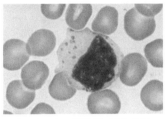

Lymphocytes. (Carr and Rodak, 1999)

lymphocytopenia (lim'·fō·sī'·tō·pē'·nē·ə), *n* an abnormally low number of lymphocytes in the blood due to malignancy, malnutrition, drugs, infectious mononucleosis, or a primary hematologic disorder.

lysine (lī'·sēn), *n* Scientific name: 2,6-diaminohexanoic acid. An essential amino acid found in dairy and meat products, wheat germ, and brewer's yeast. Used to treat cold sores and herpes simplex infections, Bell's palsy, and rheumatoid arthritis. Not for use during pregnancy or lactation or by infants or children.

Lysine. (Mosby's Medical, Nursing & Allied Health Dictionary, ed 6, 2002)

lysinurea (lī·sin'·yōō·rē'·ə), *n* the presence of lysine in the urine.

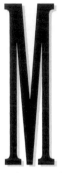

ma huang (mä hwäng), *n* Latin name: *Ephedra sinica;* parts used: seeds, leaves; uses: asthma, headache, bronchitis, inflammation, joint pain, pulmonary congestion; precautions: pregnancy, lactation, children, sympathomimetic hypersensitivity, seizure disorder, narrow-angle glaucoma, diabetes mellitus, hyperthyroidism, arrhythmias, heart block, psychosis, hypertension, angina pectoris, chest pain, palpitations, tachycardia, arrythmias, myocardial infarction, stroke, cardiac arrest, seizures, dizziness, anxiety, insomnia, hallucinations, nervousness, poor concentration, confusion, headache, tremors, nausea, constipation, diarrhea, anorexia, vomiting, urinary retention, dysuria, exfoliative dermatitis, dyspnea, uterine contractions. See also ephedra.

maceration (ma·sə·rā'·shən), *n* the process in which the skin is softened and broken down by extended exposure to wetness or moisture, as in a postterm infant or a dead fetus because of prolonged exposure to the amniotic fluid.

macrobehaviors (ma'·krō·bə·hā'·vyərz), *n.pl* in the context of hypnosis therapies, refers to instances of conduct involving intended actions and movements.

macroglossia (ma'·krō·glä'·sē·ə), *n* an increase in the size of the tongue due to congenital defects such as Down syndrome.

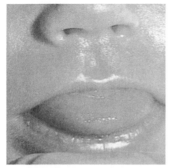

Macroglossia. (Zitelli and Davis, 1992; Dr. Christine L. Williams, New York Medical College)

macrominerals (ma'·krō·mi'·nə·rəlz), *n.pl* one of three classifications of minerals; includes calcium, chloride, magnesium, phosphorus, potassium, silicon, sodium, and sulfur.

macromolecules (ma'·krō·mô'·lə·kyōōlz), *n.pl* large molecules that are made up of many repeating units.

macronutrients (ma'·krō·nōō'·trē·ənts), *n.pl* nutrients—including proteins, fats, and carbohydrates—that are required by the body in large amounts.

macrophages (ma·krō·fā'·jəz), *n.pl* white blood cells (activated monocytes) that protect the body against infection and foreign substances by breaking them down into antigenic peptides recognized by circulating T cells.

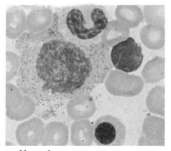

Macrophages. (Carr and Rodak, 1999)

macula (ma·kyu·lə), *n* a region within the retina of the eye; is responsible for clear and defined vision. Macular degeneration is the leading cause of loss of vision in elderly populations. Smoking, hypertension, aging, and atherosclerosis are implicated in macular degeneration.

macular degeneration (ma'·kyə·ler də·je'·nə·rā'·shən), *n* an eye condition characterized by deterioration of the macula (the central portion of the retina) and concomitant decrease of vision. This deterioration may be classified as either "dry" or "wet." See also macula.

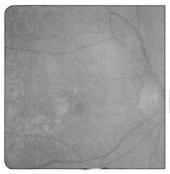

Macular degeneration. (Kanski and Nischal, 1999)

macule (mak'·yool), *n* a nonelevated region of skin that is distinguished by an alteration in color. Also called *macula*.

madder (ma'·dər), *n* Latin name: *Rubia tinctorum;* part used: roots; uses: kidney stones, paralysis, menstrual problems, jaundice; precautions: pregnancy, lactation, children; possible hepatotoxicity. Also called *dyer's madder, garance, krapp, madder root,* or *robbia.*

magnesium, *n* an element/mineral found in nuts, seeds, grains, and green vegetables that has been used in reducing noise-induced hearing loss and in treating coronary artery disease, painful menstruation, the symptoms of PMS, migraines, high blood pressure, autism and preeclampsia. Magnesium supplementation may also be needed in patients taking cisplatin, cyclosporin, or loop and thiazide diuretics. Caution is advised for children and patients taking sulfonylurea-based antidiabetic medications or potassium-sparing diuretics.

magnetic field (MF), *n* the lines of force that surround a moving charged particle or a magnet.

magnetic moment, *n* the twisting force experienced by a magnet located inside a magnetic field.

magnetic reciprocity (mag·ne'··tik res'·ə·prô'·si·tē), *n* in mesmerism, the mental or emotional rapport established between patient and therapist that enables them to sense each others' thoughts. See also mesmerism.

magnetic unruffle, *n* practice in which the therapist keeps his hands hovering just above the client's body while slowly moving down to the toes. Repeated on both sides of the body until the congested energy is dispersed.

magnetobiology, *n* the study of how magnetism within an organism (biomagnetism) affects other living creatures.

magnetocardiography, *n* the mapping of the electromagnetic field surrounding the heart.

magnetoencephalography (MEG) (mag·nē'·tō·en·se'·fə·lä'·grə·fē), *n* noninvasive method of measuring magnetic fields created by the electrical activity in the brain.

magnetotherapy (mag·ne'·tō·the'·rə·pē), *n* the therapeutic application of magnetic fields.

mahabhutas (mä·hä'·bhōō·täs), *n.pl* in Ayurveda, the five basic elements comprising all matter in the Universe—space, air, fire, water, and earth. The three body types or doshas are based on the predominance of one or more elements. See also doshas.

mahad (mə·häd'), *n* in Ayurvedic philosophy, the "cosmic intellect,"

from which is derived the substance of the universe.

Maharishi Amrit Kalash (MAK) (mä·hä·rē'··shē äm·rēt kä·läsh), *n* an Ayurvedic herbal mixture that is a commonly used antioxidant estimated to be 1000 times more effective in fighting free radicals than vitamins E and C. See also rasayanas.

Maharishi Ayur-Veda (MAV) (mä'·hä·rē'·shē ä''·yōōr-vä'·də), *n* an adaptation of Ayurveda, India's traditional healthcare system, refined and modernized by Maharishi Mahesh Yogi to include his understanding of the field of consciousness and how consciousness is expressed in nature and human physiology.

Mahesh (mə·häsh'), *n.pr* in Ayurvedic philosophy, the god who represents the destructive force of the universe.

Mahonia aquifolium, n See Oregon grape.

maintainable, *adj* a broad category used to describe patients with illnesses which, although not fully curable, can be mitigated or managed with proper treatment.

maitake (mī·tä'·kē), *n* Latin name: *Grifola frondosa;* part used: fruiting body (mushroom); uses: adaptogen, chemopreventive effects, immunomodulator, high blood pressure, diabetes mellitus, cholesterol, obesity, cancer, AIDS; precautions: pregnancy, lactation, children. Also called *dancing mushroom, king of mushrooms, monkey's bench,* or *shelf fungi.*

majja (mäj'·jə), *n* in Ayurveda, bone marrow and nerve tissue as a fundamental tissue (dhatu). See also dhatus.

majjavahasrotas (mäj'·jä·vä'·häs·rō'·təs), *n.pl* in Ayurveda, one of the 13 srotas, or body channels, the function of which is to carry marrow components; originates in the joints and bones. See also srotas.

Makko-Ho (mäk·kō·hō), *n.pr* Makko's series of basic stretching techniques; used by Shiatsu practitioners to cultivate, express, and improve the health of meridian pairs.

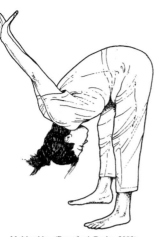

Makko-Ho. (Beresford-Cooke, 2003)

mal aire (mäl´ ī´·rā), *n* according to Curanderismo, the Mexican folk healing system, bad air (the spirits of dead people who died in a violent manner and attack passersby) that results in disease.

mal de ojo (mäl dā ō·hō), *n* "evil eye," an ethnomedical condition common to Latin America (with roots in the Mediterranean), is a childhood illness characterized by fever, headache, and irritability. An envious gaze, typically from a nonrelative and often accompanied with compliments, is considered to be the cause of this malady and the immediate cure is for a family member or care giver to touch the child being complimented. Also called *ojo.*

mal puesto (mäl pwes´·tō), *n* according to Curanderismo, the Mexican folk healing system, a mental disorder resulting from a hex in which the individual engages in abnormal behavior.

malabsorption, *n* improper absorption of nutrients, characterized by deficiency of carbohydrates, fats, minerals, proteins, and vitamins and excess fat in the stool.

malaria, *n* illness caused by infected female Anopheles mosquito (which harbors the protozoan parasite Plasmodium) bite. Studying the treatment of this illness with cinchona bark sparked Hahnemann to consider "like curing like," which became the fundamental tenet of homeopathy. Also called *marsh fever.*

malas (mə·läs´), *n.pl* in Ayurveda, the waste products of the body, which include urine, stool, and sweat. Effective elimination of malas is said to be important for maintaining good health.

male fern, *n* Latin name: *Dryopteris filix-mas;* parts used: dried rhizomes, roots; uses: anthelmintic; precautions: abortifacient, pregnancy, lactation, children, kidney disease, cardiovascular disease, liver disease, hepatotoxicity, toxic. Also called *bear's paw, erkek egrelti, helecho macho, knotty brake, marginal shield-fern, shield fern, sweet brake,* or *wurmfarn.*

malignant (mə·lig´·nənt), *adj* type of cancerous growth with a tendency to metastasize and grow unchecked. See also metastasis.

malillumination, *n* an environmental condition characterized by the absence of full-spectrum light. See also illnesses, environmental.

mallow, *n* Latin name: *Malva sylvestris;* parts used: dried flowers and leaves; uses: respiratory disorders, teething, constipation; precautions: pregnancy, lactation, children. Also called *blue mallow, cheeseflower, cheeseweed, field mallow, fleurs de mauve, high mallow, malve,* or *zighli.*

Malva sylvestris, *n* See mallow.

mamsa (mäm´·sə), *n* in Ayurveda, muscle as a fundamental tissue (dhatu). See also dhatus.

mamsavahasrotas (mäm´·sä·vä´·häs·rō´·təs), *n.pl* in Ayurveda, one of the 13 srotas, or body channels which carry muscle tissue components; originates in skin, tendons and ligaments. See also srotas.

manas (mä·nəs), *n* in Ayurvedic philosophy, the mind. A sound body,

M

mind, and soul are essential for maintaining good health.

manda (mun'·də), *adj* in Ayurveda, "slow" or "dull" as a guna, one of the qualities characterizing all substances. Its complement is tikshna. See also gunas and tikshna.

mandibular drainage, *n* a technique for soft tissue manipulation in which passively induced motion of the mandible is used to increase lymph drainage from the middle ear via the lymph system and the eustachian tubes.

mandrake, *n* Latin name: *Podophyllum peltatum;* part used: rhizome; uses: snakebite, poisoning, condyloma acuminata, weakness, tumors, and lymphadenopathy; precautions: pregnancy, children, gallbladder disease, elderly, hypersensitivity, intestinal obstruction, diabetes. Can cause confu-sion, headache, dizziness, vomiting, anorexia, diarrhea, abdominal pain, hepatotoxicity, thrombocytopenia, leukopenia, orthostatic hyptension, ataxia, apnea, shortness of breath, altered consciousness, numbness. Also called *American mandrake, devil's-apple, ground lemon, mandrake, wild mandrake, wild lemon, Indian apple, racoon berry, umbrella plant, duck's foot,* and *hog apple.* See also mayapple.

maneuver, *n* a skillful procedure or manipulation.

manganese, *n* an element/mineral found in cereal grains, nuts, and tea; a component of many enzymes. Has been used to treat painful menstruation and osteoporosis and as a dietary adjunct to alleviate deficiencies associated with seizure disorders and diabetes. Concurrent use of antacids may impair absorption of manganese. No known precautions in moderate doses.

Mangifera indica, n See tree, mango.

manic phase, *n* phase during bipolar depression; marked by disproportionate feelings of self-esteem, decreased need for sleep, excessive talking, and decrease in concentration.

manipulation, *n* in massage therapy, osteopathic medicine, chiropractic, and traditional Chinese medicine, the use of varied manual techniques to adjust the joints and spinal column, improve the range of motion of the joints, relax and stretch connective tissue and muscles, and promote overall relaxation.

mansa (män'·sə), *n* the root or rhizome of *Anemonopsis californica,* used in northern Mexico and southwestern United States to relieve colds, indigestion, and as a blood purifier.

manslaughter, *n* the act of causing the death of another person; categorized as involuntary or voluntary. Involuntary manslaughter indicates that the death occurred during the course of a crime or as a result of negligence, whereas voluntary manslaughter involves a suicide pact, incitement, or diminished responsibility.

mantra (män'·trə), *n* "mind protection;" in Hinduism and Buddhism, a pure sound that is used in meditation and rituals.

manual lymph drainage, *n* a style of massage that stimulates circulation of lymph through the lymphatic system using light, rhythmic techniques.

manual manipulation, *n* therapies that stimulate or manipulate the body to arrest disease and improve health. Manual manipulation therapies include massage, chiropractic, and osteopathic treatments.

manual neurotherapy (man'·yōō·əl nur'·ō·the'·rə·pē), *n* a method of manipulative therapy that incorporates foot reflexology (focused on reflexes in the nervous system), neuromuscular massage treatments, and modified techniques of joint mobilization. Also called *MNT.*

manuka honey (mə·nōō'·kə hu'·nē), *n* honey gathered from flowers of the manuka bush, *Leptospermum scoparium,* a wild plant found in New Zealand. The active honey, in the nonpasteurized form, contains a potent antibacterial compound called unique manuka factor (UMF). Manuka honey is used to treat sore throats, skin ulcers, heartburn, peptic ulcers, to fight *Helicobacter pylori* bacteria, and as a wound dressing. Also called *active manuka honey.*

Marcrocystis pyrifera, *n* See kelp.

margas (mär'·gəs), *n* in Ayurveda, three pathways—internal, intermediate, and deep—through which doshas travel. A dosha employs these pathways when a disease enters the third stage. See also doshas.

marigold, *n* See calendula.

marijuana (mar'·ə·wä'·nə), *n* Latin names: *Cannabis sativa; Cannabis indica;* parts used: dried flowers, leaves, and stems; uses: illegal in most countries; it has been used to treat nausea associated with chemotherapy, glaucoma, appetite loss, pain relief; precautions: increases heart rate and systolic blood pressure; impairs complex motor activities; alters mood and self perception; memory and cognitive ability. A synthetic marijuana medication called *Marinol* is available in the U.S. Also called *dank, pot, ganja, dope, grass, reefer,* or *weed.*

marjoram (mär'·jə·rəm), *n* Latin name: *Origanum majorana* L.; parts used: dried leaves, flowers; uses: diuretic, snakebite, motion sickness, dysmenorrhea, muscle pain, arthritis, headache, bruises, insomnia; precautions: pregnancy, lactation, children. Also called *garden marjoram, knotted marjoram,* or *sweet marjoram.*

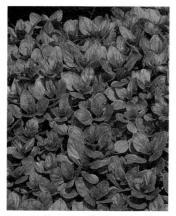

Marjoram. (Tiran, 2000)

Marlowe-Crowne score, *n.pr* a measurement obtained upon completion of the Marlowe-Crowne scale of social desirability, an evaluation that measures defensiveness or the inclination of an individual to promote himself or herself. A high measurement obtained from this evaluation has the potential to influence the development of somatic symptoms or indicators like irritable bowel syndrome, chronic pain, and insomnia if threatening beliefs are being blocked from one's consciousness.

marmas (mär'·məs), *n.pl* in Ayurveda, the 107 subcutaneous pressure points in the body that are believed to connect mind and body. Each marma influences a specific organ system and an injury to a marma damages the related organ. Many of the marmas correspond to the Japanese Shiatsu system. See also Shiatsu.

Marrubium vulgare, *n* See horehound.

Marsedenia condurango, *n* See condurango.

marshmallow, *n* Latin name: *Althaea officinalis;* parts used: dried flowers, leaves, and roots; uses: coughs, sore throats, stomach disorders, minor skin conditions; precautions: pregnancy and lactation, infants and children, liver disease, kidney disease. Also called *althaea root, althea, mortification root, sweetweed,* or *wymote.*

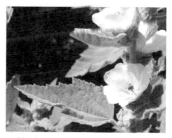

Marshmallow. (Scott and Barlow, 2003)

MASc, *n.pr* See Master of Ayurvedic Science.

mass number, *n* the total number of protons and neutrons within the nucleus of an atom. This number represents the atom's approximate mass.

mass spectrometry (MS) (mas'spek·trô'·nə·mē), *n* a method of identifying and analyzing substances by fragmenting substances with a bombardment of high-energy electrons. Each molecule has a specific pattern of fragmentation, and these patterns are recorded on a mass spectrum. This technique is often combined with gas-liquid chromatography.

massage, *n* the application of diverse manual techniques of touch and stroking to muscles and soft tissue to achieve relaxation and to improve the client's well-being. See also bodywork and massage therapy.

Benefits of massage	
Physical	**Psychological**
Muscle relaxation	Mental relaxation
Sudorific	Revitalizing
Lowers blood pressure	Releases emotions
Stimulates circulation	Facilitates communication
Increases diuresis	Aids sleep
Stimulates lymphatic drainage	Time for oneself
Reduces oedema	
Pain relieving	

Massage. (Tiran, 2000)

massage chair (mə·säj'·cher'), *n* portable, padded chair designed to fully support the relaxed weight of the massage client.

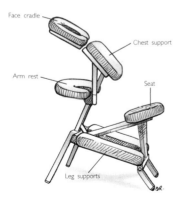

Face cradle
Chest support
Arm rest
Seat
Leg supports

Massage chair. (Fritz, 2004)

massage table (mə·säj'·tā'·bəl), *n* padded table designed specifically for massage in a recumbent position.

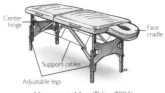

Center hinge
Face cradle
Support cables
Adjustable legs

Massage table. (Fritz, 2004)

massage, Aston, *n.pr* gentle tissue work that provides tension relief, evens body tone, and integrates structural change.

massage, Bindgeweb (bīn'·dəj·web'·mə·säzh'), *n* a style of massage applied to the connective tissue system in the body according to the areas of tenderness that correspond to certain acupuncture points. Treatment is given with the middle finger in a series of strokes without a lubricant.

massage, classical Western, *n* method of therapeutic friction, kneading and stroking of the body derived from European anatomic and physiologic concepts.

massage, connective tissue (CTM), *n* a diagnostic and therapeutic treatment that involves stroking and pulling deep connective tissues to release the existing tension and return them to a natural alignment. May be uncomfortable and produce vasodilatation and sweating.

massage, deep-tissue, *n* a style of massage that uses strong pressure; slow, deep strokes; and friction across the muscle grain to release chronic muscle tension.

massage, electrovibratory, *n* technique in which vibrations are applied to the body through electrical means.

massage, intercompetition (in'·ter·käm'·pə·ti'·shən mə·säzh'), *n* sports massage given at an athletic event.

massage, neuromuscular, *n* a style of massage used to relieve pain, stimulate circulation, and loosen trigger points. This form of massage focuses on individual muscles rather than muscle groups and uses deep pressure.

massage, orthopedic, *n* a therapeutic approach to injury and pathology treatment of the locomotor system; uses multiple techniques.

massage, recovery, *n* massage designed to address the needs of an uninjured athlete directly after a competition or a vigorous workout. The focus is on minimizing fatigue or soreness and cleansing tissues to shorten recuperation time.

massage, rehabilitation, *n* massage used specifically to speed recovery after surgery or in cases of injury.

massage, remedial, *n* massage designed to help recovery from mild to moderate injuries.

massage, sports, *n* a style of massage that works specifically on problems resulting from athletic performance, training, and injury. This form of massage uses techniques similar to those of Swedish and deep-tissue massages. See also massage, deep-tissue and massage, Swedish.

massage, Swedish, *n* systematic soft tissue manipulation applied directly to the skin via effleurage, petrissage, friction, tapotement, and vibration. Developed by Swedish physiologist and gymnast Per Henrik Ling (1776–1839).

massage, Swiss reflex, *n* conceived by Shirley Price in 1987 and based upon the principles of reflexology, according to which energy flow lines in the body connect at certain reflex points. Essential oils are blended with a bland cream that the therapist massages into the reflex points of the body. Method involves at-home patient preparation as well as ongoing client-therapist dialogue during treatments. Therapists must be accredited.

massage, systemic, *n* a structured form of massage used to enhance one organ system, usually the circulatory or lymphatic system.

massage, Thai, *n.pr* a style of bodywork that incorporates aspects of Ayurveda, Chinese medicine, and Thai Buddhist meditation. Its form is similar to like facilitated yoga because of its emphasis on opening and stretching the body. It uses acupuncture meridians to move energy, and its slow pace is conducive to of contemplative states of consciousness. Also called *noad bo-rom, Thai yoga-massage, Thailand medical massage,* or *traditional Thai massage.*

mastalgia (mas·tal´·jē-ə), *n* a painful sensation originating in the breast due to congestion that occurs during lactation, fibrocystic disease, or infection, especially during or before menstrual period or in advanced stages of cancer. Also called *mastodynia.*

Master of Ayurvedic Science, *n* in India, degree awarded to an individual after completion of a graduate program in Ayurveda. To earn this degree, an individual must complete a Bachelor of Ayurvedic Medicine and Surgery program, perform research, write a thesis based on the research subject, and pass a series of exams. In general, earning this degree takes nine or ten years after primary school. Also called *MASc.*

mastery tasks (mas´·tə·rē tasks´), *n.pl* in biofeedback therapy, assignments given to an individual in order to achieve mastery of a necessary skill. A biofeedback therapist directing a patient to use self-regulation skills in response to a stressful stimulus is an example.

mastika (mä·stē´·kə), *n* in Ayurveda, brain as described in the Atharvaveda. See also vedas.

mastitis (mas·tī´·tis), *n* an inflammation within the mammary glands; caused by staphylcoccal or streptococcal infection; treated with warm soaks, rest, analgesia, and antibiotics. Also called *mammitis.*

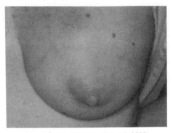

Mastitis. (Lemmi and Lemmi, 2000)

mastoid process (mas'·toid prô'·ses), *n* bony prominence located behind the ear at the base of the skull.

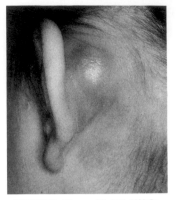

Mastoiditis. (Stone and Gorbach, 2000; Dr. N. Blevins, New England Medical Center, Boston)

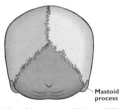

Mastoid process

Mastoid process. (Chaitow, 1999)

mastoiditis (mas·toi'·dī'·tis), *n* infection and inflammation of the honeycomb-like air cells of the mastoid bone, located behind the ear; usually results from an untreated ear infection (otitis media). See also otitis media.

masturbation (mas'·tər·bā'·shən), *n* manual stimulation of the genitals (one's own or those of another). Also called *onanism*.

materia medica (mə·tir'·ē·ə me'·di·kə), *n* a volume or volumes of collected information about the origins, effects, methods of preparation, and uses of therapeutic plants, minerals, and other substances in medicine.

Materia Medica Pura (mə·ti'·rē·ə me'·di·kə pyu'·rə), *n.pr* the complete published list of homeopathic remedies proved by Samuel Hahnemann, the founder of homeopathy.

material safety data sheet, *n* an informational form detailing the chemical and physical properties, hazards, and ways of safely handling a toxic chemical.

Matricaria chamomile, *n* See chamomile.

Matteuccia struthiopteris, *n* See ostrich fern.

maxilla (mak·sil'·ə), *n* the upper jaw bone. It encloses the maxillary sinus and other cavities and projections.

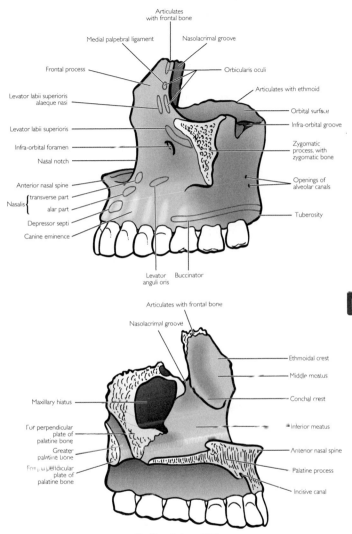

Maxilla. (Chaitow, 1998)

M

maxillae-frontal junction (mak·sil´· ē-frun´·təl junk´·shən), *n* meeting place of the upper jaw bones and the bone that forms the forehead and the top of the orbit.

maxillary-nasal junction (mak´·sə· le·rē-nā´·zəl junk´·shən), *n* meeting place of the maxillae (upper jaw bones) and the nasal bones.

maxillary sinus, *n* the air cavity that runs behind the cheek.

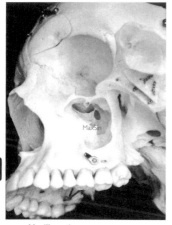

Maxillary sinus. (Carreiro, 2003)

may apple, *n* See Indian apple.

mayapple (mā´·a´·pəl), *n* Latin name: *Podophyllum peltatum;* part used: rhizome; uses: snakebites, poisoning, laxative, wart removal; precautions: pregnancy, children, gallbladder disease, elderly, hypersensitivity, intestinal obstruction, diabetes; can cause confusion, headache, dizziness, vomiting, anorexia, diarrhea, abdominal pain, hepatotoxicity, thrombocytopenia, leukopenia, ataxia, apnea, shortness of breath, altered consciousness, numbness. Also called *American mandrake, devil's-apple, ground lemon, mandrake, wild mandrake, wild lemon, Indian apple, racoon berry, umbrella plant, duck's foot,* and *hog apple.* See also mandrake.

MbOCA, *n.pr* methylenebis (orthochloroaniline); used as a curing agent for epoxy and polyurethane resins. Considered carcinogenic.

MCS, *n.pr* See multiple chemical sensitivity.

MCTs, *n.pr* See medium-chain triglycerides.

MDA, *n.pr* methylenedioxyamphetamine; a highly addictive hallucinogenic substance.

MDR, *n* See multidrug resistance.

meadow saffron (me´·dō sa´·frän), *n* Latin name: *Colchicum autumnale;* parts used: bulb, seeds; uses: pain, severe bowel evacuation, induction of vomiting, gout, nausea, diarrhea, rheumatism, leukemia, Beçhet's syndrome; precautions: kidney disease; can cause violent purging, stomach and bowel inflammation, and allergic skin reactions. Also called *cigdem, colchicum, colquico, herbstreitlose, naked boys, wilde herfsttijloos,* and *autumn crocus.*

meadow windflower, *n* Latin name: *Pulsatilla vulgaris;* part used: whole plant; uses: prevent or relieve cramps or spasms, induce perspiration, diuretic, promote menstrual flow, expectorant, eye disorders, relaxant, nettle rash, toothache, earache, bilious indigestion, measles, premenstrual syndrome, inflammations of the reproductive organs, tension headaches, neuralgia, hyperactivity, bacterial skin infections, septicemia, spasmodic coughs in asthma, whooping cough, bronchitis; precautions: upper respiratory tract infection, skin irritation, kidney irritation, urinary tract irritation, diarrhea, and vomiting. Also called *european pasqueflower, kuchenschelle, pulsatila, wildemanskruid,* and *pasque flower.*

meadowsweet, *n* Latin names: *Filipendula ulmaria, Spiraea ulmaria;* part used: dried flowers; uses: analgesic, antipyretic, anticoagulant, antidiabetic, anticancer, antioxidant, gastrointestinal conditions, urinary infections, rheumatism, colds; precautions: pregnancy, lactation, children, asthma, salicylate hypersensitivity, anticoagulants. Also called *bridewort,* *dolloff, dropwort, fleur d'ulmaire, flores ulmariae, gravel root, meadow queen, meadowort, mede-sweet, queen of the meadow,* or *spierstaude.*

meágica (mā·ä´·jē·kə), *n* in Curanderismo, the Mexican healing system, a healer who combines spiritual practices, including chanting, praying, burning incense, lighting candles, and sprinkling holy water, with herbal remedies.

mean corpuscular volume (MCV) (mēn kŏr·pus´·kyə·lər väl´·yōōm), *n* determination of the average volume of a single red blood cell, derived from the ratio of the hematocrit to the total number of red blood cells. The normal MCV range is 32% to 36% for adults and children and 32% to 34% in infants.

meaning response, *n* See placebo effect.

measles, *n* viral disease characterized by the release of toxins that affect the central nervous system, red rash, fever, and white spots (Koplik's spots) on the tongue. Serious complications arising from measles include encephalitis, diarrhea, impaired vision, and pneumonia.

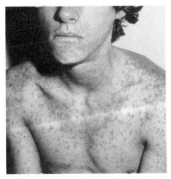

Measles. (Zitelli and Davis, 1997; Dr. M. Sherlock)

meatus (mē´·təs), *n* a natural channel or opening within the body.

mechanism, *n* the path whereby a treatment works.

mechanoreceptor (mi·kan´·ō·ri·sep´·tər), *n* a sense receptor activated by mechanical pressure (e.g., touch, massage) or distortion (e.g., muscle tension).

meda (mā´·də), *n* in Ayurveda, body fat (adipose tissue) as a fundamental tissue (dhatu). See also dhatus.

medica (mā´·dē·kə), *n* practitioner from New Mexico, of Curanderismo, the Mexican-American healing system. See also Curanderismo.

medical gymnastics, *n.pl* an older term for Per Henrik Ling's massage techniques. See massage, Swedish.

medical herbalist, *n* in England, an individual who has completed a four-year degree course in herbal medicine, studying botanical therapeutics as well as biomedical sciences.

medical homeopath, *n* a licensed doctor who also practices homeopathy. See also lay homeopath, half homeopath, and professional homeopath.

medical iridology (me´·də·kəl ir´·i·dô´·lə·jē), *n* a form of iridology (eye diagnosis) concerned with identifying pathologic dispositions.

medical optimism, *n* principle according to which doctors should advise patients to integrate creativity into their lives and to engage in responsible pleasures that do not harm society or themselves.

medicinal product, *n* a substance administered to humans or animals through injection, application, oral ingestion, inhalation, and so forth, whose purpose is to ultimately restore health or eliminate disease in an individual.

medicine, *n* the art and science of preventing, diagnosing, treating, and managing illness.

medicine family/clan, *n* the family or a group of families of healers within each Native American Nation who pass along their knowledge intergenerationally. These healers may have formal societies or work informally.

medicine, allopathic, *n* method of medical treatment in which drugs are administered to counter symptoms of the disease.

M

medicine, alternative, *n* therapeutic practices not considered integral to conventional medicine. Used instead of conventional therapies.

medicine, anthroposophical, *n* holistic, humanistic model of health care that combines allopathic medicine with the spiritual teachings of Rudolf Steiner. Also called *Anthroposophically Extended Medicine (AEM).*

medicine, arts, *n* the study of relationship between human health and the arts, in which arts and artistic activities are explored for their therapeutic benefits.

medicine, behavioral, *n* combined treatment strategies that employ both cognitive-behavioral therapies and meditation.

medicine, biochemic (bī·ō·ke'mik me'·dis·in), *n* a therapy designed to correct a disparity of essential inorganic salts in an organism by using low-potency (homeopathic) tissue salts. See also Schüssler cell salts and tissue salts.

medicine, China's traditional, *n* ancient healing system with references to the five cosmic elements that dates to 3000 BCE. It includes the use of herbal treatments, massage (tuina), acupuncture, and qi gong to maintain the balance of qi, the vital energy in the body. Also called *traditional medicine of China.* See also qi gong and qi.

medicine, complementary, *n* therapeutic practices not considered integral to conventional medicine. Used in conjunction with conventional therapies. Often used interchangeably with the term *alternative medicine,* encompasses the wide array of therapies not generally offered by MDs and not usually covered by health insurance. Complementary is considered a more accurate term because in practice, patients do not replace allopathic treatment but instead supplement it with complementary medicine.

medicine, constitutional, *n* homeopathic categorization based on Grauvogl's 1865 definition of oxygenoid, hydrogenoid, and carbonitrogenoid constitutions. Similar alterations occur within each constitution during breathing and in blood. The three constitutions were later replaced by Nebel's carbonic, fluoric, and phosphoric constitutions. See also constitution, constitutional prescribing, morphology, and typology.

medicine, conventional, *n* the model of currently established Western medicine. This paradigm was designated as *conventional* because of its prevalence. What is considered conventional is always in flux. See also allopathy; model, biomedical; and orthodox.

medicine, eclectic, *n* healing system that employs a combination of approaches. See also homeopathy, complex; homeopathy, pluralist; and homeopathy, unicist.

medicine, empirical, *n* practice of medicine based on experience rather than theory.

medicine, energy, *n* a group of medical approaches that use biological, psychological, and spiritual "energy" for diagnosis, treatment and to promote health and well-being. The term *energy* in energy medicine is understood in different terms depending upon the context; therefore energy medicine includes many different modalities. See also acupuncture, biofeedback, homeopathy, meditation, Qi gong, reiki, and therapeutic touch.

medicine, environmental, *n* medical practice that focuses on environmental exposures and health. The environment of the patient is tested for disease precipitators; living habits are evaluated; and a treatment protocol is created based on the findings.

medicine, evidence-based, *n* a medical approach in which the physician or therapist evaluates the clinical evidence supporting or refuting the claims of a particular modality as a basis for making care decisions.

medicine, folk, *n* any complementary/alternative system of medicine derived from oral, traditional, or unofficial sources (including spiritual practices and beliefs)—often though not exclusively associated with specific ethnic groups.

medicine, frontier, *n* classification of those alternative and complementary therapies for which no biomedical explanation currently exists.

medicine, functional, *n* name for an approach in medicine that aims at preventing illness and at optimizing physical and mental health function, often with supplements and lifestyle modification.

medicine, Galenic, *n.pr* the medicine of Galen, the second century Greek physician whose theories were authoritative in Europe for 1400 years. Health and disease are understood in terms of the balance and imbalance of humors (body fluids), and herbs were classified in terms of their effects on the humors. See also medicine, humoral.

medicine, herbal, *n* treatment of disease with herbs and medicinal plants; the major form of medicine used by 7 out of 10 people worldwide.

medicine, Hispano-Arabic, *n.pr* the medicine of the medieval Spanish, Moors, and Arabs. It was heavily informed by the Hellenistic medical thought of Galen and the diet therapies of India; also included the inno vations of public hygiene and surgery.

medicine, humanistic, *n* an interdisciplinary approach to the art and science of medicine that takes into account the view of the practitioner; the experiences of the patient, family, and the particular situations; and the societal role of healing and health care.

medicine, humoral, *n* medicine deriving from the Hellenistic concept of the four bodily humors that aims to restore health by maintaining their proper balance. See also medicine, Galenic.

medicine, integral, *n* holistic system of medicine based on the integral philosophy of Ken Wilber; attempts to integrate the physical, mental, emotional, spiritual, environmental, cultural, and social aspects of each patient.

medicine, integrated, *n* holistic system of medicine that uses conventional and alternative therapies to treat each patient biographically by situating their health concerns in the context of their lives and environments.

medicine, integrative, *n* holistic system of medicine that combines the best treatments and approaches from various disciplines—including traditional medicine, natural healing, phytotherapy, and Eastern modalities—so that treatments complement one another resulting in safer and effective care.

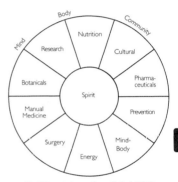

Medicine, integrative. (Rakel, 2003)

medicine, Japanese herbal, *n.pr* See kampo.

medicine, magnetic, *n* a seventeenth-century theory that asserted that good health could be restored by magneti cally transferring the patient's illness to animals and plants.

medicine, mechanistic, *n* an approach to healing that views disease as a disruption of the complex chemical and physical processes that make up a living organism. Removal of these disruptions leads to elimination or suppression of the disease.

medicine, mind-body, *n* therapeutic practices that recognize the ways in which emotional, psychosocial, and spiritual factors interact with the body to influence health. Emphasizes techniques for developing self-awareness and self-care.

M

medicine, mindfulness, *n* medical model that integrates mindfulness meditation practices to speed healing and recovery, cultivate relaxation, and increase acceptance.

Medicine, Native American (NAM), *n.pr* a system encompassing the botanical, ritual, and spiritual knowledge, beliefs, and practices of all North American indigenous peoples.

medicine, Native American herbal, *n* a therapeutic approach to healing in the Native American tradition that relies on herbal remedies.

medicine, natural, *n* therapy for curing illness via organic means—such as diet, exercise, nutrition, herbs, light, and heat—to boost the patient's self-regulating systems.

medicine, naturopathic (na'·chər·ə·pa'·thik me'·də·sin), *n* philosophy of treatment that encompasses the following seven ideas: nature's healing power; physicians should do no harm; physicians should seek to find the cause of illness; physicians treat the whole person when the cause is discovered; they prescribe preventive medicine; promote the patient's overall wellness, and, when warranted, teach the patient. In the US, naturopathic physicians (NDs) must have completed a four-year course of graduate study at an accredited institution.

medicine, oriental, *n* a general term that typically refers to Chinese traditional medicine or to one of its components, such as acupuncture or herbal medicine.

medicine, orthomolecular (ōr'·thō·mə·lek'·yə·ler me'·di·sin), *n* systematic approach to medicine using micronutrients and macronutrients, enzymes, amino acids, and friendly bacteria in optimal amounts to prevent and treat illness.

medicine, osteopathic, *n* See osteopathy.

medicine, physical, *n* the analysis and treatment of neuromuscular and musculoskeletal conditions which may interfere with mobility and function. Also called *physical therapy*.

medicine, preventive, *n* health care that aims at preventing disease in individuals and populations.

medicine, synthesis (sin'·thə·sis me'·də·sin), *n* philosophy used in diagnostic analysis and therapeutic approach. Specifically, a patient is not seen as an aggregate or compilation of parts functioning together but rather as a unit that comprises body and mind.

medicine, traditional, *n* See traditional systems of health.

medicine, traditional Chinese (TCM), *n* an ancient system of medicine developed in China, based on the concept of qi, or vital energy, that flows throughout the body. Other components include herbal medicines, restorative physical exercises, meditation, acupuncture, acupressure, and remedial massage. See also qi.

medicine, transpersonal, *n* the science and art of fostering well-being through sources beyond the patient's logical and conscious self.

medicine, ultramolecular, *n* an alternate name sometimes used for homeopathy, referring to the extreme dilutions used in preparing homeopathic remedies.

medicine, vibrational (vī·brā'·shə·nəl me'·di·sin), *n* treatment of disease through the manipulation of a person's energy fields and application of electromagnetic frequencies.

medicine, wilderness, *n* the treatment of injuries and trauma in locations, such as in national forests or parks, where traditional medical care may be inaccessible. Training in wilderness medicine includes the treatment of environmental injuries, response to plant and animal poisons, and basic backwoods transport methods.

medicines, stability of, *n* the state of a remedy wherein its active attributes remain constant. The standard for the length of time over which a remedy is likely to retain its curative ability averages 5 years for source materials and tinctures. High potencies, when sheltered from light and heat, may remain stable indefinitely. See also potency, destruction of.

medicines, status of, n the classification of relative importance of homeopathic remedies as polychrests, often used remedies, major remedies, and then minor remedies. These categories are based on the breadth of their function instead of their usefulness for a specific patient and are also determined by how much is known about a given remedy.

medicine for a small planet, n See medicine, sustainable.

medicine makers, n.pl in herbalism, those who process medicinally beneficial plants for therapeutic purposes and prescribe safe dosages for human use. In certain healing traditions, it is considered a spiritual honor and responsibility to hold such a position.

Medicine Man Society, n.pr the organization of healers within the Navajo nation. Most Native American reservations have at least one medicine man or woman, and many large indigenous nations have similar societies of healers.

meditation, n directing one's attention toward a symbol, sound, thought, or breath to alter the state of consciousness to attain a state of relaxation and stress relief; used for spiritual growth, healing, deepening concentration, and unlocking creativity.

meditation break, n employment policy in which employees are provided time and space to meditate during the course of the workday.

meditation, concentration, n any form of meditation in which peace and relaxation are effected through focused attention upon a word, image, sound, or sensation.

meditation, mindfulness, n a form of meditation in which participants practice being aware of but not responding to their thoughts or mental images. Used to help participants reduce the effects of stress and to cope with pain.

meditation-based stress reduction, n therapeutic program of group and individual meditation techniques practiced to reduce stress levels and improve a number of disorders.

medium-chain triglycerides, n.pl fats consisting of eight to ten atoms of carbon that are not broken into smaller units; they then get transferred through the lymphatic system (as are long-chain triglycerides) but are transported intact to the liver and metabolized without first being stored in fatty tissue. This ease in metabolism helps those with fat absorption problems and may also be of use in weight loss. There are no known precautions.

MEDLINE, n.pr a computer database maintained by the United States National Library of Medicine that provides access to articles in biomedical journals currently published and the preceding twenty-plus years.

medovahasrotas (mā'·dō·vä'·häs·rō'·təs), n.pl in Ayurveda, one of the 13 srotas, or body channels, which convey components for fat tissues; originate in the abdominal fat tissues and kidneys. See also srotas.

Melaleuca alternifolia, n See tree, tea.

melanin (me'·lə·nin), n a substance produced by melanocytes found in the deepest layer of the epidermis; protects the skin from the effects of the sun's harmful rays. Variations in skin color are a result of the level of melanin produced by each individual.

melatonin (me'·lə·tō'·nin), n hormone secreted from the pineal gland thought to regulate circadian rhythms. Also used in supplement form as a sleep aid.

melena (mə·lē'·nə), n dark stools with a tarlike consistency and a distinct odor comprised of digested blood; results from bleeding in the upper gastrointestinal tract; usually a sign of peptic ulcer or small bowel disease.

melilotus (me·li·lō'·shəs), n Latin name: *Melilotus officinalis* L.; parts used: leaves (dried), flowers (dried); uses: antiedema, antiinflammatory, antitumor, immunomodulator, emollient, digestive aid, flatulence, diarrhea, general pains, lymphoedema, cancer, arthritis; precautions: patients with liver disorders or on blood thinners; can cause possible hepatotoxicity. Also called *melilot, Meliloti herba,* and *sweet clover.* See also coumarin.

Melilotus officinalis L., *n* See melilotus.

Melissa officinalis L., *n* See lemon balm.

membranous balance, *n* optimally balanced tension within the dura mater.

meningitis (me·nin·jī'·tis), *n* an infection or inflammation of the membranes that cover the spinal cord and brain because of a virus or a bacterium. Bacterial infection is usually more life-threatening and is indicated by the sudden onset of a stiff neck, headache, fever, and vomiting; may cause stupor, confusion, and convulsions if untreated. Antibiotics for the specific causative agent are prescribed to treat bacterial meningitis.

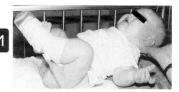

Meningitis. (Zitelli and Davis, 1997)

menopause, *n* the changes and symptoms that occur when a woman's body ceases to have ovulation and a menstrual cycle. May be gradual or abrupt due to surgery or illness. Most women begin to present menopausal symptoms by age 47; symptoms, if present, may include hot flashes, sleeplessness, irritability, depression, and libido changes. Natural or artificial hormone replacement therapy is often prescribed.

menorrhagia (men·ə·r rā'·gē·ə), *n* heavy or too-frequent menstrual periods.

mens rea (menz' rē'·ə), *n* the intent of a crime—that is, the perpetrator's mental state regarding the act committed.

menstrums, *n.pl* solvents, such as water, acetone, or alcohol, used for extraction.

mental body, *n* See mental field.

mental component, *n* the activities and influences of the mind, or consciousness. Inquiring, intending, visualizing, focusing, and transmitting are the elements of the mental component.

mental field, *n* in energy medicine, one of the ethereal layers associated with conceptualization, thought, rationalization, and event interpretation. This energy level encircles the emotional field, as is evident in the connection between thoughts and emotions.

mental image, *n* visual thought of a thing or event.

mental level, *n* See mental field.

mental telepathy, *n* a form of anomalous cognition in which an individual may receive information or thoughts directly from the mind of another.

Mentastics (men·tas'·tiks), *n.pr* mental gymnastics; term coined by Milton Trager, MD, to describe mind-guided movements that are meant to manifest freely and with little effort.

Mentha pulegium, *n* European pennyroyal. See pennyroyal.

Mentha spicata, *n* spearmint. See mint.

Mentha x piperita, *n* peppermint. See mint.

Menyanthes trifoliata, *n* See bogbean.

MEP, *n* muscle energy procedure; diagnostic and therapeutic technique. Pulsed muscle energy techniques (MET) and integrated neuromuscular inhibition technique (INIT) are two examples.

mercury, *n* a toxic heavy metal most often found in contaminated fish, dental amalgam, and some Ayurvedic and Chinese herbal medicines. Has been linked to neurological disorders, liver damage, and kidney diseases.

mercury-free, *adj* patients who have received mercury-free replacement of dental amalgams though they may still carry a "body burden" of mercury.

meric (mer'·ik), *n* chiropractic approach that emphasizes the HVLA, or thrust-oriented treatment of the third thoracic vertebra because it is believed to be the main center of subluxation.

meridian channels, *n.pl* in acupuncture, the lines of energy that connect acupoints and are conduits for qi. See also acupoints, acupuncture, and qi.

meridians, *n.pl* See channels.

mesmerism (mez'·mə·ri'·zəm), *n.pr* the therapy advanced by the German Doctor Franz Mesmer, which involved using the power of "animal magnetism" to put people into trance; considered the predecessor of modern hypnosis. See also animal magnetism.

mesomorph, *n* one of the three somatotypes described by WH Sheldon; characterized by a square, rugged,

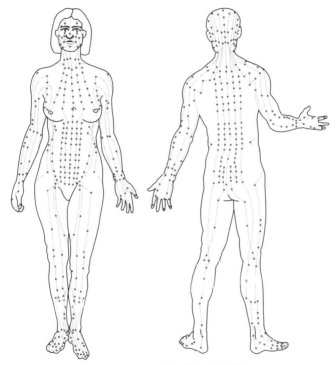

Meridians. (Beinfield and Korngold, 1991)

mesentery (mez'·ən·ter'·ē), *n* the fan-shaped, double layer of peritoneal membrane; responsible for supporting the small intestine.

hard body without body mass concentrated centrally. See also somatotype.

mesomorphy, *n* according to the Heath-Carter model of somatotypology, this body type is characterized by robust muscles and skeletal structure. See also Heath-Carter somatotype.

MET, *n* muscle energy technique; therapy that primarily targets soft tissues and uses the intrinsic strength of muscles to mobilize the joints. Applications of MET include relaxing, stretching, strengthening or restraining muscular function, disabling active trigger points, augmenting circulation throughout the body, loosening an inhibited joint, or preparing adjacent tissues for joint manipulation.

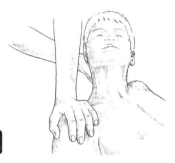

MET. (Chaitow, 1996)

metaanalysis (meˈ**·tə-ə·na**ˈ**·lə·səs),** *n* a statistical method for analyzing a large body of separate studies; aims to integrate the conclusions of those studies.

metabiosis (meˈ**·tə·bī·ō**ˈ**·sis),** *n* a mode of existence in which an organism depends on another to produce a favorable environment for its survival.

metabolic regeneration, *n* the process by which the body continually recreates itself in order to maintain life.

metabolism (mə·taˈ**·bə·li·zəm),** *n* the combined sum of the chemical processes occurring in a living organism. It is separated into anabolism, a process that results in the consumption of energy, and catabolism, a process that releases energy.

metal, *n* one of the five phases, or elements, in Chinese cosmological and medical theory, whose characteristic manifestations include analysis, logic, morality, pessimism, precision, and self-control.

metalloenzyme (meˈ**·tə·lō·en**ˈ**·zīm),** *n* an enzyme containing a metal in its active site.

metallothionien (MT) (meˈ**·tə·lō·thī**ˈ**·ə·nen),** *n* a small, intracellular, metalbinding protein. While excessive levels of MT have been associated with poor prognoses in many cancers, including those of the prostate and breast, MT is also used as a protective adjunct to chemotherapy and radiation treatments.

metals, *n* a fundamental grouping of elements such as sodium, gold, copper, and iron in the periodic table that have similar chemical and physical properties, including high density, ductility, malleability, and conductivity (of electricity and heat).

metaplasia (meˈ**·tə·plā**ˈ**·zhē·ə),** *n* abnormal cell growth in which cells become unlike the normal cells in the tissue of which they are a part.

metastasis (mə·tasˈ**·tə·sis),** *n* growth and movement of cancer cells from one area of the body to another.

method, *n* a systematized means for accomplishing a purpose.

method, **active,** *n* an osteopathic manipulative technique in which the patient performs motions directed by the physician.

method, azeotrophic **(ə·zē**ˈ**·ō·trō**ˈ**·fik me**ˈ**·thəd),** *n* a technique for processing glandular extracts in which the material is frozen, purified with a strong solvent, distilled, dried, and crushed into a powder.

method, **combined,** *n* **1.** an osteopathic treatment that begins with indirect movements and then switches to direct forces as the technique is completed. **2.** an osteopathic treatment that combines two or more different techniques.

method, **Cyriax,** *n.pr* a "pinching" technique developed by James Cyriax to promote stretching and relaxation of tissues and to decrease the amount of blood within the tissue.

method, energy diagnostic and treatment, *n* psychotherapy practiced on the foundations of acupuncture meridian theory; also employs music, visualization, song, thought recognition, and core belief analysis to correct psychologic and psychoenergetic problems.

method, exaggeration, *n* any osteopathic treatment in which the affected physical component is moved beyond the range of voluntary motion, away from the restrictive barrier, to a point where the patient feels increased tension.

method, Feldenkrais, *n.pr* therapeutic learning approach in which participants learn functional movement and self-awareness through sensory experiences. Taught one-on-one and in large class settings. Helps participants discover natural, intuitive movement.

method, functional, *n* an indirect osteopathic technique in which the physician locates the dynamic balance point, to which is applied one of the following techniques: applying indirect guiding force, holding the position, or exaggerating the position through added compression. This is done to decrease the sense of tissue resistance.

method, horn, *n* in traditional Chinese medicine, therapeutic approach that involves warming the air inside a glass, metal, or wooden cup and inverting it over a part of the body to treat various health conditions; animal horns, from which the method derives its name, were used originally.

method, Krieger/Kunz, *n.pr* the five-step, energy-based therapeutic method formerly called therapeutic touch. The five steps are centering (calming the self and client to a point of open readiness), assessment (discerning the symmetry of the energy fields surrounding the client), unruffling (the practitioner moves his hands in a clearing motion to the edges of the client's energy field), and directing and modulating energy (the practitioner channels and transfers energy to the client).

method, Mitchell, *n.pr* a technique used for relaxation in which one assumes body postures opposite to those related to stress and anxiety.

method, Morrell, *n.pr* a form of reflexology that emphasizes extremely light touch instead of applying deep pressure. Also called *Morrell Reflexology.* See also reflexology.

method, multiglass, *n* Hahnemann's process for developing homeopathic remedies; uses a clean glass receptacle for each successive dilution. See also potency, Hahnemannian; potency, Korsakov; and method, single glass.

method, negative affect–erasing (NAEM), *n* a meridian-based procedure in which a patient is instructed by the practitioner to recall a traumatic event and then is systematically tapped on specific points of the body to resolve the trauma.

method, overall examination, *n* in a pulse examination, a thorough diagnostic method that uses nine standard locations to examine the pulse. These nine locations consist of three points at each section of the body (upper— the head, center—the hands, and lower—the feet) and three points per section—one each for heaven, man, and earth. See also pulse examination.

method, passive, *n* osteopathic technique in which the patient does not engage in any voluntary contraction of the muscles.

method, respiratory one, *n.pr* a form of meditation in which participants repeat the word *one* with each exhale. Used to create an awed relaxed state.

method, Rosen, *n.pr* somatic education method created by Marion Rosen in which easy, deliberate body movements are set to music to improve flexibility, alignment, and range of motion. They also ease breathing, and deepen awareness of the body. May be performed individually, with partners, or in a circle.

method, salt precipitation, *n* technique for processing glandular extracts in which the glandular material is soaked in salt and water and then sep-

M

arated into high-density, water-soluble material and low-density, fat-soluble material by centrifugation. The water-soluble material is then dried and crushed into a powder.

method, single-glass, n procedure for developing potencies in one glass receptacle only. Fluxion is a form of this procedure. See also potency, Korsakov and fluxion.

method, three-section examination, n in a pulse examination, a diagnostic method that is used in emergencies. The three points are the ren ying (near the Adam's apple), the cun kou (wrist pulse), and fu yang (instep) points. See also pulse examination.

methods, brief, n.pl 1. relaxation techniques that can be used effectively with little or no practice. Deep breathing and paced respiration are examples. 2. in psychotherapy, abbreviated therapeutic approaches often used in crisis situations or when long-term therapy may be inappropriate.

methods, deep, n.pl relaxation techniques that often take time and practice to cultivate. Autogenic training, meditation, and progressive muscle relaxation are examples.

methods, four, n.pl in Chinese traditional medicine, four diagnostic methods—inspection, olfaction, auscultation, inquiry, and palpation— used to collect patient information.

methyl sulfonyl methane, n See MSM.

methylation, n a phase-II detoxification pathway in the liver; methyl groups combine with toxins to rid the body of various substances.

methylsalicylate (me'·thəl·sə·li'·sə·lāt), n a liquid ester with the chemical formula $C_8H_8O_3$ that is derived from the bark of a birch, *Betula lenta* or the leaves of wintergreen, *Gaultheria procumbens;* used as an antiinflammatory, counterirritant, or flavoring agent and to treat pharyngitis, chorea, lumbago, orchitis, mumps, neuralgia, and rheumatism—chronic and acute; precautions: highly toxic. In children a directly ingested dose of less than one teaspoon has been lethal. In rare cases, it has also been linked with allergic skin reactions.

metrorrhagia (mē·trə·rā'·gē·ə), n heavy uterine blood flow occurring between regular menstrual periods; usually associated with pain.

Mexican scammony (mek'·sə·kən ska'·mə·nē), n Latin name: *Convolvulus scammonia;* part used: roots; uses: bowel evacuation; precautions: may cause severe or watery bowel evacuation. Also called *heleblab, jalap, mahmude, squmania, syrian bindweed,* and *scammony.*

mezereum (mə·zēr'·ē·əm), n dried bark from *Daphne mezereum,* which causes severe intestinal tract irritation and blisters on the skin. Homeopathic preparations used to treat psoriasis, eczema, and herpes zoster.

MFR, n See myofascial release.

miasm, n 1. genetic or social predisposition to succumb to certain diseases. 2. the core source of disease, which Hahnemann divided into three types (i.e., psora, sycosis, and syphilis). These miasms are categories of diseases in which a variety of symptoms can be manifested in a specific individual. See also constitution, diathesis, predisposition, psoric miasm, sycotic miasm, syphilitic miasm, and terrain.

MIC, n an abbreviation for minimal inhibitory concentration, the lowest concentration of an antibiotic that is needed to hinder the growth of bacteria.

microarray (mī'·krō·ə·rā'), n a method of evaluating a large number of DNA changes on a slide which has RNA fragments attached.

microbehaviors (mī'·krō·bə·hā'·vyərz), n.pl in the context of hypnosis therapies, refers to the body systems.

microcephaly (mī'·krō·se'·fə·lē), n a congenital disorder characterized by an abnormally small head relative to the rest of the body and an underdeveloped brain; may result in mental retardation; caused by a chromosomal anomaly or exposure to trauma or toxic stimulus during prenatal development.

microcosmic orbit, n a form of Qi gong in which the qi cycles through the body, moving up the spinal column and down the chest and abdomen. See also Qi gong.

microcurrent (mī'·krō·ker'·ənt), *n* small current used in a noninvasive electrotherapy technique where electrodes are applied at acupuncture points.

microdose (mī'·krō·dōs'), *n* extremely small dose of highly diluted medicinal substance used in homeopathic medicine. Also called *homeopathic dose.*

microgenesis, *n* a theory about the way thoughts and messages move through the brain. Thoughts and messages percolate through the various regions of the brain (reptilian, limbic, and neomammalian cortex), thus mimicking evolution, before being perceived by the organism.

microgenetic moment, *n* when an organism is healed instantaneously.

microliter (mī'·krō·lē'·ter), *n* a metric unit of measure defined as one millionth of a liter (0.000001) and written as *μl.*

micronutrients (mī'·krō·nōō'·trē·ənts), *n.pl* substances such as vitamins and minerals needed in small amounts for normal body function.

microscopy (TSEM) (mī·kros'·kə·pē), *n* a technique that uses transmission scanning electron microscope to generate highly magnified clear three-dimensional images.

middle note, *n* a category of aromatic components of essential perfumes and oils with intermediate permanence and volatility properties. The category includes lavender and geranium. See also note.

midewewin (me·dā·wā'·wēn), *n* in Native American medicine, an Ojibway term for the society or "university" responsible for educating and training novices in the ways of healing and communing with spiritual powers and energies. An invitation to join is only given to a male or female candidate after an extensive period of assessing one's character. Accreditation is only awarded after the initiate passes through the four orders. See also four orders.

midheel line, *n* a vertical line running between the heels equidistant from both—that is used as a reference in postural evaluation and in standing front-back radiographs.

midmalleolar line (mid'-mal·lē'·ō'·lər līn'), *n* a vertical line that runs through the lateral malleolus and is used as a reference in postural evaluation and in standing side-view radiographs.

midsagittal plane (mid'·sa'·ji·təl plān'), *n* a vertical plane through the midline of the body; divides the body into right and left halves. Also called the *median* plane.

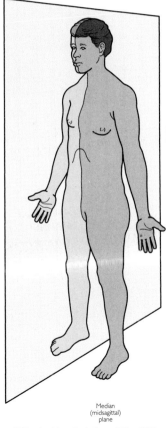

Median (midsagittal) plane

Midsagittal (median) plane. (Salvo, 2003)

midwife, *n* a woman who attends another woman during pregnancy and labor, an expert practitioner in the care of expectant women and the delivery of uncomplicated pregnancies.

migraine, *n* a type of severe headache; often recurring and characterized by sudden onset on one side of the head or face, with acute pain and sensitivity to light and noise.

migraine, atypical **(ā'·ti'·pi·kəl mī'·grān),** *n* a headache without an aura and tending to be less unilateral than classical migraines. Also called *common migraine.*

migraine, classic, *n* a condition characterized by painful headache often accompanied by an aura (a visual, motor, or cognitive phenomenon that prefaces the headache).

migraine, common, *n* a condition characterized by painful headache that is not accompanied by an aura. See also migraine, classic.

migraine with aura, *n* See classic migraine.

migraine without aura, *n* See common migraine.

migrating motor complex, *n* the coordinated response of the body to the ingestion of food, which includes peristaltic motion and secretomotor activity. This response also balances fluid and electrolyte levels in the gastrointestinal tract.

mild cognitive impairment (MCI), *n* memory loss generally associated with aging; does not affect normal independent functioning of an individual.

mild traumatic brain injury, *n* disruption of brain function by trauma characterized by but not limited to a loss of consciousness, memory loss surrounding the trauma, confusion during the incident, loss of consciousness for no more than thirty minutes, and posttraumatic amnesia lasting less than 24 hours.

miliary, *adj* pertaining to a condition, such as miliary tuberculosis, marked by the appearance of a multitude of small lesions that resemble millet seeds.

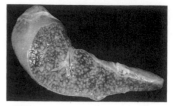

Miliary. (Kumar, Cotran, and Robbins, 1997)

milliliter (mi'·lə·lē'·ter), *n* a metric unit of measure defined as one thousandth (.001) of a liter and written as ml. See also liter.

mimic therapeutic touch (mi'·mik the'·rə·pyoo'·tik tuch'), *n* a technique used to test the efficacy of therapeutic touch by imitating the movements without directing energy, assisting the patient, centering, or attuning to the patient; used for blind studies.

mind-body healing system, *n* a patient-oriented, proactive approach to health and healing that values personal responsibility and self-motivation. Lifestyle and personal attitudes are the focus to bring about personal transformation and gain mastery over the mind and body.

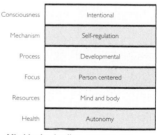

Consciousness	Intentional
Mechanism	Self-regulation
Process	Developmental
Focus	Person centered
Resources	Mind and body
Health	Autonomy

Mind-body healing system. (Micozzi, 2002)

mind clearing, *v* releasing all thoughts in order to more fully benefit from the treatment to follow; a practice in the healing touch philosophy.

mind cure, *n* healing system according to which feelings or thoughts are the most important factor in human health. Negative thinking is believed to cause disease, whereas good health results from positive thoughts.

mindcolor, *n* Australian color therapy practice designed to communicate with the subconscious.

mindfulness, *n* the capacity to maintain nonjudgmental attentiveness to the present moment.

mindfulness-based stress reduction (MBSR), *n* meditation technique that promotes relaxation through the nonjudgmental awareness of moment-to-moment sensations, experiences, and reactions.

mind-matter interactions, *n.pl* correlations between a subject's mental activities and noticeable effects in the external, physical environment, typically investigated using random event generators or other devices. See also random event generator and random number generator.

mineral, *n* an inorganic substance.

minim (mi'·nəm), *n* a small measure of liquid, roughly 1/480th of a fluid ounce, or the size of a drop of water.

mint, *n* Latin names: *Mentha x piperita, Mentha spicata;* parts used: leaves, oil; uses: antiseptic, antiemetic, diarrhea, gallbladder conditions, indigestion, topical analgesic, aromatherapy; precautions: pregnancy, lactation, children, gallbladder inflammation, GERD, severe liver conditions, kidney disease, ulcers, irritation of mucosae. Also called *balm mint, brandy mint, green mint, lamb mint* or *our lady's mint.*

miosis (mī·ō'·sis), *n* an ocular condition characterized by excessive constriction of the sphincter muscles of the iris; results in small pupils; stimulation of the pupillary reflex by an increase in light and certain drugs may result in temporary miosis.

misapplication, *n* the use of incorrect or improper procedures while administering treatment; results from inadequacy in experience, training, skills, or knowledge. May also result from impairment or incompetence.

miscibility (mi'·sə·bi'·lə·tē), *n* the ability of two liquids to mix with each other.

misdiagnosis (mis'·dī·ag·nō'·sis), *n* an inaccurate assessment of a patient's condition. Harm may be inflicted on the patient as the result of an incorrect therapeutic approach.

mislabeling, *n* **1.** the inaccurate identification of a product in which the label lists ingredients or components that are not actually included within the product. **2.** the inaccurate identification of a product in which actions claimed by the product are not truly achieved.

misrepresentation, *n* when one party purposefully exaggerates the anticipated positive results to gain another party's confidence and thereby enter into a legal agreement.

mistletoe, *n* Latin names: *Viscum album, Viscum abietis, Viscum austriacum;* parts used: branches, fruits, leaves; uses: anxiolytic, high blood pressure, seizure disorders, immunomodulator, depression, gout, insomnia, cancer; precautions: pregnancy, lactation, children, protein hypersensitivity, antihypertensive medications, cardiac glycosides, depressants, immunosuppressant medications, HIV, toxic plant. Also called *all heal, birdlime, devil's fuge, European mistletoe, golden bough,* or *mystyldene.*

mitakuye oyas'in (mē·tä'·kōō·yä ō·yä'·sə·ēn), *n* Lakota Indian philosophy according to which all humans come from one source. All are related, and everyone should identify the good and bad and strive to do good.

Mitempfindungen, *n* See referred itch.

mixer approach, *n* a school of thought associated with chiropractic medicine in which other therapeutic approaches such as physical therapy, nutritional supplements, homeopathy, acupuncture, biofeedback, and herbal remedies are used in addition to manipulation of the spine. Adherents to this school of thought believe subluxation is one of several origins of disease. Debate between the concepts associated with straight chiropractic and mixer approach are ongoing. See also subluxation and straight chiropractic.

mixture, *n* a chemical substance containing more than one type of molecule. The components of a mixture may be separated through physical means.

mkweta (m·kwā'·tə), *n* a term for an apprentice healer. From the South African language Xhosa.

MM, *n* See meditation, mindfulness.

mmHg, *n* millimeters of mercury; unit of pressure measurement.

MMI, *n.pr* See mind-matter interactions.

mobility, *n* the proficiency to organize and accomplish the act of moving.

mobilization with impulse, *n* See HVT.

mobilization with movement, *n* an emerging, manual therapy technique developed by Brian Mulligan, for the treatment of musculoskeletal dysfunction in which the therapist applies a passive glide mobilization to a joint while the patient performs physical activity using the limbs. See also NAGS, SNAGS.

mobilizing, *v* **1.** freeing or making loose and able to move. **2.** observing any ongoing movements in a client's body, whether small or large, assisted or not, that identify strengths and weaknesses, as well as the client's physical and emotional readiness for the therapy.

modak (mō'·dək), *n* in Ayurveda, pills that are derived from plant or mineral substances.

modality, *n* **1.** the technique of applying a therapeutic regimen or agent. **2.** a particular sense, such as the sense of vision.

model, *n* **1.** a concept that represents how things work together. Used to explain how theories and observations fit together, such as an explanatory model. **2.** a method for testing a specific theory that can be used repeatedly for examining dimensions and validity of that theory (e.g., a laboratory model).

model of biofeedback, drug, *n* a scientific framework used in biofeedback research; attempts to remove purported placebo effects. Thus the effect of biofeedback is isolated and measured by removing the other variables. Once used in early biofeedback results, this model is now considered to be inappropriate because it assumes the particular effects are derived from the instrument being used rather than from the subject.

model of consciousness, nonlocal, *n* in mental healing, the notion that at some level, all minds are united as one; therefore the patient and the healer are not separated by distance.

model of TT, Krieger/Kunz, *n.pr* See method, Krieger/Kunz.

model, biomedical, *n* theoretical and epistimelogical basis of conventional Western medicine.

model, bio-psycho-social-spiritual (bī'·ō-sī'·kō-sō'·shəl-spi'·ri·chŏō·əl mō'·dəl), *n* in holistic nursing, a model in which persons comprise four interrelated components—biologic, psychologic, sociologic, and spiritual—that provide holistic and comprehensive understanding of the functionality of human beings and establish a diagnosis. The biological component refers to the fundamental needs that assist an individual with maintaining his or her health. These include sleep, food, water, fresh air, exercise, and a healthy environment. The psychologic component refers to perception, language, mood, cognition, symbolic images, thoughts, intellect, memory, and capability to evaluate information. The sociologic component refers to relationships or associations with friends, family, community universe, and relationship with the self. The spiritual component refers to a broad definition of one's purpose in life, meaning, and value. It also refers to traits associated with love, caring, wisdom, honesty, and imagination. It may also refer to indications of a guiding spirit, higher existence, or higher being of power. This model guides holistic clinical nursing education, research, and practice.

model, cognitive-behavioral medicine, *n* in behavioral medicine, a system of thought in which the association between cognitive processes, stressful life events, behavior, and physiologic and emotional reactions is used.

model, eclectic (of music therapy) **(e·klek'·tik mô'·dəl əv myōō'·sik the'·rə·pē),** *n* recognition that while music therapy is applied with several techniques and approaches, music itself is a powerful shared phenomenon and that its influence on human beings is important.

model, health belief, *n.pr* a description of how complex interactions between cultural beliefs, personal idiosyncrasies, past experiences with illness, and previous interactions with doctors and other health professionals inform choices regarding possible health problems.

model, high-risk model of threat perception, *n* a framework developed by Ian Wickramasekera, PhD; proposes an interaction between a set of predisposers such as low and high hypnotic ability, triggers such as significant life change, and buffers such as coping skills or support system, which can affect the risk of an individual developing stress-related disorders. Also called *HRMTP.*

model, holistic, *n* an etiologic model in which the reactions of the patient to etiological influences and agents are examined and the treatment serves to restore homeostatic balance, improve resistance, and stimulate self-healing. For instance, a patient with indications of a headache may be prescribed acupuncture therapy to restore qi balance, or a homeopathic remedy to reestablish an autoregulatory process within the body. Treatment is not directed toward the specific case. See also qi.

model, infomedical, *n* a medical framework, contrasted to the biomedical model, that recognizes the self-organizing complexity of the human organism and emphasizes the role of multiple sources of information (e.g., body, mind, society) in the healing process.

model, mastery **(mas'·tə·rē mô'·dəl),** *n* a framework used in biofeed-

back therapy; provides a fundamental structure for actively learning and mastering a necessary skill. Mastery of a necessary skill is considered indication of a successful outcome.

model, Nagi **(nä'·gē mä'·dəl),** *n.pr* developed by SZ Nagi, according to which disability is viewed as a function of the interactions between an individual and the environment (encompassing the natural environment, culture, the economic system, the political system, and psychological factors) and not as an inherent state.

model, nonmaterialist **(nôn'·mə·tē'·rē·ə·list mô'·dəl),** *n.pl* model according to which the mind (soul, spirit), comes first and animates the physical body.

model, operant conditioning **(ô'·per·ənt kun·di'·shə·ning mô'·dəl),** *n* a scientific framework used in biofeedback research, which assumes that rewards control behavior. In this framework, information received from the feedback is synonymous with a reward. Once used in early biofeedback results, the use of this model is now considered to be inappropriate because of the failure of the researchers to facilitate the act of self-control within the participants being studied.

model, Pressurestat, *n* a model according to which the craniosacral system is similar to a hydraulic and semi-closed system that rhythmically filters cerebrospinal fluid from the blood, circulates it, and returns it to the bloodstream in a constant flow.

model, specific cause, *n* an etiological model in which the prominent pathway of a specific condition is identified, and treatment is targeted so as to interfere with this pathway. For instance, a practitioner may trace the cause of chronic headache to a vasospasm and the treatment—medicine or biofeedback—is prescribed to directly interfere with the effects of the vasospasm.

model, stress-diathesis **(stres'·dī·a'·thə·sis mô'·dəl),** *n* a psychological paradigm that explains psychopathol-

M

ogy in terms of the interaction between stressors and a patient's predisposition to mental illness.

model, systems, *n* an etiologic model in which the web of influences that contribute to a specific condition as well as their associations with covert problems and risks is identified, and treatment is targeted to the foremost factors. For instance, a patient with symptoms of chronic headache and other minor indications of borderline hypertension, insomnia, and fatigue is prescribed behavioral therapy and changes in lifestyle that address exercise, diet, substance issue, and relaxation skills.

models, materialist, *n.pl* theories about the development of illness that hold that the physical body is primary and that the body gives rise to nonphysical elements such as the mind and emotions. See also models, nonmaterialist.

molarity (mō′·ler·i·tē), *n* the number of moles of a compound or element dissolved in one liter (L) of solution. See also concentration.

mole, *n* the number of grams of a substance that is equivalent to the molecular weight. A mole of any compound or mixture comprises the same number of atoms or molecules. This number is called Avogadro's number, 6.02×10^{23}.

molecular formula, *n* a representation of the numbers of all elements that comprise one molecule of a compound.

molecular mass, *n* See molecular weight.

molecular structure, *n* describes the type, arrangement, position, and direction of the bonds linking atoms within a molecule.

molecular weight, *n* the total atomic mass (weight) of all atoms within a molecule. This determines biological and physical properties of the substance.

molecule, *n* the smallest unit of a chemical compound; comprises atoms joined with chemical bonds. See also atom and compound.

moment of suspension, *n* practical technique in Aston-Mechanics movement therapy; induces the experience of weightlessness. See also Aston-Mechanics.

Momordica charantia **L.,** *n* See bitter melon.

Monascum anka, *n* See monascus.

Monascum purpureus, *n* See monascus.

monascus (mə·nas′·kəs), *n* Latin names: *Monascum purpureus, Monascum anka;* part used: whole yeast; uses: antimicrobial, antioxidant, hepatoprotection, cholesterol, vascular conditions, gastrointestinal conditions; precautions: pregnancy, lactation, children, cirrhosis, and other liver diseases. Also called *zhi tai* or *xuezhikang.*

Mongolian milk-vetch (môn·gō′· lē·ən milk′-vech′), *n.pr* Latin name: *Astragalus mongholicus;* part used: roots; uses: stimulates immune system, general tonic, influenza, common cold; precautions: none known.

monoamine-dependent system (mô′·nō·ə·mēn′-də·pen′·dənt sis′· təm), *n* in acupuncture, a model system of activating the body's endogenous opioid peptide system to influence pain regulation with high-frequency (at least 70 Hz)/low-intensity electrical stimulation. The analgesic response is usually rapid, segmented, and not increased with repeated stimulations. See also endorphin-dependent system.

monocytes, *n.pl* the largest of the white blood cells. They have one nucleus and a large amount of grayish-blue cytoplasm. Develop into macrophages and both consume foreign material and alert T cells to its presence.

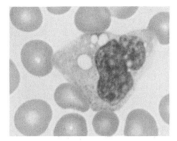

Monocytes. (Carr and Rodak, 1999)

monomer (mô'·nə·mer), *n* a single chemical compound that can join with additional, identical molecules to produce a polymer. See also polymer.

mononucleosis (mô'·nō·nōō·klē·ō'·sis), *n* an infectious disease caused by the Epstein-Barr virus and characterized by a proliferation of white blood cells (specifically mononuclear leukocytes). Symptoms include fatigue, aches, fever and chills, sore throat, swollen lymph nodes, and an enlarged spleen. Often occurs in adolescents. Also called *Epstein-Barr virus, EBV, glandular fever,* or *infectious mononucleosis.*

monoterpene (mä'·nə·ter'·pēn), *n* a member of the terpene group; comprises two units of isoprene that are linked by two carbon atoms with a single bond. Its molecular formula is $C_{10}H_8$. It has been used as an antiseptic, stimulant, analgesic, decongestant, and expectorant.

monoterpenols (nä'·nō·ter·'pə·hōlz), *n.pl* compounds found in most essential oils. They have potent antibacterial and antiviral properties and are generally nontoxic.

moon lodges (mōōn' lô'·jez), *n.pl* in Native American culture, isolated locations for women to use as sites for meditation and retreat during menstruation. This tradition was instituted to enhance the mental, spiritual, and physical health of women and the community or in some cases to isolate women during what was considered a sacred or contaminated period.

moon time (mōōn' tīm'), *n* in Native American culture, the period of menstruation; it is widely believed that women are more powerful or, in some tribes, contaminated during this particular period.

morbific influences, *n.pl* any of a number of factors that contribute to disease, including bacteria, toxins, and psychologic stress.

mordant (mōr'·dənt), *n* a chemical that fixes a dye in or on a specimen by combining with the dye. Phenol, alum, aniline, and oil are common mordants.

morinda (mō·rin'·də), *n* Latin names: *Morinda citrifolia, Morinda officinalis;* parts used: flowers, fruits, leaves; uses: immunomodulator, anticancer, anthelmintic, analgesic, sedative, arthritis, cardiac disease, diabetes, high blood pressure, gastrointestinal conditions; precautions: pregnancy, lactation, children, hyperkalemia. Also called *hog apple, Indian mulberry, mengkoedoe, mora de la India, ruibarbo caribe,* or *wild pine.*

Morinda citrifolia, *n* See morinda.

Morinda officinalis, *n* See morinda.

morphology, *n* method for classifying the body constitution type. See also constitution, carbonic; constitution, fluoric; constitution, phosphoric; and constitution, sulphuric.

mother essence, *n* flower essence therapy mixture; flowers or gemstones are placed in distilled water in direct sunlight after which the water, believed to carry imprints of the flowers or gemstones is mixed with brandy.

mother of fire, *n* in Chinese medicine, wood, one of the five elements, essential for creation of fire. See law of mother and child.

mother of metal, *n* in Chinese medicine, earth, one of the five elements, which is the source of metal. See also law of mother and child.

mother tincture, *n* in homeopathy or herbalism, any of a number of strained solutions of organic or mineral substances in alcohol or water.

motherwort (mu·ther·wōrt), *n* Latin name: *Leonurus cardiaca;* parts used: leaves, seeds; uses: cardiotonic, menstrual problems, cardiac conditions, anticoagulant, antiinflammatory, antispasmodic, anxiolytic, anticancer; precautions: pregnancy, lactation, children, thrombocytopenia, anticoagulant medications, beta blockers, cardiac glycosides. Also called *i-mu-ts'ao, lion's ear, lion's tail, lion's-tart, oman, Roman motherwort,* or *throwwort.*

motility **(mō·ti'·lə·tē),** *n* the ability to move independently and spontaneously.

motion, *n* movement.

motion barrier, *n* any limitation to motion.

motion of the spine, physiologic, *n* principles of thoracic motion that detail movements of the vertebrae in relationship to that of the vertebral column as a whole. When the spine is in a neutral position, coupled side-bending and rotation motions for a group of vertebrae happen in different directions. When the spine is bent backward or forward, these motions happen in the same direction.

motion, accessory joint, *n* See motion, secondary joint.

motion, bucket handle rib, *n* the head-ward movement of the lateral sides of the ribs during respiration; occurs mainly in the lower ribs. See also axis, anteroposterior rib axis, and axis of rib motion.

motion, caliper rib, *n* motion of ribs 11 and 12; characterized by moving as a single joint.

motion, iliosacral, *n* motion of the ilium through the sacrum along an inferior transverse axis, influenced by the movements of the pelvis, hips, and lower extremities, as in walking.

motion, inherent, *n* the spontaneous motion that characterizes all cells, tissues, etc. in the body.

motion, intersegmental, *n* the relative motion between two adjacent vertebrae, with the upper vertebra in the pair described as moving upon the lower vertebra.

motion, passive, *n* motion induced by the therapist or physician while the patient relaxes and exerts no effort.

motion, physiologic, *n* any change in the position, within a normal range, of anatomic structures.

motion, pump handle rib, *n* the head-ward movement of the anterior part of the ribs during respiration; occurs mainly in the upper ribs. See also axis of rib motion.

motion, range of, *n* the movement available to a joint. Full range of motion can be restricted by shortened muscles, connective tissue injuries, scar tissue or adhesions, pain, and other conditions. Also called *ROM.*

motion, secondary joint, *n* passive or involuntary joint motion. Also called *accessory joint motion.*

motion, segmental, *n* movement between two adjacent vertebrae; described through displacing a point at the upper front aspect of the superior vertebra.

motion, translatory, *n* movement of a body part along an axis.

motion palpation, *n* technique developed by Henri Gillet, a Belgian chiropractor, in which the practitioner's hands are used to feel the motion of specific segments of the spine while the patient moves. The purpose is evaluation of the dynamic movement of the extravertebral joints and vertebrae to assess dysfunction between the joints.

motor neurons, *n.pl* nerve cells that convey movement impulses that stimulate or inhibit muscles or glands.

mountain sun, *n* a device created by Dr. Carl Loeb to treat a variety of physical and emotional health concerns by projecting colored lights onto the patient's body.

movement empathy, *n* See kinesthetic identification.

movement-in-depth, *n* early form of dance/movement therapy incorporated into treatment plans by some therapists, now known as *authentic movement.*

movement view, *n* a philosophy that maintains that motion is learned (identical to the functional view) but narrows its study to specific frameworks, such as dance, martial arts, yoga, and so forth.

moving phase, *n* in chromatography, the gas that carries the vapors from the investigated sample all the way through the column of the gas-liquid chromatograph. Also called *mobile phase.*

moxa (mô'·ksə), *n* the powdered *Artemis vulgaris* leaves used in moxibustion. They are burned on an acupuncture needle or directly on the body at a meridian channel. The size of moxa varies, but it is used to bring heat to an area diagnosed as cold or to stimulate an acupuncture point.

moxibustion (mô'·ksi·bəs·chən), *n* a treatment similar to acupuncture in which *Artemis vulgaris* leaves are burned on an acupuncture needle or directly on a point of the body.

MPI, *n* myofascial pain index; a value that represents the level of pressure required to induce sensations of pain from a trigger point. It also facilitates the separation of absent, falsely positively, latent, or active trigger points. To determine MPI, an algometer is applied to the 18 sites on the body commonly used to assess fibromyalgia.

MPS, *n* myofascial pain syndrome, a disease nearly identical to fibromyalgia except for differences in occurrences and location of symptoms, related conditions, and available treatment options. In particular, persons diagnosed with this condition are more likely to experience pain in a localized area rather than the entire body, are less likely to have "morning stiffness," and will not fatigue easily. See also fibromyalgia.

MRT, *n* manual resistance technique, a treatment method used during the acute and recovery phases to relieve pain and rehabilitate the body's tissues and muscles. The primary goals of this treatment method are to mobilize joints, assist underactive muscles, and hinder overactive muscles. These exercises can be performed alone or with the assistance of a healthcare provider. Postisometric relaxation (PIR), hold-relax (HR), and proprioceptive neuromuscular facilitation (PNF) are examples of MRTs. See also PIR, HR, and PNF.

mrudu (mrōō'·dōō), *adj* in Ayurveda, "soft" as a guna, one of the qualities that characterizes all substances. Its complement is kathina. See also gunas and kathina.

MSM, *n.pr* methylsulfonylmethane, a sulfurous compound found in meat, dairy products, fruits, and vegetables and in supplemental form; has chemopreventive effects and is believed to treat osteoarthritis, rheumatism, and interstitial cystitis. There are no known precautions. Also called *DMSO₂.*

MT, *n* See metallothionien.

MTPJ, *n* metatarsophalangeal joint; any joint that is located between the phalanges and the metatarsals in the foot.

mucilages (myōō'·si·lô'·jəz), *n.pl* plant polysaccharide compounds that readily absorb water, becoming viscid and gelatinous. They are traditionally used as demulcents and laxatives and also provide a source of soluble fiber.

mucolytic (myōō'·kə·li'·tlk), *adj* able to loosen and release mucus.

mucopurulent (myōō'·kō·pyŏŏr'·ə·lənt), *adj* pertaining to a discharge that combines pus and mucus. See also mucus.

mucous membrane irritation, *n* **1.** inflammation and pain of the mucous membranes. Often caused by ingestion or inhalation of mold, dust, or chemical vapors. **2.** side effect of some essential oils that contain higher phenol or aldehyde levels.

Mucuna pruriens, *n* See cowhage.

mucus (myōō'·kəs), *n* a thick, slippery discharge that comprises white blood cells, mucin, inorganic salts, water, and exfoliated cells produced by the mucous membranes. Functions to moisten and protect them.

mugwort (mug'·wŏrt), *n* Latin name: *Artemisia vulgaris;* parts used: leaves, roots; uses: antiviral, antibacterial, anthelmintic, antiemetic, psychiatric disorders (depression, anxiety, neurosis), constipation, menstrual problems; precautions: pregnancy and lactation, infants and children, bleeding disorders, anticoagulant medications. Also called *ai ye, common mugfelon herb, sailor's tobacco, St. John's plant, wild wormwood,* or *wort.*

mullein (mu'·lən), *n* Latin names: *Verbascum thapsus, Verbasci flos;* parts used: dried leaves, flowers; uses: antiviral, antioxidant, expectorant, antitussive, respiratory complaints, urinary infections, ear infections; precautions: pregnancy, lactation, children. Also called *Aaron's rod, bunny's ears, candle-wick, flannel-leaf, great mullein,* or *Jacob's-staff.*

multiarticular (mul'·tē·är·ti'·kyə·ler), *adj* a muscle that crosses at least three joints.

multidisciplinary pain center (MPC), *n* treatment center where individuals suffering with chronic pain, addiction to painkillers, depression, etc., may receive treatment from multiple caregivers, all of whom cooperate with one another and the patient at a single facility.

multidrug resistance, *n* the adaptation of tumor cells or infectious agents to resist chemotherapeutic agents.

Multiple Affect Adjective Check-List, *n.pr* a checklist used to quantify the subject's mood with respect to depression and anxiety. The score results from the positive and the null items. Negative items are not counted in the score. There are various forms of this checklist, such as the today form and the general form.

multiple chemical sensitivity, *n* a disorder in which an individual reacts to multiple environmental toxins.

multiple sclerosis (məl'·ti·pul sklə·rō'·səs), *n* a disorder of the central nervous system caused by damage of the myelin sheath. Symptoms include pain, weakness, numbness, tingling, paralysis, tremors, and muscle dysfunction.

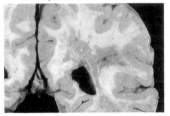

Multiple sclerosis (MS). (Kumar, Cotran, and Robbins, 1997)

multipolar magnets (mul·tē·pō'·ler mag'·nits), *n.pl* used in electromagnetic therapy to treat pain; magnets are arranged like an isosceles triangle with the poles positioned next to one another, opposite poles matching. See also therapy, electromagnetic.

multivariate analysis, *n* a statistical approach used to evaluate multiple variables.

multiwave oscillator (MWO) (məl'·tē·wāv' ä'·sə·lā'·tər), *n* device that produces a variety of radio frequencies based on the belief that each cell in the body will resonate with its own particular frequency and that this resonance will strengthen the cells against bacteria and viruses, and other diseases.

mumps, *n* a viral disease characterized by fever, fatigue, and painfully swollen parotid salivary glands. The most serious complications that can arise from the mumps occur if the disease is contracted after puberty. These include orchitis (inflammation of the testes) or ovaritis (inflammation of the ovaries).

murder, *n* the intentional termination of another human being's life through physical (violent), chemical (poisoning, illicit drugs, etc.), or neglectful (abusive) means.

muscle spasm, *n* abnormal and often painful contraction of muscle fibers commonly caused by sudden overuse or overstimulation.

muscle testing procedures, *n.pl* specific assessment tests used to determine muscle strength, neuromuscular health, and the interrelation of movement and function (applied kinesiology).

muscle tissue, *n* extremely elastic, vascular connective tissue that can shorten or elongate to effect movement.

muscular atrophy, *n* decrease in size and number of muscle fibers as a result of aging, reduction in blood supply, malnutrition, or denervation. See also innervation.

muscular dystrophy (mus'·kyə·ler dis'·trə·fē), *n* umbrella term for a group of genetically inherited diseases characterized by gradual atrophy of skeletal muscles without any neurologic damage.

muscular hypertonicity, *n* chronic contraction of a muscle in response to genetic, mechanical, chemical, or psychologic stressors. Increased tonus results in a shortened, tight muscle.

muscular hypertrophy (mus'·kyə·lər hī'·pər·trō'·fē), *n* a condition involving enlargement of muscles. May be induced pathologically or nonpathologically, as in weight training.

muscular imbalance, *n* deviation in normal facilitation or inhibition of muscle resulting from a physical, mental, or chemical stressor and often leading to further related imbalances and joint dysfunctions that may take months or years to manifest.

music therapist–board certified, *n* national examination credential awarded by the Certification Board for Music Therapists; the only currently available certification for newly trained music therapists. See also therapy, music.

mustard, *n* Latin names: *Brassica nigra, Brassica alba;* part used: seeds; uses: diuretic, emetic, anti-inflammatory, mustard plaster for topical treatment of congestive respiratory complaints; precautions: pregnancy, lactation, children, kidney disorders, ulcers, corrosive to unprotected skin, asthma. Also called *black mustard, brown mustard, California rape, charlock, Chinese mustard, Indian mustard, white mustard,* or *wild mustard.*

muti (mōō'·tē), *n* in African healing traditions, animal parts, herbs, or barks with medicinal value.

mutravahasrotas (mōō'·trä·vä'·häs·rō'·təs), *n.pl* in Ayurveda, one of the 13 srotas, or body channels that carry urine; they originate in the bladder and kidneys. See also srotas.

mutual and bidirectional, *adj* description of the relationship between mind and body in dance/movement therapy.

MVC, *n* maximum voluntary contraction, the largest amount of force that a muscle can voluntarily exert. This is typically expressed as a percentage.

MWM, *n* See mobilization with movement.

myalgia (mī·al'·jə), *n* pain in a muscle or a group of muscles that is typically accompanied by a feeling of malaise. Also called *myoneuralgia.*

myalgic encephalomyelitis (mī·al'·jik en·sef''·ə·lō·mī''·ə·lī'·tis), *n* See disease, Akureyi.

myasthenia (mī'·əs·thē'·nē·ə), *n* a condition distinguished by weakness in a muscle or a group of muscles due to a systemic myoneural disturbance.

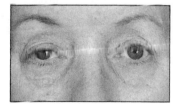

Myasthenia. (Perkin, 1998)

Mycobacterium tuberculosis **(mī'·kō·bak·tē''·rē·əm tə·ber'·kyə·lō'·sis),** *n* slim, gramnegative, rod-shaped aerobic bacterium that causes tuberculosis.

myelin (mī·lən), *n* a white fatty material that constitutes the medullary sheath that surrounds some nerve fibers.

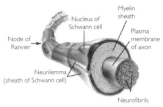

Myelin. (Mosby's Medical, Nursing & Allied Health Dictionary, ed 6, 2002)

myelinopathies (mī·lin·ô´·pə·thēz), *n.pl* **I.** any form of myelinic malignacy. **2.** in environmental medicine, forms of encephalopathy in which myelin is damaged by toxins.

myocardial infarction (mī´·ō·kär´·dē·əl in·färk´·shən), *n* necrosis of cardiac muscle tissue caused by a coronary artery obstruction linked to a spasm, thrombosis, or atherosclerosis. Also called *heart attack.*

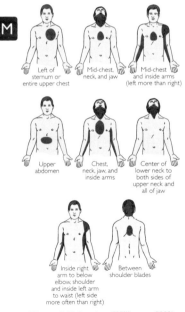

Myocardial infarction. (Williamson, 2002)

myocarditis (mī´·ō·kar·dī´·tis), *n* an inflammatory condition of the myocardium due to fungal, viral, or bacterial infection. It can also be related to a collagen disease, serum sickness, chemical agent or rheumatic fever.

myodysneuria (mī´·ō·dis·ner´·ē·ə), *n* musculoskeletal dysfunction characterized by localized functional abnormalities and multiple causes.

myoelectric biofeedback, *n* the use of an electromyogram (EMG) to amplify and feedback muscle activity and tension. Has been used to improve somatic awareness and to promote relaxation, healing, and rehabilitation. See also electromyography.

myofascial (mī´·ō·fā´·shē·əl), *n* skeletal muscles and the fascial sheaths that surround them.

myofascial meridians, *n.pl* See anatomy trains.

myofascial pain (mī´·ō·fā´·shē·əl pān´), *n* a condition characterized by localized and radiating muscle pains. Often confused with fibromyalgia. See also fibromyalgia.

myofascial release (mī´·ō·fā´·shē·əl rē·lēs´), *n* a specialized massage technique employed to treat a variety of chronic disorders in which the muscle tissue is stretched and manipulated to relieve tension in the fascia, the thin tissue covering the muscle fibers.

myofilaments (mī″·ō·fi´·lə·mənts), *n.pl* bundles of threads called myosin and actin that comprise individual fibers in a striated muscle.

myogenic tonus (mī·ō·gen´·ik tō´·nəs), *n* muscle contraction resulting from innate properties of the muscle or its innervation.

myoglobin (mī´·ō·glō´·bin), *n* oxygen- and iron-carrying compound in muscles.

myoglobilunaria (mī´·ō·glō´·bə·lōō·na´·rē·ə), *n* the presence of myoglobin, a pigment of muscle tissue that stores oxygen in urine. The condition typically develops after massive physical trauma, electrical injury, or muscle injury.

myology (mī·ŏ´·lə·jē), *n* the branch of physiology involved in the study of muscles and muscular system.

myopathology (mī´·ŏ·pə·thŏ´·lə·jē), *n* muscular dysfunction. Caused by either reduced nerve supply; weakening the muscles supporting the spine eventually, thus resulting in atrophy; or excess nerve supply, resulting in tight muscles ending in spasms.

myopathy (mī·ŏ´·pə·thē), *n* a condition of the musculoskeletal system characterized by muscle wasting, weakness, and histologic changes.

myosin, *n* one of the two proteins responsible for muscle contraction, the other protein being actin. Contraction occurs when the two protein bundles slide over one another. See also actin.

myotension, *n* a system of osteopathic techniques for diagnosing and treating somatic dysfunctions. Relaxation, stretching of muscles, and the mobilization of joints are all achieved through the use of muscular contraction and relaxation with resistance provided by the osteopathic practitioner.

myotome (mī´·ə·tōm), *n* the collection of all muscles sharing a block of mesodermal tissue as their origin and innervated by a single spinal nerve segment.

Myrica cerifera, *n* See bayberry.

Myristica fragrans, *n* See nutmeg.

myrobalan, *n* Latin name: *Terminalia chebula;* parts used: fruit, leaves, stem; uses: in Ayurveda, pacifies tridosha (light, dry), cardiotonic, anti-anaphylactic, antimutagen, antitumor, antibacterial, antiviral, immunomodulator, antiamoebic, antioxidant, apreient, astringent, carminative, fungicide, demulcent, purgative, alterative, febrifuge, antiasthmatic, bronchitis, burns, cough, inflammation, measles, prolapse, ulcers; precautions: none known. Also called *Abhay, chebulic myrobalan, hara, haritaki,* or *inknut.*

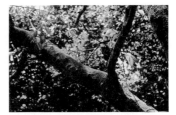

Myrobalan. (Williamson, 2002)

***myrobalan, arjun* (är·jōōn´ mī·rō´·bə·län)),** *n* See arjuna.

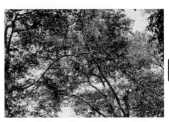

Myrobalan, arjun. (Williamson, 2002)

myrobalan, beleric, *n* Latin name: *Terminalia belerica;* part used: fruit; uses: in Ayurveda, pacifies tridosha (astringent, sweet, light, dry), antioxidant, cholinergic, hypolipidemic, antimicrobial, hepatoprotection, antiulcer, antiobesity agent, antimutagenic, antiinflammatory, tonic, purgative, immunity, coughs, eye sties, skin conditions, liver conditions; precautions: oil is purgative in large doses. Also called *bahera, bhaira, bibhitaki, vibeekaka,* or *vibitaki.*

M

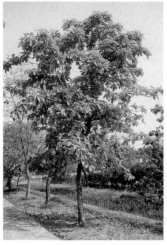

Myrobalan, beleric. (Williamson, 2002)

myrobalan, emblic, n See amla.

Myroxylon balsamum, n See balsam of Peru.

Myroxylon pereirae, n See balsam of Peru.

myrrh (mur'), n Latin name: *Commiphora molmol;* parts used: gum, oil, resin; uses: antipyretic, anticancer, upper respiratory conditions, gum disease, mouth and leg ulcers, inflamed stomach, wounds, hemorrhoids; precautions: pregnancy, lactation, children, fever, tachycardia, uterine bleeding, antidiabetic medications. Also called *African myrrh, Arabian myrrh, bal, bol, bola, gum myrrh, heerabol, Somali myrrh,* or *Yemen myrrh.*

myrtle (mur'·təl), n Latin name: *Myrtus communis;* parts used: leaves, seeds; uses: congestive respiratory conditions, urinary infections, anthelmintic, astringent, antiinflammatory, antihyperglycemic; precautions: pregnancy, lactation, children, liver conditions, gastrointestinal inflammation, diabetes mellitus, antidiabetic medication, medicines metabolized by cytochrome P-450. Also

called *bridal myrtle, common myrtle, Dutch myrtle, Jew's myrtle, mirth,* or *Roman myrtle.*

Myrtus communis, n See myrtle.

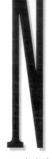

NAC, *n.pr* See *N*-acetyl cysteine.

N-acetyl cysteine (en·ə·sē'·təl sis·tēn), n a form of cysteine not found in food sources. Also an antioxidant. Has been used in chronic bronchitis, as an adjunct in nitroglycerin therapy for angina, and as a treatment for Alzheimer's disease. Can be hepatotoxic in large doses.

N-acetyl-5-methoxytryptamine (en'·ə·sē'·təl-fīv'-meth'·ôks·trip'·tə·měn), n an amino acid derivative used for insomnia, longevity, cataract formation inhibitor, jet lag, cancer, weight maintenance; precautions: pregnancy, lactation, children, melatonin hypersensitivity, cardiovascular disease, hepatic disease, depression, nervous system disorders, renal disease. Also called *melatonin* and *MEL.*

NADH, *n.pr* a coenzyme that incorporates niacin and involved in the Krebs cycle. Has been used to relieve jet lag and as a treatment for chronic fatigue syndrome. No known precautions when the daily dosage is kept at 5 mg or lower.

nadi dhatu (nä'·dē dhä'·tōō), n in Ayurveda, nervous tissue, as described in the Atharvaveda. See also vedas.

nadi shodhanam (nä'·dē shō·dhä'·näm), n See alternate nostril breathing.

nadis (nä'·dəs), *n.pl* according to yoga, the complex network of pathways or channels through which prana (life energy) passes through the physical body. Several yoga postures, pranayama techniques, and sounds are employed to open and balance the energy flow through the nadis. See also prana and pranayama.

nagi (nä·gē'), *n* Lakota Indian term for soul; one of the four constituents of the self. See also nagi la, niya, and sicun.

nagi la (nä·gē' lä), *n* Lakota Indian term for the divine spirit present in everyone; one of the four constituents of the self. See also nagi, niya, and sicun.

nagi'ksapa (nä·gē'·ǝk·sä·pä), *n* Lakota Indian term for awareness of one's own spirit or aura.

NAGS, *n* See neutral apophyseal glides.

naltrexone (nal·trek'·sōn), *n* a pharmacologic substance that increases the body's production of endorphins; used in treating narcotic addiction.

NANC, *adj* nonadrenergic noncholinergic; considered by some investigators as a third nervous system (in addition to the somatic motor and autonomic systems), believed to be involved in regulating the breathing process.

nanometer (nm) (na'·nǝ·mē'·ter), *n* a metric unit of measure defined as one billionth of a meter (0.000000001 or 10).

NAPRALERT, *n* database located at the University of Illinois at Urbana—Champaign that catalogs studies and research published in the area of natural products.

NAPT, *n.pr* See National Association of Poetry Therapy.

narcissism (när'·sǝ·siz'·ǝm), *n* excessive admiration of self, particularly of the body and sexual characteristics.

Narcissus pseudonarcissus, *n* See daffodil.

narcolepsy (när'·kǝ·lep'·sē), *n* a disorder distinguished by sudden attacks of brief deep sleep. Amphetamines and other stimulants are prescribed for treating this condition. Also called *sleep epilepsy.*

narcotic, *n* substance that relieves pain, induces sleep, and calms the body. Harmful and highly addictive if used repeatedly or in high doses.

naris (nar'·is), *n* the nostril, the external opening of the nose.

narrative analysis, *n* **1.** a method of qualitative research in which the researcher listens to the stories of the research subjects, attempting to understand the relationships between the experiences of the individuals and their social framework. **2.** in health care, the examination of patient and family stories can contribute to an understanding of factors that may assist in recovery.

nasya (nä'·syä), *n* in Ayurveda, inhalation of herbalized steam through the nose, which helps clear the nasal passages and lungs. Recommended for headaches, sinus congestions, and mental tension.

National Accreditation Commission for Schools and Colleges of Acupuncture and Oriental Medicine, *n.pr* an independent organization founded in 1982 by the Council of Colleges of Acupuncture that promotes the development and improvement of education in acupuncture and Oriental medicine programs. It establishes comprehensive institutional and educational requirements for acupuncture and Oriental medicine programs. It also acts as an accrediting agency for institutions and programs that meet particular requirements. The United States Department of Education has provided recognition for the organization as a "specialized and professional" accrediting agency. The organization is now known as the *Accreditation Commission for Acupuncture and Oriental Medicine* or *ACAOM.* Also called *NACSCAOM.*

National Acupuncture and Oriental Medicine Alliance (NAOMA), *n.pr* an organization formed to represent and promote the professional interests and priorities of licensed acupuncturists.

National Acupuncture Detoxification Association, *n.pr* membership organization formed in 1985 to train healthcare professionals to perform substance abuse acupuncture.

National Association for Holistic Aromatherapy, *n.pr* in the United

States, the organization that grants the "true aromatherapy product" certification.

National Association of Poetry Therapy, *n.pr* organization established to promote the use of poetry and other forms of literature in medical settings.

National Cancer Institute (NCI), *n.pr* U.S. government's primary agency for cancer research and education. The Institute oversees the National Cancer Program, which conducts and provides support for research, health information dissemination, training, and other resources that pertain to the prevention, diagnosis, cause, and treatment of cancer.

National Center for Complementary and Alternative Medicine, *n.pr* established in 1998 as a Center of the National Institutes of Health. Supports and conducts research on complementary and alternative medicine and informs healthcare professionals about the efficacy of different modalities. Also called the *NCCAM.*

National Heart, Lung, and Blood Institute, *n.pr* established in 1948, this division of the National Institutes of Health is responsible for research and education on cardiovascular, pulmonary, systemic diseases, and sleep disorders.

National Institutes of Health, *n.pr* an agency of the U.S. Department of Health and Human Services. Its mission is to promote medical and behavioral research and to improve health by applying the knowledge acquired to reduce disease and illness.

National Nutrition Monitoring and Related Research Act, *n.pr* legislation passed by the United States Congress in 1990 that required manufacturers of food products to reveal the fat, including unsaturated and saturated fats, sodium, cholesterol, fiber, sugar, carbohydrate, and protein carbohydrate content in their foods. As a result of this act, the Food and Drug Administration set definitions and standards for descriptions commonly applied to food, such as lean, low, reduced, light, and so forth. Labeling is required for the top 20 vegetables, fruits, shellfish, and fish. The legislation also allowed for claims originating from an endorsement or a third-party reference. Under the legislation, the United States Department of Agriculture or USDA and US Department of Health and Human Services or HHS must publish dietary guidelines for Americans at least once every five years.

natremia (nə·trē'·mē·ə), *n* the presence of sodium in urine.

natriuresis (nā'·trə·yōō·rē'·sis), *n* the secretion of increased amounts of sodium in urine. It may be due to endocrine or metabolic conditions, or due to the use of natriuretic diuretic medications.

Natrum muriaticum (na'·trəm myu'·rē·a'·ti·kəm), *n* homeopathic preparation of salt prescribed for conditions involving emotional hypersensitivity or extreme thirst. Also called *Nat mur.*

natural apophyseal glides (NAGs) (na'·chə·rəl ə·pô'·fə·sē'·əl glīdz'), *n.pl* mobilizations that can be sustained or midrange rhythmic, unilaterally or centrally applied by a practitioner in the upper thoracic and cervical spine. The practitioner is situated in a weight-bearing position, and the force's direction is applied along the facet treatment plane.

natural hygiene, *n* a school of thought that emphasizes dietary habits, such as eating raw foods, regular fasting, and food combining for maintaining health and treating disease.

natural killer cells, *n.pl* lymphocytes that are part of innate immunity that kill foreign substances and abnormal tissues. Decreased number or activity has been linked to a number of diseases, including AIDS, cancer, chronic fatigue syndrome, immunodeficiencies, and viral infections. See also innate immunity.

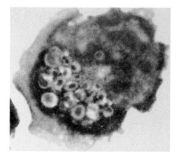

Natural killer (NK) cells. (Cotran, Kumar, and Collins, 1999; Dr. Noelle Williams, Department of Pathology, University of Texas Southwestern Medical School, Dallas, Tx)

naturalistic approach, *n* a medical philosophy that holds that illness results from external, objective causes (such as accident, infection, malformation, etc.)

Naturheilverfahren, *n* See Kneipp-kur.

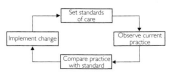

Naturheilverfahren. (Rankin-Box, 2001)

naturopathy (nā'·chə·rä'·pə·thē), *n* therapeutic system that relies on using natural agents like light, natural foods, warmth, massage, and fresh air. Naturopaths believe in the power of the body's natural processes to heal illness.

nausea, *n* an unpleasant gastrointestinal sensation, sometimes accompanied by dizziness and vomiting.

ND, *n.pr* Doctor of Naturopathy.

nebulization (ne'·byə·lī·zā'·shən), *n* a technique of administering medication by spraying it into the respiratory tract. Oxygen may or may not be used to assist carrying the medication into the lungs.

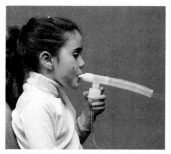

Nebulization. (Sanders et al, 2000)

neck disability index, *n* in chiropractic medicine, parameter used to monitor the progression of a patient throughout the treatment period. Specifically, this questionnaire evaluates changes in a patient's function and measures a self-evaluated disability as a result of neck pain. Each of the 10 items receives a score from 1 to 5; therefore the maximum score that can be attained is 50. It is recommended the questionnaire be administered at the initial point of contact. At least a five-point change is needed to determine a development or progression in therapy that is clinically meaningful. Also called *NDI*.

N

necrosis (nə·krō'·sis), *n* tissue death due to disease or localized injury.

neem (nēm'), *n* Latin name: *Azadirachta indica*; parts used: all parts of plant, uses: In Ayurveda, balances kapha and pitta doshas (bitter, astringent, light, pungent); astringent, antimalarial, anxiolytic, CNS depressant, hepatoprotective, immunomodulator, antiinflammatory, antipyretic, purgative, anthelmintic, dental care, antiseptic, insecticide, diabetes mellitus, contraceptive; precautions: pregnancy, lactation, children. Also called *holy tree, Indian lilac, margosa, neem treenim,* or *nimba.*

negative hallucination (ne'·gə·tiv hə·lōō'·sə·nā'·shən), *n* in hypnosis, a phenomenon that causes patients to not believe in the existence of another person or object that is right before their eyes.

neglect effect (nə·glekt'·ə·fekt'), *n* undesirable outcome of administering ineffective treatment in lieu of an existing effective treatment, thus worsening illness.

neigong (nă'·gông), *n* a form of Qi gong in which the practitioner uses the mind to move qi through the meridians. See also qi gong.

neocortex (nē'·ō·kor'·teks), *n* the outer surface of the cerebrum that is responsible for higher functions—reason, memory, cognition—in human beings.

neoplasm (nē'·ō·pla'·zəm), *n* an abnormally growing tissue in the body, such as cancer.

Nepeta cataria, *n* See catnip.

nephritis (ni·frī'·tis), *n* a chronic or acute inflammatory condition of the kidneys due to autoimmunity or infection. Different kinds of nephritis include acute nephritis, hereditary nephritis, glomerulonephritis, paren-chymatous nephritis, suppurative nephritis, and interstitial nephritis.

nephrotoxicity (ne·frə·täk·si'·sə·tē), *n* the property of harming kidney cells or causing kidney failure.

Nerium odoratum, *n* See oleander.

Nerium oleander, *n* See oleander.

neroli (nə·rō'·lē), *n* an essential oil, extracted from the petals of the bitter orange *(Citrus aurantium),* used for treating depression, frigidity, insomnia, scars and stretch marks, and stress.

nerve compression, *n* pressure on a nerve or nerves may often be caused by hypertonicity in adjacent muscles.

nerve impingement, *n* pathologic pressure placed on a nerve by connective tissue, joints, or skin.

nerve mobilization, *n* restoring movement in a nerve.

nervous system, *n* **I.** an organ system of the body consisting of the brain, spinal cord, and peripheral nerve network. **2.** a system activated by acupuncture that encompasses perivascular sympathetic fiber conduction, peripheral afferent transmis-

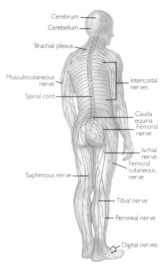

Nervous system. (LaFleur Brooks, 1994)

sion and the central neuropeptide and neurohumoral mechanisms.

nettle (ne'·təl), *n* Latin name: *Urtica dioica*; parts used: leaves, roots; uses: benign prostatic hypertrophy, allergic rhinitis, respiratory ailments, astringent, bladder conditions, expectorant, diuretic, anticancer, analgesic, antiinflammatory; precautions: abortifacient, pregnancy, lactation, children, geriatric patients, diuretic medications, skin irritations. Also called *common nettle, greater nettle,* or *stinging nettle.*

neuralgia (ner·al'·jē·ə), *n* abnormal condition that affects the nervous system and is marked by acute, stabbing pains; it is caused by a variety of disorders.

neurapraxia (ne'·rə·prak'·sē·ə), *n* nerve condition characterized by localized loss of conduction that causes short-term paralysis. There is no degeneration of the axon and complete recovery is usual.

neurasthenia (ner'·əs·thē'·nē·ə), *n* term introduced by the American neurologist GM Beard to describe a condition characterized by irritability,

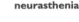

lack of concentration, hypochondria, and worry.

neuritis (ne·rī'·tis), *n* a condition distinguished by nerve inflammation; characterized by hypesthesia, neuralgia, paralysis, anesthesia, deflective reflexes, and muscular atrophy.

neuroacoustical stimulator (ne'·rō·ə·kōō'·stī·kəl stim'·yə·lā'·ter), *n* a word used for a drum; so named in a humorous response to soothe a hospital administrator's concerns about its therapeutic utility.

neurocalometer (ne'·rō·kə·lô'·mə·ter), *n* a diagnostic tool designed to detect heat variances around the spinal column. Invented by BJ Palmer.

neuroemotional subluxation complex (ner'·ō-ē'·mō'·shə·nəl səb·luk·sā'·shən käm'·pleks), *n* condition in which negative emotions induce spinal subluxation, muscle imbalance (either too weak or too strong), or acupunctural meridian imbalances.

neurolepsy (ner'·ə·lep'·sē), *n* a mental state distinguished by the obstruction of autonomic reflexes, such as that observed in hypnosis, or antipsychotic drug-induced disorders.

Neuro-Linguistic Programming, *n.pr* a technique for recognizing and transforming unconscious linguistic and conceptual patterns that limit health, self-actualization, and well-being.

neurologic muscle testing, *n* specific type of muscle testing developed to determine neuromuscular functioning.

neurology (ner·äl'·ə·jē), *n* the branch of medical science that deals with the nervous system and its disorders.

neuromagnetic stimulation, *n* a method for activating nerves by applying pulsing electromagnetic radiation to the head or another area of the body.

neuromuscular (ner'·ō·mus'·kyə·ler), *adj* term describing the feedback loop of interactions between the nervous system and muscular system.

neuromuscular junction (ner'·ō·mus'·kyə·ler junk'·shən), *n* tiny space that joins muscle tissue and nerve endings, through which impulses travel.

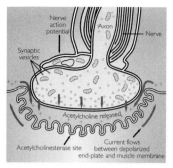

Neuromuscular junction. (Thompson et al, 1997)

neuromyelitis (ner'·ō·mī·lī'·tis), *n* a condition distinguished by the inflammation of spinal cord, peripheral nerves, and associated muscle area.

neuronopathies (ne·rōn·ō'·pə·thēz), *n.pl* in environmental medicine, forms of encephalopathy in which specific neurons or general elements of the nervous system are damaged by toxins such as adriamycin, aluminum, cisplatin, and manganese.

neuropathology (ner'·ō·pə·thô'·lə·jē), *n* study of diseases affecting the nervous system.

neuropathy (ner·ô'·pə·thē), *n* often painful change in sensation involving the peripheral nerves.

neuropeptides (ner·ō·pep'·tīdz), *n.pl* endogenous protein molecules that influence neural activity by carrying information directly to the cells and tissues. Included are VP, CCK, substance P, enkephalins, and endorphins.

neurotoxin (ner'·ō·täk'·sin), *n* a poisonous substance that damages tissues within the central nervous system; produced by certain bacteria or by the cellular deterioration of some bacteria. Other naturally occurring neurotoxins are present in the venom of some snakes, the spines of particular shells, or the skin of a shell-fish or fish. Many drugs and chemicals are also neurotoxic.

neurotransmitter (ner'·ō·trans'·mi·ter), *n* chemical messenger that modifies or affects communication across synapses or neuromuscular connections. Important neurotransmitters include dopamine, serotonin, and acetylcholine.

neurotrophy (ner'·ō·trō'·fē), *n* nutrition and metabolism of innervated tissues.

neurovascular bundle (ner'·ō·vas'·kyə·ler bun'·dəl), *n* grouping of nerve and blood vessels. Often the nerves are responsible for controlling the dilation of the blood vessels.

neurypnology (ner'·əp·nä'·lə·jē), *n* an alternate, obsolete term from the nineteenth century used to describe the practice of mesmerism, which eventually evolved into hypnotism. See also mesmerism.

neutral, *n* **1.** the extent of spinal positioning in the sagittal plane where the first principle of physiologic motion is relevant. **2.** the balance point on an articular surface from which all normal motions articulated at that joint may take place.

neutral apophyseal glides (nōō'·trəl ə·pä'·fə·sē'·əl glīdz'), *n* a highly effective, physical therapy method for treating cervical and spinal dysfunction, especially in the elderly or acute-injury patients. Smooth, sliding force is applied parallel (neutral) to the affected joints while the patient is seated upright. See also MWM, SNAGS.

neutral bath, *n* soaking of the body in water that is between 92° F and 95° F, which is the average skin temperature. Used in hydrotherapy to enhance water absorption and kidney function, or to calm an overactive nervous system (usually recommended to patients experiencing anxiety, chronic pain, exhaustion, insomnia, and nervous irritability).

neutral hypnosis, *n* an induced state, usually resembling sleep or trance, that does not involve the use of

explicit instructions to influence the patient.

neutral self-hypnosis, *n* a relaxed, unstructured state of trance induced by the patient, in which the patient is free to observe or remember images and dream sequences at will.

neutral side-bent rotated, *n* an osteopathic descriptor used to indicate vertebral position, typically used in cases of spinal dysfunction.

neutron (nōō'·trôn), *n* the neutral subatomic particle located within the nucleus of an atom. Its mass is equivalent to that of a proton.

neutropenia (nu'·trō·pē'·nē·ə), *n* an atypical decrease in the number of neutrophils circulating within the blood. The condition is associated with infection, rheumatoid arthritis, acute leukemia, chronic splenomegaly, or a deficiency in vitamin B_{12}.

neutrophils (ner·ō·trō'·filz), *n.pl* white blood cells with cytoplasmic granules that consume harmful bacteria, fungi, and other foreign materials.

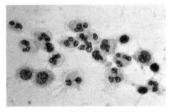

Neutrophils. (McKee, 1997)

New Age Ayurveda, *n.pr* the present form of Ayurveda that incorporates modern technology, mind-body science, quantum physics, and advanced biomedicine theory. Practiced more commonly in the West, it is making its way back to India, the place of traditional Ayurvedic origins.

new ecology of health, *n* See medicine, sustainable.

new learnings, *n.pl* new suggestions and perceptions given to the unconscious during hypnotherapy to replace old restrictive messages. See also hypnotherapy.

N

New Zealand green-lipped mussel, *n.pr* Latin name: *Perna canaliculus;* parts used: whole mussel; uses: antiinflammatory, osteoarthritis, rheumatism; precautions: pregnancy, lactation, children, shellfish allergies. Also called *NZGLM.*

Newcastle Disease virus, *n* a paramyxovirus that causes a fatal disease in birds. Both the lytic and nonlytic strains of the virus are being used in NDV-based cancer therapy.

NHLBI, *n.pr* See National Heart, Lung, and Blood Institute.

NHPA, *n.pr* See Nurse Healer's Professional Association.

niacin, *n* See vitamin B₃.

niacinamide, *n* See vitamin B₃.

nickel, *n* a toxic heavy metal found in industrial emissions; has been linked to immune system dysfunction.

Nicotiana tabacum, *n* See tobacco.

nicotinamide adenine dinucleotide, *n* See NADH.

nigella (nī·jel'·ə), *n* Latin name: *Nigella sativa;* part used: seeds; uses: carminative, stimulant, diuretic, skin eruption treatment, scorpion stings, intestinal worms in children, breast milk, insect repellent, eruption fever, puerperium, liver disease, cancer, joints, bronchial asthma, eczema, rheumatism, cough and colic, excitant, immune system support, colds; precautions: none known. Also called *small fennel, black cumin.*

Nigella sativa, *n* See nigella.

nighantus (nēg·hän'·tōōs), *n* ancient pharmacology books written between the twelfth and fourteenth centuries which have information about natural medicines used in Ayurveda.

night-blooming cereus (nīt' blōō'· ming sir'·ē·əs), *n* Latin name: *Selenicereus grandiflorus;* parts used: flowers, stems; uses: heart conditions, urinary tract conditions, hyperthyroidism, benign prostatic hypertrophy; precautions: pregnancy and lactation, infants and children, high blood pressure, severe cardiac conditions, cardiac glycosides, MAOIs. Also called *large-flowered cactus, queen of the night, sweet-scented cactus,* or *vanilla cactus.*

nightshade, black, *n* Latin name: *Solanum nigrum;* parts used: whole plant, fruit; uses: in Ayurveda, considered a rasayana, pacifies kapha dosha (bitter, light, oily), antiulcerogenic, antiinflammatory, molluscicide, hepatitis, splenitis, antiseptic gargle, burns, skin infections; precautions: teratogenic, toxicity especially unripe fruit. Also called *garden nightshade, kakamachi, makoi,* or *Solanum americanum.*

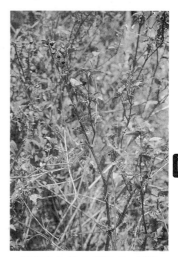

Nightshade, black. (Williamson, 2002)

nightshade, yellow-berried, *n* Latin name: *Solanum xanthocarpum*; parts used: whole plant; uses: in Ayurveda, pacifies kapha and vata doshas (pungent, bitter, light, sharp, dry), antifertility, antiasthmatic, insecticide, fever, cough, inflammation, sore throats, toothache; precautions: pregnancy; contains toxic alkaloids. Also called *cholati katheri, kateli, kantkari, laghu kantkari,* or *Solanum surattense.*

N

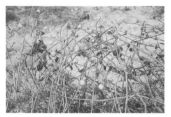

Nightshade, yellow-berried. (Williamson, 2002)

NIH, *n.pr* See National Institutes of Health.

nimmo/tonus receptor (nim´·mō/ tō´·nəs rē·sep´·tər), *n* manual therapy approach that treats trigger points by applying pressure for seven to eight seconds at a time until release is accomplished, after which the practitioner moves on to the next trigger point.

nitsch (nēts´·ch), *n* according to Apache belief, an ailment believed to result from neglecting natural entities, such as an individual who disrespects an owl may suffer from anxiety, palpitation, and sweating. Shamanic prayers and songs are required to treat the condition, which is thought to lead to suicide.

nivel espiritual (nē·vel´ es·pē´·rē· tōō·äl), *n* in Curanderismo, the Mexican-American healing system, the term for "spiritual level." Healers who work at this level invoke spirits to enable them to communicate with the physical world.

nivel material (nē·vel´ mə·te´·rē·äl), *n* in Curanderismo, the Mexican-American healing system, the term for the "material, or physical level;" therapies on this level include bone-setting and the treatment of sprains.

nivel mental (nē·vel men´täl), *n* in Curanderismo, the Mexican-American healing system, the term for the "mental level;" when called upon to work at this level, the healer channels mental vibrations toward a person to influence the person's physical or mental condition.

niveles (nē·vel´·es), *n.pl* in Curanderismo, the Mexican-American healing system, the term for "levels," with regard to the type of healing. See also nivel material, nivel mental, and nivel espiritual.

niya (nē·yä´), *n* Lakota Indian term for "the vital breath," believed to control breathing and circulation in the body; is one of the four constituents of the self. See also nagi, nagi la, and sicun.

niyama (nē·yä´·mə), *n* in Sanskrit, rules or laws, of personal conduct directed toward spiritual unfoldment, one of the eight limbs or paths of Patanjali yoga aimed at self-realization and self-knowledge. See also yama, asana, pranayama, pratyahara, dharana, dhyana, and samadhi.

NK, *n.pr* See natural killer cells.

NMM-OMM, *n.pr* certification in neuromusculoskeletal medicine and osteopathic manipulative medicine, granted by the American Osteopathic Association.

NMT, *n* neuromuscular technique; the manual application of focused strokes and pressure by the fingers or thumbs for diagnostic or therapeutic purposes.

Noad Bo-Rom, *n.pr* See massage, Thai.

NOAEL, *n* "no-observed-adverse-effect-level," the maximum concentration of a substance that is found to have no adverse effects upon the test subject.

noble gases, *n.pl* a group of very stable elements, such as neon and argon, that do not easily react with other atoms because of their filled outer electron shell. Also called *inert gases.*

nocebo (nō´·sē·bō), *n* a negative, harmful placebo effect. See also placebo and placebo effect.

nocebo effect (nō·sē´·bō ə·fekt´), *n* effect from an inert substance that causes symptoms of ill health because of the patients' beliefs. Opposite of the placebo effect.

nociception (nō´·si·sep·shən), *n* awareness of tissue injury.

nociceptors (nō´·si·sep´·ters), *n.pl* a group of cells that acts as a receptor for painful stimuli. Minor stress from a mechanical, chemical, thermal, or any other damaging stimulus may prime these cells.

Nogier vascular autonomic signal, *n.pr* an alteration in the strength and volume of the wrist pulse responding to excitation (through massage, laser pulses, or colored light) of the outer part of the ear. Also called *auricular cardiac reflex.*

nonadrenergic noncholinergic (NANC) neuron (nôn'·a·drə·nur'·jik nôn'·kō·li·nur'·jik), *n* an autonomic, efferent nerve cell, the method of transmission of which is not based upon adrenergic (e.g., epinephrine, dopamine) or cholinergic (i.e., acetylcholine) neurotransmitters.

nonaerobic exercise, *n* physical activity involving sudden, rapid motions (such as tennis, golf, or weight lifting) that produce energy without requiring oxygen. Benefits muscle coordination, strength, and flexibility—not improvement of the cardiovascular and respiratory systems.

noncontact TT, *n* See mimic therapeutic touch.

nonfeasance (nän·fē·zənts), *n* the failure to carry out an undertaking, a task or duty that a person previously agreed to perform or was legally obligated to perform.

noni, *n* See morinda.

nonlocal, *adj* having no specific space or time boundaries. A characteristic of prayer and healing intention.

nonlocal-naturalistic mechanisms, *n.pl* explanations for the efficacy of spiritual healing and prayer, particularly for healings effected at a distance, that rely on those quantum physical concepts to explain nontraditional effects.

nonmalficence (nôn'·mal·fē'·sens), *n* a principle of medical ethics according to which a person should avoid harming others.

non–medically qualified practitioner, *n* therapist who does not have a medical license of any type. See also doctor, lay homeopath, physician, professional homeopath, and half homeopath.

nonmetals, *n.pl* a fundamental grouping of elements like sulfur, carbon, hydrogen, and oxygen in the periodic table that have similar chemical and physical properties; they are insulators or semiconductors and form ionic bonds with metals and covalent bonds with other nonmetals.

nonneurotic awareness, *n* a state of mind which enables an individual to view things clearly with minimal influence by habits of perception, feeling, thought, or action and that can be enhanced by meditation. Also called *equanimity* or *mindfulness.*

nonneutral, *n* the extent of spinal positioning in the sagittal plane wherein the second principle of physiologic motion is relevant.

nonspecific effects, *n.pl* outcome other than predicted or caused by the treatment being employed. See also nocebo and placebo.

nonstatutory access, *n* informal agreement between a healthcare provider and a patient regarding the patient's rights to peruse his or her own healthcare files.

nopal (nō·päl'), *n* Latin name: *Opuntia streptacantha Lemaire, Opuntia ficus indica;* parts used: cactus pads; uses: diabetes mellitus, hyperglycemia, hyperlipidemia, constipation, and gastrointestinal conditions; precautions: none known.

noradrenaline (nōr'·ə·dren'·ə·lin), *n* See norepinephrine.

norepinephrine (nōr'·ep·i·nef'·rin), *n* a neurotransmitter released by the adrenal gland, part of the fight-or-flight response and also directly increases heart rate, blood pressure, energy release from fat, and muscle readiness.

normalization, *n* use of physiologic and anatomic mechanisms in a therapeutic context to promote the body's own health restoration and homeostatic responses.

nose, *n* an organ of the body that extends from the end of the palate to the face. Olfactory cells within the nose are responsible for detecting molecules and sending the sensory impulses along the olfactory nerve to the brain.

nosode (nō·sōd), *n* homeopathic remedy created from some element of the disease itself, such as a discharge or diseased tissue. See also autoisopathy; therapy, autohemic; autonosode; bowel nosode; and isopathy.

nosology (nō·sô'·lə·jē), *n* **1.** a list or classification of diseases. **2.** the branch of science that deals with the classification of diseases.

note, *n* a category of aromatic components of essential perfumes and oils. See also base note, body note, middle note, and top note.

notice, *n* a provision in some contracts allowing either party to inform the other that the contract must come to an end, usually by a specified date.

NSAID, *n* See nonsteroidal antiinflammatory drug.

nuchal (nyōō'·kəl), *adj* pertaining to the posterior or nape of the neck.

nucleus, *n* **1.** in chemistry, a small, closely packed, centrally located body within an atom comprised of positively charged protons and neutral particles called neutrons. The bulk of the mass of an atom is contained within the nucleus. **2.** in biology, a small, closely packed, centrally located organelle within a cell that contains the genetic material.

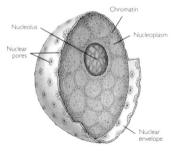

Chromatin
Nucleolus
Nucleoplasm
Nuclear pores
Nuclear envelope

Nucleus. (Thibodeau and Patton, 1999; William Ober)

null   hypothesis, *n*   theoretical assumption that a given therapy will have results not statistically different from another treatment.

Nurse Healer's Professional Association, *n.pr* the organization that comprises US nurses who perform therapeutic touch and other healing modalities. Also called *Nurse Healers Professional Associates International (NH-PAI)*.

Nursing Interventions Classification, *n.pr* a comprehensive system of classification that describes and categorizes actions and therapeutic approaches performed by nurses within all types of specialties and settings. It includes therapeutic approaches for the following categories: psychosocial, physiological, treatment of illness, prevention of illness, and promotion of health. Indirect forms of treatment, such as checking an emergency chart, are also included. Each therapeutic approach is given a specific numerical code that is used to facilitate the process of computerization. Also called *NIC*.

nutation, *n* leaning forward, the anterior movement of the sacrum around a transverse axis relative to the hip bones.

nutgrass, *n* Latin name: *Cyperus rotundus;* parts used: tubers, rhizomes; uses: in Ayurveda, pacifies kapha and pitta doshas (bitter, astringent, light, dry), antiemetic, antiinflammatory, antipyretic, antimalarial, antibacterial, tranquilizer, antiobesity, digestive disorders, cold, congestion, impotence, hypertension; precautions: none known. Also called *chido, motha, mustak, nutsedge,* or *sedge weed.*

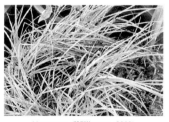

Nutgrass. (Williamson, 2002)

nutmeg, *n* Latin name: *Myristica fragrans*; part used: dried seeds; uses: gastrointestinal complaints, analgesic, toothache, nausea, antiemetic, anxiolytic, depression, antimicrobial, chemoprotective, aphrodisiac; precautions: abortifacient, pregnancy, lactation, children, severe depression, severe anxiety disorders, antidiarrheal medications, MAOI medications, psychotropic medications, toxic in large doses. Also called *mace, macis, muscadier, muskatbaum, myristica, noz moscada, nuez moscada,* or *nux moschata.*

nutraceutical (nōō′·trə·sōō′·ti·kəl), *n* any food supplement that has health benefits in addition to its nutritive value. Also called *botanical supplement, ergogenic aid, functional food, herbal, medical food,* or *nutriceutical.*

nutrient pharmacotherapy (nōō′·trē·ənt fär′·mə·kō·the′·rə·pē), *n* therapeutic use of large doses of nutrients to treat illnesses that do not arise from nutrient deficiencies.

nutrition support, *n* intravenous nutrition or orally modified formulas necessitated by inability to consume a general diet; administered to malnourished individuals who cannot consume food in its original form.

nutritional biotherapy (nōō·tri′·shə·nəl bī′·ō·the′·rə·pē), *n* the use of nutrition and diet in a clinical setting to alter the processes that cause disease within the body. Prescriptive dietetics, nutritional pharmacology, and nutrition support are examples of this approach. See also prescriptive dietetics, nutritional pharmacology, and nutrition support.

nutritional medicine, *n* **1.** use of food and nutrition as a medical approach. **2.** supplementation of diet with nutrients, intermediary metabolic products, and probiotics to prevent illness and improve health and healing. See also probiotic.

nutritional pharmacology (nōō·tri′·shə·nəl fär′·mə·kô′·lə·jē), *n* the use of minerals, vitamins, plant- or herbal-derived botanicals, and phytochemicals as nutritional supplements that affect specific functions or diseases.

nux vomica seed (nuks′ vô′·mi·kə sēd′), *n* Latin name: *Strychnos nux-vomica;* part used: root, seeds; uses: gastrointestinal tract stimulation; aperitive; digestion; constipation; atonic dyspepsia; pruritis; pain in external ear inflammations; poisoning by chloral or chloroform; surgical shock; cardiac failure; pulse rate; chronic lead poisoning; increase sensitivity of smell, touch, hearing and vision; precautions: can produce violent convulsions; increase blood pressure, deepen and quicken respiration, slow heart rate. Also called *poison nut, semen strychnos,* and *quaker buttons.*

N-VAS, *n.pr* See Nogier vascular autonomic signal.

nyctalopia (nik′·tə·lō′·pē·ə), *n* reduction in the ability to see in faint light, as at night, due to congenital defects, vitamin A deficiency, decreased rhodopsin synthesis, or degeneration of the retina. Also called *night blindness* or *day sight.*

nystagmus (nls·tag′·məs), *n* a rapid, involuntary movement of the eyes that typically occurs as a result of vertigo throughout and following the rotation of the body or following injuries to the vestibule of the ear or the cerebellum. Also called *nystaxis.*

O

OA, *n* occipitoatlantal, a region of the body located at the back of the skull. It is one of the locations in which fascial tensions may be found.

oak, *n* Latin names: *Quercus robur, Quercus petraea, Quercus alba;* parts used: bark, gall; uses: antiinflammatory, astringent, varicose veins, smoking cessation, hemorrhoids, gargle, skin conditions; precautions: pregnancy, lactation, children. Also called *British oak, brown oak, common oak, cortex quercus, ecorce de chene, eichenlohe, eicherinde, encina, English oak, gravelier, nutgall, oak apples, oak bark, oak galls, stone oak,* or *tanner's bark.*

oats, *n* Latin name: *Avena sativa*; parts used: grain, straw; uses: grain—skin irritation and itching, sedative, anticholesterolemic, laxative, antioxidant, straw—diuretic, shingles, herpes, nerve tonic, anxiolytic; precautions: intestinal obstruction, celiac disease. Also called *groats, haver, havercorn, haws, oatmeal,* or *oatstraw.*

obesity, *n* excessive body fat. Clinically, it means body fat percentage that is greater than 30% (in women) or 25% (in men) or a BMI of greater than 27. *Obesity* and *overweight* are not equivalent terms. Being overweight refers to having a disproportionate body fat level relative to a person's height.

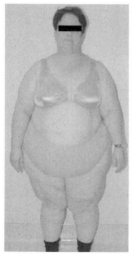

Obesity. (Lemmi and Lemmi, 2000)

obesity, hyperplastic, *n* a type of obesity that typically develops in childhood and is characterized by the increased number of fat cells within the body. See also obesity, hypertrophic and obesity, hyperplastic-hypertrophic.

obesity, hyperplastic-hypertrophic, *n* a type of obesity characterized by the increase in number and enlarged size of the fat cells within the body.

obesity, hypertrophic, *n* a type of obesity characterized by the enlarged size of fat cells within the body. An increased distribution of weight in the waist region is a typical indicator of this type of obesity. It is associated with an increased risk of hypertension, diabetes, and other metabolic disorders.

objective, *adj* easily observed and measured such that psychological and subjective factors have little influence on measurement.

objectivism (əb·jek'·ti·viz'·əm), *n* principle of modern biomedicine according to which the one observing is separate from what is being observed.

oblique axis, *n* hypothetical axis running from the upper area of sacroiliac articulation to the lower sacroiliac articulation on the opposite side of the pelvis. The right oblique axis begins at the right superior articulation and vice-versa. Proposed by osteopathic physician Fred Mitchell, Sr. Also called *diagonal axis.*

observational studies, *n.pl* an investigational method involving description of the associations between interventions and outcomes. Outcomes research and practice audits are examples of this investigational method. For instance, during a practice audit, the outcomes produced by a sampling of patients who received a specific form of treatment may be monitored. An assessment is performed before and after a regimen of therapy is administered to compare and measure the effects.

observing, *v* **1.** to look or notice through visual inspection. **2.** to quietly look at the client's inhalation and exhalation patterns to discern the breath wave and perceive areas that need therapeutic intervention.

obstetrician (ŏb'·stə·tri'·shən), *n* a medical doctor who specializes in the treatment of women's health issues, the care of expectant women, and the delivery process.

obturation (äb'·tə·rā'·shən), *n* the obstruction of a passageway within the body. An intestinal blockage is one type of an obturation.

occasion, *n* peripheral condition involved at the inception of the illness. See also precipitating factor, biopathography, etiology, and pathogenesis.

occipital (ŏk·si'·pə·təl), *adj* inferior, posterior region of the skull.

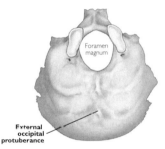

Foramen magnum

External occipital protuberance

Occipital. (Mosby's Medical, Nursing & Allied Health Dictionary, ed 6, 2002)

occiput, *n* **1.** posterior part of the head above the base of the neck. **2.** in craniosacral therapy, one of two points on the body where the therapist lays both hands and diagnoses the vitality and bounty of the cerebrospinal fluid. See also listening posts.

ocean-sounding breath, *n* in yoga, a pranayama technique that involves constricting the back of the throat while breathing to create an "ah" sound. Helps mental concentration and awareness. See also pranayama.

ochronosis (ō'·krə·nō'·sis), *n* condition marked by accumulation of black-brown pigment in cartilage, joint capsules, and other connective tissues as a result of alkaptonuria, which is a metabolic disorder result-

ing in accumulation of homogentisic acid. See also alkaptonuria.

Ocimum basilicum, *n* See basil.

Ocimum sanctum, *n* See basil, holy.

octacosanol (äk'·tə·kō'·sə·näl), *n* waxy substance derived from wheat germ and sugar cane. Has been used as an athletic performance enhancer and a potential treatment for Parkinson's disease and amyotrophic lateral sclerosis.

Od, *n.pr* See Odic force.

Odic force, *n.pr* the theorized healing energy that suffuses all life, as described by nineteenth-century scientist Baron Karl Von Reichenberg.

odontitis (ō'·dän'·tə·tis), *n* an atypical increase in the size of tooth pulp due to an inflammation of odontoblasts as a result of infection, tumor, or trauma.

odontodysplasia (ō·dän'·tō·dis·plā'·zhē·ə), *n* an anomaly in tooth development distinguished by a deficiency in the formation of dentin and enamel. The condition typically impacts the maxillary lateral and central incisors, particularly on one side of the midline. Teeth have a ghostlike appearance in radiographs. Also called *ghost teeth.*

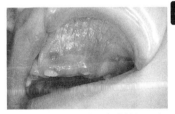

Odontodysplasia. (Regezi, Sciubba, and Pogrel, 2000)

odor, *n* the property of a substance that gives a distinguishable smell.

odorant (ō'·də·rənt), *n* a substance that has an odor.

oestrogenic (ō'·es·trə·je'·nik), *adj* ability of a substance to promote or mimic the action of female hormones.

offer, *n* often the step after an invitation to treat; involves communication leading toward a possible contract.

officinalis (ō'·fi·sē·nä'·lis), *adj* status of a substance approved of and dispensed by apothecaries.

oil, *n* 1. any of a group of organic compounds that are generally combustible, slippery, viscous, and non–water-soluble. 2. a fat that is a liquid at room temperature.

oil, carrier, *n* oil used to dilute an essential oil before it is applied on the skin to enhance lubrication for massage techniques and increase absorption by the skin. Popular carrier oils include sweet almond, avocado, evening primrose, jojoba, olive, and wheatgerm. Also called *fixed oil.*

oil, chaulmoogra (chä·ōōl·mōō·grə oil), *n* Latin names: *Hydnocarpus wightiana, Hydnocarpus anthelmintica, Taraktogenos kurzii;* part used: seeds; uses: leprosy, eczema, psoriasis, scabies, tinea, yeast infections, trichomoniasis; precautions: pregnancy, lactation, children; can cause upset stomach, subcutaneous precipitation. Also called *gynocardia oil, hydnocarpus oil,* or *krabao's tree seed.*

oil, chenopodium (che'·nə·pō'·dē·əm oil'), *n* Latin name: *Chenopodium ambrosioides;* parts used: seeds, flowering stems; uses: relieve pain, asthma, fungal infections, flatulence, appetite, anthelmintic, digestive disorders, hemorrhoids, wound healing, removal of toxins; precautions: arthritis, gout, kidney stones, hyperacidity; stimulant, can cause dizziness, vomiting, convulsions, and allergic contact dermatitis. Also called *american wormseed, apasote, chenopode, epazote, feuilles a vers, herbe a vers, meksika cayi, paico, pazote, semen contra, simon contegras, welriekende ganzenvoet, wormseed,* and *mexican tea.*

oil, croton (krō'·tən oil'), *n* Latin name: *Croton tiglium;* part used: oil; uses: induce vomiting, relieve constipation, treat rheumatism, gout, neuralgia, bronchitis; precautions: pregnancy, children, abortifacient, can cause drastic watery bowel movements with griping pain, inflammatory, can produce pustules,

tumorigenic. Also called *tiglium seeds* and *klotzsch.*

oil, essential, *n* water-immiscible medicinal substances distilled from plant materials, often used in aromatherapy.

oil, evening primrose, *n* Latin name: *Oenothera biennis, Primula elatior;* part used: seeds; uses: heart disease, arthritis, PMS, mastalgia, eczema, multiple sclerosis, coughs, bronchitis; precautions: pregnancy, lactation; patients who suffer from seizures; can cause headaches, convulsions, nausea, diarrhea, rashes, aches; and can hamper the immune system. Also called *buckles, butter rose, cowslip, fairy caps, key of heaven, king's-cure-all, mayflower, palsywort, peagles, petty mulleins,* and *plumrocks password.*

oil, fish, *n* the oils and fats from fatty, coldwater fish (e.g., albacore tuna, cod, herring, mackerel, salmon, and sardines) that contains omega-3 essential fatty acids. Has been used to promote cardiovascular health, relieve symptoms of rheumatoid arthritis, and menstrual pain, and treat depression. There are no known general precautions for fish oil supplements at low doses, but patients using cod liver oil (particularly pregnant women) should avoid additional supplementation of vitamins A and D to avoid toxicity, and those taking anticoagulants should use caution. See also acid, docosahexaenoic, acid, eicosapentaenoic, and acids, omega-3 fatty.

oil, fixed, *n* See oil, carrier.

oil, flaxseed, *n* See flax.

oil, floral, *n* oil obtained by soaking plant and floral material in vegetable oil, which is then heated gently to release the aromatic compounds from the plant into the oil. Also called *herbal oil, macerated oil,* or *infused oil.*

oil, folded, *n* 1. mixture of different batches of essential oils, thus resulting in concentration of some components and dilution of others. 2. essential oil from which a component has been removed to strengthen more desirable ingredients. Folding may also extend shelf life of essential oils.

oil, herbal, *n* a method of medicinal preparation in which chopped herbs are mixed with a vegetable oil base in clear glass and steeped in sunlight for more than two weeks, after which the herbs are strained, and the oil bottled.

oil, infused, *n* the end product obtained as a result of the process to extract essential oils via maceration. Also called *herbal oil* or *macerated oil.*

oil, Lorenzo's, *n* Scientific name: $C_{22}H_{42}O_2$ and $C_{17}H_{33}COOH$; uses: adrenoleukodystophy; precautions: can cause thrombocytopenia.

oil, reconstituted, *n* oil synthesized in a laboratory from a variety of sources and aromatic plant materials. Typically inappropriate for aromatherapy. Also called *RCO* or *synthetics.*

oil, savin (sa'·vən oil'), *n* oil extracted from the fresh tops of the shrub *Juniperus sabina,* used as a diuretic.

oil, synthetic, *n* See oil, reconstituted.

oil, terpeneless essential (ter'·pēn·ləs ə·sen'·shəl oil'), *n* an essential oil that has undergone solvent extraction or vacuum fractionation to remove some or all of the terpenes to increase the longevity of the product or increase the solubility of alcohol. Also called *folded oils.*

oil, yinergy (yi'·ner·gē oil'), *n* treatment that contains 25% magnesium chloride and raises both dehydroepiandrosterone (DHEA) and intracellular levels of magnesium.

oils, distilled, *n.pl* essential oils obtained by distillation; contain only volatile compounds.

oils, expressed, *n.pl* essential oils obtained by the process of expression, which contain compounds of all molecular sizes. See also expression.

oils, hazardous, *n.pl* oils considered dangerous to use or that require handling with extreme caution. Proper care and use of these oils is outlined in the COSHH and CHIO. See also COSHH and CHIP.

oils, macerated, *n.pl* oils prepared by adding plant material to fixed vegetable oils, thus resulting in uptake of oil-soluble molecules of the plant material by the oil. Not to be confused with essential oils.

oils, nature-identical, *n.pl* essential oils that comprise components acquired from plant sources but are manufactured from a combination of several essential oils.

ointments, *n.pl* semisolid, non–water-based treatments that are not water-soluble and that create protective films to prevent dehydration of the skin.

ojas (ō'·jəs), *n* in Ayurveda, the end product of good digestion and metabolism that is believed to connect consciousness and matter.

OKG, *n.pr* See ornithine alpha-ketoglutarate.

oleander (ō'·lē·an'·dər), *n* Latin names: *Nerium oleander, Nerium odoratum;* part used: leaves; uses: diuretic, cardiac conditions, menstrual complaints, laxative, insecticide, abortifacient, parasiticide, anthelmintic, warts; precautions: abortifacient, pregnancy, lactation, children, cardiac glycosides, toxic. Also called *adelfa, laurier rose, rosa Francesca, rosa laurel,* or *rose bay.*

oleoresins (ō'·le·ō·re'·zinz), *n.pl* a composite of oils and resins that can be found in nature or obtained by extracting resinous materials from herbs via organic solvents. Examples of oleoresins include capsicum, ginger, and paprika.

olfaction (ōl'·fak'·shən), *n* the sense of smell.

olfactory (ōl·fak'·tə·rē), *adj* relating to the perception of a scent or odor.

Olfactory. (Tiran, 2000)

oligomenorrhea (ə·li'·gə·me'·nō·rē'·ə), *n* disorder marked by irregular menstrual periods.

oligomeric proanthocyanidin complexes, *n.pl* See proanthocyanadins.

oligotherapy (ä'·li·gō'·the'·rə·pē), *n* in homeopathy, the use of remedies that comprise trace elements normally found in the human body that act as catalysts in maintaining physiologic functions.

oliguria (ō'·li·gōō'·rē·ə), *n* a decrease in the excretion of urine from the body due to dehydration, an imbalance in electrolytes or body fluids, the presence of renal lesions, the obstruction of the urinary tract, or other causes. Also called *oliguresis.*

OMD, *n.pr* Doctor of Oriental Medicine.

Omphalia, *n* See raigan.

OMT, *n* osteopathic manipulative therapy; a comprehensive, noninvasive, hands-on method used by osteopathic practitioners to diagnose, treat, and prevent bodily illnesses and treat injuries. It can be used separately or in conjunction with surgery or medicinal therapies.

onion (un'·yən), *n* Latin name: *Allium cepa;* part used: bulb; uses: antimicrobial, lowers blood glucose, diuretic, general tonic, topical wound healing, loss of appetite, thickening arteries; precautions: allergies.

ontogeny (än·tä'·jə·nē), *n* the developmental history of an organism.

ontology (ôn·tô'·lə·gē), *n* the metaphysical study of the state of being: focuses on the fundamentals of identity, disease, normalcy, and belief systems as they influence a person's existence.

OPCS, *n.pl* See proanthocyanadins.

open dissipative system (ō'·pen dis·ə·pā'·tiv sis'·təm), *n* an organized, stable system that continuously exchanges matter and energy with its surroundings to avoid thermodynamic equilibrium. Also called *dissipative system* or *dissipative structure.*

open focus, *n* feature of some meditation traditions in which the individual maintains a nonreactive awareness of thoughts, emotions, and environmental stimuli.

open system, *n* a characteristic of energy fields that allows constant interchange.

openness, *n* characteristic of energy in which individuals and the environment constantly exchange energy and matter.

operant conditioning, *n* a method of provoking a specific response by relating that response to a positive stimulus.

operator-dependent, *adj* a characteristic of esoteric forms of faith healing that cannot be verified scientifically because the healing process depends largely on the special skills of the practitioner that preclude systemic investigation.

opiate (ō'·pē·it), *n* **1.** a drug that comprises opium, an opium derivative, or a synthetic preparation that exhibits activity similar to opium. *adj* **2.** pertaining to a substance that relieves pain or induces sleep. Also called *opiod.*

opioid peptides (ō'·pē·oid pep'·tīdz), *n.pl* protein molecules found in the body that are responsible for endogenous analgesia and other functions. The three major classes are beta-endorphins, dynorphins, and enkephalins. See also endorphins and enkephalins.

opioid receptors, *n.pl* any of the several receptors to which opiates bind. Classified into three groups— delta, kappa, and mu—based on the specific substances they bind and the resulting physiologic effects.

opportunistic infections, *n.pl* the secondary infections that occur in patients whose immune systems are compromised, such as in AIDS or after chemotherapy.

optical activity, *n* the property of a substance that enables it to rotate plane-polarized light counterclockwise or clockwise.

optical isomers (ôp'·tə·kəl ī'·sə·merz), *n.pl* molecules that comprise an asymmetric carbon atom, exhibit chiral properties, and are able to rotate plane-polarized light in a counter-clockwise or clockwise direction. Also called *enantiomers*. See also stereoisomer.

optical rotation (ôp′·tə·kəl rō·tā′·shən), *n* the angle by which plane-polarized light rotates when it passes through a substance that exhibits optical activity. This is a distinguishable quality of a particular compound. See also optical activity.

optimal breathing, *n* the ideal state in which oxygen intake and carbon dioxide release are at equilibrium with the immediate metabolic needs of the body.

optimism, *n* attitude cultivated by an individual in which he or she believes in the positive resolution of a stressful event. In particular, persons with this mindset will use focused, external-ized, and nonpersisting terms to describe his or her specific situation. Studies have shown that patients who are diagnosed with a chronic disease and adopt an optimistic attitude have improved health status.

***Opuntia* (ō·pən·shē·ə),** *n* a genus of cacti; *Opuntia vulgaris* is used as a remedy in homeopathic medicine.

oral, *adj* pertaining to the mouth.

orange food, *n* group that includes oranges, apricots, carrots, pumpkin flesh and seeds, and sesame seeds.

orbit, *n* hollow space where the eyeball and its muscles, nerves, and blood vessels are located.

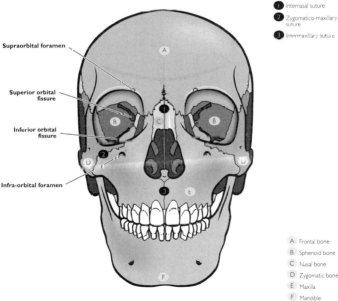

Orbit. (Chaitow, 1999)

orbitals (ōr'·bə·təlz), *n.pl* shells surrounding the nucleus of an atom; contain negatively charged electrons. The arrangement and number of electrons in the outer shells determine the stability of the atom and its ability to form a covalent or ionic bond with another atom or molecule.

oregano (ə·rä''·gə·nō'), *n* Latin name: *Origanum vulgare*; parts used: leaves (dried), stems; uses: respiratory conditions, expectorant, systemic tonic, diaphoretic, antiseptic, antioxidant, antibacterial, antifungal, oligomenorrhea; precautions: pregnancy, lactation, children. Also called *mountain mint* or *origanum*.

Oregon grape, *n.pr* Latin name: *Mahonia aquifolium*; parts used: bark, stem, roots; uses: psoriasis, acne, fungal infection, eczema, hepatitis, STDs, diarrhea, fever, gallbladder disorders, antioxidant; precautions: pregnancy, lactation, children; toxic in high doses. Also called *holly-leaved barberry, holly-leaved berberis,* or *mountain grape.*

oreoselinum (ōr'·ē·ō·se·lē'·nəm), *n* Latin name: *Peucedanum oreoselinum;* parts used: homeopathic preparations; uses: diuretic; precautions: none known. Also known as *mountain parsley.*

organ, in Chinese medicine, *n* a part of the body that is defined by the physiologic function rather than the composition. Systemic dissection was not pursued by the ancient Chinese, and observation of function formed the basis for the medical system.

organ affinity, *n* link between a remedy and the anatomy it affects. See also organotropic, affinity, disease affinity, and tissue affinity.

organ level, *n* in acupuncture, a disturbance involving the transport or metabolic functions of an organ.

organic, *adj* grown in an environment in which artificial fertilizers, herbicides, and insecticides are not utilized.

organic chemistry, *n* the study of chemistry of all carbon compounds that are primarily covalently bonded.

organic mercury exposure, *n* mercury exposure from dietary sources such as seafood.

organics profiling, *n* an analysis of organic acids (other than amino acids) and neutral compounds excreted in the urine; used to assess metabolic disorders and nutrient deficiencies.

organogenesis (ōr'·gə·nō·je'·nə·sis), *n* the origin and development of organs and organ systems during embryonic development. Also called *organogeny.*

organoleptic (ōr'·gə·nō·lep'·tik), *n* a substance that produces an effect on the senses—particularly those of smell and taste.

organotherapy, *n* See therapy, glandular.

organotropic (ōr'·gə·nō·trō'·pik), *n* in homeopathy, the strong affinity displayed by some medicines for certain tissues and organs in the body.

orgotein (ōr·gō'·tēn), *n* obtained from bovine liver, this drug has been promoted as an antiaging agent and an effective treatment for scleroderma, radiation-induced cystitis, osteoarthritis, inflammation, and urinary tract disorders. The Food and Drug Administration (FDA) has classified the parenteral formulation of the agent as an orphan drug for the treatment of familial amyotrophic lateral sclerosis; pain or allergic skin reaction at the site of injection is a commonly reported adverse effect due to the parenteral formulation. Also called *Cu Zn superoxide dismutase.*

Origanum majorana **L.,** *n* See marjoram.

Origanum vulgare, *n* See oregano.

origin, *n* the tendinous attachment of a muscle to the bone that remains fixed when the muscle contracts. In most cases, the origin is medial to the insertion.

original instructions (ō·ri'·jə·nəl in·struk'·shənz), *n* according to Native American medicine, the guidance of the great spirit, written upon the heart of every individual; these instructions are followed to lead a healthy life.

ornithine alpha-ketoglutarate (ōr'·na·thīn al'·fə-kē·tō·glōō'·tə·rāt), *n* a combination of ornithine and glutamine, two nonessential amino acids. Has been used as an athletic performance enhancer. No known precautions.

orofacial pain (ōr'·ə·fā'·shəl pān'), *n* physical discomfort associated with the mouth and face.

oropharynx (ōr·ə·far'·ingks), *n* one of the subdivisions of the pharynx that lies at the back of the mouth.

OSA, *n* obstructive sleep apnea, the most prevalent type of sleep apnea, in which breathing is interrupted for periods of 10 seconds or more during sleep. Usually caused by obesity, it affects men more often than women.

oscillation component, *n* the idea that everything vibrates in its own unique signature and that healthy beings must be in vibrational harmony to experience complete wellness.

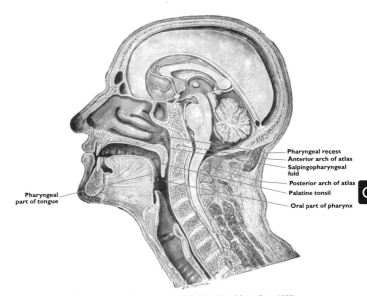

Oropharynx. (Chaitow et al, 2002; Reproduced from Gray, 1989)

orthodox, *adj* in medical practice, conventional, relating to currently accepted majority standards. See also medicine, conventional; hypothesis; and model, medical.

orthotics (ōr·thä'·tiks), *n* an external appliance used to correct a deformity of the musculoskeletal system, such as to promote a particular movement or to brace a paralyzed muscle.

oscillococcinum (ä'·si·lō·käk'·si·nəm), *n* a proprietary homeopathic preparation that comprises a 200c dilution of dissolved Barbary duck livers and model; used as a treatment for influenza.

osmium (ôz'·mē·əm), *n* 1. a hard, gray, toxic metallic element; the symbol is Os. 2. a homeopathic trituration of metallic osmium.

ostealgia (**äs'·tē·al'·jē·ə**), *n* a painful sensation related to an atypical condition of bone, such as osteomyelitis.

osteoarthritis (**ôs'·tē·ō·är·thī'·tis**), *n* degenerative disease that affects one or more joints; characterized by proliferation of bone spurs, reduced cartilage in the joints, subchondral bony sclerosis, and loss of articular cartilage. See also *DJD*.

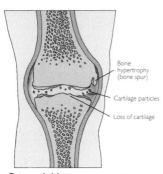

Osteoarthritis. (Ignatavicius, Workman, and Mishler, 1999)

osteokinematic movements (**ôs'·tē·ō·kin'·ə·ma'·tik mōōv'·mənts**), *n.pl* the basic joint movements, which include the extension, flexion, adduction, abduction, and rotation. Also called *physiologic movements.*

osteopath, *n* a person who is recognized by the national professional organization of his or her country as someone trained in osteopathic philosophy and techniques and who is allowed to diagnose and treat conditions based upon this training.

osteopathic lesion, *n* a technical term from osteopathy; refers to a somatic dysfunction. See also somatic dysfunction.

osteopathic manipulative treatment (OMT), *n* in osteopathic medicine, the use of the hands to diagnose and treat illness and somatic injury. Used in conjunction with other, conventional, medical procedures.

osteopathic philosophy, *n* the tenets of osteopathy that uphold the body's natural ability to heal itself without the use of external preparations—natural or pharmacological—or invasive technologies—x-rays or surgery—but in the righting of abnormalities in the body's anatomical structure through manipulation to allow the body's natural tendencies to function as the curing agent.

osteopathic physician, *n* an individual who is fully licensed to practice medicine who is trained in the principles and techniques of osteopathic philosophy.

osteopathy (**ôs·tē·ô·pə·thē**), *n* See medicine, osteopathic.

osteopathy in the cranial field, *n* a system of osteopathic techniques for balancing membrane tension and the connections between the cranium and sacrum to heal. See also somatic dysfunction.

osteoporosis, *n* bone disorder characterized by porosity, low mass, and structural deterioration, which leads to fragility and increased likelihood of fracture, especially of the spine, hip, and wrist.

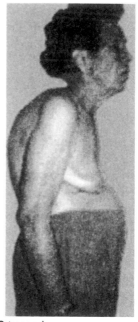

Osteoporosis. (Lemmi and Lemmi, 2000)

ostium (ô'·stē·əm), *n* an opening or passage.

ostrich fern (ôs'·trich fern'), *n* Latin name: *Matteuccia struthiopteris;* part used: leaves; uses: relieves back pain, quickens expulsion of the after-birth; precautions: contains carcinogens or thiaminase; can cause serious gastrointestinal toxicity. Also called *struisvaren.*

Oswestry instrument (ôs·wes'·trē in'·strə·ment), *n.pr* in chiropractic medicine, a questionnaire used to monitor the progression of a patient throughout the treatment period. Specifically, this questionnaire evaluates changes in a patient's function and evaluates the patient's capability to perform day-to-day activities or the level of impairment occurring as a result of the spinal condition. A score of 0 indicates the complete absence of a disability, whereas 100 indicates an incapacitating condition. It is particularly beneficial when a practitioner needs to repeatedly compare scores throughout the treatment period.

otic (ä'·tik), *adj* pertaining to the regions of the ear. Also called *auricular.*

otitis externa, *n* See ear infections.

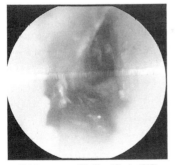

Otitis externa. (Zitelli and Davis, 1997)

otitis interna, *n* See ear infections.
otitis media, *n* See ear infections.

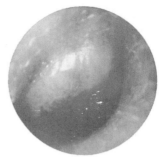

Otitis media. (Zitelli and Davis, 1997; Dr. Michael Hawke)

otorrhea (ō·tōr·rē'·ə), *n* discharge from the external portion of the ear; may be sanguineous, serous, or purulent.

outcome projection procedure (OPP), *n* a cognitive-energetic technique used in psychotherapy, in which energy treatments are administered so that the client's body and mind are confident in a challenging situation.

outflared innominate, *n* a condition in which the movement of the hip bone is unrestricted in a sideward direction and restricted in a medial direction because the anterior superior iliac spine is positioned laterally.

overfeeding, *n* feeding behavior in which infants and children are given more food than they can optimally digest. Not as common in breastfed infants, because a mother's milk production is limited naturally.

overly aggressive treatment, *n* the excessive use of a procedure, device, or medication intended to mitigate, cure, or halt the progression of a harmful disease; prescribed by some practitioners of both conventional and alternative medicine.

overpressure, *n* excessive pressure applied at the end of a physiologic joint range to confirm the severity of pain, thus helping determine the manual treatments.

oxerutins (ôk'·sē·rōō'·tənz), *n.pl* flavonoids synthesized from rutin. Has been used in conditions in which improvement of venous tone and capillary stability are required, such as varicose veins, hemorrhoids, venous insufficiency, lymphedema, and edema. Caution is advised for patients who are taking anticoagulant medications. Also called *hydroxyethylrutosides, HERs,* or *troxerutin.*

oxidation (ôk'·sə·dā'·shən), *n* **I.** a chemical reaction in which oxygen reacts with another atom, molecule, or compound to produce a new substance. **2.** a comprehensive term used to describe the loss of at least one electron from a molecule, ion, or atom.

oxidative stress, *n* an imbalance of the prooxidant : antioxidant ratio in which too few antioxidants are produced or ingested or too many oxidizing agents are produced.

oxide (ôk'·sīd), *n* a chemical compound of oxygen with another atom or molecule.

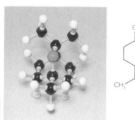

Oxide. (Clarke, 2002)

oxygen capacity of blood, *n* the maximum amount of oxygen able to combine with a given amount of hemoglobin in blood. The amount of oxygen within plasma is not included in this value.

oxygenated constituent (ôk'·sə·jə·nā'·təd kən·sti'·chu·ənt), *n* a component of an essential oil; comprises a functional group that contains oxygen, such as an aldehyde, alcohol, or a ketone.

oxytocin (ôk'·sē·tō'·sin), *n* hormone that plays a role during pregnancy, delivery, and lactation and influences other relationships such as care taking and parental or pair bonding.

PAB, *n* See PABA.

PABA, *n* paraamino benzoic acid, a substance required for synthesis of folic acid. It also absorbs ultraviolet light and is used as a topical sunscreen.

paced respiration (pāsd' res'·pə·rā'·shən), *n* a relaxation method that involves the practice of slow, deep breathing when one is faced with anxiety-provoking stimuli.

pacemaker, *n* **I.** the sinoatrial node comprises specialized tissue and is positioned at the junction of the right atrium and superior vena cava; primarily responsible for initiating the contractions of the atria which transmit the impulse to atrioventricular node resulting in contraction of the ventricles. A pacemaker that does not function properly may cause irregularities in the function of the heart. **2.** an electrical device that is temporarily or permanently implanted in the body to improve the heart rate by using electric impulses to stimulate the heart muscles. Also called *cardiac pacemaker.*

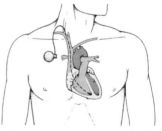

Pacemaker. (Thibodeau and Patton, 2003)

pachymenia (pa'·kə·mē'·nē·ə), *n* an atypical thickness of the skin or other membranes.

PaCO₂, *n* partial pressure of carbon dioxide in the blood. Critical in regulating breathing levels and maintaining body pH.

Paederia foetida, *n* See flower, Chinese.

pain, *n* unpleasant emotional or physical sensation, often associated with potential or actual tissue damage and classified as acute, chronic, or cancer-related. See also cancer-related pain.

pain behavior, *n* a joint test during which the patient indicates a particular point in which pain is initially experienced and/or increases while the practitioner moves the joint through the range of motion.

pain drain, *n* healing touch technique; practitioner holds one hand above an area of complaint until the pain recedes and then places the other hand near the area of relief. Used to alleviate acute and chronic pain symptoms.

PAK, *n.pr* See pyridoxal-alpha-ketoglutarate.

pakua (pə·kōō′·ə), *n* the circular diagram containing two flowing halves, one black around a white spot and the other white around a black spot. Reflects the Chinese cosmological concepts of wholeness, stillness, and movement. Also called the *Chinese monad, tai chi chuan,* or *ying-yang.* See also qi, yang, and yin.

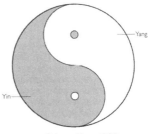

Pakua. (Cross, 2000)

palatines, *n.pl* either of the bones of the skull, which form the back of the hard palate, part of the nasal cavity, and the orbit of the eye.

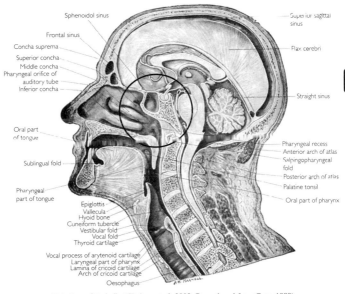

Palatines (*circled*). (Chaitow et al, 2002; Reproduced from Gray, 1989)

pale, *adj* in Chinese medicine, a facial coloration indicative of low energy, cold energy, energetic blockages, infections, and echo patterns. See also cold energy, echo pattern.

palliative care (pa'·lē·ā·tiv ker'), *n* an approach to health care that is concerned primarily with attending to physical and emotional comfort rather than effecting a cure.

palmar (päl'·mer), *adj* pertaining to the palm or anterior surface of the hand.

Palmer upper cervical (HIO), *n.pr* chiropractic technique in which a lateral thrust is administered to the C1–C2 cervicals; developed by BJ Palmer.

palpation, *n* the use of the sense of touch to assess a patient's health and to diagnose illness.

palpatory skills, *n.pl* the sensory skills developed by trained physicians and used in diagnosis and manipulative techniques.

Panax ginseng, *n* Asian ginseng. See ginseng and ginseng, Asian.

Panax quinquefolius, *n* American ginseng. See ginseng.

pancha (pän'·chə), *n* in Sanskrit, five.

panchakarma (pän'·chə·kär'·mə), *n* in Ayurveda, a five-step purification therapy that improves the ability to uptake and receive ojas by removing impurities from the shrotas and body. See also ojas and shrotas.

pancreatic exocrine insufficiency, *n* low levels of pancreatic proteases and lipases in the small intestine resulting in improper digestion of carbohydrate, fiber, and protein foods, eventually leading to malabsorption.

pancreatitis (pang'·krē·ə·tī'·tis), *n* inflammatory condition of the pancreas caused by trauma, alcohol, gall stones, and other conditions.

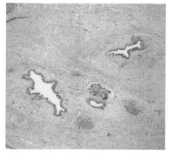

Pancreatitis. (Kumar, Cotran, and Robbins, 1997)

pandemic (pan·de'·mik), *adj* relating to the occurrence over a vast geographic region and impacting a large percentage of the population.

pandimensionality (pan'·dī·men'·shə·na'·li·tē), *n* in the science of unitary human beings, the nonlinear, nonspatial, nontemporal reality underlying the realm of everyday experience. This is where supernatural experiences such as spiritual events, astral projection, déjà vu, etc., take place.

pandits (pän·dēts), *n.pl* in Ayurveda, experts trained in Vedic knowledge, who memorize and communicate primordial sounds and relay them to others.

panesthesia (pan'·es·thē'·zhə), *n* the total of all sensations experienced by an individual at one time.

panic attacks, *n.pl* distressing episodes where an individual experiences palpitations, anxiety, apprehension, sweating, trembling, etc. Can last several minutes and recur unpredictably.

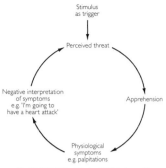

Panic attacks. (Clark, 1986 [adapted])

pan-Indian sweat lodge ceremony,
n a sacred ceremony performed in the
Native American culture used to
provide access to the realms of spirit
and deeper aspects of the self. Often
used as part of healing ceremonies.
See also realm of spirit.

pansy, *n* Latin name: *Viola tricolor;*
part used: flowers; uses: whooping
cough, inflammation, upper respiratory disorders, laxative, seborrheic
skin conditions, acne, cradle cap; precautions: pregnancy, lactation, children, salicylate sensitivity. Also called
*field pansy, heartsease, Johnny jump-
up, jupiter flower, ladies' delight,* or
wild pansy.

pantethine (pan'·tə·thēn), *n* a
derivative of pantothenic acid
(vitamin B$_5$) reported to have beneficial effects on lipid metabolism,
thus improving serum levels of
triglycerides, LDL, and HDL. No
known precautions.

PaO$_2$, *n* partial pressure of oxygen in
the blood.

papain (pə·pā'·in), *n* a proteolytic
enzyme found in the juice of the
unripe papaya fruit; used to facilitate
digestion. Allergic reaction may
occur after topical application or
oral ingestion.

Papaver bracteatum, *n* See poppy.

Papaver somniferum, *n* See poppy.

papaya, *n* Latin name: *Carica papaya;*
parts used: fruits, seeds, roots, juice,
latex; uses: in Ayurveda, pacifies
kapha and vata doshas, ripe fruit pacifies pitta doshas (pungent, bitter, light,
oily, sharp); seeds: antifertility, antiamoebic; latex: uterotonic, antiulcerogenic, anthelmintic, antifungal; roots:
diuretic; precautions: pregnancy,
coagulation disorders. Also called
chirbhita, papita, or *pawpaw.*

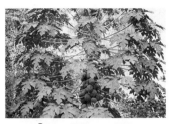

Papaya. (Williamson, 2002)

paracrine (par'·ə·krin), *adj* affecting
the cells that neighbor the cells of
origin, used in describing glandular
and hormonal action.

paradigm (par'·ə·dīm'), *n* a generally accepted model for making sense
of phenomena in a given discipline at
a particular time. When one paradigm
is replaced by another, it is called a
paradigm shift.

paradigm, scientific, *n* described by
Thomas Kuhn as a set of practices and
ways of thinking about science that
prescribes the limits and boundaries
of reality.

paraffin bath, *n* dip treatment of hot
paraffin wax, commonly used to
encourage relaxation, relieve pain,
and increase circulation in the hands
and feet. See also thermotherapy.

paranormal, *adj* **1.** outside the realm
of normal experience or scientific
explanation. *n* **2.** collective term for
anomalous phenomena.

paraphysiologic space, *n* **1.** the distance a joint can be moved beyond
the passive end range (elastic barrier)
without causing the tissue to rupture.
2. the last of three barriers to end joint
movement, distinguished by the
audible popping sound that occurs as
a gap is created in the joint.

P

paraplegia (par'·ə·plē'·jə), *n* paralysis distinguished by functional loss in the lower limbs and trunk typically due to vehicular or sporting accidents, gunshot wounds, and falls. Nontraumatic causes like spina bifida, neoplasms, or scoliosis can also cause paraplegia.

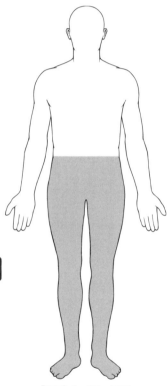

Paraplegia. (Salvo, 2003)

parapsychology, *n* the scientific study of psychic or psionic ("psi") phenomena, including extrasensory perception, precognition, psychokinesis, and telepathy.

parasympathetic autonomic nervous system, *n* that part of the involuntary nervous system which balances the sympathetic nervous system by relaxing and slowing the heart rate, digestion; causes pupil dilation and other responses to "fight or flight." Also called *relaxation response.*

parchera (pär·chā'·rə), *n* practitioner from Guatemala, of Curanderismo, the Mexican-American healing system. See also Curanderismo.

parenteral (pə·ren'·tə·rəl), *adj* pertaining to the administration of substances by other than via the oral route.

parietal bones (pə·rī'·ə·təl bōnz'), *n.pl* the two skull bones located between the frontal and occipital bones and which form the top and sides of the cranium.

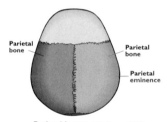

Parietal bones. (Chaitow, 1999)

parpati (pär'·pə·tē), *n* in Ayurveda, a method of medicine preparation in which metallic flakes are formed by pouring molten metal over the leaves of plants.

parsley, *n* Latin name: *Petroselinum crispum;* parts used: leaves, roots, seeds, oil; uses: diuretic, antiinfective, antiinflammatory, antioxidant, antispasmodic, coughs, menstrual complaints, gastrointestinal distress, joint pains; precautions: pregnancy, lactation, children; oil should be avoided by those with kidney inflammation, cardiac, kidney and liver disorders, high blood pressure medications, lithium, MAOIs, opiates. Also called *common parsley, garden parsley,* or *rock parsley.*

parsley piert (pär'·slē pī'·urt), *n* Latin name: *Aphanes arvensis;* parts used: aerial parts; uses: diuretic, kidney stones, kidney infections; precautions: pregnancy, lactation, children. Also called *field lady's mantle, parsley breakstone,* or *parsley piercestone.*

parteras (pär·ter'·äs), *n.pl* in Curanderismo, midwives. See pateras.

participant observation, *n* a method of qualitative research in which the researcher understands the contextual meanings of an event or events through participating and observing as a subject in the research.

partition, *n* the process of distributing an essential oil among several solvents by using the various soluble properties of the components within the essential oil.

PARTS, *n* a term used to represent and establish the diagnostic process associated with the identification and evaluation of spinal dysfunction. *P* stands for *pain/tenderness; A* stands for *asymmetry; R* stands for *range of motion abnormalities, T* stands for *tissue, tone, texture, and temperature abnormality;* and *S* for *special tests.* The conclusions act as a guide for determining the spinal regions that need manipulative adjustment.

parturient (pär·tōō'·rē·ent), *adj* having or with labor and birth.

pascal (pas·kal'), *n* a unit of pressure equivalent to one million per square meter.

Passiflora incarnata, n See flower, passion.

passion flower, *n* Latin name: *Passiflora incarnata;* parts used: flowers, fruit; uses: sedative, sleep disorders, neuralgia, tachycardia, opiate withdrawal; precautions: pregnancy, lactation, children, sedative medications, MAOIs. Also called *apricot vine, granadilla, Jamaican honeysuckle, maypop, maypot, passion fruit, passion vine, purple passion flower,* or *water lemon.*

Passion flower. (Scott and Barlow, 2003)

passive, *adj* pertaining to patients who become mere spectators as they lack the energy or interest to participate.

passive accessory intervertebral movements (pa'·siv ak·ses'·ə·rē in'·ter·ver'·tə·brəl mōōv'·mənts), *n.pl* manipulative techniques used to investigate or restore the gliding movements between vertebrae.

passive end range, *n* the distance a joint can be moved by outside force without causing a gap in the joint and an audible popping sound. The second of three barriers to end joint movement. Also called *physiologic joint space.*

passive physiologic intervertebral movements (pa'·siv fi'·zē·ə·lô'·jə·kəl in'·ter·ver'·tə·brəl mōōv'·mənts), *n.pl* manipulative techniques used to investigate or restore the physiologic movements between vertebrae.

passive physiological joint movement, *n* motion in which the practitioner produces the motion while supporting the limb to assess the joint with the muscle in a relaxed position.

passive volition, *n* the unconscious, intuitive control of physiologic processes; typically associated with biofeedback.

patch, *n* a method of medicinal preparation in which a cloth dressing is impregnated with herbal constituents and placed on the skin. Particularly used in moxibustion in Chinese medicine.

pateras (pä·te'·räs), *n.pl* in Curanderismo, the Mexican-American healing system, the term for *midwives.* See parteras.

paternalism (pə·ter'·nəl·izm), *n* a conflict between beneficence and autonomy, such as when a practitioner ignores the choice that a patient makes because he or she feels that more good can be done by the practitioner's judgment. See also beneficence and autonomy.

path of transportation, *n* in Ayurveda, the path taken by ama in combination with one or more doshas until it settles and affects a body part that is the site of disease manifestation. See also doshas and ama.

pathogenesis, *n* **1.** the course of an illness from its initial manifestation through its critical development. **2.** the process whereby disease occurs. See also symptoms, hierarchy of; proving; and homeopathic drug provings.

pathogenic (pa'·thfə·je'·nik), *adj* the ability to cause disease.

pathognomonic (pa'·thəg·nō·män'·ik), *adj* relating to characteristic symptoms of a disease that are generally used as the basis for making a diagnosis.

pathography, *n* comprehensive picture of diseases. Also called *nosography.* See also disease picture.

pathology, *n* the study of the causes and effects of disease, particularly those observable on body tissues.

pathya (pä'·thyə), *n* in Ayurveda, a specific diet prescribed during drug therapy based on the principle that drug action is influenced by dietary components.

patient cooperation, *n* **1.** complying with a prescribed succession of treatments. **2.** voluntary patient movements, performed with directions from the physician, that aid palpation and manipulation.

patient history, *n* **1.** documentation collected from the patient and further sources on the pathogenesis of the illness. **2.** patient's medical or health experiences, including illness. See also anamnesis, case taking, and catamnesis.

patient-oriented evidence that matters (POEMs), *n* an abstract of quality research that is relevant to doctors and patients.

pattern, *n* in therapeutic touch, an energy field's characteristic that gives the field its identity. Even behavior is considered evidence of a changing energy pattern.

pattern, common compensatory, *n* the preferred motion pattern of alternating fascia at the body's transitional areas, classified by osteopath J. Gordon Zink.

pattern, typical pain, *n* generally constelled sites of pain associated with a particular health condition or dysfunction.

patterns, fascial, *n.pl* systems in which the preferred directions of motion for fascia throughout the body are classified and recorded.

pattern and organization, *n* in therapeutic touch, the notion that individuals are innovative and whole in and of themselves and that a human being's energy field has pattern and organization that contributes to this idea.

pattern of disharmony, *n* in Chinese medicine, refers to disruptions in an individual's health that are caused by imbalances in interactions of organ systems with one another and with the external environment, which are believed to render the individual susceptible to future illness.

patterning, *n* an alternative technique in which neurologically impaired children are led through a series of movements that mimic the prenatal and postnatal movements of normal children. This technique is believed to assist these children in improving their neurological organization.

pau d'arco (pō' där'·kō), *n* Latin name: *Tabebuia impetiginosa;* parts used: bark, heartwood; uses: this herb is controversial. Research suggests that it has antimicrobial, antifungal, and immunostimulant effects and is useful for psoriasis and other skin conditions and as an adjunct treatment for cancer, HIV, liver conditions, diabetes mellitus, and lupus; other studies assert that it is not only relatively useless but also toxic; precautions: pregnancy, lactation, children, hemophilia, von Willebrand's disease, thrombocytopenia, liver and kidney damage at high doses, anticoagulants, active ingredient (lapachol) is possibly toxic. Also called *ipe, ipe roxo, ipes, la pacho, lapacho colorado, lapacho morado, lapachol, purple lapacho, red lapacho, roxo, tajibo, trumpet bush,* or *trumpet tree.*

Paullinia cupana, *n* See guarana.

Paullinia sorbilis, *n* See guarana.

Pausinystalia yohimbe, *n* See yohimbe.

pay-loo-ah (pā-lōō-ä), *n* a traditional preparation originating from Laos that is used to relieve fever and rash in children. There have been reports of lead and arsenic poisoning from using pay-loo-ah.

PC, *n* pericardium channel; an acupuncture channel that runs from the shoulder to the hand along the medial surface of the arm, named after the pericardium, and associated with the triple burner (TE) channel. See also TE.

PC SPES, *n.pr* anticancer herbal preparation which contains eight Chinese herbs. As of June, 2002, Botaniclab, the only lab producing PC SPES in the United States closed because of a voluntary recall of contaminated stock.

PCP, *n.pr* See primary care physician.

PCT, *n.pr* See primary care trust.

peach, *n Prunus persica;* parts used: bark, kernel oil, leaves, woody uses, bark and leaves—anthelmintic, astringent, antifungal, diuretic, insomnia, cough, constipation, minor skin conditions, peach pits (under the product name, Laetrile) are the source for the controversial and dangerous cancer treatment; precautions: pregnancy, lactation, children; pits can cause cyanide poisoning. Also called *amygdalin, Laetrile,* or *vitamin B-17.*

peak area, *n* a representation of separate substances within a mixture on a printed chart, called a chromatogram that is produced by chromatography. The size of the peak area is nearly equal to the quantity of the substance present in the mixture.

peak expiratory flow rate (pēk' ek·spī·rə·tōr'·ē flō' rāt'), *n* a simple, preliminary test that measures the maximum volume of air exhaled by the patient to assess degree of respiratory restriction.

peat, *n* in balneotherapy, a mossy plant substance used in baths and peloids. An antiinflammatory, antimicrobial, antineoplastic, antiviral substance, the effects of which include immunological stimulation, increased metabolism, and vessel dilation. See also balneotherapy and peloid.

pectenitis (pek'·tə·nī'·tis), *n* an inflammatory condition of the anal canal; hinders the activity of the anal sphincter muscle.

pectin, *n* pectin is a gummy polysaccharide constituent of the cell walls of plants that is used as a thickening agent in jams and jellies. Pectin's mucilaginous qualities are useful in treating diarrhea and high cholesterol and it may have beneficial effects on radiation sickness as well.

pectoralgia (pek'·tə·ral'·jē·ə), *n* pain experienced in the thorax or chest.

pedal (pē'·dəl), *adj* pertaining to the foot.

pedal pump, *n* a technique used to promote the drainage of lymph and venous blood from the lower extremities. Also called *Dalrymple treatment* or *pedal fascial pump.*

pediatrics, *n* the branch of medicine exclusively related to the care and treatment of infants and children.

PEFR, *n* See peak expiratory flow rate.

pejuta wicasa (pā·jōō'·tä wē·kä'·sä), *n* in Native American medicine, a Lakota term for a herbalist.

pellet, *n* **1.** mass of steroid hormones placed under the skin to be absorbed slowly. **2.** pill that comprise sucrose and saturated with medicine used in homeopathy.

peloid (pā'·loid), *n* pulp (usually from lake or sea mud, peat, or other plants) that is applied to the body for disease prevention and treatment.

pelvic, *n* inferior area of the abdominopelvic cavity.

P

pelvic declination, *n* the rotation of the pelvis around the anteroposterior axis. Also called *pelvic unleveling.*

pelvic index, *n* a radiographic measurement of the relative positions of the sacrum and the hipbones.

pelvic side-shift, *n* condition in which the pelvis deviates to the left or right of the center line.

pelvic tilt, *n* rotation of the pelvis around either a horizontal or vertical axis. The former cases would be forward or backward tilt, whereas the latter would tilt to the left or right side.

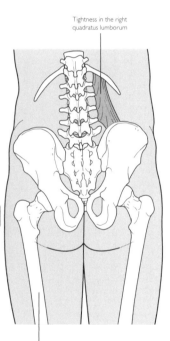

Tightness in the right quadratus lumborum

Structurally shorter left leg

Pelvic tilt. (Lowe, 2003)

pennyroyal, *n* Latin names: *Hedeoma pulegioides, Mentha pulegium*; parts used: flowers, leaves; uses: abortifacient, digestive conditions, liver conditions, gallbladder conditions, skin diseases, colic, menstrual complaints, respiratory conditions; precautions: abortifacient, pregnancy, lactation, children, seizure disorders, liver disease, kidney disease, extremely toxic; should not be ingested. Also called *American pennyroyal, European pennyroyal, mock pennyroyal, mosquito plant, pudding grass, squawbalm, squawmint,* or *tickweed.*

pepper, *n* **1.** any plant of the genus *Piper.* **2.** any plant of the genus *Capsicum.*

pepper, black, *n* Latin name: *Piper nigrum;* part used: fruit; uses: flatulence, anorexia, indigestion, heartburn, stomach cramps, colic, peptic ulcers, constipation, diarrhea; precautions: pregnancy, lactation, children; can cause apnea (in large doses). Also called *biber, filfil, golmirch, hu-chiao, kalmirch, kosho, krishnadi, lada, maricha, pepe, pfeffer, phi noi, pimenta, pjerets, poivre, the king of spices,* or *the master spice.*

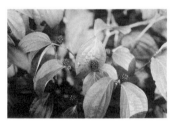

Pepper, black. (Williamson, 2002)

pepper, long, *n* Latin name: *Piper longum;* parts used: immature fruits, roots; uses: in Ayurveda pacifies kapha and vata doshas (pungent, light, oily, sharp), immunomodulator, stimulant, antiasthmatic, hepatoprotection, antiinflammatory, antiamoebic, antibacterial, bioavailability enhancer, carminative, laxative, stomachic; root: gout, back pain, rheumatism; precautions: pregnancy, lactation, barbiturates, phenytoin. Also called *pippali.*

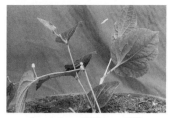

Pepper, long. (Williamson, 2002)

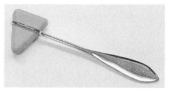

Percussion hammer. (Wilson and Giddens, 2001)

peppermint, *n* See mint.

pepsin A, *n* a gastric protease found in the stomach that breaks down proteins. Most effective at pH values between 2.0 and 3.0 and inactive at pH values higher than 5.0.

peptide hormones (pep´·tīd hōr´· mōnz), *n.pl* water-soluble hormones comprised of a few amino acids that introduce a series of chemical reactions to change the cell's metabolism. Examples include hormones of the pituitary gland and parathyroid glands

peptide T, *n* a biological substance administered intranasally, it may block the spread of HIV infection and combat related neurologic dysfunction.

percolation (per´·kǝ·lā´·shǝn), *n* a method for extracting essential oils from aromatic plant materials that strongly resembles steam distillation. As part of the process, a generator above the aromatic plant material produces steam. The steam then trickles down into the aromatic plant material, and the steam and oil are collected in the exact method used in steam distil-

lation. This process is quicker and less complex than steam distillation. Also called *hydro-diffusion*. See also steam distillation.

percussion hammer, *n* a device used in osteopathic medicine. Resembling a small-sized hammer with a soft, malleable tip, the tool is used by a practitioner to strike parts of the body to lessen restrictions in muscles and joints.

percussion movements, *n.pl* See tapotement.

percutaneous (per·kyōō·tā´·nē·ǝs), *adj* method of applying a substance through the skin.

perennial philosophy, *n* a view that sees the world as divided into two aspects: the invisible, unified, unmanifest, implicit, mystical level of reality and the visible, manifold, manifest, explicit, material level of reality (the latter is understood as derived from and secondary to the former). Some regard the perennial philosophy as the universal philosophy common to all religions and spiritual traditions. Also called *philosophia perennis*.

P

performance drinks, *n.pl* in sports nutrition, beverages used to enhance athletic performance and endurance by maintaining blood glucose levels, electrolyte balance, and hydration.

perfume, *n* a substance with fragrant properties; typically a combination of alcohols and essential oils with aromatic properties; derived from plant extracts or synthesized.

pericarditis (pe'·rē·kar·dī'·tis), *n* an inflammatory condition of the pericardium associated with malignant neoplastic disease, trauma, uremia, infection, collagen disease, or myocardial infarction.

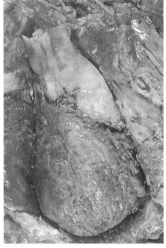

Pericarditis. (Cotran, Kumar, and Collins, 1999)

perilla (pə·ri'·lə), *n Perilla frutescens* L.; parts used: seeds, dried leaves; uses: allergies, antispasmodic, antiemetic, upper respiratory complaints; precautions: pregnancy, lactation, children. Also called *beefsteak plant* or *wild coleus.*

***Perilla frutescens* L.,** *n* See perilla.

perineal (per'·ə·nē'·əl), *adj* pertaining to the inferior pelvic cavity between the genitals and anus.

perineometer (pe'·rē·nē'·ō·mē'· ter), *n* in biofeedback therapy, an instrument that provides a measurement of the strength of contractions produced by the pelvic floor and anal sphincter muscles.

perineural connective tissue system, *n* the network of cells surrounding each of the brain's neurons.

periodic table, *n* a pictorial representation of all chemical elements arranged by increasing order of atomic numbers. Periods and groups are the primary classifications found within the table.

periodicity, *n* the quality of being periodic or recurring at definite intervals of time.

periodontitis, *n* an inflammatory disease that affects the periodontium within the oral cavity. Common symptoms include localized pain, erythema, swelling, loosening of teeth, and dental pockets. See also disease, periodontal.

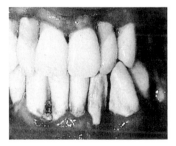

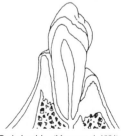

Periodontitis. (Murray et al, 1994)

periods, *n.pl* horizontal rows of elements within a periodic table. Elements within a period share similar physical and chemical properties.

peripheral (pə·rif'·ə·rəl), *adj* referring to or towards outer surrounding surfaces. Also called *superficial.*

peripheral neuropathy (pe·rif'·er· əl ner·ô'·pə·thē), *n* a degenerative condition that attacks the sensory and motor nerves, thus causing muscle atrophy, pain, decreased strength, and loss of sensation. It often accompanies the progression of a primary condition, such as AIDS or diabetes mellitus.

permanent magnets, *n.pl* magnets containing the mineral boron and the rare earth metal neodymium; often combined to create a neoprene or ceramic entity.

Perna canaliculus, *n* See New Zealand green-lipped muscle.

peroxidases (pə·räk'·sə·dā·səz), *n.pl* enzymes that use peroxide to break down bacteria and other harmful material. Located in the granules of neutrophils.

persimmon tannin (per·si'·mən ta'· nin), *n* condensed tannin derived from persimmon that in concentration-dependent doses, binds and eliminates free-radicals.

personalistic approach (per'·sən·ə· lis'·tik ə·prōch'), *n* a medical philosophy that holds that illness occurs as a result of dysfunction in intrapersonal and interpersonal relationships.

person-centered psychotherapy, *n* psychotherapeutic philosophy based on the belief that every person has an innate impulse toward growth and a desire to reach his full potential.

perturbation, *n* a small disturbance that tips a metastable system over into disorder and chaos.

Peruvian bark, *n* See calisaya bark.

pessaries, *n.pl* solid delivery method for treatments made of materials that melt at body temperature and are used to deliver medicinal substances into the vagina.

Simple ring
pessary

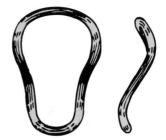

Smith Hodge pessary

Pessaries. (Wilson and Carrington, 1991)

pestilence (pes·tə·lens), *n* any epidemic of a disease that is virulent and devastating.

Petasites hybridus, *n* See butterbur.

Petasites officinalis, *n* See butterbur.

PETCO₂, *n* partial pressure of endtidal carbon dioxide; a measure of the amount of carbon dioxide present in the exhaled air.

petitgrain (pe'·tē·grān), *n* an essential oil distilled from the leaves and stems of the bitter orange (*Citrus aurantium*), useful for treating acne and oily skin, fatigue, and stress.

petition, *n* a prayer making a request on behalf of one's self.

petrissage (pe'·tri·sôzh), *n* massage technique that involves grasping and squeezing muscle tissue to relieve tension and increase circulation. Also called *kneading.*

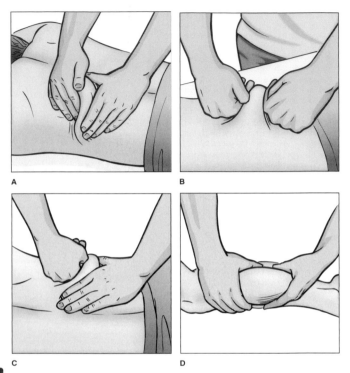

Petrissage. (Fritz, 2004)

Petroselinum crispum, *n* See parsley.

Pettibon spinal mechanics, *n.pr* an integrated system of spinal column analysis and correction developed by Dr. Burl Pettibon. Great importance is assigned to the relationship between spinal structure and function, with an emphasis on restorative therapies that create changes in soft tissue (ligaments, muscles, and discs) as well as hard tissue (the spine).

Peumus boldus, *n* See boldo.

peyote (pā·yō·tē), *n* Latin name: *Lophophora williamsii*; parts used: whole cactus; uses: traditional uses include alcohol addiction, snakebite, arthritis, rheumatism, burns, heart conditions, and as a visionary adjunct to traditional religious practices, antimicrobial, sedative; precautions: pregnancy, lactation, children, CNS stimulants, hallucinogenic, illegal in the U.S. (possible exception given to the Native American Church) and most of Europe. Also called *anhalonium, big chief, buttons, cactus, mesc, mescal, mescal buttons, mescaline, mexc, moon, pan peyote,* or *peyote button.*

Pfluger's law of generalization, *n.pr* according to which, the medulla oblongata propagates very intense irritation in one part of the body resulting in an overall increase in muscular tonus.

Pfluger's law of intensity, *n.pr* neurological law according to which, the intensity of a reflex movement is most often greater on the initial side of irritation.

Pfluger's law of radiation, *n.pr* neurological law according to which, if untreated, the discomfort increases whereby, the pain is directed to the motor nerves higher up in the spinal cord.

Pfluger's law of symmetry, *n.pr* neurological law according to which, at sufficiently intense levels of stimulation, motor reactions can be observed in similar muscles bilaterally.

Pfluger's law of unilaterality, *n.pr* neurological law according to which, mild irritation to sensory nerves produces motor activity on the irritated side only.

PFS, *n* post facilitation stretch; therapeutic approach utilized during proprioceptive neuromuscular facilitation in which the patient begins the stretch midway between the fully relaxed and fully stretched position and uses maximum level of effort to exert a strong isometric contraction. See also PNF.

pH, *n* measurement of the acidic or alkaline nature of a solution. Expressed as a numerical value, it is calculated by determining the log concentration of hydrogen ions present in the solution. A pH value of 7 indicates a neutral solution; a value less than 7 an acidic solution, and higher than 7 indicates an alkaline solution.

phanta (fän'·tə), *n* in Ayurveda, a medicinal or medicinal preparation in which herbs are infused in hot water for a brief period of time, then filtered.

phantom limb pain, *n* pain felt by an amputated individual that seems to be arise from the missing limb; often managed by learning to increase flow of blood to the residual limb.

pharmacist, *n* person trained and licensed to dispense, formulate, and educate about medications.

pharmacodynamics, *n* the division of pharmacology that studies the effects of drugs and their mechanisms of action in the body.

pharmacognosy (fär'·mə·käg'·nə·sē), *n* the study of medicinal and/or pharmaceutical substances derived from natural sources such as plants, fungi, and animals.

pharmacokinetics (far'·mə·kō·kə·ne'·tiks), *n* the division of pharmacology that studies the absorption, distribution, and localization of drugs in the body.

pharmacopeia, *n* written record of all aspects of homeopathic or herbal remedies, such as their constitutions, characteristics, specifications, and effects.

pharmacovigilance, *n* the monitoring of adverse effects of drugs and herbal remedies as they are used in the population. Also called *postmarketing surveillance*.

pharmacy, *n* **1.** place from which prescription medications are prepared and dispensed by a pharmacist. **2.** the study of the preparation and dispensing of medications.

phase I detoxification, *n* the first step in the two-step process for neutralizing toxic chemicals in the liver, during which enzymes neutralize a few chemicals but convert the majority of them into forms that can be neutralized in phase II. See also phase II detoxification.

phase II detoxification, *n* the second step in the two-step process for neutralizing toxic chemicals in the liver, during which several enzymes combine with the toxins to convert them into neutral substances or to make them easier to eliminate from the body.

phase transition, *n* the response of a system to a disturbance resulting in novel, emergent properties of order and organization.

phasic (fā'·zik), *n* a description of motor tone activity in which the muscle is actively used for movement rather than stabilization.

phenols (fē'·nôlz), *n.pl* aromatic compounds found in some essential oils; possess strong antiseptic and antibacterial properties and also act as nerve stimulants and immunostimulants; can cause hepatotoxicity and irritate the skin.

Phenol

Phenols. (Clarke, 2002)

phenomenology (fə·nä'·mə·nä'·lə·jē), *n* a philosophical approach and method of qualitative research in which the essence of an experience is sought. The researcher identifies prior assumptions and beliefs and temporarily brackets them away from the experience being researched, so that it may be understood on its own terms.

phenylpropane derivative (fē'·nəl·prō'·pān də·ri'·və·tiv), *n* phenolic compound with an attachment of a propyl chain; present in Chavicol, thymol, carvacrol, and other compounds.

pheromones (fer'·ə·mōnz), *n.pl* chemicals secreted into the environment by insects and some animals to ward off predators or to attract the opposite sex of the same species.

phlebotomy, *n* See venesection.

phlegm (flem'), *n* heavy mucus that originates in the lungs and mucous membranes of the nose and throat.

phobia, *n* an intense, irrational, and obsessive fear of a particular object, activity, or situation such as animals, heights, meeting new people, or enclosed spaces.

phonon (fō'·nôn), *n* a discrete unit of sound energy that can travel through the piezoelectric medium of connective tissue.

phosphatidylcholine, *n* See lecithin.

phosphatidylserine (fäs'·fə·tī'·dəl·sə·rēn), *n* a phospholipid that has been used to treat cognitive impairment, depression, and the symptoms of overexertion. Caution is advised for patients taking heparin. Also called *PS*.

photosensitivity, *n* an adverse skin reaction to some essential oils and other treatments, in which the skin reacts to ultraviolet rays resulting in redness, hyperpigmentation, and in severe cases, blistering.

photosensitization, *n* skin condition marked by heightened sensitivity to artificial and natural light. May occur as a side effect of some essential oils and other treatments.

photosynthesis (fō'·tō·sin'·thə·sis), *n* metabolic process by which plants and some bacteria use carbon dioxide and sunlight to produce glucose. Oxygen is a by product of this process.

phototherapy (fō'·tō·the'·rə·pē), *n* **1.** the use of light for therapeutic purposes. **2.** treatment method which uses photo-based counseling techniques by having clients consciously probe and reintegrate their insights to better understand and improve their life.

phototoxicity (fō'·tō·tôk·si'·sə·tē), *n* an adverse reaction to ultraviolet light or sunlight caused by chemicals, such as the furanocoumarins.

phrenic (fre'·nik), *adj* **1.** relating to the diaphragm. **2.** relating to the mind.

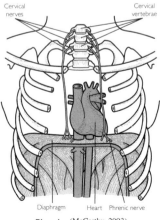

Phrenic. (McCarthy, 2003)

phyllanthus, *n* See stone breaker.

Phyllanthus amarus, *n* See stone breaker.

Phyllanthus emblica, *n* See amla.

Phyllanthus niruri, *n* See stone breaker.

phylogeny (fī·lä'·jə·nē), *n* the evolutionary history of a species. See also ontogeny.

physical field, *n* in energy medicine, one of the three etheric levels of the human energy field. This layer embodies the sense of physical sensation, vitality of the body, and the autonomic functioning of cells, tissues, and organs and is found closest to the skin surface.

physical level, *n* See physical field.

Physician's Current Procedural Terminology, *n. pr* a comprehensive system of classification developed and maintained by the American Medical Association; lists descriptive terms and identifies codes for reporting medical procedures and services. It provides a standardized language for the accurate description of diagnostic, medical, and surgical services. It is an effective method for promoting dependable communication among healthcare practitioners and third parties across the nation. Terminology contained within is the most established form of medical classification that is used to report medical services and procedures and programs of health insurance. It is employed within an administrative management process and includes claims processing and developing standards for review of medical care. Also called *CPT.*

Physician's Desk Reference (PDR), *n* an informational, scientifically validated resource that provides information relating to indications, chemical formulations, actions and potential hazards associated with most medicinal remedies currently being used. In addition to conventional medicinal remedies, a PDR related to herbal remedies is also available.

Physicians' Committee for Responsible Medicine, *n.pr* a nonprofit organization founded in 1985; promotes preventive medicine, conducts clinical research, encourages effectiveness and ethics in research efforts, and advocates to broaden the access to health care. The organization publishes a quarterly magazine called *Good Medicine.* Also called *PCRM.*

Physicians' Curriculum in Clinical Nutrition, *n.pr* a publication of the Society of Teachers of Family Medicine that provides guidelines to the most important and basic nutritional objectives. Presented in two sections, the publication examines a variety of issues related to basic care, such as nutritional assessment and screening, geriatric care, nutritional counseling, obesity, eating disorders, nutritional support, and women's health. It also contains a section dedicated to developing educational programs, and implementing a nutritional course along with methods used in caring for patients.

physiocultopathy (fi'·zē·ō·kul·tô'·pə·thē), *n* also known as the "physical culture" school of health and healing. It inspired the establishment of gymnasiums across the US and was responsible for the original development of exercise programs to empower individuals to obtain their personal health goals.

physiology, *n* in biological sciences, study concerned with the processes and functioning of organisms.

physiotherapy, *n* physical therapy; may include massage, exercise applied heat, ultrasound, electrotherapy, and short-wave diathermy.

phytoalexins (fā·tō·ə·lek'·sēnz), *n.pl* poisonous compounds that plants develop when they respond to attacks.

phytochemical (fī'·tō·ke'·mə·kəl), *n* medicinally active chemical constituents derived from plants.

phytochemistry, *n* the scientific study and classification of the chemical constituents of plants.

phytoestrogens, *n.pl* plant-derived estrogen analogs.

Phytolacca americana, *n* See pokeweed.

phytomedicine (fī'·tō·me'·di·sin), *n* the use of plants, parts of plants, and isolated phytochemicals for the prevention and treatment of various health concerns.

phytosterols (fī·tô'·ste·rôlz), *n.pl* plant-derived compounds that are structurally similar to cholesterol. These compounds may lower blood cholesterol levels, particularly LDL cholesterol, and may have uses as immunostimulants and in treating benign prostate enlargement.

phytotherapy (fī'·tō·the'·rə·pē), *n* the use of a wide variety of plants and plant extracts for the prevention and treatment of disease. Also called *herbalism.*

Picorrhiza kurroa, *n* See kutki.

picture, *n* an image of the illness. The concept that a comprehensive consideration of an illness and the individual should be used to treat malaise. See also clinical picture, symptom picture, disease picture, and drug picture.

Pierce-Stillwagon, *n.pr* chiropractic technique in which manual thrust is used in treating dysfunctions of the pelvis and cervical spine.

piezoelectricity (pē'·ā·zō·ē'·lek·tri'··si·tē), *n* electrical current produced by mechanical pressure on connective tissue and other crystals like quartz, mica, and Rochelle salt.

Pilates (pə·lä'·tēz), *n.pr* physical reeducation and exercise approach developed by Joseph Pilates (1880–1967); integrates breathing, movement, proper body mechanics, strengthening exercises, and stabilization of the pelvis and trunk.

pill-bearing spurge, *n* Latin names: *Euphorbia pilulifera, Euphorbia hirta, Euphorbia capitata*; part used: dried plant; uses: respiratory disorders, diarrhea, amebiasis, STDs, and eye conditions; precautions: pregnancy, lactation, children, bleeding disorders, ACE inhibitor medications, anticoagulants, barbiturates, cholinesterase inhibitors, disulfiram. Also called *asthma weed, catshair, euphorbia, garden spurge, milkweed, queensland asthmaweed,* or *snake weed.*

Pilocarpus jaborandi, *n* See tree, Jaborandi.

Pilocarpus microphyllus, *n* See tree, Jaborandi.

Pilocarpus pinnatifolius, *n* See tree, Jaborandi.

pilot study, *n* the early or initial study for a new medicine or method of medical treatment.

pincer compression (pin'·ser kəm·pre'·shən), *n* a compression technique in which tissues are picked up and grabbed between the thumb and finger(s). The practitioner can apply this type of compression by using curved fingers that appear similar to a "C" clamp or flattened fingers that resemble a clothespin. See also compression techniques.

pineal gland problems (pī·nē'·əl gland' prä'·bləmz), *n.pl* pathologies occurring in the pineal gland, which is responsible for gonad development, melatonin production, and biorhythms.

pineapple, *n* Latin name: *Ananas comosus*; part used: fruit; uses: antifungal, antiinflammatory, obesity, constipation, wounds, source for the enzyme complex-bromelain, known to act as a platelet aggregation inhibitor; precautions: avoid therapeutic use in pregnancy, lactation, or for children, ACE inhibitor medications, anticoagulants. Also called *ananas, golden rocket,* or *smooth cayenne.* See also bromelain.

pingala (pēng·gä'·lə) *n* according to ancient Indian philosophy, the male or positive energy, one of the two components of prana (life force), the other being ida. Good health is indicative of balance between pingala and ida, while an imbalance between the two leads to disease. See also prana and ida.

pinna, *n* See auricle.

pipe fast, *n* See Hanbleceya.

Piper longum, *n* See pepper, long.

Piper methysticum, *n* See kava.

Piper nigrum, *n* See pepper, black.

pipsissewa (pip·si'·sə·wô), *n* Latin name: *Chimaphila umbellata*; part used: dried herb; uses: astringent, antispasmodic, anxiolytic, seizures, kidney stones, skin ulcerations, diabetes, urinary infections; precautions: pregnancy, lactation, children, ulcers (peptic and duodenal), Crohn's disease, ulcerative colitis, diabetes mellitus, GERD, iron deficiency. Also called *ground holly, prince's pine, spotted wintergreen,* or *wintergreen.*

PIR, *n* postisometric relaxation; a manual resistance technique that is commonly used to treat the neuromuscular segment of a shortened, stiff, or taut muscle.

piracetam (pir'·ə·sē'·təm), *n* nootropic drug that has been used for treating dementia, dyslexia, stroke, vertigo, and sickle-cell anemia.

Piscidia erythrina, *n* See Jamaican dogwood.

pisti (pis·tē), *n* in Ayurveda, a method of medicine preparation in which gems and other minerals are finely ground and macerated in plant juices, then dried into a fine powder.

pitpapra (pit·pä'·prə), *n* Latin name: *Fumaria indica*; parts used: whole plant; uses: in Ayurveda, pacifies kapha and pitta doshas (bitter, light), hepatoprotective, anticonvulsant, anthelmintic, analgesic, antiinflammatory, antipsychotic, antifungal, antiemetic, hypotensive, hypoglycemic, pain relief, diarrhea, fever, influenza, liver conditions, skin conditions, jaundice; precautions: none known. Also called *fumitory, khetpapra,* or *parpata.*

pitta (pit·tä), *n* in Ayurveda, one of the three organizing principles (doshas) responsible for maintaining homeostasis. Formed by a combination of fire and water, pitta is involved in metabolic activities of digestion and biochemical reactions. See also doshas.

pitta sama **(sä·mɔ pit·tə),** *n* in Ayurveda, ama in combination with a pitta imbalance, manifesting as a yellow tongue, loss of thirst, and anorexia. Remedied with bitter and

some pungent herbs. See also ama and pitta.

pitta, alochaka **(ä·lō·chä'·kə pit'·tə),** *n* in Ayurveda, a subdivision of the pitta dosha whose influence is evident in the eyes. It promotes healthy vision; when unbalanced, bloodshot eyes and problems with vision may result. See also doshas.

pitta, bhrajaka **(bhrə'·jə·kə pit'·tə),** *n* in Ayurveda, a subdivision of the pitta dosha the influence of which is evident in the integument. It promotes healthy skin, and imbalance may result in skin conditions such as acne and rashes. See also doshas.

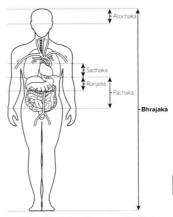

Pitta, bhrajaka. (Sharma and Clarke, 1998)

pitta, pachaka **(pä'·chə·kə),** *n* in Ayurveda, a subdivision of the pitta dosha the influence of which is evident in the stomach and small intestine. It promotes healthy digestion and elimination of ama; when unbalanced, it results in gastric conditions such as heartburn or ulcers. See also doshas.

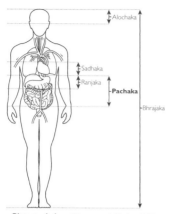

Pitta, pachaka. (Sharma and Clarke, 1998)

pitta, ranjaka (rən'·jə·kə), *n* in Ayurveda, a subdivision of the pitta dosha the influence of which is evident in the liver, spleen, and erythrocytes. It promotes red blood cell formation and balances blood chemistry; and when unbalanced, blood disorders, liver conditions, and anger-management problems result. See also doshas.

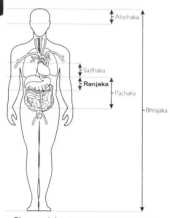

Pitta, ranjaka. (Sharma and Clarke, 1998)

pitta, sadhaka (sä'·dhə·kə), *n* in Ayurveda, a subdivision of the pitta dosha the influence of which is evident in the heart. It promotes emotions and memory; when unbalanced, cardiac disease, memory loss, and depression may result. See also doshas.

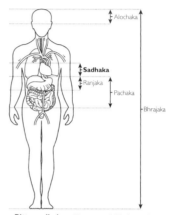

Pitta, sadhaka. (Sharma and Clarke, 1998)

pituitary dysfunction (pi·tōō'·ə·te'·rē dis·funk'·shən), *n* abnormality in the pituitary gland, a part of the endocrine system. See also therapy, craniosacral.

placebo (plə·sē'·bō), *n* **1.** inert substance used in control groups of clinical studies to maintain blinding. **2.** beneficial effects of the meaning and context of treatment independent of the treatment itself. See also meaning effect.

placebo effect, n **1.** the effect of any therapeutic technique that has no objectively determinable action on the illness for which it is prescribed. **2.** the patient's innate healing, defense and survival processes that are elicited through the meaning and context of a treatment.

placebo response, *n* changes in a patient's condition from the meaning and context of the treatment and not from an active agent.

placebo sag, *n* the reduction in the efficacy of a particular placebo therapy due to prolonged absence of an active stimulus.

placebo therapeutics, *n.pl* treatments in which a physician attempts to engage the patient's own healing processes by prescribing physiologically inactive stimuli.

plagiocephaly (plā'·jē·ə·se'·fə·lē), *n* a medical condition occurring in infants; distinguished by the reshaped, flattened, or deformed appearance of the skull. It develops as a result of constant pressure being placed on one area of the thin and flexible skull of the infant. Can be corrected if treated early; techniques involving direct cranial molding often provide the best results.

plaintiff, *n* an aggrieved party who brings a complaint to the civil court system.

plane, *n* any imaginary two dimensional surface.

plane, coronal, *n* See frontal plane.

plane, frontal, *n* imaginary plane passing through the body longitudinally, from side to side, dividing the body into two halves—front and back, or anterior and posterior.

plant gatherers, *n.pl* individuals who collect medicinally beneficial plants to use them in herbal remedies.

plant growers, *n.pl* individuals who cultivate medicinally beneficial plants for use in herbal remedies.

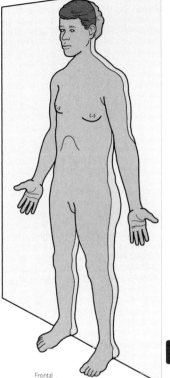

Frontal
(coronal)
plane

Plane, frontal. (Salvo, 2003)

P

plant gums, *n.pl* noncellulose polymers that provide dietary fiber and have laxative properties. Produced by cutting plants and collecting the fluid extract. Used as emulsifiers, stabilizers, and thickeners in food industry.

Plantago lanceolata, *n* See plantain.

Plantago major, *n* See plantain.

Plantago ovata, *n* See psyllium and plantain.

Plantago psyllium, *n* See plantain.

plantain, *n* Latin names: *Plantago lanceolata, Plantago major, Plantago ovata, Plantago psyllium*; parts used: husks, leaves, seeds; uses: bulking laxative, cough, urinary conditions, diarrhea, antiinflammatory; precautions: pregnancy, lactation, children, carbamazepine, cardiac medications, lithium. Also called *blond plantago, broadleaf plantain, buckhorn, cart tract plant, common plantain, English plantain, flea seed, French psyllium, greater plantain, Indian plantago, lanten, narrowleaf plantago seed, plantain seed, ribwort, ripple grass, snakeweed, Spanish psyllium, tract plant, way-bread, white man's foot, wild plantain,* or *wild saso.* Please note that this is not the same plantain as the starchy type of banana of the same name. See also psyllium, blonde and psyllium.

plantar (plan´·ter), *adj* pertaining to the sole of the foot.

plantas medicinales (plän´·täs me¹·dē·sē·nä´·les), *n.pl* in Curanderismo, the Mexican-American healing system, the medicinal herbs.

plaques, *n.pl* **1.** brain lesions found within the vacant areas between nerve cells. **2.** deposits of cholesterol in artery walls that characterize arteriosclerosis.

plasma fatty acid profile, *n* an analysis of the fatty acids present in the bloodstream.

plasters, *n.pl* cloth dressings saturated with medicinal substances, placed over skin for rubefacient or analgesic treatments.

plastic deformation, *n* any irreversible deformation of tissues.

plasticity, *n* **1.** the correlation between the physical structure of an object and the way it moves. **2.** the ability of a tissue or organism to change and adapt.

PLB, *n* pursed-lips breathing; an osteopathic manipulative therapy technique that improves lung condition and breathing efficiency by increasing the use of the diaphragm. With lips pursed, the dominant hand resting on the stomach and the weaker hand on the chest, the patient inhales through the nose and exhales through the mouth.

pleura (pler´·ə), *n* one of the two thin, serous membranes that comprise a singular layer of flat mesothelial cells that encloses and lines the lungs. The outer layer, the parietal pleura encases the diaphragm and lines the wall of the chest. The inner layer, the visceral pleura, encases the lungs. Minute amounts of fluid are present between the two layers and serve as a lubricant while the lungs contract and expand during respiration.

pleurisy (pler´·ə·sē), *n* inflammatory condition of the pleural membranes marked by stabbing pain during inspiration. Possible causes include pneumonia, viral infections, cancer, tuberculosis, and other conditions.

pleuritis (plə·rī´·tis), *n* condition characterized by inflammation of the membrane that surrounds the lungs. Also called *pleuritic chest pain.* See also pleurisy.

Plumbago zeylanica, *n* See white leadwort.

pluralist prescribing (ple´·rə·list pri·skrī´·bing), *n* homeopathic practice, popular in France, Germany, and Italy, of prescribing at least two remedies to be given concurrently or alternately to treat two or more aspects of a condition at the same time.

plussing, *n* the procedure of additional dilutions for supplemental doses of a remedy. This procedure is thought to reduce the negative consequences and augment the potency of the given remedy. See also potency, LM; dynamisation; potentization; and succussion.

PMF, *n.pr* See proprioceptive neuromuscular facilitation.

pneuma (nōō´·mə), *n* πνευμα, the ancient Greek word for vital energy, usually translated as *breath* or *soul.* See also ki, odic force, qi, and vis medicatrix naturae.

***Pneumococcus* (nōō´·mō·kô·kəs),** *n* a pathogenic bacterium often found in the lungs and upper respiratory tract.

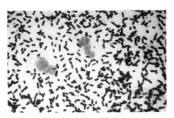

Pneumococcus. (Stone and Gorbach, 2000)

pneumonia (nə·mōn´·yə), *n* infection of the alveoli most often caused by *Streptococcus pneumoniae*, but other infectious agents can be responsible.

Type	Percentage
Viral	20
(influenza)	(3)
Mycoplasmal	10-20
Bacterial	12
Bacterial superimposed on viral	6
Chlamydia	10
Unknown cause (legionnaires' toxic)	38

Pneumonia. (Pizzorno and Murray, 1999)

pneumotaxic center (nōō´·mō·taks´·ik sen´·ter), *n* a region in the pons that regulates the quantity of air inhaled with each breath.

pneumothorax (nōō´·mō·thō´·raks), *n* an abnormal condition characterized by the buildup of air within the space between the lungs and the chest wall; as a result, the lung is unable to expand properly during respiration and eventually collapses because of the increased pressure. Symptoms include chest pain and shortness of breath; although rare, it is a potential complication of acupuncture treatments.

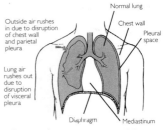

Pneumothorax. (Thibodeau and Patton, 1999; Rolin Graphics)

pneumovax (nōō´·mō·vaks¹), *n* a vaccine for bacterial pneumonia that comprises polysaccharide compounds derived from 23 species of *Pneumococcus* bacteria. Also called *pneumococcal polysaccharide vaccine, pneuomococcal vaccine, pneumococcal vaccine polyvalent, Pneumovax II,* or *Pneumovax 23.*

PNF, *n* proprioceptive neuromuscular facilitation, a manual resistance technique that works by simulating fundamental patterns of movement, such as swimming, throwing, running, or climbing. Methods used in PNF oppose motion in multiple planes concurrently. Initially used for stroke victims and children with cerebral palsy, it is now commonly used to treat a broad range of orthopedic conditions.

po (pô), *n* in Chinese medicine, one of the five spirits, housed by the lung and translated as *corporeal soul.* Po is related to the body's capacity for movement, coordination, and physical sensation and is understood to be closely linked to the essence or foundation principle. See also five spirits.

Podophyllum peltatum, *n* See mayapple.

podophyllum resin (pô¹·də·fi´·ləm re´·zən), *n* powdered mixture of resins derived from podophyllum; used to treat papillomas and other epitheliomas. See also mandrake and mayapple.

point, *n* **1.** in acupuncture, a place where the channels run near the surface of the body. These points are stimulated by acupuncture theory and experience. **2.** a location defined by a set of coordinates along a line.

point, boiling, *n* the temperature at which liquid changes to a gas at atmospheric pressure; the temperature at which a liquid boils.

point, distal (dis´·təl point´), *n* **1.** a point on the body away from the center. **2.** a referred or nearby area of pain, (as opposed to the primary, or most painful area) that acupressurists apply deep pressure to in order to release the tension.

point, extrameridian, *n* in acupuncture, a point that does not fall on a channel.

point, flash, *n* the lowest temperature at which the vapor of a liquid is flammable. Typical flash point values for essential oils are between 33° C and 77° C.

point, injection (in·jek´·shən point´), *n* the site on a gas-liquid chromatograph in which small amount of sample material being analyzed is introduced. See also gas-liquid chromatography.

point, local, *n* in acupressure, the area of acute pain.

point, melting, *n* the temperature at which a substance under normal atmospheric pressure changes from a solid phase to a liquid phase.

point, motor, *n* the muscle entry point for the motor nerve which innervates it.

point, nei guan (nā gwän point), *n* acupuncture point located just above the inner wrist; useful in the treatment of nausea and vomiting. Also called *P6* and *"inner gate."*

point, sedation, *n* area of an acupuncture meridian that induces sedation when stimulated by the insertion of a fine needle.

point, singular, *n* a place in which minute variation in one specification causes enormous change in another.

point, source, *n* area of an acupuncture meridian that activates the entire meridian.

point, still, *n* in craniosacral therapy, a short interruption in the rhythm created through fluctuation of the cerebrospinal fluid, achieved when tension of membranes or ligaments

has been balanced. See also therapy, craniosacral.

point, tonification, *n* area in an acupuncture meridian that stimulates the meridian when a filiform needle is inserted into it.

point, trigger, *n* hypersensitive spot on the body that responds to stimulation by reflexively producing pain or an other manifestation.

point, wei, *n* one of a family of acupuncture points that are stimulated when energy stimulation is needed.

points, ah shi (ä shē points), *n* points other than the classical acupuncture points that could become sensitive during illness and that could be needled to bring relief. Also called *oh yes! points.* See also points, trigger.

points,   akabane   (ä·kä·bä´·nā points), *n.pl* key points used in traditional acupuncture that are located along the toes and fingers and are considered the terminal points of the body's   meridians.   Any   marked sensitivity in these points indicates a presence of energy imbalance and dysfunction.

points, alarm, *n.pl* diagnostic and treatment tools in acupressure. Painful areas on the chest and abdomen that signify that associated organs are out of balance. Also called *front collecting points* or *mo points.*

points, Bennett's neurovascular, *n.pl* See neurovascular (NV) reflex points.

points, clearance, *n.pl* points generally positioned away from the center of the body that a practitioner can palpate to identify tension, tautness, vacancy, tenderness, or nonresilience and diagnose bodily dysfunctions.

points, command, *n.pl* special acupoints that lie on the extremities, specifically between the fingers and elbows and the toes and knees that are known for their influence over the whole body and the flow of qi. See also acupoints, acupressure, acupuncture, and qi.

points, great, *n.pl* acupoints on each meridian believed to be particularly efficacious in manipulating energy. See also acupoints, acupressure, acupuncture, meridians, and qi.

points, hypersensitive acupuncture (hī'·per·sen'·si·tiv a'·kyōō·punk'·chər), *n.pl* acupuncture sites on the body that are so sensitive to pain that needle insertion is impossible.

points, Jones tender, *n.pl* small, inconspicuous areas located throughout the body, which serve as sensory indications of a somatic disturbance or dysfunction. The system of evaluation that uses these regions as reference guides was discovered and developed by Lawrence Jones, DO. Dr. Jones also developed the strain/counterstrain or SCS approach as a method of correcting these dysfunctions. See also SCS.

points, latent, *n.pl* acupuncture points on the body that are healthy and do not present any indications of point pathology.

points, mu (mōō points), *n.pl* in medical acupuncture, reflex points located on the anterior side of the body, used for diagnostic and therapeutic purposes. Each is located on top of the organ for which it is named (e.g., the gallbladder or lung). All except two are found on the abdomen or chest. These two are located on the eleventh and twelfth rib and correspond with the kidney and spleen. Also called *alarm points.*

points, myofascial trigger (mī'·ō·fā'·shē·əl tri'·ger points'), *n.pl* areas of tenderness and spasm within tight bands of skeletal muscle.

points, neurovascular (NV) reflex (ner'·ō·vas'·kyə·ler rē'·fleks points'), *n.pl* numerous points situated all over the anterior side of the body that are used by a practitioner to

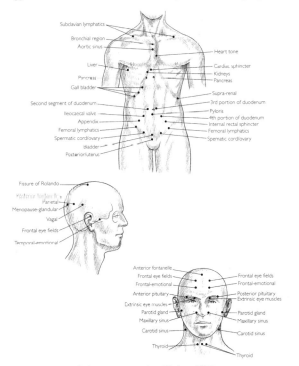

Points, neurovascular. (Chaitow, 2003)

indicate a specific diagnosis, impact functions of specific muscles, or relieve symptoms. The practitioner locates these points while performing neuromuscular techniques on the abdomen. If active, these regions will have an increased sensitivity to light pressure.

points, passive, *n.pl* points that exhibit tenderness upon application of mechanical stimulation techniques like palpation.

points, sishencong (shē·sən·tsông points), *n.pl* four acupuncture points, grouped on the most superior aspect of the scalp; useful for tranquilizing the mind and regulating the central nervous system to encourage sleep.

points, tender, *n.pl* hypersensitive points in the muscles and fascia.

points, trigger, *n.pl* tender areas localized to a specific region of the body that is able to transmit sensations of pain into a "target" tissue. Pressure can also bring about painful sensations. These areas can be located in any soft tissues, particularly fascia and/or muscle, and are described as either "active" or "latent." Palpation may be necessary to locate individual areas of tenderness.

poise, *n* in the Alexander technique, the term given to the expansive movement resulting from practice of the technique. See also technique, Alexander.

pokeweed, *n* Latin name: *Phytolacca americana*; parts used: fruit, leaves, stems, roots; uses: laxative, emetic, rheumatism, pruritus, upper respiratory ailments, antifungal, antiviral, antitumor; precautions: pregnancy, lactation, children, ulcers (stomach and duodenal), possible toxicity; known to cause respiratory depression, coma, and death. Also called *cancer jalap, cancer root, changras, coakum, crowberry, garget, pigeonberry, pocon, pokeberry, poke salad, redink plant, redwood, scoke, txiu kub nyug,* or *Virginia poke.*

polarimeter (pō'·lə·ri'·mə·ter), *n* an instrument used to measure optical rotation of a translucent solid or liquid.

polarity, *n* an eclectic, holistic therapy developed by Randoll Stone, based on traditional Asian health care systems. The polarity practitioner determines the energy imbalance in an individual and restores balance to the energy poles in the body with gentle techniques including gentle rocking, stretching, and touch.

polarity agent effect, *n* a resonance property of permanent magnets achieved by mixing various metals, namely copper, silver, gold, among others believed to have clinical benefits.

polarity tea (pō'·lar'·i·tē tē'), *n* tea made from fennel, fenugreek, flax, licorice, and peppermint boiled briefly in water that is used in polarity therapy. Also called *PolariTea.* See also therapy, polarity.

polarization, *n* a process wherein the direction of electromagnetic radiation or light is limited to a particular plane.

polarized light, *n* electromagnetic radiation within the range of visible light that has a specific plane of polarization.

policosanol (pō'·lē·kō'·sə·nôl), *n* a waxy derivative of sugar cane or beeswax. Has been used to reduce cholesterol levels, to treat intermittent claudication, to enhance athletic performance, and as a possible adjunct in treating Parkinson's disease. Caution is advised for patients taking antiplatelet medications, anticoagulants, levodopa, and nitroprusside. See also octacosanol.

pollenosis, *n* See hay fever.

polychrest, *n* homeopathic remedy (i.e., Arnica, belladonna, calcarea carbonica, and sulphur) with extensive assortment of uses to treat a variety of illnesses. See also remedy, major; remedy, minor; and medicines, status of.

Polygala senega, *n* See senega.

***Polygala* spp. (pə·li'·gə·lə),** *n* part used: root; uses: increase bronchial secretions, antibacterial, break down red blood corpuscles to separate hemoglobin, uterine stimulant, promotion of menstrual flow, nervousness, antiinflammatory, cramps or convulsions, blood pressure; precautions: gastritis, gastric ulcers. Also called *yuan zhi.*

Polygonum aviculare, *n* See wireweed.

Polygonum bistorta, *n* See bistort.

Polygonum multiflorum (pə·li˙·gə·nəm məl·tē·flō˙·rəm), *n* parts used: root, stem, leaves, extracts; uses: antibacterial, anticholesterolemic, antipyretic, muscle relaxant, softening of irritated tissue, removal of obstruction from natural ducts within body, hypoglycemic, antitumor activity, gentle stimulation of bowel movements, sedative, virility, vitality, elimination of toxins, menstrual dysfunction, menopausal symptoms, swollen lymph glands, promotion of wound healing, tonify liver and kidneys, fortify blood, strengthen muscles, prevent premature greying of hair, insomnia, relieve neurasthenia; precautions: rheumatism, arthritis, gout, kidney stones, skin irritation, photosensitivity, mineral deficiency, and hepatitis; may produce numbness in the extremities. Also called *ho chou wu, ho shou wu, she chien ts'ao, turu-dokudami,* and *he shou wu.*

polymenorrhea (pô˙·lē·me·nō·rē˙·ə), *n* disorder in which menstrual cycles are abnormally frequent and brief in duration.

polymer (pö˙·lə·mer), *n* compound that comprises several repeating units of monomers. See also monomer.

polymyalgia rheumatica (pô˙·lē·mī˙·al˙jē·ə roo·ma˙·ti·kə), *n* a condition in older patients whose symptoms include quick onset of pain or loss of motion in the shoulder or pelvic region, anemia, fever, weight loss, and malaise. Elevated erythrocyte sedimentation rate accompanies the symptoms. See also erythrocyte sedimentation rate.

polymyositis (pö˙·lē·mī˙·ə·sī˙·tis), *n* an inflammatory condition that involves multiple muscles accompanied by edema, deformity, pain, insomnia, tension, and sweating.

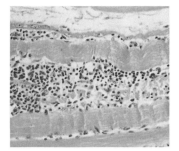

Polymyositis.

polyneuritis (pö˙·lē·nə·rī˙·tis), *n* an inflammatory condition that involves multiple nerves.

polypharmacy, *n* the practice of prescribing multiple drugs to patients suffering from more than one malady.

polypragmasy (pô˙·lē·prag˙·mə·sē), *n* application of multiple remedies simultaneously. See also homeopathy, pluralist, and polypharmacy.

polysaccharide krestin (PSK) (pô˙·lē·sa˙·kə·rīd kres˙·tin), *n* polysaccharide used in cancer treatment. PSK consists primarily of glucan with tightly bound protein extracted from the mushroom *Coriolus versicolor,* (f. Basidiomycetes).

polyunsaturated, *n* a chemical compound that comprises at least one double or triple bond. Vegetable oils and some vitamins are polyunsaturated.

polyvalent action (pô˙·lē·vā˙·lənt ak˙·shən), *n* an element's ability to combine with two or more atoms.

pomade (pō·mād˙), *n* a substance that comprises the fat that contains fragrant materials produced by enfleurage.

pomegranate, *n* Latin name: *Punica granatum*; parts used: bark, fruit, peel, roots, stem; uses: antibacterial, anthelmintic, abortifacient, diarrhea, hemorrhoids, sore throat, antimicrobial, diabetes; precautions: abortifacient, pregnancy, lactation, children, liver disease, asthma, carcinogenic, overdose can be fatal. Also called *granatum.*

P

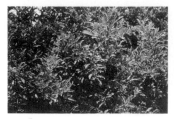

Pomegranate. (Williamson, 2002)

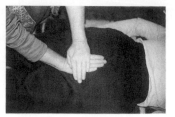

Position, T-hold. (Coughlin, 2002)

poplar, *n* Latin names: *Populus alba, Populus termuloides, Populus nigra*; part used: bark; uses: arthritis, diarrhea, urinary infections, colds, gastrointestinal complaints; precautions: pregnancy, lactation, children younger than twelve, asthma, coagulation disorders, anticoagulant disorders, salicylate sensitivity, nasal polyps, hepatoxicity. Also called *American aspen, black poplar, quaking aspen,* or *white poplar.*

poppy, *n* Latin names: *Papaver somniferum, Papaver bracteatum*; part used: seeds; uses: diarrhea, sedative, antitussive, smooth muscle relaxant; analgesic; precautions: pregnancy, lactation, children, addiction, CNS depression, respiratory depression, overdose. Also called *great scarlet poppy, opium poppy, poppyseed,* or *thebaine poppy.*

popular health care, *n* wide array of home remedies popularized through general interest magazines and television talk shows. Examples include treating a cold with chicken soup or treating a bladder infection with cranberry juice.

Populus alba, n See poplar.

Populus nigra, n See poplar.

Populus termuloides, n See poplar.

position, T-hold, *n* in reiki treatments, the therapist's hand arrangement forms a letter T with the lower hand's fingertips on the client's coccyx and palm on rectum, while the other hand lies adjacent and on top of the first hand, pressing down on the knuckles of the foundation hand.

positional isomer (pə·zi′·shə·nəl ī′·sə·mer), *n* one of two or more compounds with identical chemical composition but having a different functional group location. See also isomerism.

positional release variations, *n. pl* methods used to relieve pain and ease acute musculoskeletal dysfunction.

positional treatment, *n* an osteopathic technique in which a fulcrum, leverage, and ventilatory movements are used to effect mobilization of dysfunctional body segments.

positioning for comfort, *n* a technique developed to ease the treatment of preverbal pediatric patients; a secure physical contact between the child and attending caregiver is established before a potentially painful procedure is undertaken by the physician, thereby limiting patient mobility and promoting relaxation.

positive interactions, *n.pl* **1.** consequences occurring when multiple substances taken concurrently complement each other, for example, when one nutrient supplement alleviates a deficiency created by another medication or supplement. **2.** interpersonal situations characterized by caring, kindness, respect, and trust.

positivism, *n* the notion that all desired information can be obtained through data that are physically measurable.

positron emission tomography (PET) (pô′·zi·trôn ē·mi′·shən tə·mô′·grə·fē), *n* diagnostic exam in which physiologic images are acquired by detecting subatomic particles emitted from a radioactive substance, administered to the patient before the scan. Also known as *PET imaging* or *PET scan.*

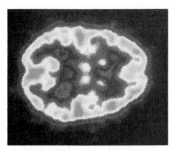

Positron emission tomography (PET). (Black, Hawks, and Keene, 2001)

posology (pō·sô·'·lə·gē), *n* the study of dosage quantity and prescription. See also dosage and effective dose.

post–antibiotic era, *n* refers to a time when a number of infectious diseases will be unresponsive to antibiotic treatments.

postcoital contraception, *n* various contraceptive methods used by women to prevent pregnancy after unprotected sex. Examples include hormone-based treatments, RU-486 (a synthetic steroid), and copper IUDs. Also called *emergency postcoital contraception* or *morning-after pills.*

posterior component, *n* a description of the position of one side of a vertebra after it has rotated. In left rotation of the spine, the anterior component is the left side and vice versa.

posthypnotic suggestion, *n* technique used during a hypnotic session to control the future behavior of the patient. The patient may be directed to act in a particular way under a given set of circumstances. See also hypnosis.

postsuggestion component (pōst·'sug·jes·'chən kəm·pō·'nənt),

n the post-session continuation of behaviors and/or goals introduced during the suggestion phase of hypnosis. See also hypnosis.

postural analysis (pôs·'·chər·əl ə·nal'·ə·sis), *n* in chiropractic, the process of evaluating a patient's positioning of his or her body and limbs to determine directly observable physical abnormalities.

postural balance, *n* optimally distributed body mass relative to the force of gravity.

postural decompensation, *n* the nonoptimal distribution of body mass resulting from the maladaptation of the mechanisms of postural homeostasis.

postural imbalance, *n* any condition wherein optimal distribution of body mass is not achieved or maintained.

posture, *n* body mass distribution in relation to the force of gravity.

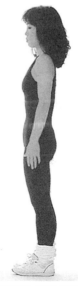

Posture. (Aloia, 1993)

potassium, *n* an element/mineral that acts as an electrolyte and functions in nerve signal transmission, muscle contraction, blood pressure regulation, and maintenance of pH balance. Side effects of potassium deficiency include cardiac arrhythmia, diarrhea, moodiness, nausea, and weakness. Dietary sources include animal products, beans, lentils, peas, squash, watermelons, raisins, bananas, and spinach.

potence, *n* the intangible agent with the ability to alter the biological condition of an organism.

potency, **1.** a measure of the efficacy of a substance or treatment. **2.** the dilution levels of homeopathic remedies.

potency complex, *n* a homeopathic remedy with more than one potency of the same medicine in dosage form. Also called *potency chord.*

potency energy, *n* the energetic field of a homeopathic remedy that theoretically resonates with the life force of the recipient.

potency homeocord, *n* in homeopathy, a combination of more than one attenuation of the same remedy in a single preparation. Also known as *potency spectrum.*

potency, centesimal, *n* one part source material combined with 99 parts liquid suspension medium. This relationship is denoted as "c" for the potency or as "cH" for Hahnemannian potency; created using Hahnemann's method of trituration. This is then serially diluted by vigorous shaking in ratios of 1:99. The relative amounts of the liquid and the source material vary depending on which pharmacopeia is used. Dilutions of 1/10,000 are 2c or 2cH, 1/1,000,000 are 3c or 3cH and so on. See also trituration, centesimal; potency, LM; potency, millesimal; and potency scale.

potency, cH, *n.pr* See potency, centesimal or potency, Hahnemannian.

potency, cK, *n* Korsakov method used to prepare a centesimal potency. See also potency, cH; potency scales; and potency, Korsakov.

potency, D, *n.pr* See potency, decimal.

potency, decimal, *n* one-part source material or the previous solution diluted with nine parts liquid suspension medium. The resulting solutions are vigorously shaken and serial dilutions repeated. This relationship is denoted as x or D. The relative amounts of the liquid and the source material vary depending on which pharmacopeia is used. Dilutions of 1/100 are 2× or D2; 1/1000 are 3× or D3 and so on. Also called *DH potency* and *x potency.* See also potency, D; potency, centesimal; potency, Hahnemannian; potency, millesimal; serial dilution; and potency scale.

potency, destruction of, *n* the neutralization of healing power of a homeopathic remedy. Contributing conditions during storage or creation of the remedy, such as heating, improper dilutents; may cause partial or complete loss of the remedy's effect. Also called *inhibition of potency.* See also antidote and drug, stability of.

potency, DH, *n.pr* See potency, decimal.

potency, fifty millesimal, *n* See potency, LM.

potency, Hahnemannian, *n.pr* Hahneman's technique for the creation of homeopathic remedies which involves serial dilution of one part of the preparation from the previous step in the process with a predetermined number of parts of dilutent in a new, clean glass receptacle (1 to 9 or 1 to 49,999 for example), which is then vigorously agitated. Repeated as desired with a new clean glass receptacle each time. See also fluxion; potency, Korsakov; potency, LM; method, multiglass; and method, single glass.

potency, high, *n* preparation usually above 30c or 12c or 9c potency depending on the country or remedy. The difference between high, medium, and low potencies is subject to debate. See also potency, medium; potency, low; and potency scale.

potency, Korsakov, *n.pr* process designed by Korsakov to produce a potency using only one glass receptacle. The initial potency is created and the liquid is either sucked out or poured out of the glass leaving only the droplets stuck to the sides of the container, which form the basis for the following serial dilutions. See also method, single glass; potency, cK; and potency, millesimal.

potency, liquid, *n* a homeopathic remedy given in liquid form.

potency, LM, *n.pr* homeopathic method of preparing remedies, in which one part source material or the previous solution is diluted with 49,999 parts liquid suspension medium. The resulting solutions are vigorously shaken and serial dilutions repeated. Believed to be effective in curing disease without causing therapeutic aggravation. Also called *Q potency* and *x potency.* See also potency, Hahnemannian; potency, Korsakov; potency, millesimal; and plussing.

potency, low, *n* in homeopathy, a preparation usually below 24c or 12c potency.

potency, M, *n.pr* See potency, millesimal.

potency, medicating, *n* fluid potency poured on sugar cube or other solid or vehicles for the remedy.

potency, medium, *n* preparation usually between 12c to 30c potency. In some countries, the range may be lower.

potency, millesimal, *n* a 1 to 999 dilution most commonly made using the single-glass Korsakov process, often commencing with an initial C3 trituration. This produces an inexact remedy and the process is not widely accepted. See also potency, Korsakov and trituration, C3.

potency, Q, *n.pr* See potency, LM.

Potentilla anserina, *n* See silverweed.

Potentilla erecta L, *n* See tormentil.

Potentilla tormentilla, *n* See tormentil.

potentization, *n* in homeopathy, the progressive process of diluting and succusing the remedy.

pouce, *n* See cun.

poultice (pōl'·tis), *n* herbal matter that is wrapped in a soft cloth and moistened for topical application.

powder, *n* in homeopathy, a dosage form, often lactose, that has had a small amount of homeopathic remedy poured on it. This powder can then be consumed by the patient.

power analysis, *n* statistical technique used to determine the number of subjects required to detect differences between experimental or control groups.

power objects, *n.pl* **I.** in shamanic traditions, natural objects such as stones or bones that are imbued with sacred meaning or power. **2.** according to the Pima Indian healing system, items such as roadrunners, buzzard feathers, and jimson weed, which are considered sacred. Nonrespect can lead to sickness known as staying sickness. See also staying sickness.

power sickness (paw'·er sik'·nǝs), *n* in Native American medicine, a condition that occurs when a spiritual power possesses a person who is ill, in distress, or needs to be initiated to a higher level of being. The spirit manifests in the form of fainting spells, restlessness, heavy breathing, or crying that cannot be controlled. Through the initiation of song, dance and ceremony, the affected person is taught to "bring out" the spiritual power.

practitioner, *n* a healthcare povider.

pragya-aparadh (prä'·gyǝ-ä·pǝ·rädh'), *n* in Ayurveda, the mind's error, results from the loss of unity of consciousness—of rishi, devata, and chhandas—manifested in the form of memory loss and ill health. Reversal of this error leads to overall well-being. See also rishi, devata, and chhandas.

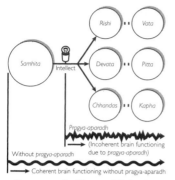

Pragya-aparadh. (Sharma and Clarke, 1998)

prakruti (prä·krŏŏ'·tē), *n* in Ayurveda, an individual's distinctive constitution. According to Ayurvedic principles, to live a lifestyle that is preventive and proper, it is vital to understand one's unique nature and the means of maintaining equilibrium despite stress and challenge.

prana (prä·nə), *n* vital energy as articulated in the spiritual and healing systems of India. Similar to the Chinese qi, the Japanese ki, and the Greek pneuma. See also ki, Odic force, pneuma, qi, and vital force.

pranavahasrotas (prä'·nä·vä'·häs·rō'·təs), *n.pl* in Ayurveda, one of the 13 srotas, or channels of the body, the function of which is to carry vital breath (prana) throughout the body. They originate in the alimentary tract and heart. See also srotas.

pranayama (prä'·nə·yä·mə), *n* in Ayurveda, the yogic art of breathing that is believed to unify an individual's consciousness with the universal consciousness rendering multiple health benefits for mind and body.

prashnam (präsh'·nəm), *n* in Ayurveda, questioning or inquiry; it provides a fundamental basis for the eight classical markers—urine, pulse, tongue, feces, voice and speech; assessment of the eyes, evaluation by touch, and general physical assessment used throughout the examination process. See also darshanam and sparshanam.

pratyahara (prä'·tyə·hä'·rə), *n* to withdraw or restrain; the practice of controlling one's senses, one of the eight limbs or paths of Patanjali yoga aimed at self-realization and self-knowledge. See also yama, niyama, asana, pranayama, dharana, dhyana, and samadhi.

prayer, *n* communication with the spiritual or ultimate reality, which may be understood as transcendent or immanent, and described in theistic or nontheistic terms.

prayer, conversational, *n* type of prayer, in which one speaks like a friend to one's god, sharing problems, thoughts, feelings, and concerns.

prayer, directed, *n* a prayer in which a specific effect or goal is expected and requested.

prayer, intercessory, *n* a variation of petitionary prayer, in which the individual praying makes a request on behalf of someone else.

prayer, meditative, *n* type of prayer, in which one focuses on a word, phrase, or sound to still the mind or to allow one to listen for the "still, small voice" of the divine. Also called *centering prayer, contemplation, contemplative prayer,* or *listening prayer.* See also mantra and meditation.

prayer, petitionary, *n* type of prayer, in which one makes a request of one's god.

prayer, ritualistic, *n* type of prayer, in which one repeats standardized prayers as an established part of one's specific spiritual traditions.

prebiotics (prē·bī·ô'·tiks), *n.pl* nondigestible food components that support overall health by promoting the activity of probiotic bacteria in the large intestine. Also called *oligosaccharides.*

precipitating factor, *n* the catalyst for an illness, symptom, or episode. This may not be the underlying cause of the illness, rather it is what elicits it. Also called *provoking factor.* See also aggravation, modality, and therapeutic aggravation.

preclinical studies, *n.pl* a term used to describe research done before a clinical study. May be laboratory or epidemiologic research.

preclinical toxicology (prē′·kli··ni·kəl tôks′·ə·kô′·lə·jē), *n* studies of the toxicology of a substance on animals and cells to prepare parameters for Phase I human subject clinical studies. These include determination of acute, subacute, and chronic toxicity, carcinogenicity, mutagenicity, teratogenicity, and effects on the reproductive system.

predigestion, *n* a method for preparing glandular extracts in which the glandular material is partially digested or hydrolyzed by using plant or animal enzymes and then filtered to separate fat-soluble and large molecules followed by freeze-drying the purified material.

predisposing cause, *n* any one of the factors that contribute to susceptibility to a disease by weakening the body's ability to defend itself, such as stress and dietary deficiencies.

pregnancy, *n* the gestational process that lasts approximately forty weeks in humans, during which a fertilized egg develops into a distinct individual within the mother's uterus.

pregnenolone (preg·ne′·nə·lōn), *n* a precursor to steroid hormones that is synthesized (endogenously) from cholesterol or (exogenously) from soybeans. Has been used in a host of conditions including Alzheimer's disease, menopausal complaints, Parkinson's disease, osteoporosis, fatigue, stress, memory loss, and other conditions. May interact with the use of supplemental steroid hormones.

premorbid conditions, *n.pl* conditions preceding the onset of disease.

prescribing strategy, *n* approach to disease treatment that considers the homeopathic remedies, their order of application, and the reasoning behind those selections. See also remedies, alternating; homeopathy, classical; homeopathy, complex; homeopathy, pluralist; second prescription; and homeopathy, unicist.

prescription (pri·skrip′·shən), *n* a written directive by an authorized person (e.g., a medical doctor) to an authorized agent (a pharmacist) to dispense a medication, device, or therapy to a specific patient for a specified period of time.

prescriptive dietetics (pri·skrip′·tiv dī·ə·te′·tiks), *n* the use of certain diets and foods designed for specific diseases in which the combination of foods is customized to fit the individual needs of the patient.

presence, *n* **1.** a state of fully being in the present moment. Thought to be important in many healing practices that cultivate a "healing presence" of depth. **2.** in holistic nursing, a perception of consciously "being with" a client in an emotional and psychologic sense. One of the three principal concepts of holistic nursing, it lets the holistic nurse guide a patient into revealing personal stories. The purpose of this exercise is to facilitate the process of the client's discovery regarding new health choices and behaviors, meaning and purpose within life, and insights into effective ways to cope. As a result, the holistic nurse is able to make a more accurate diagnosis and prescribe an appropriate therapeutic approach.

presenting problem, *n* initial symptom motivating the patient to consult a practitioner. See also anamnesis; symptom, guiding; and symptom, keynote.

preservation, *n* something that maintains the potency of a remedy or herb. An example of this would be using alcohol along with water.

preservatives, *n.pl* food additives that hinder spoilage by reducing the growth of microorganisms. Include nitrates and nitrites, benzoates and sulfites, and many others.

pressing and pushing, *n* pressing implies compacting an area, while pushing literally involves moving something from one place to another, no matter how small the distance. Both are variations of compression techniques used in manual therapy.

pressure bars, *n* in manipulation therapy, a tool used by a practitioner to safeguard thumbs from an excessive amount of pressure and facilitate access to crevices that may be difficult to reach with thumbs alone.

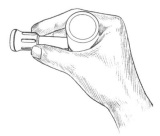

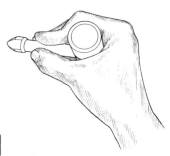

Pressure bars. (Chaitow, 2003)

pressurestat (pre'·sher·stät'), *n* model developed by John E. Upledger, according to which, a sound craniosacral system is important for normal body functioning.

preste (pre'·ste), *n* a festive ceremony performed in the Kallawaya system of healing practiced in Bolivia, to offer the assistance of a group to a person afflicted with disease, used especially for treating susto. See also susto.

presuggestion component (prē'·sug·jes'·chən kəm·pō'·nənt), *n* the use of imagery and relaxation to focus attention and induce hypnotic suggestibility. See also hypnosis.

prevention, *n* the management of those factors that could lead to disease so as to prevent the occurrence of the disease.

prickly ash, *n* Latin names: *Zanthoxylum americanum, Zanthoxylum clavaherculis*; part used: bark; uses: flatulence, fevers, circulatory conditions, antiinflammatory; precautions: pregnancy, lactation, children, ulcers (peptic and duodenal), gastrointestinal inflammation, anticoagulant medications. Also called *angelica tree, Hercules' club, northern prickly ash, southern prickly ash, suterberry, toothache tree,* or *yellow wood.*

prima facie (prī'·mə fā'·shē), *n* at first site; the minimum amount of evidence required from one party that compels another party to defend itself in court.

Primary Care Certificate in Homeotherapeutics (prī'·me·rē ker' ser·ti'·fi·kit in hō'·mē·ō·the'·rə·pyōō'·tiks), *n.pr* a designation granted to medical and osteopathic doctors of homeopathy by the American Board of Homeotherapeutics. To receive this certification, a homeopathic physician is required to complete between 60 and 100 hours of training in homeotherapeutics, and pass an oral and a written exam.

primary care physician, *n* the first medical doctor a patient will seek for care. A specialist for general conditions.

primary care trust, *n* an organization legally established in the United Kingdom whose purpose is to develop health services for a particular community.

primary control, *n* in the Alexander technique, the innate relationship of the head, neck, and spine to poise and balance. See also technique, Alexander.

primary drug action, *n* the initial influence of a medicine on a person. See also secondary drug action, taxic drug action, biphasic activity, and therapeutic aggravation.

primary machinery of life, *n* a term coined by physiologist IM Korr to describe the neuromusculoskeletal system that he believed transmitted and modified the force and motion through which life is lived.

primary respiratory impulse, *n* See cranial rhythmic impulse.

primary somatic dysfunction, *n* **I.** any somatic dysfunction whose existence maintains an entire dys-functional pattern. **2.** the initial somatic dysfunction in a pattern of dysfunction.

prime mover, *n* that muscle which is primarily responsible for producing a particular movement.

Primula elatior, *n* See oil, evening primrose.

Primula veris, *n* See cowslip.

primum non nocere **(prē′·mum nōn′ nô·kā′·rā),** *n* "first do no harm." One of the fundamental principles of medicine according to which the physician should not cause harm to the patient.

principal meridians, *n.pl* in acupuncture, energy channels that pass through the body's muscles and serve as a source for nourishment to all tissues. These channels also provide vitality for physical activity and animation.

principle of infinitesimal dose, *n.pr* in homeopathy, the assertion that the most effective remedies are the most diluted.

principle of similars, *n.pr* in homeopathy, the assertion that a substance known to cause the symptoms of disease will induce a cure of those symptoms if administered in a small amount.

principle of specificity of the individual, *n.pr* in homeopathy, the assertion that treatments must be designed for the specific symptoms of specific individuals and must take into account all of the physical as well as psychologic conditions of the patient.

prior probability, *n* the extent of belief held by a patient and practitioner in the ability of a specific therapeutic approach to produce a positive outcome before treatment begins. This level of belief should be taken into consideration by the patient and practitioner to make a decision as to

whether the treatment should be used or to permit the therapy to continue.

Pritikin longevity programs, *n.pr* residential programs that teach Pritikin diet principles, stress management, and exercise in 1 to 4 week courses.

privity, *n* the association and knowledge between parties engaged in a legal agreement, especially private information pertinent to the relationship and contract.

proanthrocyanadins (prō·an′·thrō· sī·an′·ə·dēnz), *n.pl* antioxidants found in grape seeds, red wine, and maritime pine bark. Has been used in treating venous insufficiency, post-surgical edema, postinjury edema, atherosclerosis, asthma, cirrhosis, smoking-related platelet aggregation, and reduction of cholesterol levels. No known precautions. Also called *PCOs* or *procyanidolic oligomers.* See also pycnogenol.

probiotic (prō′·bī·ô′·tik), *n* **I.** product that simultaneously encourages beneficial bacteria to flourish in the body while hindering the growth of harmful microorganisms. **2.** beneficial bacteria such as Lactobacillus used to colonize the gastrointestinal tract.

procedural learning, *n* term used in the Feldenkrais method; refers to the preverbal stage of knowledge acquisition in which a baby relates to the surroundings in an essentially non-verbal, nonanalytical fashion. See also method, Feldenkrais.

professional herbalist (pro·te′·shə· nəl er′·bə·list), *n* a formally trained individual who has experience in either plant/medical studies or in spiritual healing/plant studies and has extensive knowledge of plants—including identification, preparation, therapeutic uses, precautions, and dosage.

professional homeopath, *n* non-medically trained homeopathic practitioner. See also doctor, lay homeopath, nonmedically qualified practitioner, and primary care physician.

professional misconduct, *n* conduct inappropriate to the practice of health care.

professional touch, *n* skilled healing touch given as part of a professional relationship between a client and therapist.

professionalized systems, *n.pl* medical systems in which practitioners are formally trained and licensed or certified to practice.

progesterone, *n* hormone responsible for preparing for and maintaining pregnancy in females. A drop in progesterone levels can result in spontaneous abortion (miscarriage) or labor and delivery.

progesterone cream (prə·ges′·tə·rōn), *n* a form of the steroid hormone progesterone delivered transdermally in a cream base. Has been used to alleviate menopausal complaints and to help treat osteoporosis. Caution in patients with liver or kidney disease. Also called *natural progesterone.*

prognosis, *n* expected path of the illness.

proinflammatory prostaglandin (PGE2) (prō′·in′·fla·mə·tōr′·ē prô′·stə·glan′·din), *n* an unsaturated fatty acid in the body that causes inflammation.

prolactinemia (prō·lak′·ti·nē′·mē·ə), *n* condition characterized by a deficiency or excess of the hormone prolactin, usually caused by prolactinoma, a benign tumor in the pituitary gland, or hormone replacement therapy.

prolactinoma (prō′·lak·tə·nō′·mə), *n* a noncancerous tumor of the pituitary gland, most often in women, that leads to excess production of prolactin, the hormone responsible for modulating lactation. Also called *secreting adenoma.*

proliferant, *n* a mildly irritating substance used in sclerotherapy to strengthen weakened connective tissues. Also called *Ongley solution.* See also sclerotherapy.

prolotherapy, *n* See sclerotherapy.

pronation, *n* medial rotation of the radioulnar joint to face the palm down.

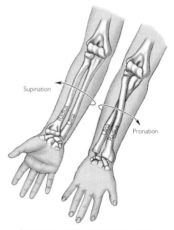

Pronation. (Herlihy and Meabius, 2000)

prone, *n* recumbent face down position.

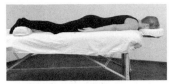

Prone. (Salvo, 2003)

prooxidant (prō·ôk´·sə·dənt), *n* cell oxidation agent.

proper nutrition, *n* in Tibetan medicine, a therapeutic concept that begins with a digestive formulation because it is believed that a medical condition is primarily the result of a nutritional dysfunction or disturbance in the process of delivering nutrients.

prophylactic, *adj* serving to prevent or defend against disease.

prophylactic, *n* **1.** intervention that prevents or defends against disease. **2.** a condom.

prophylactic strategies (prō´·fə·lak´·tik stra´·tə·jēz), *n.pl* **1.** subcategory of prescriptive dietetics and nutritional pharmacology that is intended to prevent genotype related to a disease from expressing itself by selecting certain foods and food preparation methods. **2.** general concept of behavioral and medical approaches meant to prevent disease or its consequences.

propolis (prä´·pə·ləs), *n* a compound made by bees by mixing balsams and resin collected from certain trees with saliva and digestive enzymes. Used for its antioxidant, antiviral, antibacterial, antitumor, and antiinflammatory properties and to promote the healing of wounds.

proprietary product, *n* any medicinal or herbal preparation whose formulation is owned exclusively by an individual or business.

proprioception, *n* the kinesthetic sense. The sense that deals with sensations of body position, posture, balance, and motion.

proprioceptive neural facilitation (prō·prē·ō·sep´·tiv ner´·əl fə´·si·li·tā´·shən), *n* a form of treatment of neuromusculoskeletal dysfunction that uses verbal and visual prompts with manual contact.

proprioceptive neuromuscular facilitation (prō´·prē·ō·sep´·tiv ner´·ō·mus´·kyə·ler fə·si´·li·tā´·shən), *n* techniques designed to call into action the body's receptors that influence relaxation, muscle tone, and muscle lengthening.

proprioceptor, *n* sensory organs located in joint capsules, muscles, and tendons that receive information on posture, body position, and motion and send this information to the central nervous system.

proprioceptors (prō´·prē·ō·sep´·terz), *n.pl* neuromuscular receptors that register stimuli, such as stretch, tonicity, and movement within muscles.

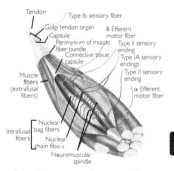

Proprioceptors. (Thibodeau and Patton, 1999; Christine Oleksyk)

proptosis (präp·tō´·səs), *n* a protrusion or bulging of a bodily region or organ, such as the eye.

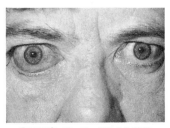

Proptosis. (Kanski and Nischal, 1999)

prostaglandins (prŏ'·stə·glan'· dinz), *n.pl* a family of lipid compounds found in various tissues, associated with muscular contraction and the inflammation response.

prostate, *n* a small doughnut-shaped gland in the pelvis that is a part of the male reproductive system and is responsible for lubricating the urethra with a thin, milky, alkaline fluid (semen), which increases the mobility of sperm and prevents infection.

prosthesis (präs·thē'·sis), *n* **1.** an artificial device that is used to replace a part of the body that is missing, such as an arm, leg, or joint. **2.** an artificial device used to improve the function of a part of the body, such as a hearing aid.

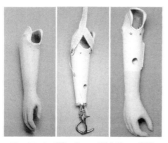

Prosthesis. (Monahan and Neighbors, 1998; Otto Bock Orthopedic Industry, Inc., Minneapolis, MN)

protease inhibitors (prō'·tē·ās in· hi·bi'·terz), *n.pl* a class of drugs used in antiretroviral therapy against HIV, which prevent the cleavage of viral proteins.

protection, *n* **1.** contraceptive barrier which lowers risk of pregnancy or sexually transmitted disease. **2.** in therapeutic touch, the practitioner's ability to guard against receiving negative energy. **3.** protection by a vaccine.

proteins, *n.pl* macromolecules made of up of amino acids joined by peptide linkages and that provide essential life functions. Major sources of dietary proteins include meat, fowl, fish, eggs, beans, seeds, nuts, legumes, and dairy products.

proteolytic enzymes (prō'·tē·ō· li·tik en'·zīmz), *n.pl* enzymes involved in the digestion of proteins; supplemented in cases of pancreatic insufficiency. Have been used for their antiinflammatory, antiedema, immunomodulatory, and fibrinolytic actions, to speed the healing of injuries, to treat herpes zoster, and to relieve the pain and inflammation of osteoarthritis. Caution is advised for patients who are taking anticoagulants or antiplatelet medications. See also bromelain, pancreatin, and trypsin.

proticity (prə·ti'·si·tē), *n* a form of electricity characterized by the flow of protons instead of electrons. Typically generated by the mitochondria of cells.

protobiotics, *n.pl* See probiotic.

proton, *n* positively charged subatomic particle that is located in the nucleus of an atom. Its mass is equivalent to that of a neutron. The number of protons is equivalent to the atomic number.

protopathic sensitivity, *n* the general, deep sensitivity that is the first to return to injured parts of the body. See also epicritic sensitivity.

protraction, *n* forward movement.

prover, *n* a healthy person who takes a homeopathic remedy and then reports its effects. Also called *volunteer.*

provider practice acts, *n.pl* health care provider licensing/certification requirements and scope of practice descriptions enacted through state legislatures.

provings, *n.pl* a method for determining the effects of a homeopathic remedy by giving it to healthy individuals and recording the symptoms.

provisional tolerable weekly intake, *n* the acceptable level of toxic metal that can be ingested on a weekly basis, as determined by the World Health Organization and the Food and Agriculture Organization. Also called *PTWI.*

proximal, *adj* closer to the referent, commonly the trunk or midsagittal plane.

prsthavamsa (prəs·thə·väm'·sə), *n* in Aryuveda, the vertebral column as described in the Atharvaveda. See also Vedas.

Prunus africana, *n* See pygeum.

Prunus persica, *n* See peach.

Prunus serotina, *n* See wild cherry.

Prunus virginiana, *n* See wild cherry.

prurigo (prŏŏ·rī'·gō), *n* a chronic inflammatory condition of the skin distinguished by the presence of several, itchy papules shaped like domes that are topped with small vesicles. Lichenification and crusting may develop as a result of repetitive scratching. A specific drug, allergy, malignancy, parasite, or endocrine abnormality may cause the inflammation.

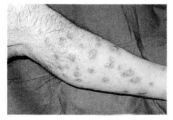

Prurigo. (Lawrence and Cox, 1993)

pruritus (prŏŏ·rī'·tis), *n* itching. An uncomfortable sensation that leads to scratching a portion of the body; caused by infection, allergy, chronic renal disease, jaundice, skin irritation, lymphoma, or other conditions. Treatment is related to the specific cause; starch baths, antihistamines, cool water, topical corticosteroids, or an application of alcohol may relieve symptoms.

pseudoparesis (sŏŏ'·dō·pə·rē'·sis), *n* false paralysis. A psychologic condition in which the patient appears and acts paralyzed.

PSG, *n* polysomnograph; polygraph performed during sleep. Physiological variables such as pulse, blood pressure, and respiration are monitored and charted.

PSIS, *n* posterior superior iliac spine; the hip bones located towards the back of the body.

psoralens (sōr'·ə·lenz), *n.pl* polycyclic molecules with the ability to absorb ultraviolet photons.

psoriasis (sə·rī'·ə·sis), *n* a skin condition marked by a development of red, patchy blemishes and more extensive regions covered with silver-colored scales.

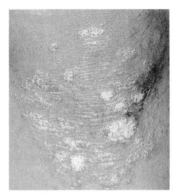

Psoriasis. (Habif, 1996)

psoric miasm (sōr'·lk mī''·a·zəm), *n* in homeopathy, one of the three basic chronic illnesses. Symptoms and susceptibility often characterized by itchy skin. See also miasm, sycotic miasm, syphilitic miasm, itch diathesis, and diathesis.

psyche, *n* nonphysical attributes of a being, such as the soul and the mind. See also life force.

psychedelic, *adj* **1.** pertaining to a mental state distinguished by the presence of hallucinations and an alteration in the sensation of perception. The affected person may also report feelings of fear or euphoria. *adj* **2.** pertaining to a specific substance or drug, such as mescaline; known to produce mood-altering effects.

psychiatry (sī'·kī'·ə·trē), *n* the modern medical specialty that focuses on understanding; diagnosing; and treating emotional, mental, and behavioral dysfunctions or disorders.

psychic body (sī'·kik bô'·dē), *n* the transformed body of energy that is carried by the subtle body and controls and overrides the somatic functions of the physical body.

psychic energy, *n* the subjective force responsible for causing change and motion in the noumenal world. Also called *mental energy.*

psychic force, *n* in psychoanalysis, the libidinous energy of the id. This is regarded as the primary motivating force in the human personality. Also called *psychic energy.*

psychic surgery, *n* a form of psychic healing that involves physical and spiritual surgery, practiced primarily in several indigenous cultures.

psychoanalysis, *n* form of mental and emotional therapy that aims to discover and resolve the causes of conflicts in a client's relationships.

psychoaromatherapy (sī'·kō·ə·rō'· mə·the'·rə·pē), *n* use of fragrances to manipulate mood, with the goal of bringing about an enhanced sense of well-being.

psychoeducational (sī'·kō·ed·jə· kā'·shə·nəl), *adj* adjunct health programs that address stress management and health education.

psychologic hardiness, *n* a predisposition that allows an individual to accept the challenges and changes in life with good humor and resilience, which in turn influences behavior that prevents illness.

psychoneuroimmunology (sī'·kō· ner'·ō·im'·yōō·nô'·lə·gē), *n* the study of the integrated interactions of the immunologic, neurologic, and psychologic systems and their effects on health.

psychopharmaceutical (sī'·kō·fär'· mə·sōō'·ti·kəl), *adj* concerns drugs that affect the mind or emotional state.

psychophysiological self-regulation (sī·kō·fi'·zē·ə·lô·ji·kəl self-re'·gyōō· lā'·shən), *n* in biofeedback therapy, the process by which a patient learns and employs emotional, mental, and physiological skills and strategies to attain self-regulation of internal autonomic states.

psychophysiology (sī'·kō·fi'·zē·ô'· lə·jē), *n* study of the interrelationship between the human body functions and the mind.

psychosis, *n* a mental condition marked by a significant inability of an individual to correctly assess the accuracy of his or her thoughts as well as perceptions. The person may also make erroneous statements about external reality despite the presence of opposing facts. Can be characterized by mood and affect that is not appropriate, regressive behavior, and a decrease in impulse control. Symptoms may also include delusions and hallucinations

psychosocial body, *n* a concept of human existence held by certain shamanic healers and psychotherapists; refers to the individual's mind, emotions, or essence, which interact with the outside world.

psychosocial resources, *n.pl* emotional and cognitive states—including self-esteem, optimism, and self-mastery—that may affect behavior and health.

psychosynthesis (sī'·kō·sin'·thə· sis), *n* an approach in psychology developed by Roberto Assagioli, in which the goal is to help individuals accomplish a fusion of the various parts of their personality into a more cohesive self. A great deal of emphasis is placed on the person's spiritual dimension or higher self as a source of inspiration, wisdom, unconditional love, and meaning in life. Also found in psychosynthesis is the idea that the universe is orderly and structured to promote the evolution of consciousness. Similarly, individual lives have purpose and meaning, and each individual can discover this.

psychotherapy, *n* a family of related treatments for emotional and mental disorders that use psychologic, rather than biologic or pharmacologic methods. Mosby's Medical, Nursing & Allied Health Dictionary, 1430.

psychotropic (sī'·kō·trō'·pik), *adj* concerns drugs that affect the mind and influence behavior.

psyllium (sil'·ē·əm), *n* Latin names: *Plantago ovata, Plantago psyllium,* or *Plantago indica;* parts used: husks, leaves, and seeds; uses: laxative, dietary aid, hypercholesterolemia, urinary tract conditions, and diarrhea; precautions: individuals with intestinal obstruction. May cause vomiting, anorexia, flatus, diarrhea, and bloating. Also called *blond plantago, broadleaf plantain, buckhorn, flea seed, French psyllium, snakeweed, way-bread, white man's foot, wild plantain, lanten,* or *ripple grass.*

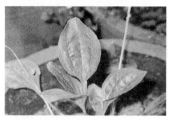

Psyllium, blond. (Williamson, 2002)

PT, *n.pr* See physiotherapy.

pterion (te′·rē·ôn), *n* point of convergence of sutures between the frontal, sphenoid, parietal bones and temporal squama.

puberty, *n* the period of development in which the body becomes physically capable of reproduction, distinguished by the maturity of the gonads and appearance of secondary sexual characteristics.

pubic, *adj* pertaining to the pubic symphysis or the genital region.

pubic compression, *n* a condition in which the pubic bones are constricted in the pubic symphysis, characterized by tenderness at the symphysis, restricted pelvic motion, and an absence of pelvic asymmetry. Also called *pelvic adduction.*

pubic gapping, *n* a condition in which the pubic bones are pulled apart in the pubic symphysis. Also called *pubic abduction.*

pubic hair, *n* hair in the pubic region; secondary sexual characteristic that develops during puberty.

Pueraria lobata, *n* See kudzu.

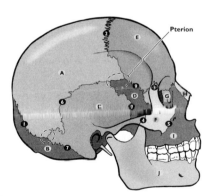

A Parietal bone
B Occipital bone
C Temporal bone
D Sphenoid bone
E Frontal bone
F Zygomatic bone
G Lacrimal
H Nasal
I Maxilla bone
J Mandible bone

❶ Lambdoidal suture
❷ Coronal suture
❸ Fronto-zygomatic suture
❹ Tempoo-zygomatic suture
❺ Zygomatico-maxillary suture
❻ Parieto-temporal suture
❼ Occipito-temporal suture
❽ Spheno-temporal suture
❾ Spheno-frontal suture

Pterion. (Chaitow, 1999)

pulling, *v* **1.** to draw toward oneself. *n* **2.** technique used in massage therapy to stretch and lengthen muscle fibers and to increase elasticity of soft tissues. Also used to assess elasticity and to test rebound response of soft tissues.

Pulmonaria officinalis, *n* See lungwort.

pulmonary embolism, *n* the obstruction of a pulmonary artery due to the presence of air, fat, blood clot, or a tumor. In general, the obstruction originates from a peripheral vein, which is most frequently located in the legs. Symptoms such as labored breathing, shock, chest pain, and cyanosis appear and are similar to those of pneumonia or a myocardial infarction. Also called *PE.*

pulsatilla (pəl·sə·til´·lə), *n* Latin name: *Anemone pulsatilla*; parts used: dried leaves, stems, flowers; uses: diuretic, sedative, insomnia, cough, genitourinary complaints, menstrual complaints, ear infection, eye conditions; precautions: abortifacient, pregnancy, lactation, nephrotoxicity, seizures, toxic—not advised for self-medication. Also called *crowfoot, Easter flower, kubjelle, meadow anemone, meadow windflower, pasque flower, prairie anemone, smell fox, stor,* or *wind flower.*

pulsatilla nigricans (pəl·sə·til´·lə ni´·gri·kanz), *n* a homeopathic preparation of the meadow anemone that is used to treat many conditions, including arthritis, bronchitis, chickenpox, cold, fevers, headaches, measles, mumps, and menstrual disorders. Also called *queen of homeopathic remedies.*

Pulsatilla vulgaris, *n* See meadow windflower.

pulsation, *n* a traditional Chinese medicine in which the practitioner examines the pulse at each wrist in order to make a diagnosis.

pulse reading, *n* in Tibetan medicine, Chinese medicine, Ayurveda, and other systems, a tool of diagnosis employed by practitioners to obtain information related to major systems within the body, including the cardio-vascular system, and other organs. The practitioner uses his or her ring, middle, and index fingers to read the pulse at the radial artery on each wrist. The amount of pressure exerted should vary from finger to finger, and the fingers should not touch one another. For male patients, a practitioner will first examine the left wrist with his or her right hand. For female patients, a practitioner will first examine the right wrist with his or her left hand.

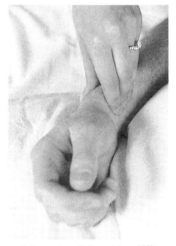

Pulse reading. (Potter and Perry, 1993)

pulsed electromagnetic fields (PEMF), *n.pl* a type of electromagnetic therapy in which small electrical currents are intermittently applied to the body. Has been used to induce bone formation, help incontinence, and treat swelling, inflammation, and arthritis. See also therapy, electromagnetic.

pumpkin, *n* Latin names: *Cucurbita pepo, Cucurbita maxima, Cucurbita moschata;* part used: seeds; uses:

anthelmintic, tapeworms, benign prostatic hypertrophy, childhood enuresis, bladder irritation; precautions: pregnancy, lactation. Also called *cucurbita, pumpkinseed,* or *vegetable marrow.*

punarnava (pōō·när·nä·və), *n* Latin name: *Boerhaavia diffusa;* parts used: roots, leaves, flowers; uses: in Ayurveda, pacifies all three doshas (sweet, bitter, astringent, light, dry), antifibrinolytic, diuretic; precautions: hypertension, heart conditions. Also called *gadahpurna, pigweed,* or *spreading hogweed.*

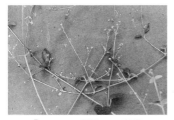

Punarnava. (Williamson, 2002)

Punica granatum, n See pomegranate.

pure consciousness, *n* in the Vedic tradition and Ayurveda, the ground of being that manifests as the totality of creation.

purgative, *n* substance that promotes bowel loosening and movement.

purishvahasrotas (pŏŏ'·rĭsh·və·hȧs·rō'·təs), *n.pl* in Ayurveda, one of the 13 types of srotas (body channels) that function in conveying feces. They originate in the rectum and colon.

Purshiana bark, *n* See chittem bark.

purusha (pŏŏr·rŏŏ'·shə), *n* in Ayurvedic philosophy, male energy, one of the two manifestations of cosmic consciousness; an energy that has passive awareness but is without form or attribute. See also prakriti.

purvakarma (pŏŏr'·vä·kär'·mə), *n* in Ayurveda, the two-step preparation of the body before Panchakarma, which includes a specially prescribed diet and ingestion of oil, followed by an oil-based massage, and sweating by heat treatment. Purvakarma is performed to loosen ama, cool the irritated doshas, open blocked srotas, and lubricate the passages of malas. See also Panchakarma, ama, doshas, srotas, and malas.

putrefaction (pyōō'·trə·fak'·shən), *n* the decomposition of protein compounds.

***p*-value,** *n* in statistics, the probability that a random variable will be found to have a value equal to or greater than the observed value by chance alone. This value provides an objective basis from which to assess the relative change in the data.

pycnogenol (pīk'·nə·ge'·nôl), *n* a combination of bioflavonoids obtained from the bark of the *Pinus maritima* pine tree, known for their antioxidant properties. Has been used to treat hypoxia, tumors, and inflammation. Contraindicated for use during pregnancy or lactation and by infants and children.

pygeum (pī·gē'·əm), *n* Latin names: *Prunus africana, Pygeum africanum;* part used: bark; uses: urinary tract conditions, benign prostatic hypertrophy, male impotence; precautions: pregnancy, lactation, children. Also called *African plum tree.*

Pygeum africanum, n See pygeum.

pyridoxal-alpha-ketoglutarate (pī'·ri·dô·ksəl-al'·fə-kē'·tō·glōō'·tə·rāt), *n* a supplement used in sports nutrition, claimed to improve the endurance performance of athletes by enhancing the generation of ATP, GTP, and other high-energy phosphate bonds and by suppressing the formation of lactic acid.

pyridoxine, *n* See vitamin B_6.

pyruvate (pī·rōō'·vāt), *n* a biochemical involved in the Krebs cycle that facilitates ATP production. Has been claimed to assist in weight reduction by enhancing metabolism. No known precautions. Also called *sodium pyruvate, calcium pyruvate, potassium pyruvate, magnesium pyruvate,* or *dihydroxyacetone pyruvate.*

P

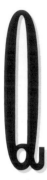

qi (chē), *n* the body's life force. In Chinese philosophy, qi is the force that flows through channels in the body and enlivens all living beings. An imbalance in qi is believed to cause illness. See also prana and pneuma.

qi cultivation, *n* in traditional Chinese medicine, practices derived from Chinese martial arts and Buddhist and Daoist meditation aimed at increasing the free flow of qi and strengthening the body. See also qi.

qi, defensive (chē), *n* one of two forms of qi that true qi assumes; it is yang in nature, and its function is to take a protective, exterior role and position in the body. It is not believed to be able to enter the channels, so it flows under the skin and between muscles, where it is diffused over the abdomen and chest and turns to vapor between membranes.

qi, food (chē), *n* the initial phase of transformation that food undergoes on its way to becoming qi. After entering the stomach, where it "rots and ripens," the spleen processes the food and makes food qi. This type of qi is not yet usable to the body. The middle burner then sends it to the chest and lungs to continue the process. Also called *gu qui* or *qui of food.*

qi, gathering (chē), *n* the product of the second step of the process after which digested food becomes food-qi and is sent by the middle burner to the chest and lungs. After food-qi is combined with air, it creates gathering qi, which is usable by the body. Its primary functions are to nourish the lungs and heart, encourage the lungs to direct respiration and control qi, and promote the heart's responsibilities of regulating the blood and blood vessels. See also qi, food.

qi, nutritive (chē), *n* one of the two forms of qi that true qi assumes; yin in nature, it nourishes the internal organs as well as the entire body. It moves in the body through the blood vessels along with the blood and in the channels of the body. During acupuncture, this is the qi being activated. See also true qi.

qi, original (chē), *n* in traditional Chinese medicine, the form of qi, or life energy, manifested as essence—that is, a hereditary energy that establishes an individual's constitution.

qi, true (chē), *n* the last stage of qi transformation after food-qi and gathering qi, it is the result of the catalytic efforts of original qi; true qi originates in the lungs and circulates through the channels to provide nourishment to the organs. True qi manifests in two different forms: defensive qi and nutritive qi. See also food qi, gathering qi, original qi, defensive qi, and nutritive qi.

qi gong (chē gông), *n* cultivation of qi. The general term for all Chinese techniques of breathing, visualization, and (often) movement, the purpose of which is the promotion of balanced qi flow. Hundreds of forms exist, many of which overlap with martial arts practices, such as taijiquan or spiritual/meditative disciplines. qi gong can be divided into internal qi gong, in which the practitioner uses these techniques for self-care, and external qi gong, wherein a master practitioner identifies and releases the energetic blockages of another. Also called *Chinese energy medicine, chi gong, chi gung, qigong, qi gung, qigung,* or *traditional Chinese qigong (TCQ).* See also qi and taijiquan.

qi gong anesthesia (QA), *n* the practice of releasing qi through the palm of the practitioner onto the skin of a patient suffering from pain or to a patient preparing to undergo surgery; produces an analgesic effect. See also qi.

qi gong master, *n* experienced practitioner of qi gong. See also qi gong, external.

qi gong, external, *n* Also called *medical qi gong* and *qi therapy*.

qi gong, internal, *n* practices that accumulate and circulate qi within the individual. See also qi gong.

qi transformation (chē trans'·fōr·mā'·shən), *n* encompasses all the functional activities of qi in the body, including blood circulation, essence transformation, body fluid movement, waste excretion, skin moistening, nutrient absorption, sinew and bone moistening, and resistance to external pathogens. More specifically, it refers to work of transformation by the triple burner. See also qi and triple burner.

qianghuo (chē·äng·hwō), *n* Latin name: *Notopterygium incisum;* parts used: rhizome and root; uses: pain reliever, rheumatism, common cold; precautions: not to be used with weak or anemic individuals. Also called *notopterygium* and *qiang Huo.*

qie (chē·ə), *n* in traditional Chinese medicine, the fourth aspect of diagnosis; includes the examination of a client's pulse and palpation of the client's body and acupuncture points. See also wang and wen.

qihua (chē·hwä), *n* in traditional Chinese medicine, transforming—metabolizing qi, blood and body fluids which is one of the five functions of qi, vital energy that sustains activities pertinent to life. See also qi.

QL, *n* quadratus lumborum; an abdominal muscle that is shaped like a quadrilateral. Its primary functions include laterally flexing of the body trunk.

QOL, *n* quality of life, a subjective assessment of one's emotional and physical well-being.

quadriplegia (kwä'·drə·plē'·jē·ə), *n* paralysis distinguished by the loss of motion, reflexes, and sensation in the trunk of the body in addition to both legs and arms. Also called *tetraplegia.* See also paraplegia.

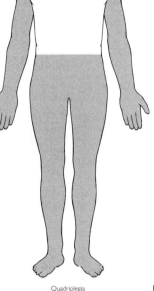

Quadriplegia

Quadriplegia. (Salvo, 2003)

quaker button, *n* See dog button.

qualitative research, *n* method of investigation that includes patient interviews and detailed case studies. Extensively used in the nursing profession, the method is increasingly used in the primary care setting.

quality control, *n* standards and procedures used to ensure the proper identification and quality level of a product.

quantum mechanics, *n* the application of quantum theory to statistical mechanics to explain the properties of matter when examined at the subatomic level. See also quantum.

Quassia (kwä·shə), *n* a genus of the trees that belong to the family *Simaroubaceae,* wood of which is used as a fever reducer.

Queen Anne's lace, *n* Latin name: *Daucus carota;* parts used: leaves, seeds, roots; uses: hepatoprotectant, antibacterial, tonsillitis, intestinal parasites, skin conditions; precautions: pregnancy, lactation, cardiac depression, high blood pressure medications, cardiac glycosides, CNS depressants, diuretics. Also called *bee's nest, bird's nest, carrot, devil's plague, mother's die, oil of carrot, philatron,* or *wild carrot.*

quenching, *n* in aromatherapy, an aspect of synergetic combinations of oils in which undesired results arising from one component are neutralized by another component.

quercetin (kwer'·sə·tən), *n* flavonoid derived from red wine, citrus, onions, parsley, and tea. Has been used as an antioxidant, antiviral, and reported to help allergies, prostate inflammation, interstitial cystitis, atherosclerosis, and cataracts. Caution in patients taking anticoagulant or antiplatelet medications. Also called *quercetin chalcone.*

Quercus alba, *n* See oak.

Quercus petraea, *n* See oak.

Quercus robur, *n* See oak.

questionnaire, *n* a series of questions used to gather information.

questionnaire, McGill pain, n.pr a measure of the subject's pain sensations on several dimensions. There are 11 questions regarding the sensory component of pain and four questions concerning the affective component of pain. A scale with a Likert format collects responses ranging from 3 (severe) to 0 (none).

questionnaire, menstrual distress, n.pr a feedback form that results in a score for total menstrual symptoms. The eight subsets of symptoms being evaluated are pain, arousal, autonomic reactions, behavioral change, concentration, control, negative affect, and water retention. Each set of symptoms is assessed on a scale with six points ranging from having no effect at all to being partially disabling.

Quillaja (kwē·lä'·hä), *n* Latin name: *Quillaja saponaria;* part used: bark; uses: astringent, antiinflammatory, expectorant, antimicrobial, immunostimulant; precautions: none known. Also called *quillaia, kilaya, soapbark tree, murillo bark,* and *panama wood.*

quillay bark (kwi·lā' bärk'), *n* the dried inner bark of *Quillaja saponaria* used as an antiinflammatory, astringent, expectorant, immunostimulant, and surfactant.

quince (kwins), *n* Latin name: *Cydonia oblonga;* parts used: seeds, fruit; uses: diarrhea, gonorrhea, dysentery, thrush, sore throat, canker sores, gum conditions, possible treatment for cancer; precautions: pregnancy, lactation; seeds are toxic. Also called *common quince* or *golden apple.*

quinine, *n* Latin name: *Cinchona succirubra;* part used: bark; uses: malaria, nighttime leg cramps; precautions: pregnancy, lactation, severe gastrointestinal illness, neurological disorders, severe liver disease, psoriasis, tinnitus, cardiotoxic, kidney damage, aluminum salts, anticoagulants, cardiac glycosides, neuromuscular blocking medications, sodium bicarbonate. Also called *cinchona, Jesuit's bark,* or *Peruvian bark.*

quinquina (kwin'·kwi'·nə), *n* bark from the root or stem of the *Cinchona* tree; formerly was used to treat malaria. Also called *Jesuit's cinchona,* and *Peruvian bark.*

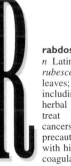

rabdosia (rab·dō'·sē· ə), *n* Latin name: *Rabdosia rubescens;* part used: leaves; uses: multiple, including in Chinese herbal formulas used to treat hormone-sensitive cancers of the prostate; precautions: patients with high blood pressure, coagulation disorders, thrombosis, or gallstones. Also called *dong ling cao* or *rubescens.*

Rabdosia rubescens, *n* See rabdosia.

racemic (rā·sē'·mik), *n* a combination of both levorotatory and dextrorotatory isomers in an optically active substance. See also dextrorotatory and levorotatory.

racemic modification (rā·sē'·mik mô'·də·fə·kā'·shən), *n* the synthesis of an equivalent number of both levorotatory and dextrorotatory isomers in an optically active substance in a laboratory. Also called *racemic mixtures* or *racemates.*

racephedrine hydrochloride (rä'·sə·fe'·drin hī'·drō·klō'·rīd), *n* a sympathomimetic drug used as a decongestant and bronchodilator for allergy and asthma treatment.

radiculopathy (rə·di'·kyə·lô'·pə·thē), *n* a form of acupuncture similar to segmental and trigger point acupuncture techniques, in which intramuscular stimulation is used to relieve muscles and viscera of supersensitivity. See also intramuscular stimulation and supersensitivity.

radioallergosorbent procedure, *n* a diagnostic test for identifying reactive substances that cause hypersensitivity of the immune system. Like the modified radioallergosorbent test (RAST), RASP uses a solid-phase radioimmunoassay to detect the presence of IgE reactions but is more sensitive than either the RAST or the modified RAST. See also test, modified radioallergosorbent.

radiology (rā·dē·ô'·lə·jē), *n* **1.** the science of radiation; the sources of radiation; and the biological, physical, and chemical effects of radiation. **2.** medical imaging using radiation, radionuclides, nuclear magnetic resonance, and ultrasound for treating illness.

radiolucency (rā'·dē·ō·lōō'·sen·sē), *n* the capability of a substance with a relatively small atomic number to let a large amount of x-rays pass through it, thus producing darkened images on x-ray films.

radionics (rā·dē·ô'·niks), *n* healing system that uses symbolic and energetic correspondences to diagnose and deliver treatment.

radiopacity (rā'·dē·ō·pas'·i·tē), *n* the capability of a substance to hinder or completely stop the passage of x-rays, such as lead and bones, thus producing a light image on film. Also called *radiodensity.*

ragweed, *n* Latin names: *Ambrosia artemisifolia, Ambrosia trifida.* An annual weed that blooms in the fall and is implicated as the primary cause of hay fever.

ragwort, *n* Latin name: *Senecio jacoboea;* parts used: seeds, leaves, flowers; uses: menstrual complaints; topically applied to stings and skin ulcers; precautions: no internal use in pregnancy, lactation or for children, hepatotoxicity, liver conditions, toxic if ingested. Also called *cankerwort, cocashweed, coughweed, dog standard, false valerian, golden ragwort, golden senecio, liferoot, ragweed, St. James wort, staggerwort, stammerwort, stinking nanny, squaw weed,* or *squawroot.*

raigan (rä·ē·gän), *n* in Chinese medicine, dried form of the mushroom *Omphalia lapidescens,* which is used to kill parasitic worms.

rajas (rä·jəs), *n* in Ayurveda, the primordial quality of matter responsible for action and activity. This guna is considered positive when in balance.

rajasic manipulation (rä·jä'·sēk mə·ni'·pyə·lā'·shən), *n* in Ayurveda, one of three types of touch therapies. Corresponds to effleurage and myofascial release and is beneficial for individuals with pitta constitution. See also effleurage and pitta.

rakta (räk'·tə), *n* in Ayurveda, blood as a fundamental tissue (dhatu). See also dhatus.

rakta moksha (räk'·tə mōk'·shə), *n* in Ayurveda, one of the five steps of panchakarma that refers to the purification of blood by bloodletting to eliminate toxins that are absorbed into the bloodstream through the gastrointestinal tract; used to relieve skin disease, gout, and treat spleen or liver enlargement. It should not be administered to children, elderly, and in

R

cases of anemia or edema. See also panchakarma.

raktavahasrotas (räk'·tä·vä'·häs·rō'·təs), *n.pl* in Ayurveda, one of the 13 types of srotas (body channels) whose function is to convey red blood cells. They originate in the spleen and liver. See also srotas.

random assignment, *n* a method of allotting membership in research groups that tends to factor out any confounding variables so that any remaining differences can be attributed to the variable being researched.

random event generator, *n* any system, such as coin flipping or dice throwing, that exhibits random behavior. Such random systems are useful in studying mind-matter interactions. See also mind-matter interactions and random number generator.

random number generator, *n* a specific kind of random event generator that uses an electronic circuit to produce a random string of numbers. Such circuits are useful in studying mind-matter interactions. See also mind-matter interactions and random event generator.

randomization (ran'·də·mə·zā'·shən), *n* a method based on chance in which participants of a clinical study are assigned to comparison and/or control and treatment groups. Randomization minimizes the differences among groups by equally distributing people with particular characteristics among all the trial groups. Randomization can also be done in laboratory and observational studies.

randomized clinical trial, *n* a clinical study where volunteer participants with comparable characteristics are randomly assigned to different test groups to compare the efficacy of therapies.

randomized clinical trial evidence, *n* See clinical experimental evidence.

randomized controlled clinical trials, *n.pl* medical research studies in which one or more groups are formed by random assignment to treatments and controls. Allows groups to be more equivalent when comparing he effects of treatment.

Raphanus sativus **var.** *niger,* *n* See black radish.

rapid eye movement, *n* recurring phase of sleep associated with dreaming, characterized by the rapid motion of the eyes beneath the eyelids. Also called *paradoxical sleep, rapid eye movement sleep,* or *REM sleep.*

rapid eye technology, *n* a psychotherapy technique used to treat trauma by having the client recall the event while moving his or her eyes in various patterns. See also technique, EMDR.

rapid induction of protective tolerance, *n* the induction of resistive and reparative mechanisms using low-dose toxins to biological, chemical, and nuclear exposures.

rare earth magnets, *n.pl* magnets made from materials such as samarium, cobalt, neodymium, and boron. These magnets generally produce relatively strong magnetic fields.

rare gases, *n.pl* a group of very stable elements, such as neon and argon, that—because of their filled outer electron shells—do not easily react with other atoms. Also called *inert gases* or *noble gases.*

rasas (rä'·səz), *n.pl* in Ayurveda, the six tastes: sweet, sour, salty, bitter, pungent, and astringent. These tastes are intimately bound up with doshas, so that individuals crave the tastes they need to restore balance in the doshas. See also doshas.

Rasa	Predominant mahabhutas
Sweet	Prithivi and jala
Sour	Prithivi and tejas
Salty	Jala and tejas
Pungent	Vayu and tejas
Bitter	Vayu and akasha
Astringent	Vayu and Prithivi

Rasas. (Sharma and Clarke, 1998)

rasashastra (rä'·sä·shäs'·trə), *n* branch of Ayurveda that deals with the preparation of mineral- and inorganic-based drugs, their properties, and therapeutic uses.

R

rasavahasrotas (rä'·sä·vä'·häs·rō'· təs), *n.pl* in Ayurveda, one of the 13 types of srotas (body channels); their function is to carry lymph, plasma, and chyle. They originate in the heart and in the vessels that emanate from the heart.

rasayanas (rä·sä'·yä·näs), *n.pl* Ayurvedic herbal preparations used to promote general health and well-being by increasing disease resistance, stimulating tissue repair mechanisms, and slowing the aging process.

RASP, *n.pr* See radioallergosorbent procedure.

raspberry, *n* Latin name: *Rubus idaeus;* parts used: berries, leaves, roots; uses: antidiabetic, antimicrobial, diuretic, antiinflammatory, cough, kidney stones, urinary infections, morning sickness, eases labor; precautions: pregnancy, lactation, antidiabetic medications. Also called *bramble, bramble of Mount Ida, hindberry,* or *red raspberry.*

RAST, *n.pr* See test, modified radioallergosorbent.

rattlesnake meat, *n* a Mexican folk remedy available in pill, powder, or capsule form; believed to treat a variety of medical conditions. Since rattlesnake is known as a source of *Salmonella Arizona,* its use has been associated with severe systemic infections. Used primarily in El Salvador, Mexico, and the southwestern region of the United States. Also called *vibora de cascabel, carne de vibora,* and *polvo de vibora.*

Rauvolfia serpentina, n See rauwolfia.

rauwolfia (rô·wul'·fē·ə), *n* Latin name: *Rauvolfia serpentina;* parts used: roots; uses: high blood pressure, snake bite, fever, dropsy, nervousness, insomnia; precautions: pregnancy, lactation, children, depression, suicidal tendencies, peptic ulcers, ulcerative colitis, Parkinson's disease, seizure disorders, kidney disease, amphetamines, heart medications, cardiac glycosides, CNS depressants, ephedrine, L-dopa, MAOIs. Also

called *Indian snakeroot* or *snakeroot.*

raw cabbage juice, *n* juice extracted from an uncooked cabbage. A remedy used for the treatment of peptic ulcers.

RDA, *n.pr* See recommended dietary allowance.

reaction, *n* a process of changing the chemical properties of a substance through the interaction between different molecules. A catalyst, such as heat or enzymes, may alter the rate of reaction.

reaction, stress, n See fight-or-flight response.

reactive oxygen species, *n* molecules and ions of oxygen that have an unpaired electron, thus rendering them extremely reactive. Many cellular structures are susceptible to attack by ROS contributing to cancer, heart disease, and cerebrovascular disease.

reactivity, *n* the degree to which a being responds to a stimulus. The degree may be affected by the receptivity of the being. See also receptivity.

readiness potential, *n* a change in the electrical activity of the brain that occurs before the subject's conscious decision to move a muscle.

reagent, *n* a substance used in a chemical reaction.

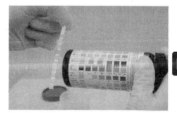

Reagent strips. (Zitelli, 1995)

realm of Spirit, *n* according to Native American culture, a term that refers to the unconscious world that belongs to an individual or a group of people. Pertinent information is passed from this world to the patient and the healer. Persons can gain access to this otherworldly region through dreams and during the Sweat Lodge and other ceremonies, Cree Kosāpahcikéwin or "shaking tent" or Lakota Yuwipi, during which spiritual beings are believed to communicate with the healer. See also Sweat Lodge Ceremony and Lakota Yuwipi.

reasonable doubt, *n* a standard of proof in court proceedings in which the prosecution must convince those in court that the accused is more than likely guilty of the offense with which he is charged.

receptivity, *n* the state of being open to the action of a drug or homeopathic remedy. See also reactivity.

reciprocal inhibition (rē·si´·prə·kəl in´·hə·bi´·shən), *n* muscle energy technique (MET) used to remedy joint and muscle dysfunction. This technique is used when the agonist muscles in need of stretching have experienced trauma or are otherwise painful when contracted. The stronger, antagonist muscles are manipulated instead to create a give-and-take toning effect in both the groups.

reciprocal tension membranes, *n.pl* soft tissues which, because of their connection between the sacrum and the occiput, play a key role in sequential craniosacral movement.

recoil, *n* chiropractic technique where a thrust is applied with the force produced from the practitioner's arms, chest, and hands. Once delivered, the practitioner's hands recoil from the client's vertebra.

recommended dietary allowance, *n* a guideline developed by the National Research Council's Food and Nutrition Board to aid in adequate nutritional intake of specific vitamins and minerals. Aimed at preventing nutritional deficiencies and does not define the optimum intake levels for an individual.

recommended optimum nutrient intakes, *n.pl* guidelines developed to aid individuals in determining the optimal levels of specific vitamin and mineral intake.

recovery, *n* **1.** the return to a healthy state. **2.** the self-regulation and life force of a patient being returned to a normal balanced status. The patient is considered healthy again. See also cure, entelechy, and healing.

recruitment, *n* **1.** the use of adjunct muscles to assist an overburdened muscle or group of muscles during movement. **2.** in clinical studies, the process of soliciting and selecting patients for participation.

rectification (rek´·tə·fə·kā´·shən), *n* a process such as redistillation, by which undesired components are removed from an essential oil.

red, *adj* in Chinese medicine, a facial coloration indicative of hot energy, poor digestion, and possible respiratory inflammation. See also energy, hot.

red bush tea, *n* See rooibos tea.

red clover, *n* Latin name: *Trifolium pratense;* part used: flowering tops; uses: blood purifier, chemoprevention, menopausal complaints, skin conditions; precautions: patients at risk for hormone-sensitive cancers; those taking anticoagulants or undergoing hormone therapy. Also called *wild clover, purple clover,* or *trefoil.*

red food, *n* warming foods that increase circulation and yang energy; include radishes, red cabbage and peppers, hot peppers, tomatoes, cherries, watermelon, cranberries, wheat, and rye.

Red Road Approach, *n* the incorporation of traditional Native American methods of healing, such as wiwang wicipi, inipi, and hanbleceya, into the treatment process for the people living on the Cheyenne River Indian Reservation at Eagle Butte. See also wiwang wicipi, inipi, and hanbleceya.

red yeast rice, *n* See monascus.

reductionism (rē·duk´·shə·ni´·zəm), *n* a tenet of the modern bioscientific approach to knowledge—according to which anything complex can be explained primarily in terms of its simpler components.

referred itch, *n* an itch that results from scratching an itch on another part of the body.

referred pain, *n* pain experienced in a part of the body away from the diseased or injured part (often a trigger point), such as the pain in left shoulder, which is caused by angina pectoris.

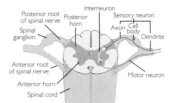

Reflex arc. (Chipps, Clanin, and Campbell, 1992)

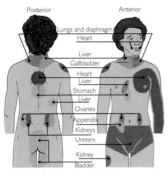

Referred pain. (Lewis, Heitkemper, and Dirksen, 2000)

reflex, *n* an automatic, predictable and adaptive neuromuscular response to a stimuli.

reflex analysis, contact, *n* technique in which a health professional studies a client's reflexes through a series of tests.

reflex arc, *n* the smallest functional unit of the nervous system that consists of two or more neurons (afferent and efferent) and can react to a stimulus.

reflex sympathetic dystrophy, *n* a complex neuromuscular disorder of the limbs that may result from trauma.

reflex, arterial trunk, *n* in hydrotherapy, one of the five principles used to improve blood circulation. The response of the trunk and branches of an artery to contract when the trunk is exposed to long periods of cold and to dilate when exposed to long periods of heat.

reflex, cervicolumbar **(ser'·vi·kō'·lum'·bar rē'·fleks),** *n* shortening of the lumbar paravertebral muscles as an automatic response to the shortening of the neck's postural muscles.

reflex, Chapman, *n.pr* a system of reflex points first used by osteopath Frank Chapman and described by osteopath Charles Owens. These reflexes manifest as predictable abnormalities in fascial tissue, which are thought to reflect visceral pathologies and are discernable as stringy textured tissues upon palpation.

R

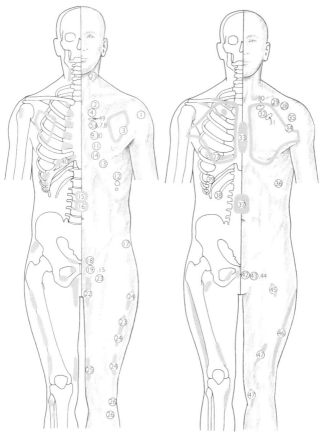

Reflex, Chapman. (Chaitow, 2003)

reflex, conditioned, n any reflex that does not naturally occur in an organism but learned through the regular association of an unrelated, external stimulus with a physiologic response until the response occurs whenever the stimulus is present.

reflex, deep tendon, n sharp muscle contraction after a rapid stretch; occurs in response to a tap on the tendon of the muscle.

reflex, Hering-Breuer, n.pr a biologic reaction that prevents the lungs from overexpanding when inhaling and from expelling too much air during exhalation.

reflex, inhibition, n in osteopathy, application of constant pressure to soft tissues to normalize and relax reflex activity.

reflex, oculocephalogyric (ôk'·yə·lō·se'·fə·lō·gī'·rik   rē'·fleks), *n* automatic head movement leading or accompanying eye movement. Also called *oculogyric reflex* or *cephalogyric reflex*.

reflex, red, *n* **1.** the red reflection from the fundus created when light is shined upon the retina of the eye. **2.** biochemical reaction in which the skin reddens in response to the application of friction. The reaction is greater, both in degree and duration, in an area in which somatic dysfunction is acute rather than chronic.

reflex, somato-somatic, *n* reflex patterns in somatic structures; produced by stimulating segmentally related somatic structures.

reflex, somatovisceral (sō·ma¹·tō·vi¹·se·rəl rē¹·fleks), *n* reflex patterns in visceral structures; produced by stimulating segmentally related somatic structures.

reflex, tonic vibration, *n* toning response of a muscle to vibratory methods applied to the tendon.

reflex, viscero-visceral (vi¹·se·rō·vi¹·sə·rəl rē¹·fleks), *n* reflex patterns in visceral structures; produced by stimulation to segmentally related visceral structures.

reflexes, neurolymphatic, *n* an applied kinesiology term (also referred to as *Chapman's reflexes*); refers to specific areas of the body that encourage lymphatic drainage in various glands and organs when stimulated.

reflexology (rē¹·fleks·ō¹·lə·jē), *n* a natural healing system based on the principle that reflexes in the hands and feet correspond to various organs and organ systems in the body; stimulating such reflexes by applying pressure on hands and feet improves circulation, thereby promoting bodily functions.

reflexology, holistic multidimensional, *n* practice of treating specific disorders by applying pressure to specific points on the soles of the feet or palms of the hands.

reflexology, vacuflex (va¹·kyu·fleks¹ rē·flek·sō¹·lə·jē), *n* two-phase treatment that links meridian rebalancing and reflex stimulation. As part of the technique, the patient has suction

boots on his or her feet and suction cups on other parts of the body; these are attached to a suction pump that stimulates reflexes.

refractive index (RI) (rē·frak¹·tiv in¹·deks), *n* a measurement of the bending of a light ray when moving from a less dense substance to a higher dense material. Measured by a refractometer.

reframing (rē·frā¹·ming), *n* the revisiting and reconstruction of a patient's view of an experience to imbue it with a different—usually more positive—meaning in the patient's mind.

REG, *n.pr* See random event generator.

region, *n* an anatomical section of the body defined by arbitrary, functional, or natural boundaries.

region, cervicothoracic (CT) (ser¹·vi·kō·thə·ra¹·sik rē¹·jən), *n* the back region that encompasses the seventh cervical vertebra through the first thoracic vertebra.

region, lumbosacral (LS) (ləm·bō·sā¹·krəl rē¹·jən), *n* the back region that encompasses the fifth lumbar vertebra through the first sacral segment.

region, occipitocervical (OA) (ôk·si¹·pi·tō·ser¹·vi·kəl rē¹·jən), *n* the back region that encompasses the occipital bone, the atlas, the axis, and the second cervical vertebra.

region, thoracolumbar (TL) (thōr¹·ə·kō·lum¹·bar rē¹·jən), *n* the back region that encompasses the tenth thoracic vertebra through the first lumbar vertebra.

regions, transitional, *n.pl* areas of the skull, spinal column, pelvis, and ribs where changes in structure lead to changes in function. See also region, cervicothoracic (CT); region, lumbosacral (LS); region, occipitocervical (OA); and region, thoracolumbar (TL).

regional cerebral blood flow (rCBF), *n* the amount of blood flow to a specific region of the brain.

regional flexion, *n* bringing the ends of the spinal curve (in the sagittal plane) closer together. Also called *Fryette regional flexion*.

registered music therapist, *n* certification formerly awarded by the

National Association for Music Therapy, based on education and training requirements. The National Music Therapy Registry lists therapists who wish to maintain the designation.

regular compression pattern, *n* after an observation of active and combined movements, a classification given to describe symptoms that are indicated on the identical side of the movement's direction.

regular stretch pattern, *n* after an observation of active and combined movements, a classification given to describe symptoms that are indicated on the opposing side of the movement's direction.

rehabilitation, *n* physical therapy or training specially designed by a health professional to assist an individual recover physical skills lost or compromised as the result of illness or injury.

rehabilitation, integrative, *n* the use of both conventional and complementary rehabilitation methods in a unified, coordinated approach.

rehabilitation counseling, *n* counseling started in the United States in 1920 to assist individuals disabled by industrial accidents; originally included physical, psychologic, and occupational training; expanded over the next 70 years and laid the groundwork for the Americans with Disabilities Act.

rehabilitation sequence, *n* the relative order of therapeutic priorities after the acute inflammation of an injury subsides—namely, to reduce ischemia and spasm, promote drainage, neutralize trigger points, increase flexibility, restore muscle tone, facilitate cardiovascular health, mend proprioceptive coordination and function, and renew the patient's breathing as well as posture and movement capabilities.

rehmannia (rē´·mə·nē´·ə), *n* Latin name: *Rehmannia glutinosa* (Gaertn.) Libosch.; part used: roots ; uses: antiinflammatory, antipyretic, antihemorrhagic, laxative, skin rashes, diabetes, rheumatoid arthritis, urticaria, anemia, bleeding disorders, asthma, chemotherapy damage; precautions: can cause possible mutagen (cured root); diarrhea with excessive doses. Also called *Chinese foxglove, di huang, shojio,* or *glutinous rehmannia.*

Rehmannia glutinosa **(Gaertn.) Libosch.,** *n* See rehmannia.

Reiki (rā·kē), *n* a system of spiritual healing/energy medicine developed by Japanese physician Dr. Mikao Usui.

reishi (rā·shē), *n* Latin name: *Ganoderma lucidum;* part used: fruiting body (mushroom); uses: adaptogen, antiviral, chemoprevention, immunomodulator, asthma, bronchitis, cardiovascular conditions, cognitive enhancement, ulcers, altitude sickness; precautions: no known precautions. Also called *ling zhi.*

relationship-centered care, *n* health care that honors and focuses on relationships—including those between the practitioner and self, practitioner and patient, practitioner and practitioner, and practitioner and community.

relaxants, *n.pl* medicinal substances that alleviate stress related to emotional and physical tension and strain.

relaxation, *n* the release of tension from muscles, physically lengthening the muscles and leading to a state of reduced stress and anxiety.

relaxation training, *n* method that teaches specific techniques for producing the relaxation response. See also relaxation response.

relaxation, active, *n* repeated tensing and releasing of individual muscles or groups of muscles for the purpose of inducing relaxation. Also called *progressive relaxation.*

relaxation, cognitive, *n* in relaxation therapy, the use of prolonged conscious attention combined with a nonjudgmental attitude; may be a sound, a word, a thought, or the sound and rhythm of breathing.

relaxation, differential, *n* minimal exertion of muscle tension required to accomplish a task while allowing the muscles not directly involved in the activity to remain relaxed.

relaxation, mini-relaxation, *n* a type of differential relaxation; relaxation of the muscles or a muscle group not involved in any particular activity.

relaxation, passive, *n* any technique in which one focuses attention on the breath; physical sensations in various muscles; or a word, phrase, or sound to induce a state of relaxation.

relaxation, postcontraction, *n* active technique (in which the patient does the work) in manual therapy; used to treat individual muscles and muscle groups. Also known as *postisometric relaxation.*

relaxation, postisometric (pōst'·ī·sō·me'·trik rē'·lak·sā'·shən), *n* a state of greater ease in a muscle following an isometric contraction. Transmitted by the golgi tendon bodies. See also contraction, isometric.

relaxation, progressive, *n* a technique used to achieve relaxation in which the muscles (beginning at the head and moving down) are systematically contracted and relaxed. Used to relieve anxiety and stress.

relaxation, progressive muscle (prō'·gre'·siv mus'·əl rē'·lak·sā'·shən), *n* a method of inducing deep relaxation through sequential tensing and releasing of major muscle groups, sometimes accompanied with deep breathing, calm music, or visualization exercises. Also called *PMR.*

relaxation, somatic, *n* a method of relaxation in which the participants identify and physically relax specific muscles.

relaxation response, *n* the physiologic counterbalance to the fight-or-flight response, in which a deep state of mental and physiological rest may be elicited.

relaxed, *adj* freed from tension, being at ease, as applied to muscles and the mind.

relaxin, *n* hormone responsible for softening and relaxing muscles, tendons, and ligaments during pregnancy in preparation for labor and delivery.

release, *n* in bodywork, the letting go of muscle tension and associated emotional stress.

release, direct myofascial, *n* an osteopathic technique for myofascial release in which a constant force is applied to a restrictive barrier until the tissue releases.

release, emotional stress, *n* procedure developed by George A. Goodheart, Jr., in which a practitioner addresses the emotional factors underlying an illness by using the emotional neurovascular reflexes located in the forehead.

release, indirect myofascial, *n* an osteopathic technique for myofascial release in which the therapist guides the dysfunctional tissues along a gentle path with little resistance until the tissues release.

release, integrated neuromuscular, *n* an osteopathic therapeutic system that combines different procedures—direct and indirect—to stretch and release restrictions in the soft tissue and joints.

release, mesenteric (me'·zən·ter·ik rē·lēs'), *n* an osteopathic procedure in which the abdomen is compressed to promote the drainage of lymph and venous blood from the colon, as the tension of the mesenteric attachment to the posterior body wall is alleviated. Also called *mesenteric lift.*

release phenomenon (ri·lēs' fə·nô'·mə·nən), *n* release of a pathologic barrier, which is either inhibitory or viscous, in soft tissues; occurs as a result of manipulation, such as PIR, thrust, myofascial release, or oscillation.

religion, *n* the outward and often social articulation of belief in higher powers, often practiced in a community setting; may include attendance of public worship and participation in the rituals particular to the faith tradition being embraced.

religious coping, *n* means of dealing with stress (which may be a consequence of illness) that are religious. These include prayer, congregational support, pastoral care, and religious faith.

REM, *n* rapid eye movement; the cyclical phase of sleep that occurs roughly

R

every 90 minutes and lasts from 5 to 30 minutes; is associated with dreaming.

remedios caseros (rā·me'·dē·ōs kä·se'·rōs), *n.pl* in Curanderismo, the Mexican-American healing system, the term for "home remedies."

remedy, *n* the agent that restores a patient to health.

remedies, Bach Flower, *n.pl* a type of practice using flower essences as a means of promoting emotional well-being. Developed by Edward Bach.

remedies, combination, *n.pl* remedies derived from more than one stock joined together in one dose. Also called *complex remedies.* See also homeopathy, complex and remedies, group.

remedies, concordant **(kən·kōr'· dənt re'·mə·dēz),** *n* in homeopathic medicine, remedies of different origin that have similar actions.

remedies, cyclical, *n* a set of homeopathic preparations that are sequentially and repeatedly suggested by the symptoms of a certain patient. See also following remedies.

remedies, group, *n* a set of medicines with similar properties. See also complex homeopathy.

remedies, inimic **(i·ni'·mik re'· mə·dēz),** *n* in homeopathy, treatments with antagonistic actions.

remedies, magnetically enhanced homeopathic, *n* a combination treatment in which homeopathic and herbal preparations are exposed to magnetic fields and administered to the patient via injections targeted at precise points.

remedies, relationship of, *n* how different remedies interact, follow, and relate to each other. See also antidote; remedy, complementary; concordances; remedy, following; inimical; and synergistic.

remedies, tissue, *n* in homeopathy, the twelve remedies that form the mineral bases of the body.

remedy, acute, *n* homeopathic medicine used to treat an acute illness. These remedies often require repetition because they act quickly and do not last long.

remedy, alternating, *n* sequential or repeated use of remedies to complement each other. During the inception of homeopathy, single remedies were promulgated; however, by the late nineteenth century rotating remedies was routine.

remedy, complementary, *n* **1.** compatible or synergistic homeopathic medicine used in conjuction with another remedy. **2.** homeopathic remedy warranted by an acute symptom or by its core chronic condition. See also compatible; concordances; remedy, following; and remedies, relationship of.

remedy, constitutional, *n* homeopathic remedy that corresponds to the constitution of the patient. See also constitutional prescribing.

remedy, epidemic, *n* homeopathic cure that corresponds to an epidemic disease picture.

remedy, following, *n* a remedy that is taken after application of another medicine. See also compatible and concordances.

remedy, follow-up, *n* in homeopathy, a remedy which is given after response to the initial remedy for the patient's symptoms is not resolved.

remedy, homeopathic, *n* pharmaceutical created homeopathically (by succession and dilution) from a selection of source materials. The *British Homeopathic Journal* prefers the term *homeopathic medicine.* Also called *homeopathic medicine, homeopathic drug,* or *homeopathic prescription.*

remedy, intercurrent, *n* a homeopathic preparation used along with another but not concurrently. The symptoms indicating the use of this preparation are dissimilar to or a subset of those regulating the use of the other. See also remedy, alternating; remedy, major; remedy, minor; and homeopathy, pluralist.

remedy, ladder, *n* a set of sequential homeopathic remedies, the cumulative effect of which is successful in alleviating a chronic disease when a single remedy is not curative. See also remedy, alternating; compatible; remedy, complementary; concordances; remedy, following; and remedies, relationship of.

remedy, major, *n* the primary homeopathic medicine used that tends to have a broad or profound effect on the course of the disease. See also polychrest.

remedy, minor, *n* **1.** a homeopathic preparation that has a restricted range of applicability. **2.** a minimally tested homeopathic remedy, the whole range of abilities of which is unknown.

remedy, rescue, *n* a combination of flower essences from cherry plum, clematis, impatiens, rock rose, and star of Bethlehem. Used to calm in times of stress or crisis. See also flower essences and remedies, Bach Flower.

Remijia (rē·mi'·jē·ə), *n* a genus of the shrubs belonging to the family Rubiaceae; is a source of cuprea bark, which contains cinchona alkaloids.

remote staring, *n* a parapsychologic research context used in DMILS. An individual (the "starer") gazes at a second individual (the "staree") through a one-way mirror or closed-circuit television setup. To see whether they have a sense of being stared at, the starees are asked about their perceptions of a gaze or monitored for signs of autonomic arousal such as electrodermal response. See also direct mental interaction in living systems.

remote viewing, *n* a term used to describe the anomalous cognition that allows a subject (the "receiver") to obtain information about a distant target object or image to which the subject and the researcher are blinded. See also anomalous cognition.

ren (rən), *n* endurance and the ability to feel pain, one of five virtues in Chinese medicine. Hun is responsible for ren. See also hun.

ren shen (rən sən), *n* Latin name: *Radix ginseng;* part used: root; uses: physical and mental capacities, liver disease, coughs, antipyretic, tuberculosis, antirheumatic, morning sickness, hypothermia, dyspnea, nervous disorders, impotence, prevention of hepatotoxicity, gastrointestinal disorders such as ulcers and gastritis; precautions: diabetes; can cause nervousness, hypertension, diarrhea, irritability, insomnia, and skin eruptions. Also called *chosen ninjin, ginseng, ginsengwurzel, hakusan, hakushan, higeninjin, hongshen, hungseng, hungshen, hunseng, jenseng, jenshen, jinpi, kao-li-seng, korean ginseng, minjin, nhan sam, ninjin, ninzin, niuhuan, oriental ginseng, otane ninjin, renshen, san-pi, shanshen, sheng-sai-seng, shenshais-hanshen, shengshaishen, t'ang-seng, tyosenninzin, yakuyo ninjin, yakuyo ninzin, yehshan-seng, yuan-seng,* and *yuanshen.*

repatterning, *n* the therapeutic touch phase in which the practitioner revisits the sites of imbalance noticed in the clearing phase and modifies the localized energy reversing its status (i.e., if cold, the practitioner warms it). Also called *balancing.*

repeated movements, *n.pl* a test of the active physiologic joint movements in which the practitioner frequently applies a movement to determine whether symptoms decrease or increase.

repertories, *n.pl* in homeopathy, an index of compilations of thousands of symptoms and their remedy indications.

repertorization (re'·per·tor'·i·zā'·shən), *n* in homeopathy, the use of a lexicon of symptoms and their corresponding remedies to aid in the selection of an appropriate remedy based on detailed observations of the patient's symptoms and medical history. Computerized methods are now available.

repertory, *n* in homeopathy, an extensive reference book or computer program that lists and cross-references precise symptoms and remedies for those symptoms.

repetitive strain injury, *n* a family of conditions characterized by pain, stiffness, numbness, and inflammation in joints and muscles; caused by chronic overuse. Also called *cumulative trauma disorders, CTD,* or *repetitive motion injuries.*

replication, *n* the repetition of a scientific study to corroborate or dispute its conclusions. Multiple replications are needed in each individual study to ensure statistical reliability.

representational systems, *n.pl* a neurolinguistic programming term for the senses (visual, auditory, olfactory, kinesthetic, and gustatory).

rescission (ri·si'·zhən), *n* the termination of a contract, either by a party legally entitled to do so or by court order.

Research Institute for Fragrance Materials, *n.pr* a United States–based organization that maintains a program for research and testing ingredients in fragrances, including those found in essential oils. The research reports and test results, specifically related to safety, are published in raw materials monographs.

resilience (rə·zil'·yens), *n* the property of a tissue that allows it to resume its former position, shape, or size after being bent, compressed, stretched, or otherwise mechanically distorted.

resinoid (re'·zə·noid), *n* a highly scented, viscous, purified material obtained by extraction of plant materials using organic solvents.

resins, *n.pl* complex, insoluble, sticky substances secreted by plants. Used as astringents, antimicrobials, and anti-inflammatories, and are burned as incense. Can cause oral ulcers and epidermal irritations.

resistance strategy, *n* an exercise method that uses weights or a counterforce to increase the intensity of muscle contractions and thereby create bulkier, more powerful muscles.

resonancy (re'·zə·nən·sē), *n* **I.** resonance; the tendency for an object to begin vibrating or oscillating when exposed to oscillations of the same frequency as the object's natural vibratory frequency. **2.** in the Science of Unitary Human Beings, a principle in energy field work; indicates the ever-present movement of energy from lower to higher frequencies in the environment and in humans.

resonant frequency, *n* the specific frequency at which an object vibrates.

resorcylic acid lactones (rez'·ōr·si'·lik a'·sid lak'·tōnz), *n.pl* phytoestrogens formed by molds; often responsible for cereal crop contamination.

respiratory cooperation, *n* an exhalation and/or inhalation performed by a patient, with directions from the physician to assist manipulative techniques.

respiratory sinus arrhythmia (res'·pər·ə·tō'·rē sī'·nəs ə·rith'·mē·ə), *n* the cyclical change in heart rate that occurs in correspondence with breathing rhythm; can be used as an indicator of health. The dampening or absence of RSA may indicate stress or heart damage.

respiratory syncytial virus (sin·si'·shē·əl vī'·rəs), *n* common virus that causes mild respiratory conditions in adults but can cause more serious conditions, such as bronchiolitis, croup, and pneumonia, in infants and children.

respiratory synkinesis (res'·pər·ə·tōr'·ē sin'·kə·nē'·sis), *n* the pattern of alternating movement or restriction of different spinal segments during respiration.

response, inflammatory (in·flam'·mə·tōr'·ē ri·spôns'), *n* the healthy physiologic response to injuries and infections; caused by increased blood flow and immune system activity and characterized by fever, pain, redness, and swelling.

response to prescription, *n* **I.** reaction to a drug. **2.** homeopathic reaction to a remedy. Also called *remedy reaction.* See also adverse drug reaction, direction of cure, reactivity, second prescription, pathography, prognosis, and sensitive type.

restless, *adj* in Chinese medicine, pertaining to either an abundance of heat energy, in conjunction with redness of face or to overstimulation in which case the face will be pale or greenish.

restriction, *n* a barrier or limit to movement.

restrictive barrier, *n* a temporary physiologic motion barrier that the proprioceptive system produces to prevent muscle damage in a muscle spasm.

resuscitation (rē·sə'·si·tā'·shən), *n.pl* revival methods that maintain vital signs for a person in cardiac or respiratory failure. Cardiac massage and artificial respiration techniques are employed, and fluid and acid-base imbalances are corrected.

retention time, *n* the amount of time it takes for a vaporized compound to pass through the column in chromatography.

reticuloendothelial system (re'·ti·kyə·lō·en·də·thē'·lē·əl sis'·təm), *n* a functional system of the body primarily involved in defending the body against infection and disposing the end products of cellular breakdown. It comprises the Kupffer cells within the liver; macrophages; and the reticulum cells of the bone marrow, lungs, lymph nodes, and spleen. Gaucher's disease, eosinophilic granuloma and Niemann-Pick disease are due to dysfunctions in this system. Also called *RES.*

retinal hypothalamic pathway, *n* the physical and energetic connection between the retina of the eye and the hypothalamus in the brain. Through this pathway, different colors or frequencies of light are said to modulate emotional responses and autonomic regulatory functions, such as metabolism. See also therapy, light.

retinoids (re'·tə·noidz), *n.pl* compounds in the vitamin A family.

retraction, *n* posterior movement, removal, or pulling away.

retrolisthesis (re'·trō·lis·thē'·sis), *n* backward slippage of one vertebra onto the vertebra immediately below.

retroversion, *n* a condition in which an organ or bodily structure is turned backward, as with the uterus. Typically no indication of flexion or another kind of distortion.

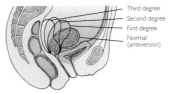

Retroversion. (Beare and Myers, 1998)

return phase, *n* in holistic nursing, the third and final segment of a ceremony or rite in which a person tries to finally disregard feelings of anger, fears, or memories that no longer provide a purpose in one's daily activities.

reversal of body morality, *n* concept advocated by John Diamond to describe a state in which individuals display resistance to a wide array of meridian-based therapies. A "reversed" person perceives good things as bad, and vice versa.

Revici Cancer Control (rə·vē'·chē kan'·sər kən'·trōl), *n.pr* a treatment based on the idea that cancer is caused by an imbalance between constructive and destructive metabolic processes. Treatment consists of taking various nutritional substances to bring the metabolism back into balance, the appropriate substances being determined through analysis of specific gravity, acidity, surface tension of the patient's urine, and other methods. Also called *biologically guided chemotherapy* or *lipid therapy.*

revulsive effect, *n* one of the physiologic principles used in hydrotherapy to modify blood circulation. The alternating applications of heat and cold increase the blood flow through a body part.

Rhamnus cathartica, *n* See buckthorn.

rhatany root (ra·tən·ē rōōt), *n* Latin name: *Krameria triandra;* part used: root; uses: chronic diarrhea, dysentery, menorrhagia, urine incontinence, hematuria, passive hemorrhage, anal fissure, prolapsus ani, leucorrhoea, sore throat, astringent, general health, clean teeth; precautions: can cause allergic mucosal reaction and irritation. Also called *rhatanhia, ratanhiawurzel, krameria root, peruvian rhatany, mapato, pumacuchu, raiz para los dientes,* and *red rhatany.*

Rheum palmatum, *n* See rhubarb; rhubarb, Chinese.

rheumatism (rōō′·mə·ti′·zəm), *n* an inflammatory condition of the joints, bursae, muscles, or ligaments; distinguished by a hindering of movement, pain, and a deterioration in at least one part of the musculoskeletal system. Examples include rheumatoid arthritis, gout, ankylosing spondylitis, or systemic lupus erythematosus.

rheumatoid arthritis (rōō′·mə·toid är·thī′·tis), *n* an autoimmune, inflammatory form of arthritis marked by periods of progression and remission; results in joint destruction and deformity; often strikes women between the ages of 36 and 50. Also called *arthritis deformans, atrophic arthritis.*

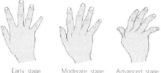

Early stage   Moderate stage   Advanced stage

Rheumatoid arthritis. (Monahan and Neighbors, 1998)

R

rhinencephalon (rī′·nen·se′·fə·lôn′), *n* the area positioned in the front of the brain in which structures relating to the perception of odor or scent are located.

rhinoplasty (rī′·nō·pla·stē), *n* surgical procedure used to alter the nose for purposes of aesthetics, function, or a combination of the two. Also called *nose job.*

rhizome (rī′·zōm), *n* root system of some perennial plants; consists of roots that grow horizontally; may also bear scales and nodes.

Rhododendron ferrugineum (rō·də·den′·drən fe·rōō·ji′·nē·əm), *n* parts used: flowers, leaves, galls, plant; uses: antirheumatic, induction of perspiration, diuretic, carminative; precautions: may cause vomiting, diarrhea; chronic use may cause poisoning. Also called *komar, rododendro, rusty-leaved alprose,* and *alpenrose.*

rhubarb, *n* Latin name: *Rheum palmatum;* parts used: roots, root bark; uses: laxative, constipation; precautions: patients with appendicitis, intestinal obstruction, intestinal inflammatory conditions; heart or kidney conditions; patients taking laxatives or heart medications; avoid long-term use. Also called *China rhubarb, Indian rhubarb, Russian rhubarb,* or *Turkey rhubarb.*

rhubarb, Chinese, *n.pr* Latin name: *Rheum palmatum;* parts used: bark, roots (dried), substructure (dried); uses: antidiarrheal, laxative, detoxifier; precautions: pregnancy, lactation, children; patients with stomach blockage or bleeding, stomach pain, nausea; Crohn's disease, and appendicitis. Can cause nausea; diarrhea; stomach cramps; hematuria; albuminuria; imbalances in mineral, vitamin, and fluid intake. Also called *Himalayan rhubarb, medicinal rhubarb, rhei radix, rhei rhizoma, rubarbo,* or *Turkish rhubarb.*

rhythm, *n* recurring pattern of waves, vibrations, or sounds.

rhythm, alpha, *n* the most prevalent pattern of brain waves, characterized by a frequency of 8 to 13 Hz. These brain waves underlie behaviors such as daydreaming.

rhythm, alpha/theta, *n* a brain wave pattern of around 8 Hz; often accompanied by a transfer of energy and a feeling of connectivity between therapist and client.

rhythm, beta, *n* normal brain wave pattern when a person is awake; characterized by a frequency of 13 to 30 Hz. These brain waves are associated with thinking, problem solving, movement, and anxiety.

rhythm, theta, *n* the brain wave pattern associated with dreaming, meditation, and hypnogogic/hypnopompic states of consciousness, characterized by a frequency of 4 to 7 Hz.

RI, *n* See reciprocal inhibition.

rib dysfunction, *n* a condition in which the position or movement of one or more ribs is changed or impeded. Also called *rib lesion.* See also exhalation rib and inhalation rib.

riboflavin, *n* See vitamin B_2.

ribose (rī'·bōs), *n* a carbohydrate constituent of nucleotides and nucleic acids involved in ATP synthesis and other functions. Has been reported to augment athletic performance and to treat coronary artery disease and myoadenylate deaminase deficiency. No known precautions.

ribosuria (rī·bō·sōō'·rē·ə), *n* increased excretion of ribose in urines; generally an indication of muscular dystrophy.

Ricinum communis, *n* See castor.

RIFM, *n* See Research Institute for Fragrance Materials.

ripple, *v* **1.** to flow or fall in waves; to undulate as a wave. **2.** during relaxation, the continuous wave of tension release that begins at the crown of the head and moves through the body to the toes.

rishi (rē'·shē), *n* in Sanskrit, one who possesses knowledge. It is one of the three components of the vedas, the ancient Hindu scriptures considered sources of pure knowledge. According to vedic sciences, interactions of rishi, devata, and chhandas give rise to matter. See also veda, devata, and chhandas.

rising liver fire, *n* hepatitis, in traditional Chinese medicine.

risk, *n* the possible peril related to a particular condition or treatment. The risk may come directly from the condition itself or indirectly from the process or method involved in the treatment application.

RIT, *n* See therapy, regenerative injection.

ritucharya (rē'·tōō·chär'·yə), *n* in Ayurveda, the time of year. An impor-

tant factor in determining an appropriate diet; aimed at preventing formation and accumulation of ama. See also ama.

RLS, *n.pr* See syndrome, restless legs.

rLung (lōōng), *n* in Tibetan medicine, wind, motion, and vital force. The Tibetan equivalent of qi.

RMSF, *n.pr* See Rocky Mountain spotted fever.

RNG, *n.pr* See random number generator.

Rocky Mountain spotted fever, *n.pr* a severe bacterial disease caused by *Rickettsia rickettsii;* characterized by the rapid onset of fever, headache, muscle pains, nausea, vomiting, and a characteristic rash. Without accurate diagnosis and antibiotic treatment, this condition can be fatal. The range for this disease is not limited to the Rocky Mountains but extends from Canada throughout the continental United States into Central and South America.

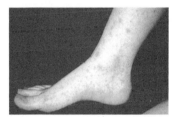

Rocky Mountain spotted fever (RMSP). (Goldstein and Goldstein, 1997; Medical College of Georgia, Department of Dermatology)

rogiparishka (rō'·gē·pä·rēk'·shə), *n* in Ayurveda, a diagnostic procedure in which the practitioner assesses the patient's physical and mental strength and establishes the patient's prakriti, or constitution.

role playing, *n* in behavioral medicine, learning exercise in which individuals assume characters different from their own. The individual may also be asked to simulate a particularly difficult situation and apply the characteristics that are common to his or her assumed role. The purpose of the exercise is to provide a strategy for coping with a difficult circumstance.

Rolfing, *n.pr* a 10-session manual therapy developed to optimize the body's movement and alignment and coordination with the forces of gravity.

Rolfing Structural Integration, *n.pr* systematic therapeutic program of soft tissue manipulation developed by Ida Rolf (1896–1979) in the 1950s. Ten-session sequences aim at rebalancing misaligned body structures and improving physical function.

rolling, *v* turning the client's limbs over so that the muscle tissue is mobilized and warmed, thus resulting in increased circulation.

ROM, *n.pr* See Respiratory One Method.

rooibos tea (rōō·ē·bōs tē), *n* Latin names: *Aspalathus linearis, Borbonia pinifolia, Aspalathus contaminata;* part used: leaves; uses: caffeine-free beverage, antioxidant, possible antitumor properties, possible antiaging effects; precautions: none known.

ropiness, *n* an abnormal, cordlike texture.

ROS, *n.pr* See reactive oxygen species.

Rosa canina, *n* See rose hips.

rosacea (rō·zā'·shə), *n* chronic disorder of the skin; marked by an increase in the size of subcutaneous blood vessels. The inflammation is most prevalent on the cheeks, eyelids, nose, chin, or forehead. Swelling, redness, an increasingly prominent appearance of blood vessels, noticeable increase in the tissue size, and skin eruptions resembling acne are common signs. Typically affects men and women with fair skin.

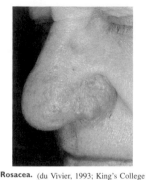

Rosacea. (du Vivier, 1993; King's College Hospital)

rose hips, *n* Latin name: *Rosa canina;* part used: hips (fruits); uses: diuretic, antioxidant, source of vitamin C, kidney and urinary disorders, arthritis, rheumatism, gout, scurvy, sciatica; precautions: pregnancy, lactation. Also called *dog brier fruit, dog rose fruit, hipberries, wild brier berries, brier hip, hip, brier rose, eglantine gall, hog seed, dog berry, sweet brier, witches brier, hip tree, hip fruit,* or *hop fruit.*

rosemary, *n* Latin name: *Turnera diffusa;* part used: leaves; uses: aphrodisiac, diuretic, antidepressant, euphoria; precautions: pregnancy, lactation, children, liver disease, rosemary hypersensitivity, hallucinations, confusion, vomiting, urethral irritation, sweating, nausea, anorexia, hepatoxicity. Also called *herba de la pastora, Mexican damiana, old woman's broom, rosemary.*

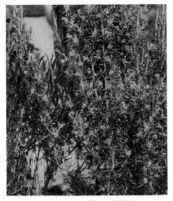

Rosemary. (Tiran, 2000)

rotated dysfunction of the sacrum, *n* condition where the sacrum has rotated around the longitudinal axis, so that movement in the direction of the rotation is freer, whereas movement in the opposite direction is restricted.

rotation, *n* circular movement of a bone around its own axis. *Lateral* and *medial rotation* are directional referents. *Upward* and *downward rotation* refer only to the scapulae.

rotation of sacrum, *n* sacral movement around a vertical axis, often in relation to the hipbones.

rotation of vertebra, *n* vertebral movement around the vertebral anatomic vertical axis.

rotation, pelvic, *n* the movement of the entire pelvis in a horizontal plane (relative to the body) around a longitudinal axis.

rotation, posterior innominate, *n* a condition in which the movement of the hipbone is unrestricted in upward and rearward directions and restricted in downward and forward directions, because the anterior superior iliac spine (ASIS) is positioned behind and above the contralateral point.

route of administration, *n* the path by which a substance is taken into the body (i.e., by mouth, injection, inhalation, rectum, or by application). See also dosage form.

royal jelly, *n* a product created by worker bees for the nourishment of the queen bee; uses: tumor prevention, antimicrobial, sexual dysfunction in males, baldness, menopause, cancer prevention, heart disease prevention; precautions: allergies, anaphylaxis.

royal touch, *n* the ancient belief in the healing power of the hands of sovereign leaders.

RRAF, *n* See Ruddy's reciprocal antagonist facilitation.

RSA, *n* See respiratory sinus arrythmia.

RSI, *n* See repetitive strain injury.

rubbing, *v* creating friction and heat by drawing the hands across the body at varying speeds, rhythms, and depths. Benefits include muscle elongation, tension release, and increased flexibility.

rubefacient   (rōō'·bə·fā'·shənt), *n* an herb or substance used to bring blood rapidly to a concentrated area of the skin, thus causing redness of skin.

rubella (rōō·be'·lə), *n* highly contagious viral disease that presents symptoms such as mild upper respiratory tract symptoms, fever, arthralgia, enlarged lymph nodes, and a fine red rash. Can cause deafness in children if it occurs in early gestation. Also called *German measles* or *three-day measles.*

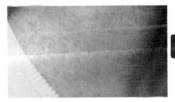

Rubella. (Zitelli and Davis, 1997; Dr. Michael Sherlock)

Rubenfeld Synergy, *n.pr* a holistic therapy developed by Ilana Rubenfeld in the 1960s; uses verbal dialogue along with gentle touch; also incorporates active listening, humor, imagery, metaphor, Gestalt process, and movement to ease the client's body into the healing process.

R

Rubeola, *n.pr* See measles.

Rubia cordifolia, *n* See Indian madder.

rubric (rōō'·brik), *n* the heading in a homeopathic repertory that labels the symptom and the medicines that induce that symptom. In addition to symptoms, syndromes and their constituent parts are also included.

Rubus idaeus, *n* See raspberry.

Ruddy's reciprocal antagonist facilitation, *n.pr* an adaptive muscle energy technique (MET) used to remedy joint and muscle dysfunction. The patient is instructed to complete a series of small, fast contractions against an applied resistance, which, over time, strengthens and conditions the muscles and facilitates more forceful, broader movements.

rue, *n* Latin name: *Ruta graveolens;* parts used: leaves, roots; uses: abortifacient, sedative, anthelmintic, analgesic, antiinflammatory, menstrual complaints, high blood pressure, gastrointestinal complaints; precautions: abortifacient, pregnancy, lactation, children, heart disease, patients taking high blood pressure medication, cardiac glycosides. Also called *herb-of-grace, herbygrass, rutae herba,* or *vinruta.*

ruksha (rōōk'·shə), *adj* in Ayurveda, "dry" as a guna, one of the qualities that characterizes all substances. Its complement is snigdha. See also gunas and snigdha.

rule of threes, *n* a procedure for approximating the location of the transverse process of a thoracic vertebra by using that same vertebra's spinous process as a landmark.

rum cherry, *n* See wild cherry.

Rumex crispus, *n* See yellow dock.

Ruscus aculeatus, *n* See broom, butcher's.

Ruta graveolens, *n* See rue.

RV, *n* residual volume; the volume of air that remains in the lungs even after maximum exhalation.

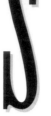

sabinol (sa'·bə·nôl), *n* chief constituent of savin oil, an acrid oil from the fresh tops of *Juniperus sabina.* It has been used in folk medicine as an anthelmintic, emmenagogue, and antirheumatic and in perfumery; may cause violent gastrointestinal irritation and hematuria when administered internally; fatal poisoning has resulted from its use as an abortifacient.

Sabul serrulata, *n* See saw palmetto.

sacral, *adj* pertaining to the sacrum.

sacral base, *n* the uppermost posterior part of the first sacral segment, which articulates with the fifth lumbar vertebral segment.

sacral base declination, *n* divergence of the sacral base from the horizontal level in the frontal plane; measured while the patient is sitting or standing.

sacral base unleveling, *n* See sacral base declination.

sacral sulcus (sa'·krəl səl'·kəs), *n* a depressed area in the sacrum next to the posterior spine iliac spine (PSIS).

sacred bark, *n* See chittem bark.

sacred space, *n* space—tangible or otherwise—that enables those who acknowledge and accept it to feel reverence and connection with the spiritual.

sacroiliac, *adj* pertaining to the immoveable joint formed by the sacrum of the inferior spinal column and the ilium of the posterior pelvis.

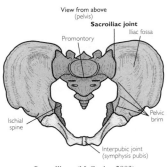

View from above
(pelvis)

Sacroiliac joint

Iliac fossa

Promontory

Ischial
spine

Pelvic
brim

Interpubic joint
(symphysis pubis)

Sacroiliac. (McCarthy, 2003)

sacrum, *n* triangular bone at the base of the spine.

sacrum, posterior, *n* condition in which backward rotation of the sacrum and side-bending to the side opposite the rotation have occurred. Resulting tissue changes may be located at the lower pole on the rotated side.

sacrum, posterior translated, *n* condition in which the whole sacrum has moved backward between the ilia. Forward motion is restricted, and backward motion is freer.

sacrum, somatic dysfunction of, *n* any somatic dysfunction affecting the sacrum; results from sacral trauma or restriction to normal motion.

SAD, *n* See disorder, seasonal affective.

S-adenosylmethionine (es-a·de¹·nō·sal·me·thī¹·ō·nēn) *n* a compound found in living cells that is involved in the synthesis of some amino acids. It has antiinflammatory properties and has been used to treat depression, Alzheimer's disease, osteoarthritis, fibromyalgia, liver disease, and migraines. Contraindicated for use by pregnant and lactating women, infants, children, and those with bipolar depression.

safety, *n* the condition of possessing freedom from being exposed to risk, danger, or harm.

safflower, *n* *Carthamus tinctorius;* parts used: seeds, flowers; uses: antiinflammatory, antioxidant, antimycotic, high blood pressure, fever, constipation, cough, menstrual complaints, massage oil; precautions: uterine stimulant, pregnancy, lactation, HIV/AIDS, lupus, immunosuppression, burns, sepsis. Also called *American saffron, azafran, bastard saffron, benibana, dyer's-saffron, fake saffron, false saffron,* or *zaffer.*

saffron (sa¹·frän), *n* Latin name: *Crocus sativus;* parts used: flowers, stigmas; uses: pain, cramps or spasms, sexual desire, flatulence, induction perspiration, promotion of menstrual flow, expectorant, relaxant, sleep induction, digestive disorders; precautions: may induce premature expulsion of a fetus. Also called *asian saffron, azafran, bulgarian saffron, crocus, fan hung hua, greek saffron, italian saffron, koema-koema, kumkum, persian saffron, po fu lan, sa fa ang, sa'faran, saffron crocus, safran, sahuran,* and *saffron.*

sage, *n Salvia officinalis;* parts used: whole plant; uses: menstrual complaints, diarrhea, sore throat, gum disease, gastrointestinal disorders; precautions: uterine stimulant, pregnancy, lactation, children, diabetes mellitus, seizure disorders. Also called *Dalmatian, garden sage, meadow sage, scarlet sage, tree sage, common sage, true sage,* or *broad-leafed sage.*

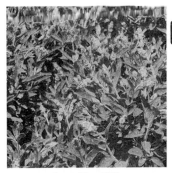

Sage. (Tiran, 2000)

S

sagittal plane, *n* the longitudinal plane that divides the body into right and left sections.

Sagittal suture. (Chaitow, 1999)

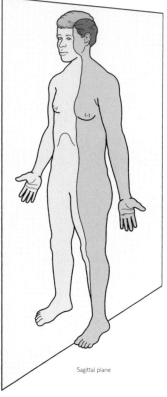

Sagittal plane. (Salvo, 2003)

sagittal plane postural decompensation, *n* nonoptimal distribution of body mass in the sagittal plane resulting in lordotic and/or kyphotic changes in posture.

sagittal suture (sa·ji·təl sōō·tcher), *n* meeting place of the parietal bones. See also parietal bones.

sahumerio, *n* See incensing.

saiko ka ryukotsu borei to (sä·ē·kō·kä-ryōō·kŏt·sōō-bō·rä·ē-tō), *n* in Japanese herbal medicine, a mixture of herbs that may help lower cholesterol.

salakya (sä·läk'·yə), *n* the branch of Ayurveda associated with surgery.

Salix spp., *n* See willow.

Salmalia malabarica, *n* See tree, silk cotton.

salt glow, *n* hydrotherapeutic treatment that involves vigorous rubbing of wet salt—often scented—on the skin.

salutogenesis (sə·lōō'·tō·je'·nə·sis), *n* the process of healing, recovery, and repair. The term was first used by Aaron Antonovsky to contrast with pathogenesis.

Salvia militiorrhiza (sal'·vē·ə mi'·lē·tē'·ə·rī·zə), *n* part used: root; uses: adaptation to stress, general health, muscle relaxant, anticholesterolemic, antirheumatic, antibacterial, cancer, menstrual dysfunction, sedative, wound healing, heart disease, irritability, insomnia, breast abscesses, mastitis, postnatal pains, respiratory conditions; precautions: none known. Also called *dan shen*.

Salvia sclarea, *n* See clary.

sama (sä'·mə), *n* in Ayurveda, an extremely rare body constitution characterized by exceptional balance and good health.

samadhi (sä'·mə·dhē), *n* bliss; union with the supreme, one of the eight limbs or paths of Patanjali yoga aimed at self realization and self-knowledge. See also yama, niyama, asana, pranayama, pratyahara, dharana, and dhyana.

samadoshas (sä·mä·dō·shəz), *n.pl* in Maharishi Ayurveda, persons with a constitutional type that integrates all three doshas: vata, pitta, and kapha. A balance of the three doshas results in flexibility and emotional and physical stability. See also vata, pitta, and kapha.

samanya (sä·män·yä), *adj* in Ayurveda, similar; similar elements or mahabhutas augment a dosha. See also mahabhutas and dosha.

Sambucus canadensis, *n* See elderberry.

Sambucus nigra, *n* See elderberry.

SAM-e, *n* See S-adenosylmethionine.

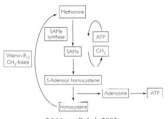

SAM-e. (Rakel, 2003)

samhita (säm·hē'·tə), *n* in Sanskrit, the elemental unity from which rishi, devata, and chhandas originate and among which a constant interaction forms the basis of diversity in creation. See also rishi, devata, and chhandas.

samkhya (säm'khya), *n* in Ayurveda, the philosophy of creation and nature of the universe. Includes the concepts of cosmic energy present in all things and that the universe contains 24 elements. Existence is seen as a manifestation of the energies of the cosmic consciousness, and human life is a universe within the universe.

samyoga (säm·yō'·gə), *n* in Ayurveda, union; the practice of administering drugs in specific combinations to increase their effectiveness.

san jiao organ, *n.pr* See triple heater.

sandra (sän'·drə), *adj* in Ayurveda, "dense," "concentrated," or "solid" as a guna, one of the qualities characterizing all substances. Its complement is drava. See also gunas and drava.

sang shen (shäng sən), *n* Latin name: *Fructus mori;* part used: fruit; uses: in traditional Chinese medicine, nourishes yin, enhances kidney essence, replenishes blood, stimulates production of bodily fluid, stops thirst, moistens intestines, and works as laxative; precautions: cannot be administered to individuals with diarrhea due to cold; deficiency of the spleen and stomach. Also called *mulberry* and *morus fruit.*

Sanguinaria canadensis **L,** *n* See bloodroot.

sanjiao (sən·jyōw), *n* Chinese term for a named, formless organ. It is found centrally in human anatomy. Also called the *triple energizer* and *triple warmer.*

Santalum album **(san'·tə·ləm al'·bəm),** *n* part used: oil; uses: chronic bronchitis, chronic cystitis, gonorrhea; precautions: can cause itching and nausea. Also called *sandalwood* and *sanders-wood.*

SaO₂, *n* the saturation level of oxygen in hemoglobin, as measured by samples obtained from arterial puncture.

saponins, *n.pl* glycosides from plants that foam in aqueous solutions. They contain adaptogenic, antiinflammatory, mucoprotective characteristics and can induce hemolysis. Also called *rapogenins.*

sara (sä·rə), *n* in Ayurveda, the quality or "essence" in development and functioning of each tissue (dhatu); differs from individual to individual. The quality of the tissues is directly related to the quality of ingested foods and the efficiency of digestion.

sarcode (sar·kōd), *n* in homeopathy a remedy whose source material came from a healthy tissue or organ of a human or an animal. See also isopathy, nosode, and organotherapy.

sarcoma (sar·kō'·mə), *n* malignant tumor of the soft tissues originating in

S

fatty, fibrous, synovial, muscular, or vascular tissue.

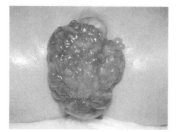

Sarcoma. (Zitelli and Davis, 1997)

Sarothamnus scoparius, n See broom.

sarsa (sär´·sə), *n* group of plants of the *Smilax* genus, the roots of which are used to flavor beverages, in homeopathic remedies, and to treat skin conditions.

sarsasapogenin (sär´·sə·sa´·pə·je´·nin), *n* steroid obtained by hydrolysis of sarsasaponin from the plant sarsaparilla. See also sarsaparilla.

sarsparilla (sär´·spə·ri´·lə), *n* Latin name: *Smilax officinalis;* part used: root; uses: antiinflammatory, antiseptic, antifungal, antibiotic, stimulant, stomachic, tonic, carminative, diuretic, antipyretic; precautions: may cause gastrointestinal upset. Historically used to make root beer, a common soft drink in the United States. Also called *salsaparrilha, khao yen, saparna, smilace, smilax, zarzaparilla,* and *jupicanga.*

sassafras (sa´·sə·fras), *n* Latin name: *Sassafras albidum;* parts used: root, stem; uses: pain reliever, flatulence, induction of perspiration, diuretic, vasodilator, gastrointestinal disorders, colds, kidney disorders, liver disorders, rheumatism, skin inflammations, blood purification, eye disorders, lice, insect bites; precautions: may cause carcinogenic activity, dilated pupils, vomiting, stupor, kidney damage, and liver damage. Also called *sassahura.*

Sassafras albidum, n See sassafras.

sattwa (sät´·twə), *n* in Ayurveda, the primordial quality (guna) of matter responsible for creation and creativity. Rasayanas, both herbal and behavioral, promote this quality. Also called *sattva.* See also rasayanas.

saturated compound, *n* a chemical compound that is comprised of single bonds with no double or triple bonds.

satva (sät´·wə), *n* in Ayurvedic philosophy, the essence; one of the three attributes of prakriti; the inactive, creative potential in the universe, represented by Brahma.

satvic manipulation (sät´·vēk mə·ni´·pyə·lā´·shən), *n* in Ayurveda, one of three types of touch therapies. Corresponds to chiropractic, cranial osteopathy, and the Feldenkrais method and benefits individuals with vata constitution. See also vata.

sauna, *n* full-body dry heat treatment. Benefits include relaxation, perspiration, and cleansing. See also thermotherapy.

Sauropus androgynus, n part used: extract; uses: reduce body weight; precautions: can cause bronchiolitis obliterans. Also called *chekkurmanis.*

saw palmetto, *n* Latin names: *Sabul serrulata, Serenoa repens;* part used: fruit; uses: benign prostatic hypertrophy, diuretic, cystitis, chronic nonbacterial prostatitis, breast augmentation, increased sperm count and sexual potency; precautions: pregnancy, lactation, children, antiinflammatories, hormone therapy, immunostimulants. Also called *American dwarf palm, cabbage palm, fan palm, IDS 89, LSESR, sabal,* or *scrub palm.*

SBS side-bending/rotation, *n* rotation of the occipital and sphenoid bones in opposing directions about parallel vertical axes combined with rotation in the same direction about an anteroposterior axis. May either be left- or right side-bending/rotation, depending on the position of the convexity. Also called *sphenobasilar synchondrosis (symphysis) side-bending/rotation.*

scabies (skā´·bēz), *n* an infectious condition caused by the human itch mite *Sarcoptes scabiei* and distinguished by persistent itching that creates a raw, irritated lesion. A

S

papular, pruritic rash may develop on the thighs, flexor region of the wrist, or the webs between the fingers approximately 2 days to 4 months after the first infection. A secondary bacterial infection is a potential complication.

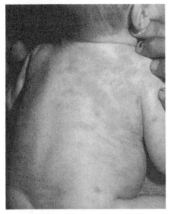

Scabies. (Weston and Lane, 1991)

scale, *n* a measuring system devised of units at regular intervals.

scale, 50 millesimal (LM) **(fif´·tē mə·le´·sə·məl skāl´),** *n* Hahnemann's potency scale for dispensing homeopathic medicines; developed by adding one part remedy to an alcohol/water solution of the rating 1:50,000. One drop is placed in 2 ml alcohol and succussed 100 times. A drop of this mixture is used to medicate 500 pellets or placed in a small amount of water for dosing.

Scale, Behavior Observation, *n.pr* an observer-scored scale that rates activity, anxiety, and positive facial expressions with a three-point continuum on four scales. The observer is unaware of the subject's group identity.

Scale, Brief Psychiatric Rating, *n.pr* a questionnaire that measures the severity of several psychiatric symptoms, such as self-neglect, hallucinations, conceptual disorganization, and suicidal tendencies.

Scale, Brief Social Phobia, *n.pr* a questionnaire that measures characteristic symptoms in three categories: avoidance, fear, and psychologic arousal. The subscale results are combined to arrive at a total score.

Scale, Center for Epidemiology Studies—Depression, *n.pr* a scale that is used to assess symptoms of depression.

scale, group environmental, *n* in rehabilitation, a tool used to assess the patient's feelings about team conference, in which he or she plays an active role rather than being passively examined by a medical group.

Scale, Hamilton Anxiety and Depression, *n.pr* commonly used rating scale to assess neurovegetative symptoms of anxiety and depression during a semistructured interview.

scale, potency, *n* range of the amount of potency for a given homeopathic remedy. Scales include the following: centesimal, Hahnemannian potency, Korsakov potency, Dunham scale, decimal potency, fluxion potency, fluxion centesimal potency, LM or Q potency, millesimal potency, and mother tincture.

Scale, Profile of Mood States, *n.pr* a measurement tool used to establish a person's frame of mind at a particular point in time. Used in clinical research, this self-report screening instrument specifically measures the following dimensions of mood: fatigue, anxiety, depression, confusion, vigor, and anger. Used for clinical research purposes, it only takes 3 to 5 minutes to complete. The participant is asked to assess how he or she has felt over a particular period of time on 65 adjectives, such as anxious, grouchy, or guilty. A higher score indicates a higher level of disturbance or distress on the dimension described. Also called *POMS.*

Scale, Profile of Mood States Depression, *n.pr* a questionnaire with 14 items to have subjects rate their current mood based on the adjectives listed.

Scale, Roland-Morris, *n.pr* in chiropractic medicine, a parameter used to

S

monitor the patient's progress throughout the treatment period. Specifically, the questionnaire evaluates changes in a patient's functions and focuses on activity intolerances associated with a patient's lower back problem. Versions with 18 or 24 questions are available. It is administered at the initial point of contact with a patient, with follow-up every 2 to 4 weeks. See also Oswestry instrument.

Scale, Stanford Hypnotic Susceptibility, Form C, *n.pr* a standardized test used to measure an individual's ability to be hypnotized. Unlike the Harvard Group Scale of Hypnotic Susceptibility, Form A, this test is not recommended for use in routine clinical practice, and a skilled technician can administer the assessment to an individual within an hour. A larger percentage of participants also report the development of undesirable side effects—including nausea, disorientation, or headache—than those persons who take the Harvard Group Scale of Hypnotic Susceptibility, Form A. See also Harvard Group Scale of Hypnotic Susceptibility, Form A.

Scale, StateTrait Anxiety, *n.pr* a self-report screening instrument used to assess a person's feelings of overall tension, apprehension, worry, and nervousness at a particular point in time. A higher score indicates a higher level of anxiety.

Scale, Touch Sensitivity, *n.pr* a 22-item scale used to collect feedback to various types of touch, such as dislike of being touched unintentionally.

Scale, visual analog **(vi'·zhoo·əl a'·nə·lôg skal'),** *n* an instrument used to quantify the subjective experience of pain and other conditions and to communicate this information to a healthcare provider, usually in values rating on a 100 cm line with 0 indicating no pain and 100 indicating the most severe pain possible. Also called *VAS.*

Scale, Vitas Pain, *n.pr* scale used to indicate intensity of pain from headaches. The scale starts at zero with no pain and increases in intensity to 10, indicating the worst pain. Graphically represented faces are

associated with the even numbers on the scale corresponding to the amount of pain with the faces indicating very happy, happy, contented, somewhat distressed, distressed, and very distressed.

Scales, Beck Anxiety and Depression, *n.pl* a questionnaire that assesses severity of anxiety and depression in adolescents and adults.

scan, *n* **1.** the image produced by computer use of radiographic information. *v* **2.** to pass the focus of attention (e.g., over a particular muscle or group of muscles); to check or feel a particular part of the body or the body as a whole (e.g., to take note of tension present).

scaphocephaly (ska'·fō·se'·fə·lē), *n* transverse compression of the skull resulting in a midsagittal ridge. Also called *hatchet head* or *scaphoid head.*

scapular, *adj* pertaining to the region of the scapulae.

scarification (skar·'ə·fi·kā'·shən), *n* the process of repeatedly scratching or puncturing the skin superficially before the introduction of a vaccine.

scarlet fever, *n* an infection characterized by high fever and a red rash caused by *Streptococcus.*

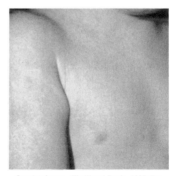

Scarlet fever. (Zitelli and Davis, 1997; Dr. Michael Sherlock)

schara (schä·rä), *n* in Tibetan medicine, willpower, one of the three functions of the mind, which symbolizes the function required to fulfill actions by an individual and also plays an important role in spiritual development. See also chi and badahan.

schara type (schä·rä tĭp), *n* in Tibetan medicine, a unique psychosomatic set of characteristics; on a physical level, a schara type will have a well-proportioned figure, robust muscles; medium-sized height; brawny, medium-sized neck; straight, medium-sized shoulders; well-built chest; small, muscular abdomen; strong extremities; medium-sized feet and hands; square, elastic, medium-sized nails; and a pink-colored skin tone covered with acne, freckles, or moles. Moderately gray hair covers the small, balding head. Facial qualities include wide, folded forehead; fine eyelashes and eyebrows; medium-sized, attentive eyes with a typically bloodshot appearance; medium-sized nose; and well-developed, proportionate ears. On a psychological level, this person may have qualities similar to a corporate or political leader with a strong will. A critical, intelligent, and penetrating mind can put into action ideas that are fully defined. However, this person may care more about the implementation of ideas than about people. The susceptibility to neoplastic disease, venereal disease, infectious disease, and the resulting infectious psychoses is high. Typically, every individual is a combination of all three types—chi, schara, and badahan. One or two of the types prevail over the others. See also chi type and badahan type.

schemas (skē'·məz), *n.pl* basic organizing themes deeply embedded within one's cognitive processes. This includes basic assumptions or rules that provide a template for selecting, sorting, processing, and assessing the importance of a particular experience. A person may or may not be consciously aware of such assumptions. Situations associated with high levels of stress—such as an illness or medical emergency—may trigger underlying fundamental assumptions and beliefs that may affect one's attitude, thoughts, or views.

schisandra (shə·san'·drə), *n* Latin name: *Schisandra chinesis;* parts used: fruit, stems, kernels; uses: antioxidant, immunostimulant, hepa-

toprotection, athletic performance, chemoprevention, respiratory complaints, liver conditions, kidney conditions; precautions: pregnancy, lactation, children, possible CNS depression. Also called *fructus schizandrae, gomishi, magnolia vine, omicha, schizandra, TJN-101,* or *wu-wei-zu.*

Schisandra chinesis, *n* See schisandra.

school, *n* the practice of therapeutic practitioners developing and passing on their specific theoretical tenets and techniques.

Schumann resonance, *n.pr* the sum total of all electromagnetic vibrations and waves between the earth and the ionosphere. The energy originates from lightning strikes.

Schussler Cell Salts, *n.pl* salts of minerals such as calcium, sodium, potassium, iron, and magnesium; used to treat a variety of conditions according to a variation of the homeopathic system founded by Wilhelm Heinrich Schuessler.

sciatica, *n* inflammation or compression of the sciatic nerve; causes dull aches and tenderness or numbness to sharp or severe radiating pain through the buttock region and down the posterior of the thigh, sometimes to the foot.

scientific health care, *n* the rational, intellectual body of knowledge and practice based on the scientific method for the prevention and treatment of human disease.

scientific medicine, *n* a term used to describe the form of medicine derived from the Flexnerian reformation of medical education and the germ theory in the early 1900s.

scilla, *n* See squill.

scillitic (ski·lĭ'·tĭk), *adj* of or pertaining to scilla or squill. See also white squill.

sclerotherapy (sklə·rō·the'·rə·pē), *n* a treatment in which a mildly irritating substance (a proliferant) is injected into osseus-ligamentous junctions or into weak connective tissues. The body's response to the irritant includes increased blood flow and tissue strengthening. Also called *reconstructive therapy.* See also proliferant.

sclerotome (sklə·rō·tōm´), *n* an area of bone innervated by a single spinal nerve and its branches.

sclerotome pain (skler´·ō·tōm pān´), *n* pain that radiates into various tissues but that does not have a pattern of radiation corresponding to specific areas of nerve supply. See also type-A pain.

SCM, *n* sternocleidomastoid; a thick, prominent muscle located towards the front of the neck. Its primary functions include bending, rotating, flexing, and extending the head.

scoliosis, *n* abnormal lateral curvature of the spine, primarily affecting the thoracic vertebrae.

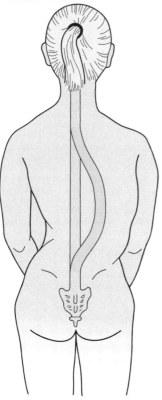

Scoliosis. (Salvo, 2003)

scopola (skō´·pə·lə), *n* dried rhizome of the plant *Scopolia carniolica*; blocks nerve impulses in the muscular walls of the digestive and urinary tracts, thereby relieving spasms. Also used to relieve muscular tremors and rigidity and to speed up heart rate.

screen, *n* initial examination to determine the existence of a disease or disorder.

script, *n* the set of instructions or suggestions communicated to a patient during hypnosis to direct the process and bring about the desired outcomes. See also hypnosis.

Scrophularia ningpoensis, *n* See figwort.

Scrophularia nodosa, *n* See figwort.

SCS, *n* strain/counterstrain, an approach of applying pressure to certain tender points in the muscles or joints to decrease or remove the pain sensed at the point of palpation.

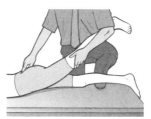

SCS. (Chaitow, 2002)

Scutellaria baicalensis, *n* See skullcap.

Scutellaria laterifolia, *n* See skullcap.

SDF, *n.pr* See segmental dysfunction.

seasonal allergic rhinitis, *n* See hay fever.

seborrheic dermatitis (se·bə·rē´·ik der·mə·tī´·tis), *n* a disorder of the skin; characterized by loose white or yellowish scales that may feel oily or dry and are located on the scalp, eyelids, eyebrows, or lips. It may also develop inside or outside the ears and the skin of the trunk, specifically in the areas that cover the sternum and near the folds of skin. The origin is unknown, but hereditary factors and fatigue, stress, weather, other disor-

S

ders of the skin, and poor hygiene seem to increase the risk.

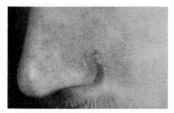

Seborrheic dermatitis. (Huether and McCance, 2000; Department of Dermatology, School of Medicine, University of Utah)

sebum (sē´·bəm), *n* substance with an oily consistency produced by the sebaceous glands. It lubricates hair, is an antifungal/antibacterial, and imparts waterproofing properties to the skin.

second messengers, *n* intracellular substances that translate chemical or electrical messages from the environment into intracellular responses.

second prescription, *n* the homeopathic remedy given after the initial remedy. See also remedy, following; repetition of dose; response to prescription; single dose; and homeopathy, unicist.

secondary drug action, *n* the resultant stage during the treatment course when the aggravation initially caused by the homeopathic remedy has subsided and the curative effects of the remedy appear. See also counteraction, dose dependent reverse effect and tonic drug action.

secondary somatic dysfunction, *n* any dysfunction developed as a consequence of somatic responses to other causes.

secretory immunoglobulin A, *n* protein found in bodily secretions; can protect against antigen overload by binding the antigens and transporting them through the liver into the bile to be eliminated. In some cases it can prevent the absorption of antigens.

sedative, *n* a substance that reduces excitability and calms the nervous system.

segment, *n* **1.** a section into which something may be divided. **2.** a part of a larger structure delineated through arbitrary or naturally occurring boundaries, often corresponding with a spinal segment. Also used to describe single vertebra (i.e., as a "vertebral segment").

segmental dysfunction, *n* a motion theory concept that states that two articulating joint surfaces cannot interact optimally if they are misaligned. Basis of vertebral subluxation and theory of illness. See also subluxation, vertebral.

seiki (sā·ē·kē), *n* a form of or development from Shiatsu in which the practitioner waits until the client's energy expresses itself. Touch may or may not be used; if used it may involve deep or light pressure depending on the client's needs. See also Shiatsu.

selected vegetables, *n* a proprietary mixture of herbs and freeze-dried vegetables marketed as a nutritional supplement and adjunct for treating various health concerns, especially cancer and AIDS. Also called *DSV, freeze-dried SV,* or *SV.* See also sun's soup.

selegiline (se´·lə·gi·lēn´), *n* an MAO-B inhibitor used to treat Parkinson's disease. It also acts as an antioxidant and an immunostimulant, protects nerve tissue from degeneration, and has positive effects on cognition. Also called *deprenyl* or *l-deprenyl.*

Selenicereus grandiflorus, *n* See cactus grandiflora, night-blooming cereus.

selenium (sə·lē´·nē·əm), *n* an essential element/mineral found in most vegetables, breads, and meats. Has been used in AIDS, asthma, cardiovascular conditions, cataracts, cervical dysplasia, multiple sclerosis, osteoarthritis, and rheumatism. No known precautions, but selenium supplementation is toxic at daily doses greater than 750μg.

self-directed imagery, *n* process in which individuals seek to influence their minds by reaching a deep meditative state to integrate healthy images into their thinking.

self-efficacy (self'-e''fi·kə·sē), adj positive subjective assessment of one's ability to cope with a given situation; sense of personal power.

self-healing qi gong movement exercises, n.pl See qi gong, internal.

self-hypnosis, n the process by which patients cause themselves to enter into a state of trance.

self-monitoring exercises, n.pl in behavioral medicine, exercises by which an individual records behaviors or thoughts in a journal or on a tape. The purpose is to increase an individual's awareness of distorted, negative thoughts and dysfunctional self-talk, thereby allowing him or her to make the appropriate modifications to these behaviors. See also self-talk.

self-talk, n in behavioral medicine, internal monologues that can have a positive or negative influence upon the individual.

Semecarpus anacardium, n See tree, marking-nut.

semiconductor, n an object that conducts electricity less than a conductor does but more an insulator does.

semiotics, n See symptomatology.

Senecio jacoboea, n See ragwort.

senega (se'·ni·gə), n Latin name: *Polygala senega;* part used: dried root; uses: hypoglycemic, emetic, immunostimulant, sedative, snakebite, respiratory disorders, skin disorders; precautions: pregnancy, lactation, children, salicylate sensitivity, ulcers (peptic or duodenal), anticoagulants, antidiabetic medications, CNS depressants. Also called *milkwort, mountain flax, northern senega, polygala root, rattlesnake root, seneca, seneca root, seneca snakeroot, senega root, senega snakeroot,* or *seneka.*

senile cataract, n disease of the eye; associated with old age and characterized by clouding of the eye lens; ultimately results in loss of vision.

senna (se'·nə), n Latin name: *Senna alexandrina, Cassia* spp.; part used: leaves; uses: presurgery laxative, acute constipation; precautions: pregnancy, lactation, children, intestinal obstruction, ulcerative colitis, nausea, vomiting, congestive heart failure; do not use longer than 7 to 14 days without consulting a doctor; cardiac glycosides, other laxatives. Also called *Alexandrian senna, black draught, Dr. Calwell dosalax, Fletcher's Castoria, Gentlax, Khartoum senna,* or *tinnevelly senna.*

Senna alexandrina, n See senna.

señora (se·nyōr'·ə), n in Curanderismo, the Mexican-American healing system, a practitioner from San Antonio. See also Curanderismo.

sense of coherence, n a view that recognizes the world as meaningful and predictable. The coherence of a worldview may have a positive correlation to health and longevity. See also worldviews.

sensing, v receiving stimuli, both internal and external. Used by client and practitioner alike, often in concert to detect areas of pain and discomfort.

sensitive type, n one who is highly susceptible to a given stimulus, such as an environmental chemical or homeopathic remedy. See also adverse drug reaction, constitution, receptivity, and typology.

sensitization, n **1.** a reaction in which exposure to an antigen produces antibodies; can be induced by immunization, in which an attenuated pathogen is introduced into the body. **2.** a photodynamic method of killing microbes by the use of fluorescent dyes that emit energy at wavelengths damaging to them.

sensory, adj pertaining to the senses (smelling, tasting, touching, hearing, or seeing).

sensory denial or negation, n a test for hypnotic susceptibility in which a client tends to negative hallucination and analgesia.

sensory nerve action potential (SNAP), n the electrical impulse that carries information along a sensory neuron.

sensory stimulation, n in acupuncture, the practice of inserting needles into skin and tissue to coax the body into using its energy to heal itself.

sentience and thought (sen'·shens and thôt'), n the functions of language, emotion, thought, abstraction, imagery, and sensation.

separation, *n* skeletal pathology in which the joint structure is stretched but the bone is not displaced out of the joint capsule.

separation phase, *n* in holistic nursing, the first segment of a ceremony or rite, in which a person makes a symbolic gesture of removing himself or herself from the busy and demanding activities of life. A person may adjourn to a sacred area for a period of time—which may be any place, including a room in one's house—but it can become more personal by adding an object of special importance such as a religious symbol or a burning candle. A feeling of calmness can be brought about by focusing on that particular object.

septicemia (sep'·tə·sē'·mē·ə), *n* the presence of virulent microorganisms or their toxins in the bloodstream; characterized by chill, fever, prostration, hypotension, headache, or pain. Also called *blood poisoning.*

sequela (si·kwe'·lə), *n* an abnormality that develops after a specific injury, disease, or treatment, such as scar formation after a laceration or paralysis after a poliomyelitis attack.

Serenoa repens, *n* See saw palmetto.

seroconversion (sir'·ō·kən·ver'·zhən), *n* change of serologic test results from negative to positive because of antibodies that develop in reaction to a vaccine or infection.

serotonin (sir'·ə·tō'·nin), *n* neuroendocrine chemical responsible for reducing irritability, depression, and brain function.

serum glutamic oxaloacetic transaminase (sir'·əm glōō·ta'·mik ôk'·sə·lō'·ə·si'·tik tranz·a'·mə·nās'), *n* an enzyme found in the heart and liver, elevated blood levels of which may indicate heart or liver damage. Also called *aspartate aminotransferase (AST).*

serum glutamic pyruvic transaminase (sir'·əm glōō·ta'·mik pī·rōō'·vik tranz·a'·mə·nās'), *n* an enzyme found in the heart and liver, elevated blood levels of which may indicate heart or liver damage. Also called *alanine aminotransferase (ALT).*

sesquiterpene (ses'·kwə·ter'·pēn), *n* a member of the terpene group; comprises three units of isoprene. Its molecular formula is $C_{15}H_{24}$. It may be used as an antiseptic, antibacterial, or antiinflammatory and as a calming agent by aromatherapists.

sesquiterpenoid (ses'·kwə·ter'·pə·noid), *n* a derivative of a chemical compound found in the sesquiterpene group; contains a functional group such as alcohol.

sesquiterpenols (ses'·kwə·ter'·pə·nôlz'), *n.pl* organic compounds found in many essential oils. They nave decongestant and tonic properties and also act as heart and liver stimulants.

SF-36 Health Survey, *n.pr* a widely used, valid, and standardized questionnaire used to measure an individual's overall subjective health status. The eight concepts measured by the survey are body pain, general mental health, perception of general health, physical functioning, role limitations caused by mental condition, role limitations caused by a physical condition, social functioning, and vitality.

SG, *n* substantia gelatinosa. Sensory neurons found in the spinal cord; transmit information about tissue damage to the brain.

SGOT, *n.pr* See serum glutamic oxaloacetic transaminase.

SGPT, *n.pr* See serum glutamic pyruvic transaminase.

shaking, *n* massage technique of holding and loosely, rhythmically moving a muscle mass or area of the body. Also called *rhythmic mobilization.*

shamanic state of consciousness, *n* alternate state of consciousness in which shamans attain knowledge, information, and insights used for healing or harmful purposes.

shamanism (shō'·mən·izm), *n* a diverse set of ritual healing practices that use trance and spiritual practices for therapy.

shanka bhasma (shän'·kə bhäs'·mə), *n* a traditional Ayurvedic preparation derived from the calcinated conch shell of *Turbinella pyrum*, which comprises magnesium, calcium, and iron. With well-known digestive and antacid properties, its use is indicated for sprue, hyperchlorhydria, hepatosplenomegaly, and colic. Also called *conch shell calx, conch shell ash,* and *shankh bhasma.*

Shankhapushpi (shän·khä·pōōsh'·pē), *n* an Ayurvedic syrup prepared from *Convulvus pluricaulis, Centella asiatica, Nepeta elliptica, Nardostachys jatamansi, Onosma bracteatum,* and *Nepeta hindostana.* It is used to relieve mental fatigue and improve concentration and memory power. Also called *shankpushpi* and *shankapushpi.*

shao yang (sōw yäng), *n* in Chinese medicine, one of the six principle meridians through which the vital force qi flows; further subdivided into yin division (gallbladder) and yang division (triple heater). The balance of yin and yang components and the proper flow of qi in an individual indicate sound health. See also qi, tai yang, yang ming, tai min, shao yin, and jue yin.

shaoyin (sōw yin), *n* in Chinese medicine, one of the six principle meridians through which the vital force qi flows; further subdivided into yin division (kidney), and yang division (heart). The balance of yin and yang components and the proper flow of qi in an individual indicate sound health. See also qi, tai yang, shao yang, yang ming, shao yin, and jue yin.

shark cartilage, *n* cartilage obtained from the hammerhead and dogfish sharks, used as an anticancer, antiinflammatory, and antiangiogenic treatment. Precautions for those with liver disease.

shatavari (shə·tä'·və·rē), *n* Latin name: *Asparagus racemosus;* parts used: roots, leaves; uses: in Ayurveda, promotes kapha dosha, pacifies pitta and vata doshas (sweet, bitter, heavy, oily), lactation, infertility, impotence, menopause, chronic fevers, cough; precautions: none known. Also called

abhiru, satavari, sparrow-grass, or *wild asparagus.*

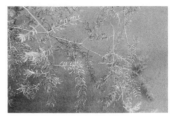

Shatavari. (Williamson, 2002)

shavasana (shä·vä'·sə·nə), *n* "corpse pose," a component of yoga practice that promotes a state of homeostasis, thus allowing the person to release emotional and physical tension; performed at the end of all the asanas. See also asanas.

shear, *n* any force that causes slippage between a pair of contiguous articulated parts in a direction that parallels the plane in which they contact.

shear, inferior innominate, *n* a condition in which the movement of the hipbone is restricted in upward and unrestricted in downward directions because the posterior and anterior superior iliac spines (PSIS and ASIS, respectively) are positioned below the contralateral points.

shear, inferior pubic, *n* a condition in which one pubic bone is displaced below its normal mate.

shear, posterior pubic, *n* a condition in which one pubic bone is displaced rearward of its normal mate.

shear, sacral, *n* complex nonphysiologic translational sacral motion relative to the hipbones.

shear, superior innominate, *n* a condition in which the movement of the hipbone is unrestricted in upward and restricted in downward directions because the posterior and anterior superior iliac spines (PSIS and ASIS, respectively) are positioned above the contralateral points.

S

shear, superior pubic, *n* a condition in which one pubic bone is displaced above its normal mate.

shear, symphyseal (sim·fə·sēl' shēr'), *n* condition in which the two halves of the symphysis slide over one other in a direction parallel to the plane in which they contact.

shegan (shā·gän), *n* Latin name: *Belamcanda sinensis;* part used: rhizome; uses: expectorant, antiinflammatory, asthma, cough, pain; precautions: none known.

shelf life, *n* the amount of time that a product can be stored and still be considered safe and effective for use.

shell shock, *n* a colloquial term for the dysfunction that sometimes manifests itself in war or in survivors of other violent traumatic events. See also disorder, post–traumatic stress.

shen (sən), *n* in Chinese medicine, one of the five spirits. Shen is housed by the heart and is associated with consciousness and memory, awareness, and expression. See also five spirits.

sheng cycle (səng sī'·kəl), *n* in traditional Chinese medicine, one of the two cycles of the five elements, considered the creative cycle representing the relationships between the five elements where one element nourishes or creates the next element in the cycle. The sheng cycle may be compared to the relationship between a mother and child in terms of nurturing. A therapeutic application of the sheng cycle could be a situation in which a patient's liver energy is disproportionate to the kidney energy.

shenmen (sən·mən), *n* in traditional Chinese medicine, an acupuncture point located within the small depression between the ulna and pisiform on the outer edge of the wrist. Treatment involving this point nourishes and regulates the heart in addition to calming tension. Also called *HE7*.

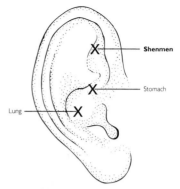

Shenmen. (Campbell, 2002)

shiatsu, *n* a type of massage developed in Japan. It consists of the application of pressure with the palms and thumbs.

shiatsu treatment, vibrational, n type of shiatsu treatment in which the client's energetic needs are tuned into on all levels—physical, emotional, mental, and spiritual. See also shiatsu.

shiatsu, five-element (fīv' el'·ə·ment shē·ä'·tsōō), *n.pr* a variant of shiatsu in which each of the five elements, (wood, fire, earth, metal, and water) correspond to a pair of human organs in yin-yang relationship to one another. An assessment is made after conducting back palpation and a radial pulse survey of the body to find areas of disharmony. See also shiatsu.

shiatsu, five principles of Zen (zen shē·ä'·tsōō), *n* the fundamental guidelines for practice of Zen shiatsu. First, Zen shiatsu should be relaxed, spontaneous, and egoless, like a child playing. Second, energetic penetration arising from this relaxation is preferred to conscious pressure. Third, penetration should be stationary and perpendicular to the tsubos. Fourth,

S

the practice always uses two hands. Fifth, the practitioner works with continuous meridians instead of upon discrete tsubos. See also shiatsu; tsubos; and shiatsu, Zen.

shiatsu, macrobiotic, *n* a noninvasive touch therapy that emphasizes the philosophy that individuals are inextricably linked to nature. Many techniques are employed to increase the client's strength and balance, including palm healing, postural rebalancing, dietary advice, breathing techniques, corrective exercises, and self Shiatsu, among others.

shiatsu, namikoshi style (nä·mē·kō·shē stīl shē·ä·'tsōō) , *n* a style of shiatsu common in Japan but theoretically founded in Western medicine instead of in meridian or kyo-jitsu theories. It emphasizes neuromuscular work and points. Also called *nippon shiatsu.*

shiatsu, tao (dä·ō shē·ä·tsōō), *n* style of shiatsu in which proponents believe that there are 24—not 12—meridians in the body and the means of contacting the body's meridian energy differs from that used in other Shiatsu methods.

shiatsu, Zen (zen' shē·ä·'tsōō), *n.pr* a variant of shiatsu that emphasizes the energy meridians as opposed to points used in acupuncture for treating several ailments. See also shiatsu.

shiitake, *n* See lentinan.

shilajit (shē·lä·'jēt), *n* Sanskrit name for asphaltum, a mineral used in Ayurveda as an analgesic, antiinflammatory, antibacterial, cholagogic, diuretic, wound cleaner, expectorant, mild stimulation of bowel movements, expulsion of stones from kidney and bladder, respiratory stimulant, general health, asthma, cystitis, diabetes, dysuria, edema, epilepsy, hemorrhoids, insanity, jaundice, obesity, skin diseases, menstrual disorders, uterine contractions, paralysis, genitourinary diseases, enlarged spleen, digestive disorders, tuberculosis, hypertrophy, increased red blood cells, anorexia, bone fracture; precautions: increased uric acid count, febrile diseases. Also called *mineral*

pitch, vegetable asphalt, shilajita, guj, jowr' pitch, kalmadam, perangyum, rel-yahudi, and *silaras.*

shin splints, *n* anterior or posterior tibial muscle strain characterized by pain along the length of the shin bone.

shingles (shing'·gəlz), *n* painful lesions along a nerve dermatome caused by the virus Varicella zoster, which also causes chickenpox.

shirah shoolah (shē'·räh shō·ō'·ləh), *n* in Ayurveda, a headache.

shleshman, *n* See Kapha.

sho (shō), *n* See akashi.

shonishin (shō·nē·shēn), *n* pediatric acupuncture techniques such as tapping, scraping, or rubbing with rounded or blunt instruments rather than needles. "Children's needle" was developed in Japan in the mid-1700s in the Osaka region and remains popular today. See also acupuncture.

sho saiko to (shō·sä·ē·kō·tō), *n* mixture of seven medicinal Chinese herbs used to treat some forms of cancer.

SHQE, *n.pr* See Qi gong, internal.

shrira (shrē'·rə), *n* in Ayurveda, the body. A sound body, mind, and soul are all necessary for good health.

shrotas (shrō'·täs), *n.pl* in Ayurveda, the 13 types of channels used to convey dhatus and malas. Any injury to the shrotas leads to poor circulation, thus resulting in disease. See also dhatus and malas.

shu (sōō), *n* in traditional Chinese medicine, the five transporting acupuncture points that originate in the tip of the four limbs and continue all the way to the elbows or knees.

shudhi (shōō'·dhē), *n* in Ayurveda, purification; a technique used to remove toxins from plants and minerals used in medicines.

shukra (shōō'·krə), *n* in Ayurveda, semen and reproductive tissues as a fundamental tissue (dhatu). See also dhatus.

shukravahasrotas (shōōk'·rä·vä'·häs·rō'·təs), *n.pl* in Ayurveda, one of the 13 types of srotas (body channels) that carry components of the female and male reproductive tissues.

They originate in the ovaries and testicles. See also srotas.

si jun zi tang (shī djōōn zī täng), *n* in traditional Chinese medicine, an herbal formula used to treat fatigue, decreased appetite, pale tongue, weak pulse, and loose stools. These symptoms indicate a qi deficiency in the stomach and spleen. Also called *four-gentleman decoction.*

si zhen (sē dzən), *n* in traditional Chinese medicine, the four types of examination used to diagnose an illness; include observation (visual examination to look for abnormalities in the complexion, tongue, facial expression, gait), listening (to detect abnormalities in the patient's voice and respiration), questioning (about diet, sleep, excretion, and symptoms), and palpation and touch (involves taking six pulses on each wrist to determine the depth and quality of each).

SI, *n* small intestine channel; an acupuncture channel running from the hand to the face along the ulnar surface of the arm and associated with the heart (HT) channel. See also HT.

SI(J), *n* See sacroiliac joint.

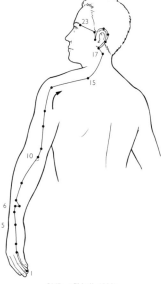

SI(J). (Chirali, 1999)

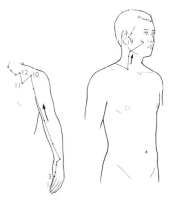

SI. (Chirali, 1999)

sick role, *n* an unconscious adoption of characteristic attitudes and behaviors by a sick individual. As a result he or she is temporarily granted certain advantages and privileges and is relieved from particular responsibilities.

sickness, *n* condition in which an individual experiences bodily malfunction or discomfort.

sicun (sē·kōōn'), *n* Lakota Indian term for intellect; considered one of the four dimensions of self. See also nagi, nagi la, and niya.

side-bending, *n* movement around an anterior-posterior axis in a frontal plane. Also called *flexion left, flexion right, lateral flexion,* or *lateroflexion.*

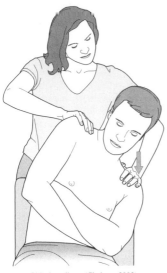

Side-bending. (Chaitow, 2003)

S

side-bent, *n* the position of one or more vertebrae during side-bending. See also side-bending.

side-bent left, extended rotated, *n* spinal dysfunction in which the vertebra(e) involved is ERS to the left. See also extended rotated side-bent.

side-bent left, flexed rotated, *n* spinal dysfunction in which the vertebra(e) involved is FRS to the left. See also side-bent, flexed rotated.

side-bent right, extended rotated, *n* spinal dysfunction in which the vertebra(e) involved is ERS to the right. See also extended rotated side-bent.

side-bent right, flexed rotated, *n* spinal dysfunction in which the vertebra(e) involved is FRS to the right. See also side-bent, flexed rotated.

side-bent, extended rotated, *n* an osteopathic description of a combination (extended, rotated, side-bent) vertebral position in cases of spinal dysfunction.

side-bent, flexed rotated, *n* an osteopathic description of a combination (flexed rotated side-bent) vertebral position in cases of spinal dysfunction.

SIDS, *n* See syndrome, sudden infant death.

SIJ, *n* sacroiliac joint; the joint located between the ilium and the sacrum. Also called *sacroiliac* or *sacroiliac articulation.*

sikor (sē′·kōr), *n* a traditional preparation from Asia; relieves indigestion and acts as a tonic during pregnancy. The preparation contains concentrations of lead and arsenic and mercury, cadmium, and other potentially risky metals.

silicea (si·lə·kā′), *n* homeopathic remedy derived from silica; used for chronic health problems and for general weakness and anemia. Also used in cases of vertigo, numbness in legs, dizziness, and mental confusion.

silicon, *n* a mineral/element (Si) that has been used for osteoporosis to increase the integrity and strength of the connective tissue matrix of bone.

silverweed (sil·ver·wēd), *n* Latin name: *Convolvulus scammonia;* part used: plant; uses: pain reliever, contract bodily tissues, diuretic, hemorrhoids, diarrhea, sore throat, ulcers; precautions: may cause gastrointestinal disturbances. Also called *common silverweed, eged's pacific silverweed, genserich, gumusu besparmak, silverweed cinquefoil, wild tansy, yerba plateada,* and *zilverschoon.*

Silybum marianum, *n* See thistle, milk.

silymarin (sil·ē·mär′·ən), *n* a type of flavonoid compound found in milk thistle. Extracts are used to protect the liver from environmental toxins.

similia principle, *n* the founding concept behind homeopathy that diseases can be cured by something that induces the same symptoms as the disease itself—thus "like cures like" or *similia similibus curentur.* See also cinchona and simillimum.

similia similibus curantur (si·mi′·lē·ä si·mi′·li·bŏŏs kōō·rän′·tŏŏr′), *n* the homeopathic doctrine of similars, in which "likes are cured by likes," so that a substance producing symptoms in a healthy individual can alleviate similar symptoms originating from illness. See also similia principle.

simillimum (si·mil'·lə·məm), *n* the homeopathic remedy that produces the set of symptoms most like that which the disease produces; ideally exactly congruent. See also clinical picture, drug picture, and symptoms, totality of.

Simmondsia californica, n See jojoba.

Simmondsia chinensis, n See jojoba.

simple carbohydrates, *n.pl* sugars— including dextrose, fructose, lactose, maltose, sucrose, white sugar, corn syrup, honey, and turbinado sugar— that are quickly and easily absorbed into the bloodstream.

single essence, *n* the essence of a single plant or gemstone contained in a bottle.

single photon emission computer tomography, *n* the recording of internal body images at a fixed plane with radiographic equipment to observe physiologic and biochemic processes and the volume and size of target organs.

sinking, *n* a process to relax by focusing attention on points of contact between the body and the surface it lies or stands on and imagining the body sinking down into the support surface, with the rhythmic modulation of breath.

Sinomenium acutum (sī'·nō·mē'·nē·əm a·kyōō·tam) *n* part used: root; uses: relieve pain, carminative, edema, moisture-related beriberi, rheumatoid arthritis; precautions: may cause systemic edematous erythema with itching. Also called *snailseed.*

sinusitis (sī'·nə·sī'·təs), *n* an infecting or inflammatory condition that develops in sinuses. Can be caused by a dental infection, upper respiratory tract infection, allergy, or a defect in the structure of the nose. As a result, the mucous membranes in the nasal passage swell, and the channels from the nose to the sinus cavities can be blocked; characterized by pain,

pressure, fever, headache, local tenderness, and an increase of sinus secretions.

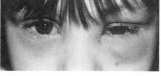

Sinusitis. (Zitelli and Davis, 1997; Dr. Ellen Wald, Children's Hospital of Pittsburgh)

sita kasaya (sē'·tə kə·sä'·yə), *n* in Ayurveda, a method of medicine preparation in which herbs are infused in cold water for a period of time (typically overnight), then filtered.

site of disease manifestation, *n* in Ayurveda, the location in a person's body in which doshas and ama settle and cause illness. See also doshas and ama.

sitz bath, *n* hydrotherapeutic treatment that involves immersion bath of the hips, buttocks, and abdominopelvic region. The legs are generally supported outside the water. See also hydrotherapy.

six pathogens (siks' pa'·thə·jənz), *n.pl* damp, wind, cold, dryness, summer heat, and fire. In traditional Chinese medicine, the external causes believed to cause disease (in severe conditions or when the corresponding qi is less resistant). Fire is believed to cause fever; summer heat is responsible for thirst and dizziness; damp is connected with edema; cold with stiffness and contractions; and wind assaults the face and head and also facilitates entry of fire, heat, damp, cold, and dryness into the body. See also qi.

skeletal formula, *n* representation of the bonding between two carbons in an organic compound. One line represents a single bond, two lines represent a double bond; and three lines indicate a triple bond.

skin drag, *n* a comparative measure of resiliency of the fascia and tissues positioned near the surface of the skin. The purpose of obtaining this information is to determine the functional quality of these structures. The practitioner acquires this finding with fundamental palpatory skills.

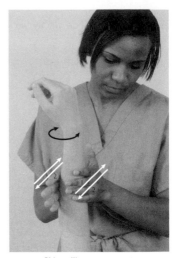

Skin rolling. (Salvo, 2003)

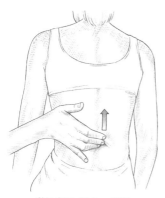

Skin drag. (Chaitow, 2003)

skin irritation, *n* reaction to a particular irritant that results in inflammation of the skin and itchiness.

skin rolling, *n* a therapeutic approach in which the hands lift, stretch, and squeeze bodily tissues. During the technique, a practitioner uses one or both hands to draw tissue in his direction while using the thumbs to roll over the gathered tissue. This technique is best applied in bodily regions in which the tissue is positioned tightly to the structures that lie underneath (e.g., directly above the shoulder joint).

skin sensitization, *n* an allergic reaction to a particular irritant that results in the development of skin inflammation and itchiness. Unlike skin irritation, the skin becomes increasingly reactive to the substance as a result of subsequent exposures. Ylang ylang and cinnamon bark may increase the risk of this type of reaction.

skinfold thickness measurement, *n* a noninvasive, quantitative technique for determining a person's body fat composition by measuring the width of the subcutaneous fat with calipers at various skinfold sites on the body, such as the triceps, suprailiac, biceps, and subscapular.

skull fracture, *n* a rupture or break in the cranial bones.

skullcap, *n* Latin names: *Scutellaria laterifolia, Scutellaria baicalensis;* parts used: leaves, roots; uses: antiinflammatory, sleep disorders, seizure disorders, spastic disorders, high cholesterol; possible uses as antiviral, anticancer (lung cancer), strokes, embolism; precautions: pregnancy, lactation, children, patients on immunosuppressant medications; may cause hepatotoxicity. Also called *blue pimpernel, helmet flower, hoodwort, huang-qin, mad-dog weed, madweed, Quaker bonnet,* or *scullcap.*

slakshna (släk'·shnə), *adj* in Ayurveda, "slimy" as a guna, one of the qualities that characterize all substances. Its complement is khara. See also gunas and khara.

slapping, *n* massage technique that uses the flat palms of the hands percussively; a form of tapotement. See also tapotement.

sleep hygiene (slēp' hī'·jēn), *n* education with the goal of effecting behavior modification, thus leading to a healthy sleep pattern. Behaviors that support healthy sleep include daily exercise, daily exposure to natural light, a regular sleep schedule, and relaxation exercises in the evening.

slippery elm, *n* Latin names: *Ulmus rubra, Ulmus fulva;* part used: bark; uses: coughs, gastrointestinal irritation, skin irritation, poultice for wounds or burns; precautions: spontaneous abortion, pregnancy, lactation, children. Also called *American elm, Indian elm, moose elm, red elm,* or *sweet elm.*

SLR, *n* straight leg raise. **I.** a position used to assess the potential shortened length of the upper and lower hamstrings. The patient flexes his hip and knee while the practitioner, using minimal force, straightens the leg to test for a restriction barrier. The other leg should be straight or flexed and remain on the table. **2.** evaluation procedure in back pain to assess disk disease.

smell, *n* a distinguishable odor released by a substance and recognized by the body's olfactory system.

smell brain, *n* term for the limbic system in lower vertebrates, which must rely for survival on their sense of smell.

SMT, *n.pr* See therapy, spinal manual.

smudging (smu'·jing), *n* in Native American medicine, the ritual of purifying the location, patient, healer, helpers and ritual objects by using the

smoke obtained by burning sacred plants, such as sage, sweetgrass, and cedar. It alters the state of consciousness and enhances sensitivity. This altered sensitivity to imbalances in the spiritual and energetic realms is necessary for the healer to assess and treat an illness. Cleansing often initiates healing sessions.

SNAGS, *n.pl* See sustained natural apophyseal glides.

snakeweed, *n* Latin name: *Euphorbia hirta;* parts used: whole plant; uses: in Ayurveda, pacifies pitta dosha (sweet, oily), antiamoebic, antispasmodic, antidiarrheal, antiinflammatory, anticancer, antibacterial, immunomodulator, antifungal, galactogenic, antifertility, antiasthmatic, female disorders, respiratory disorders, worms, dysentery, jaundice; precautions: none known, but many other species of genus *Euphorbia* contain toxic compounds and should be avoided. Also called *dudhi* or *dugadhika.*

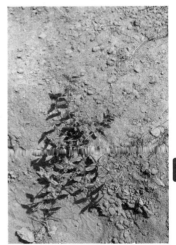

Snakeweed. (Williamson, 2002)

sneha (snā'·hə), *n* in Ayurveda, a method of medicine preparation in which lightly heated oil or ghee is infused with herbs and/or herbal extracts.

snehan (snā·hän), *n* in Ayurveda, medicated oil massage. Performed before beginning panchakarma. See also Panchakarma.

snehana (snā·hä·nə), *n* in Ayurveda, a purification therapy that involves cleansing the body of impurities. Performed over 4 days. Each day, the patient ingests prescribed amounts of ghee on an empty stomach, avoids fats and consumes few calories. After the 4 days, the person takes a hot bath and more laxatives and undergoes purgation for the next 12 hours.

snigdha (snēg·dhə), *adj* in Ayurveda, "oily" as a guna, one of the qualities that characterizes all substances. Its complement is ruksha. See also gunas and ruksha.

soap bark, *n* See quillay bark.

SOAP charting, *n.pr* abbreviation for a healthcare charting system that considers four variables: the **S**ubjective experience of the client, the **O**bjective discoveries of the healthcare professional, the **A**ssessment of the patient's condition, and the **P**lan for further treatment.

sobadores (sō·bä·dō·res), *n* in Curanderismo, the Mexican-American healing system, healers who work on the material level and specialize in the treatment of tense muscles and sprains.

Society for Clinical and Experimental Hypnosis, *n.pr* an organization founded in 1949 to promote hypnosis. Specifically, the group works to encourage and provide support for research on hypnosis and areas related to hypnosis. It offers standardized training and education for practitioners and establishes standards of ethics and practice. The organization publishes *International Journal of Clinical and Experimental Hypnosis* and *FOCUS,* the newsletter. Also called *SCEH.*

sodium, *n* an element/mineral that acts as an electrolyte and functions in nerve signal transmission, blood pressure regulation, cell function, and maintenance of pH balance. Side-effects of sodium deficiency include cramps, lethargy, nausea, and weakness. Dietary sources include fruits; vegetables (particularly sea vegetables and celery); processed foods; and, of course, table salt.

soft sciences, *n.pl.,* slang term for the body of research that often uses more subjective and difficult-to-control measures and designs, such as psychology and the social sciences.

soft tissue, *n* a system of osteopathic techniques for diagnosing and treating somatic dysfunctions within tissues other than bones or joints. See also somatic dysfunction.

soft-tissue manipulation (STM), *n* all methods that use a manual approach, such as massage, to treat muscle and soft tissues.

Solanum nigrum, *n* See nightshade, black.

Solanum xanthocarpum, *n* See nightshade, yellow-berried.

solid extract, *n* in herbal medicine, a substance derived from mixing an herb with a solvent (usually a mixture of alcohol and water) and then removing the solvent. May be soft (viscous) or dry (powdered), depending on the plant, part of the plant, and the process used for extraction.

soliton (sō·lə·tôn), *n* a type of highly coherent wave that does not readily disperse. These solitary waves are sometimes used to explain the effects of energy medicine.

solute, *n* in homeopathy, the portion of the source material used to create a liquid remedy. See also source material, mother tincture, and stock.

solvation structures, *n* in theory, the reorganization of molecular lattice of water and water-ethanol mixes during the potentization procedure. This reorganization is postulated to carry the medicinal features of the mixture. See also clathrate.

solvent, *n* a dissolving agent of a solution.

solvent extraction, *n* a method of extracting essential oils in which chemical solvents dissolve plant resins and produce absolutes. Because trace amounts of the solvent remain in the oils so produced, many aromatherapists do not use solvent extracted absolutes. See also absolute.

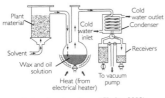

Solvent extraction. (Clarke, 2002)

soma (sō'·mə), *n* Greek word, meaning "body."

somatic cranial work (sō·ma'·tik krā'·nē·əl werk'), *n* gentle, hands-on technique in which light touch is used to encourage proper movement of all the elements within the cranial sacral system, following which the self-healing mechanism of the body takes over and completes the correction.

somatic dysfunction, *n* **1.** in psychology, embodied neuroses. The physical manifestation of psychologic defenses. **2.** in neuromuscular therapy, an area of limited motion and physical tenderness. Formerly called *neuromuscular lesion.*

somatic education, *n* mind-body learning approaches that are kinesthetic and somatosensory in nature—that is, motion and awareness are taught to return the patient to intuitive, natural movement.

somatic memories, *n pl* memories of trauma that are stored in an organism's body.

somatic nervous system, *n* voluntary system that controls impulses conveyed to the skeletal muscles from the central nervous system.

somatic recall, *n* the release of powerful, buried memories and emotions that may occur during a bodywork session.

somatics, *n* a neuromuscular system of education developed by Thomas Hanna; assists students in release and reversal of pain patterns due to past injuries, repetitive motion patterns, learned postural misalignment, and stress.

somatoemotional release (sō·ma'·tə·ē·mō'·shə·nəl rə·lēs'), *n* technique developed in the 1970s as an offshoot of craniosacral therapy that releases residual negative energies from past traumatic experiences. See also therapy, craniosacral.

somatogenic (sō·ma·tə·je'·nik), *adj* produced by actions, reactions, and changes within the musculoskeletal system.

somatosensory event related potentials (SERP) (sō·ma'·tə·sen'·sə·rē ē·vent' rē·lā'·təd pō·ten'·chəlz), *n.pl* diagnostic tests that assist researchers in determining the correlates of brain-mind activity.

somatosensory noise, *n* the background level of sensory input generated by tense muscles, joint compression, etc. Massage therapy helps alleviate the resulting muscle tension by helping the client develop somatic awareness.

somatotonia (sō·ma·tə·tō'·nē·ə), *n* one of the three temperaments described by WH Sheldon—characterized as active, energetic, assertive, sometimes aggressive, and not openly affective.

somatotype, *n* a person's physique or body type. The importance of the somatotype toward health has been recognized since the time of Hippocrates, and the somatotype is currently regarded as the physical expression of lifelong interaction between a person's genotype and his or her environment. See also ectomorph, endomorph, and mesomorph.

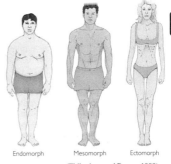

Endomorph   Mesomorph   Ectomorph

Somatotype. (Thibodeau and Patton, 1999)

S

somatotype, Heath-Carter, *n.pr* a modern model for determining soma totypes; used by sports educators and anthropologists and has some clinical use in identifying predisposition to physical and psychologic illness. See also ectomorphy, endomorphy, mesomorphy, and somatotype.

sophrology (sō·frô'·lə·jē), *n* an alternate term for the field of hypnosis; still in limited use in some countries. See also hypnosis.

sorcerer (sōr'·ser·er), *n* in several traditional cultures, a person who employs knowledge and prayer to bring about negative ends for a personal purpose. This person may propel forces of negativity, such as spirits that cause disease and embody destructive thoughts, or remove a victim's life energy. Stones, herbs, charms, and physical objects taken from the person being victimized are used to cast spells. Also called *dida:hnese:sg(i).* See healers.

sortilegio (sōr'·ti·lā'·hē·ō), *n* in Curanderismo, the Mexican-American healing system, a ritual in which ribbons are used to tie up the negative influences due to excessive drinking, infidelity, or problems arising from antisocial magic.

soul loss, *n* in Lakota Indian philosophy, a condition in which a patient's nagi (soul) becomes detached from his or her body because of neglect, abuse, or rejection. Ceremonies are performed by a healer to find the nagi and bring it back to unite the spirit and the body.

source material, *n* the substance used as a basis for a homeopathic remedy. This substance could be chemical substance, human, animal, vegetable, or mineral in origin or even magnetism, x-rays, or sunlight. Also called *basic product, crude material, crude substance, raw material,* and *starting material.* See also mother tincture; drugs, standardization of; and stock.

soy, *n* Latin name: *Glycine max;* part used: seeds (beans); uses: high cholesterol, analgesic, antipyretic, anorexia, hyperactivity, liver conditions; possible use in menopausal symptoms,

osteoporosis, cancers (breast, prostate, colon); precautions: none known. Also called *soya, soybean,* or *soy lecithin.*

SP, *n* spleen channel; an acupuncture channel running from the feet to the chest and associated with the stomach (ST) channel. See also ST.

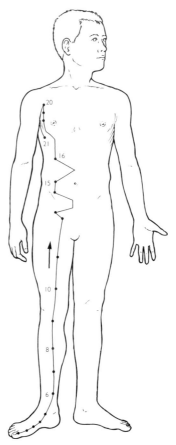

SP. (Chirali, 1999)

Spanish fly, *n* a preparation made from the crushed, dried bodies of the *Cantharis vesicatoria,* the blister beetles. Claimed to have aphrodisiac properties, its effects are derived from the irritant effects upon the body's genitourinary tract. Toxic doses of the preparation lead to priapism in men and pelvic congestion with occasional uterine bleeding in women. Formerly used as a counterirritant, it is no longer used (except in homeopathic doses) because of its high toxicity. Also called *cantharides*.

sparshanam (spär·shä'·nəm), *n* in Ayurveda, touch; it provides a fundamental basis for the eight classical markers—urine, pulse, tongue, feces, voice and speech, assessment of the eyes, evaluation by touch, and general physical assessment—used throughout the examination. See also darshanam and prashnam.

spasm, *n* sudden, involuntary contraction of muscle tissue accompanied by pain and interference with normal functioning.

spasmolytic (spaz'·mə·li'·tik), *n* a substance that relieves cramping, spasms, and convulsions.

spasmolytic, *adj* providing relief to cramping, spasms, and convulsions.

spasticity, *n* hypertonicity of muscles associated with increased tendon reflexes.

spearmint, *n* See mint.

specific, *n* a homeopathic medicine that is the precise remedy for a given symptom or illness. For example, soft-tissue trauma calls for *Arnica montana*, which is considered to be a specific for that symptom. See also homeopathic pathological prescribing.

specific gravity (SG), *n* a measurement calculated by dividing the mass of the desired volume of a substance by the mass of an equivalent volume of water. Both measurements must be taken under identical pressure and temperature conditions. Used to determine the presence of impurities within an essential oil. Also used in diagnostic analysis of fluids such as urine.

specifism, *n* curative technique that advocates selecting homeopathic remedies without regard to a particular person's reactions to the illness but simply by the organ or tissue to which the remedy has an affinity. This application of these remedies does not

follow the basic tenants of homeopathy. See also homeopathic pathological prescribing and specific.

SPECT, *n* See single photon emission computer tomography.

spectrochrome system (spek'·trə·krōm' sis'·təm), *n* color-therapy technique introduced by Ghadiali Dinshah in 1920. Spectrochrome uses colored filters to affect change in the electromagnetic field surrounding the body.

spectrogram (spek'·trə·gram), *n* a pictorial representation in the form of a graph or diagram that illustrates the results produced by the spectroscopic analysis of a particular substance.

spectroscopy (spek·trôs'·kə·pē), *n* practice of using spectroscopes and spectrometers to obtain qualitative and quantitative information about substances.

sphenobasilar synchondrosis (sfē'·nō·ba'·zi·ler sing'·kôn·drō'·sis), *n* the cartilaginous junction of the posterior surface of the body of the sphenoid bone and the anterior end of the basal portion of the occipital bone.

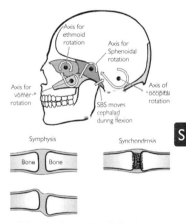

Sphenobasilar synchrondosis. (Chaitow, 1999)

sphenoid (sfe'·noid), *n* the hollow bone structure, located in the middle of the skull, which encases the sphenoid air sinuses.

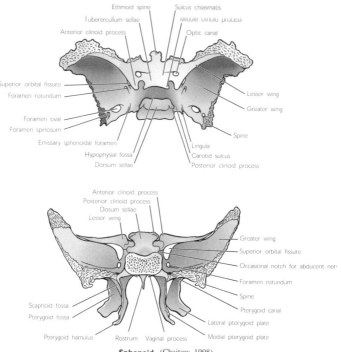

Ethmoid spine   Sulcus chiasmatis
Tuberercullum sellae   Middle clinoid process
Anterior clinoid process   Optic canal
Superior orbital fissure
Foramen rotundum   Lesser wing
Greater wing
Foramen oval
Foramen spinosum   Spine
Emissary sphenoidal foramen   Lingula
Hypophysial fossa   Carotid sulcus
Dorsum sellae   Posterior clinoid process

Anterior clinoid process
Posterior clinoid process
Dosum sellae
Lesser wing
Greater wing
Superior orbital fissure
Occasional notch for abducent nerv
Foramen rotundum
Spine
Scaphoid fossa   Pterygoid canal
Pterygoid fossa   Lateral pterygoid plate
Pterygoid hamulus   Rostrum   Vaginal process   Medial pterygoid plate

Sphenoid. (Chaitow, 1998)

sphenoid sinus, *n* Located beneath the nasal bridge, one of the passages through which air flows.

spina bifida (spī´·nə bi´·fi·də), *n* a congenital defect of the neural tube marked by absence of vertebral arches, through which the spinal cord and membranes may protrude; symptoms are few unless several vertebrae are affected. Also called *spinal dysrhaphia*.

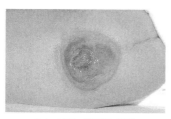

Spina bifida. (Newton, 1995)

spinal anesthesia illusion (spī´·nəl a·nəs·thē´·zhə i·lōō´·zhən), *n* form of hypnosis used to induce numbness in individuals undergoing surgery; the individual is instructed to focus on counting or on a specific image, and as deep relaxation sets in, the practitioner suggests that numbness will gradually take over the patient's body. Once the surgical procedure is complete, another suggestion is given that sensation will gradually return to the patient's body.

spinal kinesiopathology (spī´·nəl ki´·nē·zē·ô´·pə·thô´·lə·gē), *n* atypical positioning or motion of the spinal bones.

spinal locking (spī´·nəl lô´·king), *n* the positioning of adjacent spinal segments by using ligamentous myofascial tension or facet apposition or a combination of the two techniques. See also HVT.

spinal reflex effect, *n* one of the physiologic principles used in hydrotherapy to improve blood circulation by intense heat and cold applications. This affects both the local and remote physiologic areas and is mediated by spinal reflex arcs.

spinal stenosis (spī'·nəl stə·nō'·sis), *n* an abnormal narrowing of the spinal canal, nerve root canals, or intervertebral foramina of the lumbar spine; may be congenital or acquired.

spinous process (spī'·nəs prô'·ses), *n* the median process, which resembles a plate or spine, of a vertebra's neural arch. In chiropractic medicine, Daniel David Palmer was the first to use this specific process as a lever in the manual adjustment of a spine.

Spiraea ulmaria, *n* See meadowsweet.

spiritual healing, *n* healing systems based on the principle of spirituality and its effect on well-being and recovery.

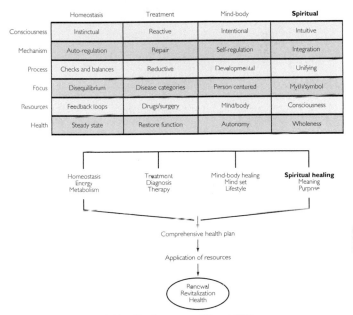

	Homeostasis	Treatment	Mind-body	**Spiritual**
Consciousness	Instinctual	Reactive	Intentional	Intuitive
Mechanism	Auto-regulation	Repair	Self-regulation	Integration
Process	Checks and balances	Reductive	Developmental	Unifying
Focus	Disequilibrium	Disease categories	Person centered	Myth/symbol
Resources	Feedback loops	Drugs/surgery	Mind/body	Consciousness
Health	Steady state	Restore function	Autonomy	Wholeness

Homeostasis
Energy
Metabolism

Treatment
Diagnosis
Therapy

Mind-body healing
Mind set
Lifestyle

Spiritual healing
Meaning
Purpose

Comprehensive health plan

Application of resources

Renewal
Revitalization
Health

Spiritual healing system. (Micozzi, 2002)

S

spiritual well-being, *n* a sense of peace and contentment stemming from an individual's relationship with the spiritual aspects of life.

spirituality, *n* an individual's quest for understanding the true meaning of life and the desire to integrate with the transcendent or sacred. May or may not arise from or lead to community formation or ritual observance.

spirulina (spī'·rə·lē'·nə), *n* Latin name: *Spirulina* spp.; parts used: whole plant (algae cells); uses: nourishment, weight loss, antiviral, antiallergy, antitumor, cholesterol, chemoprevention, immunomodulator, hepatoprotection; precautions: pregnancy, lactation, children; patients with thyroid conditions, thyroid medications; may cause possible heavy metal poisoning. Also called *blue-green algae, DIHE,* or *tecuitlatl.*

***Spirulina* spp.,** *n* See spirulina.

splenomegaly (sple'·nō·me'·gə·lē), *n* an abnormal increase in the size of the spleen; often associated with hemolytic anemia, mononucleosis, leukemia, portal hypertension, or malaria.

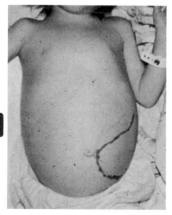

Splenomegaly. (Jorde et al, 1999)

SpO₂, *n* the saturation level of oxygen in hemoglobin; can be determined by noninvasive method of pulse oximetry.

spondelitis, *n* See spondylitis.

spondylitis (spôn·də·lī'·təs), *n* condition marked by inflammation of the vertebrae.

spondylolisthesis (spôn'·də·lō·lis'·thə·sis), *n* anterior slippage of a vertebra relative to the vertebra immediately below.

spondylosis (spôn'·də·lō'·lə·sis), *n* **1.** fusion of adjacent vertebraeh. **2.** condition characterized by the breakdown of the pars interarticularis (the thin strip of bone that connects the inferior and superior facets of a vertebra), maldevelopment of the vertebral arch, or flattening and breakdown of the vertebra. Also called *prespondylolisthesis.*

spondylotherapy (spôn'·di·lō·the'·rə·pē), *n* therapeutic approach in which the practitioner places the middle finger on the spinous process while using the other hand to strike the finger with blows that rapidly rebound. Typically, the practitioner applies one or two cycles per second. This approach is generally applied to at least three vertebrae adjacent to each other. Also called *percussion technique.*

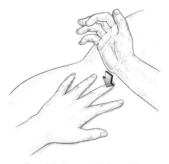

Spondylotherapy. (Chaitow, 2003)

spontaneous remission, *n* phrase used by medical professionals to describe a patient's complete recovery that is inexplicable by medical means.

sprain, *n* an acute injury to ligamentous tissues that results from overstretching, ranging in severity from tissue microtrauma to total disruption of the tissues.

spring nutrition, *n* in Tibetan medicine, the adjustment of an individual's eating habits to spring weather. Specifically, between the winter and summer solstice, the digestive processes within the gastrointestinal tract are believed to progressively decrease in comparison to the activity during the winter. The change in atmospheric conditions diminishes the demand for energy provided by the absorptive and digestive functions. As a result, because the functions associated with badahan and schara gradually weaken, they become quite vulnerable to errors in dietary habits. As a rule, individuals are instructed to consume foods with bitter, rough, pungent, and astringent tastes that are characteristic of spring fruits and vegetables or to fast occasionally to decrease the amount of burden placed on the digestive processes within the body. See also schara and badahan.

springing (spring·ing), *v* soft tissue manipulation in which the practitioner gradually applies slow, repetitive pressure; often used as a diagnostic tool.

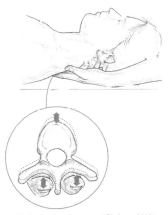

Springing/spring test. (Chaitow, 2003)

squalene (skwä'·lēn), *n* a popular traditional Asian remedy derived from the liver oil of sharks. Available as an over-the-counter agent, it is widely used for cosmetic purposes—particularly the regeneration of the skin. Oral administration of squalene has been associated with lipoid pneumonia due to aspiration.

squeezing and pinching, *v* squeezing is tightly enclosing the flesh between two opposing forces, whereas pinching is squeezing even more tightly between the finger and the thumb. Allows the therapist to assess overall tissue quality.

SQUID, *n.pr* acronym for superconducting quantum interference device. A device used to record the brain's biomagnetic fields.

squill (skwil'), *n* Latin names: *Urginea maritima, Drimia maritima;* part used: bulb; uses: diuretic, cardiac glycoside effects, heart conditions, cough; precautions: pregnancy, lactation, children, patients with hypokalemia, hypertropic cardiomyopathy, sick sinus syndrome, ventricular tachycardia, heart block (second- and third-degree), patients using cardiac medications, CNS stimulants, glucocorticoids, laxatives. Also called *European squill, Indian squill, Mediterranean squill, red squill, scilla, sea onion, sea squill,* or *white squill.*

srotas (srō'·tas), *n.pl* in Ayurveda, the thirteen internal body channels that convey elements crucial to physical functioning throughout the human body. Examples include veins, arteries, the small intestine, and the large intestine.

ST, *n* stomach channel; an acupuncture channel running from the head to the feet on the front of the body and associated with the spleen (SP) channel. See also SP.

S

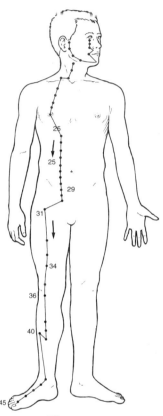

ST. (Chirali, 1999)

S

St. John's wort, *n.pr* Latin name: *Hypericum perforatum* L; part used: flowers; uses: depression, anxiety, topical antiinflammatory, hemorrhoids, vitiligo, possible antiviral; precautions: patients taking amphetamines, immunosuppressants, indinavir, MAOIs, paroxetine, SSRIs, trazodone, or tricyclic antidepressants; avoid alchohol and tyramine-containing foods. Also called *amber, goatweed, hardhay, John's wort, Klamath weed,* *mellipertuis, rosin rose,* or *witches' herb.*

stabilizing, *v* to hold a limb motionless in order to ground its energy; a standard isometric resistance technique, it releases tension and lengthens muscle fibers.

Stachys officinalis, *n* See betony.

standard sample, *n* a small portion of a substance that conforms to the specification for that particular material. It is used for evaluating other samples.

standard solution, *n* solution containing known concentration of a solute in a known volume of solution. See also concentration.

STAR, *n* an acronym used in osteopathic medicine that represents "sensitivity," "tissue texture change," "asymmetry," and "range of motion reduced." STAR prompts practitioners to remember the indications of somatic dysfunction, including those associated with myofascial trigger points.

star anise (stär´ a˙·nis), *n* Latin name: *Illicium verum;* parts used: fruit, oil, seeds; uses: bronchitis, carminative, colic, cough, diuretic, loss of appetite, rheumatism, stimulant; precautions: pregnancy, cancer, liver disease. Also called *Chinese anise.*

starvation, *n* condition in which prolonged (for weeks or months) lack of nourishment depletes most of the body's fat stores and causes it to use protein for fuel.

State Trait Anxiety Inventory, *n.pr* a questionnaire form concerning the subject's current anxiety feelings based on the responses to 40 items on a frequency scale that ranges from 1—meaning not at all—to 4—indicating almost always or very much so.

state-bound, *adj* continuous or powerful novel memories synchronously encoded in the limbic system with the emotions and behavior becoming inseparable.

state-dependent memory, *n* memory that, along with its state-bound reponses, is triggered by a similarly perceived situation. See also statebound.

static compression, *n* massage technique in which direct pressure is applied to an area of muscle and held until the tissue relaxes.

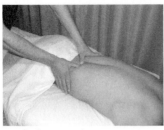

Static compression. (Lowe, 2003)

static palpation (sta'·tik pal·pā'·shən), *n* in chiropractic treatment, a technique of using one's hands to feel and assess several parameters that govern the mobility and health of tissues located near or on the body's surface. The purpose of this particular examination is to facilitate the analysis of soft or bony tissue structures within the body.

staying sickness, *n* according to the Pima Indian healing system, an illness caused by not respecting sacred power objects. Characterized by weakness and exhaustion. Can only be relieved through a shamanic ceremony. See also power objects.

steam bath, *n* a device used in the Kallawaya system of healing, practiced in Bolivia, in which a mixture of herbs is heated to produce steam that is used to eliminate toxins from the body.

steam room, *n* a room used to provide superficial, full body moist heat treatment to facilitate relaxation and detoxification through sweating. See also thermotherapy.

steam-and-vacuum distillation, *n* a speedy method of extracting essential oils that uses both steam and partial vacuum.

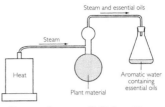

Steam-and-vacuum distillation. (Tiran, 2000)

Stellaria media, *n* See chickweed.

stenosis (stə·nō'·sis), *n* a decrease in the size of a channel, passageway, or opening within a structure, such as pyloric stenosis or aortic stenosis.

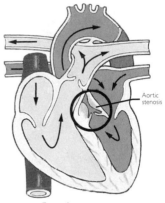

Stenosis. (Wong, 1999)

step, *n* a phase in the dilution process or a specific degree of dilution. Also called *lift-in potency.* See also dilution, dynamisation, and potentization.

stereochemistry (ste'·rē·ō·ke'·mi·strē), *n* area of chemistry dealing with the three-dimensional arrangement of atoms that make up a molecule.

stereoisomers (ste'·rē·ō·ī'·sə·merz), *n.pl* compounds with identical chemical composition and atomic bonding that differ in the spatial arrangement of atoms.

Sthapathya Veda (st·hä·pə·t·hyä vä·də), *n.pr* ancient Indian architectural discipline, which aims to create dwellings that promote good health by taking into consideration the orientation of dwellings, the materials used to build them, ventilation, light, and the natural settings.

sthira (sthē'·rä), *adj* in Ayurveda, "static" as a guna, one of the qualities that characterizes all substances. Its complement is chala. See also gunas and chala.

sthula (sthōō'·lə), *adj* in Ayurveda, "gross" as a guna, one of the qualities that characterizes all substances. Its complement is sukshma. See also gunas and sukshma.

still, *n* an apparatus used for steam or water distillation. It comprises a vessel that contains water and aromatic plant material, a condenser that cools the vapor produced from heating the plant material, and a receiver for collecting the condensed products.

stimulant, *n* **1.** a substance that temporarily increases the physiologic activity of an organ or organ system. **2.** a substance that increases nervous excitability and alertness.

stock, *n* initial material used to create a homeopathic remedy via dilution or trituration.

stomachic (stə·ma'·kik), *n* product that serves to increase stomach secretions.

stone breaker, *n* Latin name: *Phyllanthus niruri;* parts used: herb, leaf, root; uses: in Ayurveda, pacifies kapha and pitta doshas (bitter, astringent, sweet, light, dry), diuretic, hypoglycemic, antimicrobial, antioxidant, choleretic, kidney stones, gall stones, liver conditions, jaundice, diabetes, diarrhea, inflammation; precautions: none known. Also called *bahupatra, bhuinanvalah, bhumyaamlaki,* or *shatter stone.*

storax (stōr'·aks), *n* Latin name: *Liquidambar orientalis;* parts used: bark, gum, leaves; uses: diuretic, expecto-

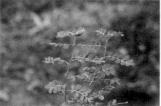

Stone breaker. (Williamson, 2002)

rant, diarrhea, sore throat, possible antibacterial properties; precautions: pregnancy, lactation, children. Also called *alligator tree, star-leaved gum, sweet gum tree, balsam styracis, liquid amber, opossum tree, red gum,* or *white gum.*

story line, *n* an inner dialogue often instigated by the onset of meditation-related mindfulness; may include thoughts, history, and painful emotions associated with chronic physical pain.

strabismus (strə·biz'·məs), *n* a condition wherein the two visual axes of the eyes are not aimed at a single object. In paralytic strabismus the muscles in the eyes are unable to move because of infection, tumor, or injury. In nonparalytic strabismus, there is a defect in the location of the eyes in relationship to their focal point. Also called *squint.*

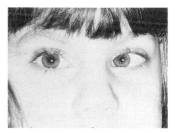

Strabismus. (Zitelli and Davis, 1997)

S

straight chain, *n* series of carbon atoms found in acyclic organic compounds that are successively linked without any branches.

straight chiropractic (strāt´ kī´·rō·prak´·tik), *n* a fundamentalist school of thought associated with chiropractic medicine in which manipulation of the spine is used as the primary therapeutic approach. Adherents to this school of thought emphasize the concept of innate intelligence and believe subluxation is the primary origin of disease. An ongoing debate exists between the concepts associated with straight chiropractic and mixer approach. See also subluxation and mixer approach.

strain, *n* **1.** an injury to muscle tissue resulting from overstretching. **2.** deformation and distortion of tissues. **3.** mental distress.

strain, ligamentous, *n* asymmetric position and/or motion correlated with elastic deformation of ligaments, fascia, and other connective tissues.

strain, ligamentous articular **(li·gə·men´·chəs är·tik´·yu·ler stran´),** *n* any condition that results in excessive or otherwise abnormal tension or strain on the ligaments.

strain, membranous articular, *n* any cranial condition that results in excessive or abnormal tension in the membranes of the dura mater.

strain, muscle, *n.pl* mild, moderate, or severe tearing of the muscle tissue in response to overstretching or trauma.

strain, muscular, *n* mild, moderate, or severe tearing of muscle fibers in response to overstretching.

strain, role, *n* stressful life event that occurs as a result of the struggle between the different demands of life. Throughout the lifetime, a person may simultaneously adopt several functions, including that of a parent, caretaker, or employee, and the competing demands of these roles may produce stress in affecting a person's health.

strain, SBS lateral, *n* rotation of the occipital and sphenoid bones in the same direction about parallel vertical axes. May either be left or right lateral strain, depending on the basisphenoid's position. Also called *sphenobasilar synchondrosis (symphysis) lateral strain.*

strain, SBS vertical, *n* rotation of the occipital and sphenoid bones in the same direction about parallel transverse axes. May be either superior or inferior, depending on the position of the basisphenoid. Also called *sphenobasilar synchondrosis (symphysis) vertical strain.*

strain/counterstrain (SCS) (strān/ kawn·ter·strān), *n* soft-tissue manipulation technique in which the practitioner seeks to locate and alleviate nonradiating tender points in the patient's myofascial structures. The practitioner positions dysfunctional tissue at a point of balance in a direction opposite the restrictive barrier. The position of ease is held for 90 seconds, after which the patient is gently returned to the original position where the tender point is rechecked. Also called *positional release therapy.*

stramonium (strə·mō´·nē·əm), *n* See thorn apple.

strength testing, *n* assessment procedure to determine the contractile strength of a muscle.

streptococcal pharyngitis (strep· tō·kô´·kəl far·in·jī´·tis), *n* an inflammation of the pharynx caused by infection from *Streptococcus.* Spread by direct contact from person-to-person. It is typically indicated by the presence of a sore and/or red throat, an impaired ability to swallow, sudden onset of fever, and the swelling of the lymph nodes. Also called *strep throat.*

Streptococcus (strep·tō kô´·kəs), *n* a pathogenic bacterium often found in the mucosae of the mouth, nose, and throat and occasionally in skin, muscle, or heart tissue.

stress, *n* any factor (environmental, chemical, physical, or emotional) that contributes to the "stress response" (physiologic reactions to tension). Has been implicated in a number of diseases—including asthma, autoimmune disease, cancer, cardiovascular disease, diabetes, depression, irritable bowel syndrome, premenstrual tension syndrome, rheumatoid arthritis, and ulcers.

stress hardiness, *n* mindset exhibited by an individual that makes him or her resistant to the negative impacts of stressful circumstances and events. Three attitudes are associated with this concept: control, challenge and commitment. See also control, challenge, and commitment.

stress management, *n* activities of all types that serve to release the mind and body from undue tension, such as fitness programs, mind-body methods, lifestyle modifications, and relaxation techniques.

stress response, *n* physiologic response to stress; comprises three phases. The fight-or-flight response is the first phase, in which the sympathetic nervous system is activated, increasing heart rate, respiration, and blood pressure. In the second phase the organism adapts to the source of stress. The third and final phase is exhaustion. Also called *general adaptation syndrome.*

stress-induced analgesia (stres´-in·dōōsd´ a´·nəl·jē´·zē·ə), *n* a numbness to pain that the body generates itself as a protective mechanism in response to mental anxiety or trauma.

stretching (stre´·ching), *n* mechanical lengthening of myofascial fibers. Muscles and fascia lengthen longitudinally and cross-directionally.

strict liability, *n* a case in which responsibility for breaking the law is enforced without proving intent, or *mens rea*. In civil law, a case in which negligence does not have to be proven in order to be found legally liable.

stridor (strī´·dər), *n* an abnormal, high-pitched, whistling sound heard during inspiration due to a blockage in the larynx or trachea. The condition may indicate inflammatory and neoplastic conditions, such as asthma, glottic edema, laryngospasm, diphtheria, papilloma, or other causes of swelling or laxity.

striking, *v* applying drumming-type rhythms and strokes to the body;

an oscillation procedure in manual therapy sessions that serves to decongest the lungs, stimulate the nervous system, create rhythms, and loosen attachments.

stringiness, *n* an abnormal texture of myofascial tissues; characterized by a stringy feeling.

stroke, *n* **1.** a massage technique that involves pressure or movement of the therapist's hand or arm across the body's surface. **2.** a condition in which hemorrhage or occlusion of a cerebral blood vessel leads to ischemia and tissue damage to the brain. May result in changes in speech or sensation, weakness, paralysis, and death.

stroking, *n* manual touch employed by a massage therapist to treat a client. Stroking comprises techniques such as effluerage (gliding), petrissage (kneading), friction (warming), tapotement (percussion), and vibration (shaking). (MTPAP, 152)

structural and postural integration approaches (struk´·chur·əl and pôs´·chur·əl in·tə·grā´·shən ə·prō´·chez), *n.pl* terms applied to bodywork methods influenced by postural alignment and biomechanics and that focus primarily on connective tissues.

structural equations, *n.pl* statistical approach that comprehensively addresses multidimensional, complex relationships among research variables.

structural integration, *n* See Rolfing.

structural view, *n* philosophy that sees the body and its components in the context of its relationship to the forces of gravity. Observes the body's fascial planes to assess its condition.

Strychnos nux-vomica, *n* See nux vomica seed.

stupor, *n* lethargic state of consciousness characterized by reduced response to stimulation.

styptic (stip´·tik), *adj* ability to quickly contract tissues to stop heavy bleeding.

Styrax benzoin, *n* See benzoin.

Styrax paralleloneurus, *n* See benzoin.

Styrax tonkinesis, *n* See benzoin.

suanzaoretang (sōō·än·zä·ō·rä·täng), *n* herbal remedy used in China since ancient times for irritability, weakness, and insomnia. Used today in the treatment of anxiety disorders.

subclinical deficiency, *n* in orthomolecular medicine, a nutritional deficiency not yet displaying classical deficiency symptoms.

subcutaneous tissue (sub'·kyōō·tā'·ne·əs ti''·shōō), *n* the layer of tissue between the dermis and muscle, consisting of adipose and connective tissues, blood vessels, and nerves.

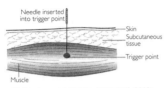

Subcutaneous tissue. (Campbell, 2002)

subjective health status, *n* an analysis of an individual's concerns and attitudes about health and illness and predictions about treatment outcome.

subjective units of distress (SUD), *n.pl* measurements used to describe an individual's level of suffering or grief associated with painful memories.

subluxation (sə·bluk·sā'·shən), *n* the atypical anatomic positioning of any joint that exceeds the physiologic but not the anatomic limit.

subluxation, vertebral **(ver·tə·brəl sub·luk·sā' shən),** *n* structural misalignments in the spinal column that interrupt normal neural transmissions.

submolecular, *adj* See ultramolecular.

subspecies, *n* an intermediate taxonomical category in biology. Immediately subordinate to species, it usually denotes geographically isolated or morphologically different populations that may interbreed with other subspecies. Abbreviated as *subsp.*

substance abuse, *n* misuse of mood-altering drugs; negatively influences the user's life.

substantia gelatinosa, *n* See SG.

substantia nigra (səb·stan'·shē·ə nī'·grə), *n* the portion of the mesencephalon (midbrain) whose degeneration is implicated in Parkinson's disease.

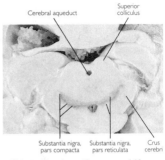

Substantia nigra. (Crossman and Neary, 1995)

subtle body (su'·təl bô'·dē), *n* in Tibetan medicine, a network of energy channels that transport energy derived from oxygen-, sensory-, and food-derived nutrients. This network lies parallel to the blood vessels and nerves in the body; it facilitates and coordinates the movement of the flow of blood and neural impulses. It is not an anatomical system such as the cardiovascular or nervous system and cannot be viewed conventionally. Instead, it is accessed through practice of imagination and visualization that can be accomplished through meditation.

succussion (sək·kə'·shən), *n* the forceful agitation between each dilution step during the preparation of the homeopathic remedy. See also fluxion and trituration.

sucrose, *n* $C_{12}H_{22}O_{11}$, a sugar whose source is sugarcane or sugarbeet, commonly found in solid preparations.

sudorific (sōō'·də·ri'·fik), *adj* causing perspiration.

suggestability, *n* a state of easy influence by suggestion.

suggestion phase, *n* the stage in a session of hypnosis in which behavioral changes are introduced. See also hypnosis.

suggestive therapeutics, *n.pl* philosophy developed by Sidney Weltmer according to which mind and the body are equal determinants of good health. A faltering belief by the mind can lead to lowered resistance to disease and physical discomfort can influence the person's thoughts, both of which result in the state of disease.

sukha (soō'·khə), *n* in Sanskrit, ease; the manner in which yoga postures are to be performed.

sukshma (soōk'·shmə), *adj* in Ayurveda, "subtle" as a guna, one of the qualities that characterize all substances. Its complement is sthula. See also gunas and sthula.

sulcus (sul'·kəs), *n* any of the narrow grooves in an organ or tissue, such as those that separate the convolutions of the cerebral hemisphere; used interchangeably with *fissure,* although a sulcus is not as deep as a fissure.

sulfation, *n* a phase-II detoxification pathway that occurs in the liver and in which compounds that contain sulfur combine with components to remove them from the body.

sulfoxidation, *n* a phase-II detoxification pathway that occurs in the liver and in which sulfite oxidase converts sulfites, such as those found in food preservatives and colorings, garlic compounds, and chlorpromazine into sulfates so they can be safely eliminated from the body.

summary judgment, *n* a legal course of action in which a judgment can be made against a defendant without hearing any testimony from said defendant.

summer nutrition, *n* in Tibetan medicine, the purposeful adjustment of an individual's eating habits to summer weather. During the warm months, the peak amount of energy exerted by the sun is thought to place a minimal amount of stress on the digestive processes that pull out energy for the body's use. The gastrointestinal tract's dormant state increases its vulnerability to foods that taste strong. As a rule, individuals are encouraged to eat foods that are cool and light. Predominantly, these foods should also have a sweet taste. Warm tea with lemon is preferable to cold drinks to prevent disturbing thermoregulation, a process that is dependent on schara. The individual is discouraged from eating foods that have a pungent, bitter, or astringent taste. Heavy, greasy, and canned foods are also not to be consumed. See also schara.

sun style (swən stīl), *n.pr.* variant of tai chi developed by Sun Lutang and characterized by its quickness and compact moves; Sun was among the first to teach tai chi to the general public.

Sun's soup, *n.pr* a proprietary mixture of herbs and vegetables, developed by Dr. Alexander Sun and marketed as a nutritional supplement and adjunct for treating various health concerns, such as cancer and AIDS. Also called *Sun Farms Vegetable Soup* or *Sun Soup.* See also selected vegetables.

sunburn, *n* injury to the skin caused by prolonged exposure to the sun characterized by mild tenderness to severe pain, heat, redness, and occasional blistering.

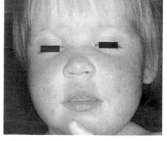

Sunburn. (Weston, Lane, and Morrelli, 1996)

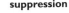

sunflower, *n* Latin name: *Helianthus annuus;* parts used: leaves, flowers, roots; uses: diuretic, expectorant, febrifuge, appetite stimulant, contraction of bodily tissues; wound healing, malaria, lung conditions, rheumatism; precautions: may cause allergic reactions. Also called *a'bbad al shams, a'in ash shams, aycicegi, common sunflower, fleur soleil, flor de sol, girasol, gula barbaroza, guna baqan, gundondu, helianthe, himawari, tournesol, ward ash shams,* and *zonnebloem.*

superbugs, *n.pl* infectious diseases that are unresponsive to known antibiotic treatments.

superficial, *n* **1.** in massage therapy, external, or outer surface. **2.** in psychotherapy, the primary use of such techniques as persuasion, counseling, reeducation, and inspiration. Also called *supportive psychotherapy* or *suppressive psychotherapy.*

superficial fascia (soo'·per·fi'·shəl fā'·shē·ə), *n* loose connective tissue that is located under the skin which contains fat.

superior, *adj* **1.** positioned toward the head or above the referent. Also called *cranial* or *cephalic.* **2.** being of higher quality.

supernatural mechanisms, *n.pl* explanations for the efficacy of spiritual healing and prayer that refer to a force, which is outside nature and natural laws altogether, such as God, gods, or spirits.

superoxide dismutase (soo·per· ōk'·sīd dis·myoo'·tār), *n* an enzyme that comprises metalloproteins and clears the body of superoxide radicals by converting them into less toxic substances.

supersensitivity, *n* a condition in which structures innervated by a dysfunctional peripheral nerve behave abnormally, with tightening of muscles and development of trigger points.

supination (soo'·pə·nā'·shən), *n* lateral rotation of the radioulnar joint to face the palm upwards.

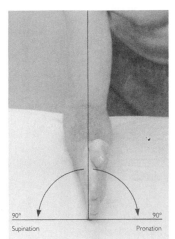

90°   90°
Supination   Pronation

Supination. (Seidel et al, 1999)

supine (soo'·pīn), *adj* face up or back down position assumed by the client during a bodywork session.

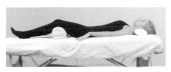

Supine. (Salvo, 2003)

supportive care, *n* medical and other interventions that attempt to support and make comfortable rather than to cure.

suppositories, *n.pl* solid capsules made of materials that melt at body temperature and are used to deliver medicinal substances into the rectum.

suppression, *n* **1.** in naturopathic medicine, the successful relief of symptoms without curing the underlying illness or disease. **2.** in homeopathy, the elimination of symptoms, often with topicals, without curing deeper aspects of the disease. Thought

S

to result in more serious inner disease later.

supreme master, *n* in Chinese medicine, the heart, as it "presides" over other organs of the body. The decisions of the heart strictly dictate the behaviors of the other organs within the body and the health of the heart reflects the general health of an individual.

surgery, *n* medical procedure in which the body is manually cut open to treat medical conditions.

surma (sŏŏr´·mə), *n* a traditional preparation originating from India and Pakistan used for cosmetic purposes. Available in a black powder, it is applied to the inner surface of the eyelid. It is also used as a teething powder. Reports of lead poisoning and fatal encephalopathy from surma have been published. See also al kohl.

surrogate, *n* **1.** a replacement. **2.** in homeopathy, a substitute medicine for the exact remedy. See also simillimum.

Suryanamaskar (sŏŏr´·yə·nä´·mə·skär), *n.pr* ancient Indian yogic exercise, ("salutation to the Sun"), which is a combination of 12 positions performed sequentially. Improves physical and mental flexibility and vitality. Said to help weight loss.

Sushruta Samhita (sŏŏ·shrŏŏ´·tə säm·hē´·tə), *n.pr* ancient text of Ayurveda on surgery, written by sage Sushruta; includes description of surgical operations done to remove obstructions in the intestines, bladder stones, cataracts of the eye, and rhinoplasty.

suspension, *n* a fluid with particles floating within it. See also colloid.

sustained movement, *n* movement held at end of range of motion to determine its effects on the symptoms. This position allows for lengthening of the soft tissue being stretched resulting in increased range of motion.

sustained natural apophyseal glides (sə·stānd´ na´·chrəl ə·pä´·fə·sē´·əl glīdz´), *n pl* a physical therapy method for treating cervical and spinal dysfunction, especially in the elderly or patients with acute injuries. Smooth, sliding force is applied continuously and parallel (neutral) to the pain-free limit of the affected joints while the patient is seated upright. See also MWM, NAGS.

sustaining cause, *n* factors that develop in the course of an illness, prolonging the condition and forestalling a healthy resolution.

susto (sŏŏ·stō), *n* "soul loss," an ethnomedical condition common to Latin America, an illness caused when the soul is displaced after a traumatic emotional or physical event. Can be a life-threatening illness characterized by lethargy, lack of motivation, insomnia, and diarrhea and is usually treated through spiritual means, ritual cleansings, and herbal teas. Also called *espanto.*

susumna (sŏŏ·sŏŏm´·nə), *n* in Ayurveda, spinal cord as described in the Atharvaveda. See vedas.

Sutherland fulcrum, *n.pr* axis around which the dural membranes, the tentorium, and falx move and also the point at which all the tension in these membranes is focused. Because these membranes are directly connected to cranial bones, their tension patterns are thought to have significant effect on the movement of the cranial bones.

Sutherland wave, *n.pr* See cranial rhythmic impulse.

svedavahasrotas (svā´·dä·vä´·häs·rō´·təs), *n.pl,* in Ayurveda, one of the 13 types of srotas (body channels) that convey sweat and originate in hair follicles and fat tissues. See also srotas.

swayback posture, *n* posture characterized by an exaggerated curve between the pelvis and ribs resulting in stress on the lower back.

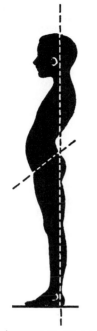

Swayback posture. (Kendall et al, 1993)

sweat bath, *n* **1.** a small shelter, made of stone or wood, which is heated with hot stones (to which water is often applied, to produce steam) and used therapeutically. Also called *sauna.* **2.** the therapeutic procedure in which individuals sit in the sweat bath for a short time to promote sweating and to increase circulation and detoxification. See also sweat lodge.

sweat lodge, *n* a particular type of sweat bath traditionally used by various Native American peoples for purposes of purification, integration, and spiritual vision quest. Also called *inipi* or *temazkal.*

Swedish gymnastics, *n.pl* active or passive joint mobilizations and stretches designed to increase flexibility, reduce pain, and maintain health.

Swedish movement cure, *n* an older term for Per Henrik Ling's massage techniques. See massage, Swedish.

sweet balm, *n* Latin name: *Melissa officinalis;* parts used: foliage, oil; uses: carminative; to counteract anxiety, insomnia, and menstrual problems; gastrointestinal complaints; sedative; wound healing; other folk medicine uses; precautions: none known. Also called *blue balm, lemon balm, cure-all,* and *dropsy plant.*

sweet flag, *n* Latin name: *Acorus calamu;* parts used: rhizomes, rootstock; uses: in Ayurveda, pacifies kapha and vata doshas (pungent, bitter, light, sharp), kidney and liver diseases, nerve tonic, sedative, diarrhea, dysentery, fevers; precautions: emetic at large doses. Also called *myrtle flag, sweet sedge, ugragandha,* or *vacha.*

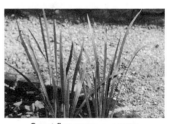

Sweet flag. (Williamson, 2002)

sycotic miasm (sā·kô'·tik mī'·a·zəm), *n* in homeopathy, a disease diathesis originally considered to stem from gonorrhea. Also called *sycosis.* See also miasm, psoric miasm, syphilitic miasm, tubercular diathesis, and diathesis.

symmetry, *n* similar arrangement of parts around a shared axis or plane.

sympathetic autonomic nervous system, *n* that part of the involuntary nervous system that balances the parasympathetic nervous system, increasing heart rate, pupil dilation, blood flow to skeletal muscles, and alertness. Also called *fight or flight.*

Symplocos racemosa, *n* See lodhra.

symptom, *n* any reported subjective attribute of an illness. See also anamnesis; case taking; symptom, complete; symptom, functional; symptom, general; symptom, local; symptom, mental; symptom, particular; modality; and symptoms, totality of.

symptom inventory, *n* a questionnaire used to record patient symptoms to assess their condition.

symptom picture, *n* account of all attributes of an illness specific to the patient. This is similar to clinical picture yet is individualized to that patient. See also clinical picture, disease picture, and symptom.

symptom selection, *n* the method of choosing the most helpful symptoms to determine the most effective homeopathic remedy. See also symptoms, hierarchy of; case taking; and symptoms, ranking of.

symptom, accessory, *n* within a group of symptoms, a less significant one. A less significant symptom. Also called *concomitant symptom*. See also symptom, incidental.

symptom, "as if", *n* subjective patient-described symptoms based on personalized perceived parallels as in "I feel as if." Primarily used in homeopathy.

symptom, benign, *n.pl* **1.** symptom associated with inconsequential or minor condition. **2.** in naturopathic medicine, indications (usually physical) of the body's response to a pathogen; symptoms that occur as part of the healing reaction as the body works to heal itself.

symptom, complete, *n* description of all aspects of a symptom—including where, when, how, how strong, how long, how often, and so forth. The plethora of variables involved in the complaint. See also symptom selection and symptoms, weighting of.

symptom, eliminating, *n* a symptom that, if not present in the listing for a given remedy in materia medica, removes that remedy from the list of those possible to treat the disease. See also symptom, guiding.

symptom, general, *n* systemic indicator of an illness. See also aggravating factors and modality.

symptom, guiding, *n* symptom that points toward a certain remedy. See also symptom, eliminating.

symptom, incidental, *n* a minor symptom of the illness that is not of primary importance. See also symptom, accessory; complaint; and concomitants.

symptom, keynote, *n* See symptom, guiding.

symptom, local, *n* a symptom limited to a specific body part, organ, or system. See also symptom, general and symptom, particular.

symptom, mental, *n* psychologic symptom of an illness. Also called *mind symptom*. See also symptoms, hierarchy of; symptom, general; and symptom, local.

symptom, paradoxical, *n* a symptom that is not consistent with the disease.

symptom, particular, *n* a symptom related to a specific anatomical part. See also symptom, local and complaint.

symptom, strange, rare, and peculiar, *n* an unusual symptom atypical for the illness. This type of symptom is important for case analysis in homeopathy as it allows for individualizing the remedy. See also symptom selection and symptoms, weighting of.

symptoms of maximum value, minimum, *n* the small number of deterministic symptoms that identify the core of the illness in an individual.

symptoms, alternating, *n.pl* two or more symptoms with only one symptom present at any given time. See also metastasis and syndrome shift.

symptoms, hierarchy of, *n* prioritization of symptoms with respect to their consequences and importance. See also symptom selection.

symptoms, morbid, *n.pl* subjective indications of pain or severe discomfort that arise directly from an injury or disease.

symptoms, new, *n.pl* novel symptoms that may be a result of the current illness or the homeopathic remedy used to treat the illness.

symptoms, proving, *n.pl* documented symptoms described by the person who is testing a homeopathic remedy. See also adverse drug reaction; disease, iatrogenic; and symptoms, new.

symptoms, ranking of, n the standing of symptoms prioritized based on their significance in developing the most efficient treatment for the illness. See also symptoms, heirarchy of and symptoms, weighting of.

symptoms, reappearance of old, n the reappearance of old symptoms after a homeopathic remedy is applied. Return of these symptoms often indicates positive progress in healing. See also suppression and therapeutic aggravation.

symptoms, resting, n.pl symptoms observed before any active physiologic movements, which help determine the effect of the movements on the symptoms.

symptoms, totality of, n one of the organizing principles of homeopathy, according to which the entire symptom profile of the patient is matched with the symptom profile of the homeopathic remedy.

Symptom Checklist 90R, n.pr self-report survey of 90 items that assesses medical and psychiatric patients for psychologic symptoms, such as interpersonal sensitivity, anxiety, depression, obsessive-compulsive symptoms, somatization, phobic anxiety, paranoid ideation, hostility, and psychoticism.

symptomatic relief (sim·tə·ma´·tik rə·lēf´), n control of symptoms rather than cure by a single or multiple therapies.

symptomatology, n **1.** all of the subjective indicators of an illness. **2.** the survey of symptoms with respect to how likely they are to correspond to specific homeopathic remedies. See also case taking; analysis; and materia medica.

synapse (si´·naps), n the junction between two neurons across which nerve impulses are conducted.

synarthrotic (si´·nə·thrô´·tik), adj joints, such as the sutures in the cranium, in which movement is absent or very limited.

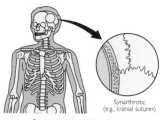

Synarthrotic. (Salvo, 2003)

Synarthrotic
(e.g., cranial sutures)

synchronicity (sing´·krən·ni´·si·tē), n the coincidence of an observer's internal state with an external event. Believed by Carl Jung to show evidence of a general acausal link between mind and matter. See also acausal.

synchronizing, n a technique that a therapist uses to coordinate his or her breath with that of the client; builds trust and establishes relationship.

syncope (sing´·kə·pē), n a sudden but temporary loss of consciousness due to insufficient blood supply to the brain; may be caused by vagal stimulation, emotional stress, blood loss, diaphoresis, or an immediate change in the position of the body or surrounding temperature. Also called *fainting*.

syndrome, n a set of disparate signs and symptoms that are not traceable to a single cause.

syndrome shift, n a change to a different set of symptoms than the previous set. This change can result from treatment or be a natural progression of the illness. In homeopathic terms the shift can also be from one level to another, such as from mental to physical. See also symptoms, alternating; direction of cure; illness, layers of; illness, levels of; metastasis; suppression; and vicariation.

syndrome X, n a syndrome of blood glucose dysregulation and intolerance and a disproportionate secretion of insulin. In turn, this causes the body to develop a decreased sensitivity to insulin and may cause other prob-

S

lems such as hypertension, obesity, increased cholesterol, and type II diabetes.

syndrome, acquired immune deficiency, *n* an infectious disease of epidemic proportions caused by the human immunodeficiency virus (HIV), which impairs the body's immune system, thus resulting in opportunistic infections and cancers. It is transmitted by bodily fluids, especially by sexual contact or contaminated needles.

syndrome, bi (pē sin´·drōm), *n* in traditional Chinese medicine, obstruction of qi and blood because of invasion of muscles, tendons, and ligaments by pathogens present in wind, cold, or dampness, thus resulting in muscle soreness and joint pain. See also qi.

syndrome, carpal tunnel, *n* pain in the hands and the arms and symptoms in which the median nerve is compressed between the carpal ligament and other elements inside the carpal tunnel. Can be caused by repetitive motion, synovitis, tumor, rheumatoid arthritis, amyloidosis, acromegaly, or diabetes.

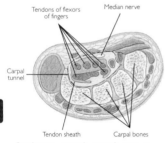

Syndrome, carpal tunnel. (Thibodeau and Patton, 1999; Rolin Graphics)

syndrome, Charcot's, *n.pr* a set of symptoms marked by weakness, cramps, and leg pain; caused by poor blood circulation in the leg muscles; brought on by physical effort and disappears upon resting. Also called *intermittent claudication* and *angina cruris.*

syndrome, Chediale-Higashi, *n* an inherited immune system disorder due to CHS1 gene mutations, characterized by neurologic disease, decreased pigment, and chronic infections resulting in early death. Children with this disorder may have light-colored eyes; a silvery sheen to their hair; nystagmus; and recurring infections in skin, lungs, and mucous membranes.

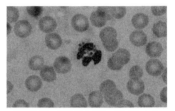

Syndrome, Chediale-Higashi. (Mosby's Medical, Nursing & Allied Health Dictionary, ed 6, 2002)

syndrome, chronic fatigue, *n* a set of symptoms marked by incapacitating fatigue and a mixture of flulike complaints such as swollen lymph glands, sore throat, headaches, low-grade fever, and muscle weakness or pain.

syndrome, compartment, *n* condition of increased pressure inside a closed chamber, usually from swelling of muscles in fascial compartments; can damage irreversibly the tissues of the chamber.

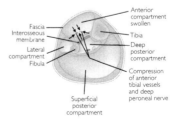

Syndrome, compartment. (Black, Hawks, and Keene, 2001)

syndrome, Cushing's, n disorder caused by the presence of excessive cortisol in the body; may be induced by the administration of high doses of glucocorticoids; occurs naturally when an individual's body cannot regulate cortisol or adrenocorticotropic hormone. Most commonly occurs as a result of a pituitary tumor. Also called *hyperadrenocorticism.*

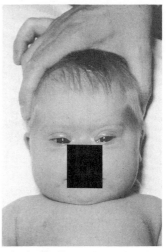

Syndrome, Down. (Zitelli and Davis, 1997)

syndrome, eosinophilia-myalgia (ē·ō·si·nə·fi'·lē·ə-mī·al'·jyə sin'·drōm), n a rare autoimmune condition characterized by muscle pains and increased production of eosinophils; associated with the consumption of contaminated *L*-tryptophan.

syndrome, fetal alcohol, n a group of physical, emotional, and behavioral characteristics present at birth; connected to maternal alcohol intake during pregnancy.

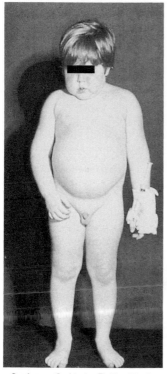

Syndrome, Cushing's. (Zitelli and Davis, 1997)

syndrome, Down, n congenital disorder caused by the occurrence of an additional twenty-first chromosome. The person is mild to moderately mentally retarded, short-statured, and has a compressed facial profile. Also called *trisomy 21.*

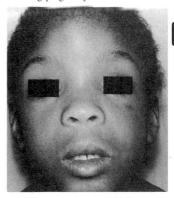

Syndrome, fetal alcohol (FAS). (Zitelli and Davis, 1997)

syndrome, general adaptation (gen'· rəl a'·dap·tā'·shən sin'·drōm), *n* the physiologic response to stressors that comprises three reactions: alarm, resistance, and exhaustion.

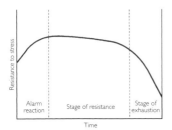

Syndrome, general adaptation. (Cox: Stress, 1978 [Adapted and used with permission from Macmillan, London])

syndrome, Gilbert's, n.pr common inherited disorder that affects the way the liver processes bilirubin resulting in jaundice. Condition is generally benign. Also called *icterus intermittens juvenilis, low-grade chronic hyperbilirubinemia, familial non-hemolytic–non-obstructive jaundice, constitutional liver dysfunction,* or *unconjugated benign bilirubinemia.*

syndrome, Guillain-Barré, n an inflammation of the nerves in the extremities; induces weakness, pain, and paralysis; often advances to the face and chest. May occur in the recovery time following a viral infection and in rare cases, after an influenza immunization. Also called *acute febrile polyneuritis, acute idiopathic polyneuritis,* or *infectious polyneuritis.*

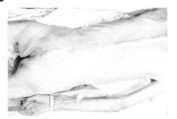

Syndrome, Guillain–Barré. (Perkin et al, 1986; Dr. P.O. Behen)

syndrome, iliotibial band (tract), n a condition characterized by pain and inflammation in the knee and caused by overexertion of the knee joint, usually through long-distance running. Also called *iliotibial band friction syndrome.*

syndrome, irritable bowel (IBS), n abnormal condition in which the small and large intestines exhibit increased motility, resulting in diarrhea and abdominal pain. Cause is unknown; thus treatments include diet changes, antidiarrheal medication, herbs, biofeedback, antispasmodics, homeopathy, and occasionally mild tranquilizers to help the patient cope emotionally.

syndrome, layer, n syndrome characterized by alternating layers of overactive and weak muscle groups that render an individual incapable of using specific muscles, resulting in poor movement patterns and poor muscular stability of the spine. Corrective measures include manual therapy and regular exercise.

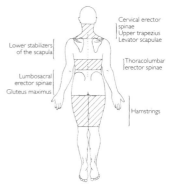

Syndrome, layer. (Petty and Moore, 2001)

syndrome, leaky-gut, n condition in which incompletely digested nutrients enter the bloodstream where they must be broken down by the immune system. This syndrome may cause a variety of health complaints including food and respiratory allergies.

syndrome, lower crossed, *n* posture characterized by increased lumbar lordosis, slightly flexed hips, and a pelvis rotated to the front. Also called *pelvic crossed syndrome.*

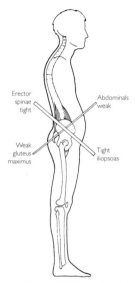

Syndrome, lower crossed. (Petty and Moore, 2001)

syndrome, Marfan's, *n.pr* a hereditary disorder that is present at birth and affects the connective tissue. The condition is characterized by atypical lengthening of the extremities, particularly hands, fingers and toes, in addition to problems in the eyes and circulatory system; caused by a defect in the gene that controls the production of fibrillin.

syndrome, nerve compression, *n* a condition in which a nerve is trapped or compressed, thus resulting in problems with motor and/or sensory function.

syndrome, overuse, *n* See repetitive strain injury.

syndrome, piriformis muscle (pi·rē·fōr'·məs mus'·əl sin'·drōm), *n* a rare disorder of the neuromuscular system that develops as a result of the piriformis muscle compressing or irritating the sciatic nerve. This can be due to injury, repetitive stress, or active trigger points located within the muscle. The pain can be described as numbness or tingling in the buttocks and down the leg. Walking, running, sitting for extended periods of time, or climbing stairs may exacerbate the pain.

syndrome, premenstrual (PMS) (pre'·men'·stəl sin'·drōm), *n* a set of physical, mental, and emotional symptoms triggered by hormonal changes from which some women suffer in the 1- to 2-week period before menstruation.

syndrome, psoas (sō'·az sin'·drōm), *n* painful condition of the lower back in which the psoas muscle is hypertonic.

syndrome, restless legs, *n* neurological condition characterized by uncomfortable sensations, deep in the leg muscles, irresistibly urging sufferers to move their legs. Symptoms worsen at night or when at rest and are ameliorated through voluntary movement of the legs, such as walking.

syndrome, sick (closed) building, *n* a set of health problems—including symptoms such as nose, eye, or throat irritation; nausea and dizziness; dry or itchy skin; headache; fatigue; sensitivity to odors; dry cough; and difficulty in concentrating—linked to the amount of time spent in specific buildings.

syndrome, Sjögren's, *n* an autoimmune disease in which the immune system mistakenly attacks the glands responsible for production of saliva and tears. May cause dryness of skin, nose, and vagina and may also affect other organs—including lungs, kidneys, blood vessels, and brain. Treatment is symptomatic and supportive. In extreme cases corticosteroids may be prescribed.

syndrome, sudden infant death, *n* unexpected and sudden death of a normal infant during sleep; cause is unknown.

syndrome, toxic shock, n syndrome resulting from a serious infection with strains of *Staphylococcus aureus* that produce a toxin known as enterotoxin F; characterized by a sudden increase in body temperature, headache, sore throat accompanied by swelling in the mucous membranes, nausea, diarrhea, and an atypical redness of the skin. Although the condition typically occurs in menstruating women who use highly absorbent tampons, it has also been observed in men, newborns, and children.

syndrome, upper crossed, n muscle dysfunction characterized by forward stance of the head, lengthening and elevation of the shoulders, and abduction and rounded scapulae, thus resulting in muscle weakness; corrected by massage and exercise. Also called *shoulder crossed syndrome.*

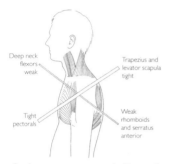

Syndrome, upper crossed. (Petty and Moore, 2001)

S

syndrome, urethral **(yu·rē'·trəl sin'·drōm'),** n a condition, that primarily affects females, in which symptoms of an irritated bladder are present, often without infection. See also interstitial cystitis.

syndrome, wasting, n a condition distinguished by a loss of weight due to diarrhea or chronic fever.

syndromes, culture bound, n.pl culturally defined conditions that cannot necessarily be correlated with any biomedical diseases and that may be psychosomatic. Symptoms of culturally bound syndromes may be alleviated using modern medicine, but the underlying causes can only be addressed through culturally specific and appropriate means. Also called *ethnomedical illnesses.*

syndromes, false-positive, n.pl medical conditions that are falsely assessed and treated as a result of therapy. A practitioner will work extensively with a patient to assess symptoms and recommend a course of action for treatment. Within a particular duration of time, many of these indications may no longer be present as a result of statistical regression, spontaneous remission, or other reasons. The patient believes that the recommended treatment was the source of the cure and returns to the practitioner for further extensive evaluation of symptoms. As before, the practitioner will prescribe a course of action for treatment. This phenomenon can lead to the development of adverse effects as the patient repeatedly visits a practitioner to seek treatment for the resolution of all symptoms assessed. The patient may become "addicted" to the treatment of these falsely classified dysfunctions. Risk is also increased because the patient may be asked to undergo treatment methods that may not be necessary for his or her condition.

syndromes, fire, n.pl in Chinese medicine, a number of illnesses distinguished by an excess or deficiency of heat. Inflammation is a general indication, and pain, fever, redness, and swelling are noticeable symptoms. Joint pain, sore throat, colitis, night sweats, burning sensations, hot flashes, and pent-up anger are also examples.

syndromes, impingement **(im·ping· mənt sin'·drōms),** n.pl pathologies caused by excessive pressure on blood vessels or nerves. See also entrapment.

synergist (si'·ner·jist), n **1.** a muscle that works in cooperation with an agonist to augment its movement. **2.** a treatment that when combined with others, has more than an additive effect.

synergistic **(si·ner·jis'·tik),** *adj* having the properties of the interaction between two or more elements that increases the effectiveness of the elements alone. Not additive only.

synergy, *n* the effects of combined components interacting to produce new and different effects than individual components. Typically used to refer to the action of whole plants, as opposed to active constituents in isolation.

synovial fluid (si·nō'·vē·əl flōō'·id), *n* viscous liquid found in synovial sheaths, bursae, and joints that delivers nutrition and provides lubrication for movement without friction. Also called *synovia.*

synovial membranes (si·nō'·vē·əl mem'·brānz), *n.pl* membranes that cover freely moving joints and secrete synovial fluid.

synovial sheath (si·nō'·vē·əl shēth'), *n* tubular covering that surrounds the tendon of a muscle that contains synovial fluid.

synthesis (sin'·thə·sis), *n* the process of creating complex compounds from simpler ones or individual elements by initiating at least one chemical reaction.

synthetic picture, *n* in Western medicine, a compilation of findings derived from an analysis of the body. A practitioner will use this information to diagnose the illness and choose an appropriate therapeutic approach.

syntonic optometric phototherapy, *n* See syntonics.

syntonics, *n* a system of therapy in which colored lights are directed into the eyes to resolve various physical and emotional health concerns. Also called *optometric phototherapy, photoretinology,* or *syntonic optometric phototherapy.* See also therapy, light.

syphilitic miasm (si·fi·li'·tik mī'·a·zuhm), *n* a disease susceptibility originally considered to stem from syphilis. Also called *lues* or *luetic miasim.* See also miasm, psoric miasm, sycotic miasm, tubercular diathesis, and diathesis.

syrups, *n* a medicinal preparation in which herbal infusions or decoctions are mixed with glycerin, honey, or sugar.

systematic care, *n* health care guided by a model that allows practitioners to address the cause of the complaint, devise a plan for therapy if necessary, and continued counsel aimed at empowering the patient to become and remain well.

systematic desensitization (sis'·tə·ma'·tik dē'·sen'·si·ti·zā'·shən), *n* **1.** the gradual eradication of a patient's phobias, which sometimes involves the introduction of coping mechanisms and can be accelerated with the use of hypnosis. **2.** stimulation of the immune system and reduction in allergic response through exposure to steadily increasing doses of substance to which the patient is allergic.

systematic review, *n* a detailed structural analysis of previously conducted research.

systemic lupus erythematosus (SLE) (si·ste'·mik lōō'·pəs er'·ə·thē'·mə·tō'·sis), *n* an autoimmune condition characterized by mouth ulcers, ruddy butterfly rash across the face, and damage to the valves of the heart.

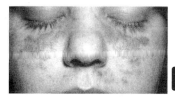

Systemic lupus erythematosus (SLE). (Goldstein and Goldstein, 1997; Department of Dermatology, University of North Carolina at Chapel Hill)

systemic memory hypothesis, *n* the theory wherein information and energy are stored by material systems with recurrent feedback processes.

systemic regulation, *n* the entire network of pathways by which the various systems of the body interact in

S

order to allow an organism to live, move, and remain healthy.

Syzygium aromaticum, *n* See cloves.

Syzygium cumini, *n* See jamun.

Syzygium cuminii, *n* See jambul.

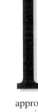

T, *adj* See thoracic.

t'ai chi (t·ä·ē dzhē), *n* Chinese movement art practiced to strengthen and develop balance, flexibility, cardiovascular functioning, and to build and circulate qi.

t'ai ch'i, *n* See taijiquan.

Tabebuia impetiginosa, *n* See pau d'arco.

tablework, *n* one of two aspects of the Trager approach, the other being mentastics; consists mainly of gentle joint movements. See also Mentastics and Trager approach.

tachycardia (ta'·kē·kär'·dē·ə), *n* rapid heart beat of more than 100 beats per minute in an adult. It occurs normally in response to fever, exercise, or excitement. It may also accompany anoxia caused by heart failure, shock, hemorrhage, or from certain arrhythmias.

tachyphylaxis (ta·kē·flak'·sis), *n* swiftly developed tolerance to a drug or toxin achieved through repeated exposure to minute doses.

tachypnea (tak'·ip·nē'·ə), *n* abnormally rapid rate of breathing, such as that associated with high fever.

tactile-kinesthetic stimulation, *n* a type of massage therapy, referring to either a tickle stimulus or a deeper pressure body massage and passive flexion/extension of the limbs.

taheebo, *n* See pau d'arco.

tai chi chuan, *n* See taijiquan.

tai chi, *n* See taijiquan.

tai min (tī min), *n* in Chinese medicine, one of the six principle meridians through which the vital force qi flows; further subdivided into yin division (spleen), and yang division

(lung). The balance of yin and yang components, and the proper flow of qi in an individual are indicative of sound health. See also qi, tai yang, shao yang, yang ming, shao yin, and jue yin.

tai yang (tī yäng), *n* in Chinese medicine, one of the six principle meridians through which the vital force qi flows; further subdivided into yin division (bladder) and yang division (small intestine). The balance of yin and yang components and the proper flow of qi indicate sound health. See also qi, tai min, shao yang, yang ming, shao yin, and jue yin.

taiji, *n* See tai chi.

taijiquan (tī'·gē·kwôn), *n* in traditional Chinese medicine, family of health-promoting exercises that provide benefits for the body, mind, and soul by maintaining balance between the yin and yang components. Developed in the fourteenth century, these exercises comprise flowing movements that imitate the motion and form of animals, all of which share fundamental elements rooted in qi gong. Such elements include continuous, fluid movements; alternation between yin and yang principles (e.g., empty and full, open and closed); and deep, conscious breathing. Taijiquan is practiced to relax, to improve balance, to promote the flow of qi, and as an interior martial art. One may practice taijiquan either as the form (solitary) or as push hands (with a partner). Also called *tai chi, ta'i ch'i, tai chi chuan, tai chi quan,* or *taiji.* See also qi and qi gong.

taila (tä'·ē·lə), *n* in Ayurveda, medicated oils that are derived from plants and minerals.

taixi (tä·zhē), *n* in traditional Chinese medicine, an acupuncture point located within the depression between the Achille's tendon and the prominence of the medial malleolus. Treatment involving this point improves the function of kidneys, increases the strength of the lumbar spine, anchors qi, and benefits the lungs. A deficiency in heat is also cleared. Also called *K13.* See also qi.

talipes, *n* a congenital deformity of the ankle and foot wherein the foot is twisted and fixed in an abnormal position.

talk-therapy, *n* psychotherapeutic approach that emphasizes verbal communication between a practitioner and patient to treat an emotional or mental disorder.

tamarind, *n* Latin name: *Tamarindus indica;* parts used: fruits, pulp, leaves, flowers, bark; uses: in Ayurveda, pacifies vata dosha; increases kapha and pitta doshas (sour, heavy, dry), immunomodulator, antioxidant, antiinflammatory, hypolipidemic, hypoglycemic, antibacterial, antifungal, mollusicide, antiviral, enhances bioavailability, carminative, laxative, digestive, constipation, fever, flatulence, appetite stimulant, nausea, conjunctiva inflammations; precautions: none known. Also called *amlika, imli,* or *tintiri.*

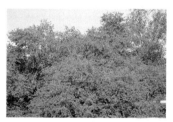

Tamarind. (Williamson 2002)

Tamarindus indica, *n* See tamarind.

tamas (tä·məs), *n* in Ayurveda, the primordial quality (guna) of matter that is responsible for inertia. This guna is considered positive when it is in balance, but too much is thought to be unhealthy.

tamasic manipulation (tä·mä¨·sēk mə·ni'·pyə·lā¨·shən), *n* in Ayurveda, one of three types of touch therapies. Corresponds to chiropractic, osteopathy, and massage techniques and benefits individuals with kapha constitution. See also kapha.

Tamus communis (tä¨·mōōs), *n* See black bryony.

Tanacetum vulgare, *n* See common tansy.

tangles, *n.pl* brain lesions that occur between nerve cells.

Tanner stages, *n.pr* an assessment system for evaluating developmental progression through puberty.

tannins, *n.pl* polyphenolic phytochemicals whose name derives from their use in tanning animal skins. Used as astringents, antioxidants, and styptics; treats burns, relieves diarrhea.

tapotement (ta·pō¨·tə·mənt), *n* massage technique that invigorates tissue by quickly and percussively tapping, cupping, hacking, slapping, or beating. Used most often during maintenance and relaxation massage.

tapping, *n* massage technique that uses the fingertips percussively. See also tapotement.

Taraktogenus kurzii, *n* See oil, chaulmoogra.

Taraxacum laevigatum, *n* See dandelion.

Taraxacum officinale, *n* See dandelion.

tardive dyskinesia (TD) (tär¨·dīv dis'·kə·nē¨·zhē·ə) *n* condition marked by repetitious and involuntary muscle movements in the trunk, limbs, and face. Often caused by antipsychotic medications.

target muscle, *n* a single muscle or muscle group on which a massage therapist focuses specific methods for specific responses.

target organ, *n* the organ or body part whose activity levels demonstrate change in the course of biofeedback.

tarsal (tär¨·səl), *adj* pertaining to the ankle.

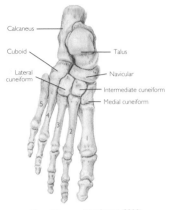

Tarsal bones. (Applegate, 2000)

TART, *n* in osteopathic medicine, a modification of the STAR acronym, which represents "tenderness," asymmetry," range of motion modified," and "tissue texture change." See also STAR.

taste groups, *n.pl* in Tibetan medicine, classifications assigned to a particular food based on its flavor; sour, bitter, and sweet are the three fundamental classifications. The three moderating tastes are astringent, salty, and pungent, respectively. Medication and foods are made by combining specific flavors. Practitioners use these flavor pairs to make meals that are suitable for a particular season. Because these particular combinations are believed to directly influence the psychosomatic components of badahan, chi, and schara, they are used to regulate the corresponding taste elements. To establish an appropriate diet for the relief of symptoms, determining a correlation between flavors/foods and eating patterns/habits is important.

tau (tou), *n* microtubule-asssociated protein, the function of which is to assemble microtubules that support nerve cell structure.

taurine (tô'·rēn), *n* an amino acid often found in nerve and muscle tissues. Has been reported as an adju-

vant treatment for congestive heart failure, viral hepatitis, alcoholism, cataracts, cerebrovascular accidents, diabetes, gallbladder conditions, high blood pressure, multiple sclerosis, psoriasis, and seizure disorders. No known precautions. Also called *L-taurine.*

taut band (tôt' band'), *n* the group of tense muscle fibers extending from a trigger point to the muscle attachments, the tension being caused by contraction knots that are located in the trigger point region. See also points, trigger.

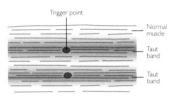

Taut band. (Campbell, 2002)

tautopathy (tô'·tä'·pə·thē), *n* See therapy, homotoxic.

taxation fatigue (tak·sā'·shən fə·tēg'), *n* in traditional Chinese medicine, the category of diseases caused by overexertion or inactivity that disrupt the balance between yin and yang and the free movement of qi, prevented by moderation. See also qi, yang, and yin.

taxic drug action, *n* the action of a medicine that is identical at standard strength and at a more diluted state. See also antitaxic drug action.

taxonomy (ta·ksô'·nə·mē), *n* **1.** any specialized method of classifying objects or events. **2.** scientific system used to classify living organisms.

Taxus baccata, *n* See yew.

Taxus brevifolia, *n* See yew.

***Taxus celebica* (tak'·səs se'·lə·bē'·kə),** *n* part used: whole plant; uses: diabetes mellitus; precautions: gastrointestinal distress, fever, and acute renal failure.

TBT, *n* See theta brainwave training.

T-cell mediated hypersensitivity, *n* a Type IV hypersensitivity reaction in which exposure to an antigen causes a delayed response. T-cells respond to specific antigens by releasing lymphokines thereby causing an inflammatory reaction within days.

TCM, *n* traditional Chinese medicine; a medical system involving acupuncture, physical therapy, herbal medicines, or a combination of these techniques.

TE, *n* triple burner channel; an acupuncture channel that runs from the hand to the face along the median surface of the arm and associated with the pericardium (PC) channel. See also PC, sanjiao, and triple burner.

technique, *n* any systematic procedure for achieving a desired result.

technique, activator, *n* a therapeutic approach associated with chiropractic medicine in which measured thrusts are delivered to the spine by using a spring-loaded device that resembles a hammer.

technique, Alexander, *n.pr* a method (named after Frederick Matthias Alexander) to become aware of posture, breathing, coordination, and balance during normal, everyday activities so that unnecessary muscular tension can be released and new methods of moving can be learned.

technique, articulatory (ar·tik'·yə·lə·tō'·rē tek·nēk'), *n* a method of osteopathic manipulation in which a restrictive barrier is reduced through gentle, repeated motion of the target body part through the restricted portion of its range of motion.

technique, aseptic (ā·sep'·tik tek·nēk'), *n* sterilization practices that decrease the likelihood of microbial infections between medical practitioners and patients.

technique, atlas orthogonality, *n* chiropractic manipulation that employs rapid accelerated force, applied either mechanically or manually.

technique, Bio-Energetic Synchronization, *n.pr* an energetic chiropractic method.

technique, Bowen (BT), *n* original system developed by Tom Bowen (1916–1982) of powerful yet subtle and painless soft tissue mobilizations.

technique, Buteyko breathing, *n.pr* a method of exercises designed to retrain patients' breathing to increase tolerance for higher levels of carbon dioxide (CO_2).

technique, compression, *n* neuromuscular technique in which the practitioner applies mild pressure to a tissue. See also flat compression and pincer compression.

technique, contract-relax-antagonist-contract, *n* See proprioceptive neural facilitation.

technique, counterstrain (kown'·ter·strān' tek·nēk'), *n* an osteopathic approach in which the afflicted joint is placed in a relaxed position to stop the erroneous proprioception underlying a somatic dysfunction. See also proprioception and somatic dysfunction.

technique, Cox flexion/extension, *n.pr* in chiropractic, an approach that aims to remove pressure from dysfunctional vertebra and nerves. To facilitate the treatment, the practitioner shifts the flexion distraction table in a variety of positions to fully release pressure on the spine and alleviate pressure away from the bulging nerves and discs. The spine is then repetitively maneuvered to increase the flow of blood, diminish the level of discomfort, and promote relaxation. The treatment is used for a variety of conditions. It was developed and taught by James M. Cox, DC, DACBR, for more than 30 years. Also called *F/D, Flexion Distraction, Cox(I) Technique,* and *chiropractic distraction.*

technique, craniooccipital (krā'·nē·ō·ōk·si'·pi·təl tek·nēk'), *n* See cranial osteopathy.

technique, diversified, *n* most common chiropractic approach; the entire spine is adjusted by using a wide variety of spinal manipulation approaches.

technique, exaggeration, *n* an indirect osteopathic technique in which the affected physical component is moved from the restrictive barrier, after which a high velocity/low amplitude technique is applied in the same direction.

technique, functional, *n* indirect manipulative technique that employs practitioner-induced movement while the area of complaint is continuously palpated. The practitioner takes the joint in all possible directions of ease (purposely avoiding directions that bind) to gradually guide it to the point of greatest ease. The practitioner's palpating hand allows him to feel the point at which the affected area is no longer in pain.

technique, Gonstead, *n.pr* chiropractic approach developed by Clarence S. Gonstead aimed at correcting spinal dysfunction resulting from displaced intervertebral discs. Specific spinal adjustments are done using static and manual palpation, instrumentation and x-ray analysis.

technique, hypnoreflexogenous (hip'·nŏ·rē'·flek·sä'·jə·nəs tek·nēk'), *n* a type of hypnosis often used during childbirth to help patients remain in control during labor and delivery. Patients are encouraged to concentrate on—rather than try to ignore—their contractions, which act as a stimulus to relax the body and mind.

technique, induration (in'·də·r ā'·shən tek·nēk'), *n* chiropractic soft tissue technique by which the practitioner pushes around the paraspinal point of concern from different directions until a reduction in pain is noted; the pressure is applied for at least twenty seconds.

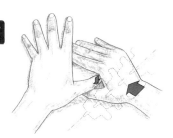

Technique, induration. (Chaitow, 2002)

technique, inhibitory pressure, *n* application of constant pressure to soft tissues to relax and to reduce the activity of reflexes.

technique, integrated neuromuscular inhibition, *n* sequential method used to disable a trigger point and the surrounding tissues. It involves the use of muscle energy techniques (MET), strain and counterstrain (SCS), and direct inhibition techniques to specifically target soft tissues that are dysfunctional. See also MET, SCS, and trigger points.

technique, ligamentous articular strain, *n* in osteopathy, a system of techniques used for myofascial release.

technique, Logan Basic, *n.pr* chiropractic technique developed by HB Logan, that comprises light, sustained pressure exerted against a specific point at the base of the spine. Also uses the surrounding muscular structure around the sacrum as a lever to balance the entire spinal structure.

technique, m, *n* touch technique used in conjunction with aromatherapy applications. See also aromatherapy.

technique, metamorphic (me·tə· mōr'·fik tek·nēk'), *n* in reflexology, a therapy approach based on the belief that a pregnant woman's foot mirrors the gestation period of her child and that early therapy—gentle rubbing of her feet, hands, and head—can avert development of problems *in utero* by relieving energy flow blockages.

technique, muscle energy, *n* method of stretching muscles by using resistance to improve the range of motion.

technique(s), myofascial release (mī'·ō·fā·shē'·əl rē·lēs' tek·nēk'), *n.pl* methods that employ prolonged pressure to stretch muscle tissue beyond its usual length to achieve better movement by reducing fascial restrictions.

technique, myofascie-soft tissue (mī'·ō·fa'·shē·ə-sôft' ti'·shōō tek·nēk'), *n* a combination of indirect and direct massage that reduces fascial tension and muscle spasm.

technique, neuroemotional (NET), *n* a chiropractic approach used to release negative emotions (conscious or unconscious) that manifest as spinal subluxations.

technique, neuroorganizational, *n* chiropractic approach that corrects misalignments in the spine and skull to improve neurologic functions.

technique, neurolymphatic reflex **(nur'·ō·lim·fa'·tik rē'·fleks tek· nēk'),** *n* procedure that involves the stimulation of neurological reflex points (neurolymphatic reflexes) located all through the body, particularly between the ribs, along the spine, and in the pelvic region; thought to influence lymphatic drainage. Activation of these reflexes results in strengthening of muscles.

technique, neuromuscular **(ner'·ō· mus'·kyə·ler tek·nēk'),** *n* method in which the practitioner uses his or her fingers to feel tissue abnormalities and gently manipulates the areas to restore normal function.

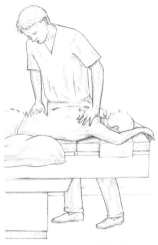

Technique, neuromuscular. (Chaitow, 2003)

technique, neurovascular reflex **(nur'·ō·vas'·kyu·ler rē'·fleks tek· nēk'),** *n* method employed to improve blood flow and muscle strength via the neurovascular circuits found in the skin by activating them with small tissue tugs.

technique, okibari **(ō·kē·bä·rē tek'·nēk),** *n* a Japanese acupuncture technique in which gold, silver, or stainless steel needles are inserted as normal, but the extended part is cut off and the remainder left in permanently. The technique is a source of iatrogenic conditions resulting from acupuncture treatments. Also called *maibotsushin.*

technique, one-eye, *n* energy-based therapy in which the patient recalls a traumatic event while moving his or her eye in various patterns; used to treat psychological problems.

technique, percussion vibrator, *n* an osteopathic manipulative procedure for treating somatic dysfunction by using specific applications of vibratory force. See also somatic dysfunction.

technique, progressive inhibition of neuromuscular structures (PINS), *n* manipulative treatment that includes application of mild pressure to two sensitive points that are related to one another.

technique, range of motion, *n* an osteopathic technique using movement (passive or active) of a body part to its full range of motion in any or all planes.

technique, receptor/tonus, *n* a system of soft tissue manipulation that involves stretching the osseous structures and applying pressure for five to seven seconds to trigger points.

technique, sacral-occipital blocking, *n* chiropractic method in which blocks of various shapes are applied to the body over a period of time to align the spine.

T

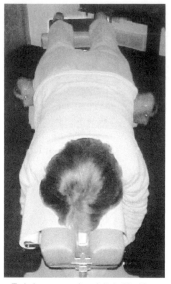

Technique, sacral-occipital blocking.
(Leskowitz, 2003; Courtesy Kalamazoo Community Chiropractic, Kalamazoo, MI)

technique, sacro-occipital (SOT) (sā'·krō-ôk·si'·pi·təl tek·nēk'), *n* method of chiropractic care in which manipulative reflex techniques are used to correct spinal, cranial, and organ-related problems.

technique, Spencer, n.pr a series of osteopathic manipulative procedures used to prevent or alleviate restrictions in the soft tissues around the shoulders.

technique, splenic pump, n an osteopathic technique for immunostimulation in which rhythmic compressions are applied to the area over the patient's spleen.

technique, springing, n an osteopathic technique for increasing free motion through repetitive applications of low-velocity/medium-amplitude force to the restrictive barrier undergoing treatment.

technique, Still, n.pr a system of osteopathic techniques for diagnosing and treating somatic dysfunctions; consists of nonrepetitive applications of direct and indirect pressure to the joints. This technique is attributed to the founder of osteopathy, Andrew Still. See also somatic dysfunction.

technique, Thompson Terminal Point, n.pr chiropractic technique developed by Dr. Clay Thompson; addresses all areas of the spine to reveal any vertebral subluxation. See also subluxation, vertebral.

technique, toggle, n a short lever osteopathic technique that uses shearing forces in combination with compression.

technique, trigger-band, n a variation of myofasical release technique in which the practitioner uses fingers or a device to apply pressure along specific pathways of connective tissue. The purpose of this approach is to change pathologic cross-linkages in fascia.

techniques, direct osteopathic manipulative, n.pl manipulative techniques for finding areas of the body in which the range of motion is limited and for releasing the blockage responsible for the limit by positioning into the blockage. Examples of such techniques include high-velocity/low-amplitude, positometric relaxation, and direct myofascial release.

techniques, friction, n a set of neuromuscular techniques in which the practitioner applies friction to myofascial tissues in a transverse direction or in the direction of the fibers. The type of technique applied depends on the condition of the affected tissues and desired results.

techniques, indirect osteopathic manipulative, n.pl manipulative techniques for finding areas of the body in which the range of motion is limited and for releasing the blockage responsible for the limit by positioning away from the blockage. Indirect techniques use the intrinsic forces of muscles, ligaments, and tendons to facilitate release.

techniques, lifestyle modification, n.pl analysis and advice that physicians offer to their patients to make health-promoting changes in their lives. May include stress-reducing strategies, exercise, and dietary modifications.

techniques, *physiotherapeutic breathing* **(fi·zē·ō·the·rə·pyōō·tik brē·thing tek·nēk's),** *n.pl* scientific term used for qi gong. See also qi gong.

techniques, refocusing, *n.pl* a group of mental techniques based on the recognition that what one chooses to focus upon defines who one is and how one experiences the world.

techniques, visceral, *n.pl* stretching and balancing methods developed to correct imbalances present in the viscera.

teething, *n* the process of baby teeth erupting through the gums; sometimes accompanied by pain, fever, inflammation, difficulty in sleeping, and irritability.

teki'ci'hilapi (te·kē'·chē·hē·lä·pē), *n* a Lakota Indian term for the ability to esteem, treasure, and cherish others in the community.

telangiectasia (te'·lan·jē·ek·tā·zhē·ə), *n* a permanent dilation of arterioles, venules, and capillaries due to actinic damage, atrophy-producing dermatoses, increased estrogen, rosacea, congenital collagen vascular conditions, or other conditions.

Telangiectasia. (Lemmi and Lemmi, 2000)

teleology (tē·lē·ô'·lə·jē), *n* in philosophy, a view that explains the universe through recourse to final goals or ends..

temperature modality, *n* the influence on a symptom from chilling or heating. See also symptom, general and modality.

temporal arteritis (tem·pôr·əl är·tə·rī'·təs), *n* an inflammatory condition that most often occurs in older patients. Symptoms include jaw claudication, scalp sensitivity, thickening or slowing of the temporal artery, throbbing headache, and visual difficulty or discomfort and are accompanied by increased erythrocyte sedimentation rate.

temporal squama (tem'·pə·rəl skwä'·mə), *n* portion of the temporal bone composed of scale like matter.

temporomandibular joint dysfunction (tem'·pə·rō·man·di'·byə·lər joint' dis·funk'·shən), *n* an abnormality marked by facial pain and mandibular dysfunction; caused by a dislocated or defective temporomandibular joint. Common characteristics are limited jaw movement, pain, and temporomandibular dislocation. Also called *TMJ.*

temu lawak (tā'·mōō lä'·wäk), *n* Latin name: *Curcuma xanthorrhiza;* part used: root; uses: general health, cholerctic, pain, antirheumatic, itching, liver problems, jaundice, gall stones, galactogogic, skin diseases, antispasmodic, menstrual dysfunction, rectum inflammation, hemmorhoids, antidiarrheal, antidysenteric, stomach disorders, antipyretic, yeast infection, leukorrhoea, gastric gas, constipation, diabetes, blood clots, antifungal, antibacterial, induction of uterine contraction, antioxidant, antitumor; precautions: pregnancy, obstruction of bile duct gallbladder disease, blood-thinning medication; can cause gastrointestinal irritation. Also called *giant curcuma, false tumeric,* and *temulawak.*

tenalgia (tə·nal'·jē·ə), *n* pain referred to a tendon. Also called *tenodynia.*

tenderness, *n* discomfort elicited through palpation indicates unusual sensitivity to pressure or touch.

tendinomuscular meridians (ten'·də·nō·mus'·kyə·ler mə·ri'·dē·ənz), *n.pl* in acupuncture, energy channels positioned closest to the body's surface that serve as a boundary between the body and the external environment.

tendinosis (ten·də·nō´·sis), *n* noninflammatory repetitive stress injury of tendon fibers. A common condition; often mislabeled as tendonitis. See also tendonitis.

tendon, *n* strong fibrous tissue that connects skeletal muscle to bone. Also called *sinew.*

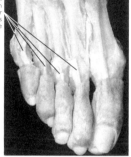

Tendon. (Vidic and Suarez, 1984)

Tendons of digitorum extensor longus muscle

tendon organs, *n.pl* protective tendinous and musculotendinous structures that sense stretch or tension in the tendons.

tendon rupture, *n* tearing of a tendon that occurs when the forces placed upon the tendon exceed its tensile strength.

tendon sheaths (ten´·dən shēthz´), *n.pl* synovial membrane-lined structures protecting tendons that cross multiple joints.

tendonitis (ten·də·nī´·tis), *n* inflammatory condition of tendon fibers. Fairly uncommon and often confused with the more common tendinosis, a repetitive stress injury of tendon fibers. See also tendinosis.

tenesmus (tə·nez´·məs), *n* a painful and persistent spasm of the bladder or rectum with an urgent desire to empty the bladder or bowel without the formation of feces; associated with irritable bowel syndrome.

tenosynovitis (te´·nō·si´·nō·vī´·tis), *n* condition marked by inflammation of the synovial sheath that surrounds a tendon.

TENS, *n* See transcutaneous electrical nerve stimulation.

tensegrity (ten·sā´·gri·tē), *n* an architectural principle in which compression and tension are used to give a structure its form. Conceived by R. Buckminster Fuller, it is used to create such structures as geodesic domes and boat sails.

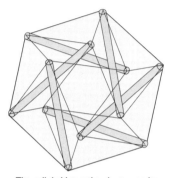

The cell, held together by tensegrity. (After Levine 1985, with kind permission from Johns Hopkins Magazine)

tensegrity system, *n* an interconnected network of structures which use tension and pressure in order to move or retain their shape.

tense-release, *n* an active relaxation process of tensing or tightening particular muscles and then releasing or letting go; often begun at the top of the head, proceeding down through the face, then neck and shoulders to the arms and hands, the chest and back, down to the stomach, hips, and legs. See relaxtion, progressive.

tension headache, *n* a condition characterized by discomfort or pain in the head and/or neck, often correlated with muscular hypertonicity in these locations.

teratism (ter´·ə·tiz´·əm), *n* **1.** any condition in which a severely deformed fetus is produced. Also called *teratosis.* **2.** a developmental or congenital abnormality that arises from environmental or inherited factors or a combination of both factors.

T

teratogen (tə·ra'·tə·gən), *n* a process, a substance, or an agent that interferes with regular, thus causing developmental abnormalities within a fetus. Examples include alkylating agents, thalidomide, and alcohol; infectious microbes like cytomegalovirus or the rubella virus; ionizing radiation such as x-rays; and environmental aspects such as the mother's age and overall health or trauma to the fetus during the gestational period.

teratogenicity (ter'·ə·tə·jə·nis'·i·tē), *n* ability to cause birth defects. See also teratogen.

Terminalia arjuna, *n* See arjuna.

Terminalia belerica, *n* See myrobalan, beleric.

Terminalia chebula, *n* See myrobalan.

termination, *n* the gradual ending of deep relaxation that allows the individual to slowly become alert to the surroundings. Also called *arousal* and *return to everyday activity*.

terpenes (ter'·pēnz), *n.pl* a large-sized group of unsaturated hydrocarbons with the empirical formula $(C_5H_8)_n$. A large number of compounds found in plants comprise this type of functional group or its derivatives.

terpenoids (ter'·pə·noidz), *n.pl* derivatives of the terpenes group comprise a functional group like a ketone, aldehyde, or an alcohol in addition to the basic, unsaturated hydrocarbon skeleton.

terrain, *n* the fertile ground for all function (i.e., physical, mental, social, and environmental) of a human being; the environment in which disease may develop. See also typology, constitution, and morphology.

test, *n* any method for critical evaluation.

Test, Ames, *n.pr* a carcinogenicity test in which the test substance is exposed to *Salmonella* bacteria, and the rate of mutations is noted so as to determine the carcinogenicity of the substance.

test, anterior superior iliac spine compression, *n* a test for ascertaining the side of the body afflicted with pelvic somatic dysfunction. Also called *anterior compression test, ilial compression test*, or *ilial rocking test*.

test, ASIS compression, *n* See anterior superior iliac spine compression test.

test, backward bending, *n* a test that determines whether sacral torsion is forward or backward and whether sacral motion exemplifies flexion or extension.

test, Fantus, *n.pr* a diagnostic evaluation used to measure the amount of chlorides in urine to determine the intake of sodium chloride, to identify and treat edema and dehydration, and to monitor symptoms of high blood pressure.

test, F-test, *n* test used in statistical analyses to compare the variance between the means of two or more groups. Used to determine whether a hypothesis has been susbstantially proven based on the observed variance between two trial populations.

test, health attribution, *n* a 22-item questionnaire that attempts to determine a patient's beliefs regarding the possible causes of his or her condition or illness.

test, Henshaw, *n.pr* old method used to select the suitable homeopathic technique for treating a certain condition.

test, hyperventilation provocation, *n* a voluntary overbreathing exercise used to reproduce a hyperventilating patient's symptoms in a clinical setting, thereby facilitating diagnosis and treatment of the condition.

test, hypnotic induction profile, *n* inventory that assesses hypnotic capacity in an individual by measuring dissociation control, absorption tendencies, and suggestibility. See also hypnosis.

test, infrared, *n* a test for measuring the quality of essential oils; involves passing infrared radiation through a small amount of oil to produce a printed spectrum for analysis.

test, Luscher color, *n.pr* diagnostic aid developed by Dr. Max Luscher in the 1940s and used widely by psychologists and color therapists. Consists of eight colors, ranked in order of preference; this ranking is used to characterize the psychologic type of the test-taker.

test, modified radioallergosorbent (rā'·dē·ō·al'·ler·gō·sor'·bənt), *n* a solid-phase radioimmunoassay used in detection of IgE (type-1) reactions.

test, provocation-neutralization, *n* a method used to identify food sensitivities. Specific dilutions of antigens are administered to determine the dilutions that cause allergic symptoms and those that relieve them.

test, purpose-in-life, *n* self-report survey based on Victor Frankl's logotherapeutic orientation; measures the extent to which the respondent has found significant meaning in life.

test, radioallergosorbent (rā'·dē·ō·ə·lər'·gō·sōr'·bənt test'), *n* method that uses radioimmunoassay to determine allergic reactions; the serum is mixed with allergenic antigen and observed for any clumping reaction, which indicates presence of antibodies.

test, seated flexion, *n* a test for determining sacroiliac (the sacrum moving on the ilium) dysfunction.

test, serial dilution titration, *n* a systematic analysis used to identify food sensitivities. Specific dilutions of antigens are administered to determine the dilutions that cause symptoms and those that relieve the symptoms.

test, sphinx, *n* See test, backward bending.

test, spring, *n* 1. test used to discern the backward rotations/torsions of the sacrum from the forward. 2. test used to discern the bilateral extension of the sacrum from bilateral flexion.

test, standing flexion, *n* a test for determining iliosacral (the ilium moving on the sacrum) dysfunction.

test, t-test, *n* a statistical measure used to determine the change difference between the mean measurements of two data sets.

tests, differentiation, *n.pl* joint movement tests done to distinguish two structures suspected to be the source of symptoms; the position that provokes symptoms is held constant while a movement that aggravates or

reduces the stress on one of the structures is added and its effect on the symptoms is observed.

tests, flexion, *n.pl* tests for determining dysfunction of the iliosacral or sacroiliac joints.

tests, hepatic function, *n.pl* a series of tests intended to evaluate the liver's performance of its multiple roles. Tests included in the hepatic function profile include serum protein electrophoresis, platelet count, and measurement of albumin and bilirubin levels. See also hepatic function.

tests, hydrogen/methane breath, *n.pl* noninvasive diagnostic tests used to identify the overgrowth of bacteria in the small intestine, especially in patients with chronic gastrointestinal disorders. After an overnight fast and a challenge dose of carbohydrates (lactulose or glucose), breath samples are collected and tested for hydrogen or methane.

tetanus, *n* a spastic/paralytic condition of the central nervous system caused by an exotoxin known as tetanospasmin produced by *Clostridium tetani,* an anaerobic bacillus that enters the body through an abrasion, puncture wound, burn, or laceration; characterized by headache, irritability, and painful muscle spasms that cause risus sardonicus, lockjaw, laryngeal spasm, and opisthotonos. Can be fatal.

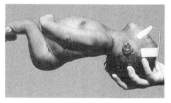

Tetanus: characteristic muscle spasms. (Farrar, 1993; Dr. T.F. Sellers, Jr.)

tetanus toxoid (tet'·nəs täk'·soid), *n* detoxified tetanus poison used to produce a permanent immune response against tetanus infections. See also tetanus vaccine.

tetanus vaccine, *n* one of several vaccinations used to immunize against tetanus (lockjaw). Varieties include DTaP vaccine (for diphtheria, tetanus, and pertussis in children), DT vaccine (for diphtheria and tetanus in children), Td vaccine and boosters (for diphtheria and tetanus in adults), and T vaccine (for tetanus alone).

tetany (te·ten'·ē), *n* a disorder consisting of muscle cramping and twitching.

tetrahydropalmatine (te'·trə·hī'·drō·päl'·mə·tīn), *n* an alkaloid derived from the tuber of corydalis, *Corydalis turtschaninovii,* and various other species of plants and acts as a pain-relieving and sleep-inducing agent. It is the active ingredient in Chinese jin bu huan anodyne capsules. Fatigue, vertigo, drowsiness, and nausea are possible side effects. In children, overdose results in respiratory depression and bradycardia. In adults, overdose leads to hepatitis. Also called *THP.*

tetralogy of Fallot, *n.pr* a congenital heart defect that comprises the following four characteristics: ventricular septic defect, pulmonary stenosis, right ventricular hypertrophy, and aortic malposition; originates from the right ventricle or septal defect. In newborns and infants, the condition manifests in hypoxia, cyanosis, inability to gain weight, marked difficulty to feed, and poor development. In older children, the condition is distinguished by clubbing of the toes and fingers and squatting. Treatment involves implementing supportive measures and surgery. Also called *Fallot's syndrome.*

Teucrium chamaedrys, *n* See wall germander.

TFL, *n* tensor fascia lata; a muscle that originates from the anterior superior iliac spine and anterior portion of the iliac crest. Its primary functions include flexing and abducting the thigh.

thanksgiving, *n* a prayer of gratefulness or appreciation.

theme, *n* a common trait among different diseases or different homeo-

pathic remedies that connects them. See also essence.

Theobroma cacao, *n* See cacao.

theology, *n* humanity's attempt to explain the nature and ways of god in a temporal framework.

theory, *n* **1.** a belief that explains phenomena and provides a certain course of action. **2.** an explanation of phenomena; supported by repeated observation and experimentation.

theory, dynamic energy systems, *n* umbrella term for many contemporary energy theories.

theory, entrainment, *n* the idea that rhythms within the body harmonize with one another. In cranial manipulation, this applies to signals that influence one another—often the stronger coaxing the weaker into its cadence—to create the cranial rhythmic impulse. Cranial treatments can be equated with the stronger signal, which can pull weaker signals into more healthy rhythms. See also cranial rhythmic impulse.

theory, five phases, *n* in traditional Chinese medicine, a complex theory of five phases—wood, fire, earth, metal, and water—that are connected to the organs of the body. Treatments can be determined by the interaction of the phases.

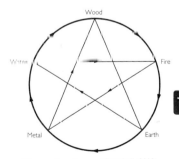

Theory, five phases. (Campbell, 2002)

theory, gate-control, *n* hypothesis that describes a pain gate-control theory that postulates a control "gate," through which afferent nerve impulses pass. In theory, pain impulses can be blocked at the "gate" by delivering pressure through rubbing, massage, or other stimulation.

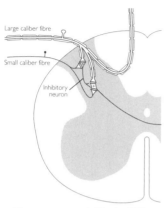

Large caliber fibre

Small caliber fibre

Inhibitory neuron

Theory, gate control. (Carreiro, 2003)

theory, grounded, *n* a method of qualitative research in which valid theories that match experiential data and are derived from localized practices are developed by interviewing and observing research subjects.

theory, memory-of-water, *n* a theory that the structure of water-alcohol solutions used in homeopathy is changed by the remedy during dilution and succussion and that the changed structure is maintained even after the chemical aspects of the remedy have been diluted away.

theory, object relations, *n* in psychology, a theory postulating that human relations are foundational and primary for the development of an individual's personality and are the principle influence for later relations with others. Psychologic philosophy that holds that human self-structure is internalized during childhood through the process of relating to people and treasured objects; these experiences create a blueprint for forming and maintaining subsequent relationships.

Psychopathology is the term used in object relations practice to describe expressions of negative self-object experiences from childhood that are being reenacted and worked out in the patient's current relationships. Psychotherapy is the proposed path for resolution of self-defeating relational patterns so that patients may mature and eventually self-actualize.

theory, pain-gate, *n* a theory of pain control used to explain the analgesic effects of acupressure and acupuncture. Stimulation of sensory nerve fibers closes the "pain gates," thereby inhibiting transmission of pain signals from afferent neurons to the brain.

theory, personal construct, *n* a set of beliefs, according to which each individual forms hypotheses about the world, tests these theories against the reality of his or her own experiences and modifies them as necessary.

theory, reflectorial effect (rē·flek·tōr'·ē·əl i·fekt' thē'·ə·rē), *n* in aromatherapy, theory that states that odors considered pleasant by a patient will allow the person to feel happier and positive and perform tasks in an efficient manner.

theory, sliding-filament, *n* theory of the sliding movements of muscle fibers to shorten or lengthen a muscle.

theory, systemic-effect, *n* in aromatherapy, theory that states that an odor functions much like a neurotransmitter and that therefore specific ailments can be treated using specific odors. Also called *lock and key theory of odors.*

theory, systems, *n* a model of medical care that attempts to take the myriad complex parts of health care and integrate them into a sum greater than its components. Each subsystem in this model is complete in itself while having a place in the larger system.

theory, triadic (trī·a'·dik thē'·ə·rē), *n* in Tibetan medicine, the three functions of the mind—chi, schara, and badahan—a practitioner uses to establish the patient's psychosomatic type and to diagnose, treat, and prevent a medical condition. See also chi, schara, and badahan.

theory, weak-quantum, *n* a modification of quantum theory; postulates the resistance of macro-entanglement that involves consciousness and that may account for anomalous, transpersonal, and healing phenomena.

therapeutic aggravation, *n* transitory exacerbation of symptoms as a result of the use of a homeopathic remedy. This aggravation is often considered constructive because it indicates a positive reaction to the remedy. Also called *healing crisis, initial reaction,* and *initial aggravation.* See also aggravation; complication; symptoms, new; and secondary drug action.

therapeutic encounter, *n* contact between at least two people designed to enhance the health of one or more of those engaged in the contact. See also therapeutic alliance.

therapeutic modality, *n* an intervention used to heal someone. See model, biomedical and homeopathy.

therapeutic riding (the′·rə·pyōō′·tik rī′·ding), *n* equine therapy in which disabled individuals ride horses to relax, and to develop muscle tone, coordination, confidence, and well-being.

therapeutic strategies, *n.pl* **1.** approaches to treatment based on principles of organization. **2.** in nutritional therapy, subcategory of prescriptive dietetics and nutritional pharmacology that addresses the imbalances in biochemistry or disturbances in physiology like tissue or organ dysfunction due to an organic disease. See prescriptive dietetics and nutritional pharmacology.

Therapeutic Touch, *n.pr* See Kreiger/Kunz method.

therapeutics, *n* medical discipline devoted to the application of treatment to illness.

therapy, *n* method used to cure an illness.

therapy localization, *n* revealing of emotional aspects of a physical dysfunction by simultaneously testing an indicator muscle with its associated emotional neuromuscular reflex(es).

therapies, being, *n.pl* in holistic nursing, therapeutic approaches that involve one's sense of peace and awareness. The patient may use prayer, meditation, quiet contemplation, and imagery.

therapies, doing, *n.pl* in holistic nursing, directed therapeutic approach that involves several conventional medicine techniques, such as traditional procedures, medications, and surgery with a specific goal or outcome.

therapies, elimination, *n.pl* in Ayurveda, the processes that patients undergo at the end of the day's treatment that serve to eliminate impurities, which have been loosened during the therapies. See also anu and naruha.

therapies, expressive, *n.pl* approaches where expressive arts are employed to promote awareness, healing, and growth.

therapies, five-sense, *n.pl* in Ayurveda, the fundamental treatments for restoring imbalances of the doshas. The therapies include diet and herbs (taste), color therapies (sight), mantras (hearing), aromatherapy (smell), and massage (touch), all of which are prescribed to balance dosha(s). Meditation is the therapy for what is considered the sixth sense, the mind. See also doshas, mantras.

therapies, mind-body, *n.pl* therapies such as hypnosis, visual imagery, yoga, relaxation, and meditation, in which the mind and body are used in conjunction to assist in facilitate the healing process.

therapies, mind-body-spirit, *n.pl* therapeutic modalities that involve body postures, breathing, movement, prayer, and/or meditation to facilitate relaxation and awareness of mental, emotional, and spiritual states.

therapies, Native American, *n.pl* various traditional and modern herbal treatments and ceremonies used to address physical complaints and psychospiritual maladies.

therapies, nature-based, *n.pl* techniques that use nature-based animals or plants that reconnect patients to the natural environment and its rhythms to improve and hasten healing and improve quality of life.

therapy, adjuvant (a'·jə·vənt the'·rə·pē), *n* the use of one therapy to boost or enhance the effect of another. See also compatible.

therapy, alleviation (ə·lē'·vē·ā'·shən the'·rə·pē), *n* in Ayurveda, the use of sesame oil or castor oil to remove vata, butter or ghee to remove pitta, and honey to remove kapha. See also dosha, vata, pitta, and kapha.

therapy, animal-assisted, *n* technique in which animals are brought into contact with patients who are recovering; provides touch, builds connection, empathy, and enjoyment.

therapy, antihomotoxic, *n* therapeutic method that elimates toxins via combination homeopathic remedies. See also homotoxicology and toxin.

therapy, antiretroviral (*ART*) (an'·tī·re'·trō·vī'·rəl the'·rə·pē), *n* a combination drug treatment used to suppress HIV virus levels and activity in AIDS patients. See also HAART.

therapy, aura-soma (ōr'·ə·sō'·mə the'·rə·pē), *n* a structured color therapy involving interpretation of the patient's choice of four out of 101 dual-colored bottles containing herbal extracts and essential oils ("Equilibrium oils"). The contents of the chosen bottle are applied to the skin. Also called *aura-soma color therapy.*

therapy, autogenic, *n* mental health therapy in which the patient concentrates on selected verbal stimuli to reach a self-induced state of relaxation. Used in pain management, panic attacks, control of nausea, and vomiting resulting from chemotherapy or radiation therapy. Not advised for patients with acute psychoses or personality disorder. See also biofeedback.

therapy, autohemic, *n* therapy that involves treating a patient with nosodes prepared from the patient's blood sample or a pooled sample from several patients. Occasionally the patient's blood is mixed with homeopathic potencies before administration. Also called *autosanguine therapy.*

therapy, autologous blood (ô·tol'·ə·gəs blud' the'·rə·pē), *n* practice of removing blood from the veins and injecting it into the muscles of the same individual to treat persistent ailments. Has been used for psoriasis, eczema, and asthma. Possible side effects include infection, bruising, and pain.

therapy, autoregulatory, *n* therapeutic method that stimulates the patient's innate ability to heal, as when a healing touch removes blockages or constrictions within the body's energy flow. Therapy that frees the body to heal itself. See also medicine, natural.

therapy, bee-sting, *n* the use of venom derived from bees for medicinal purposes; used in the treatment of skin, pulmonary, rheumatologic, cardiovascular, pulmonary, sensory, psychological, and endocrine conditions. It has also been used to treat bacterial and viral infections; administered by a variety of methods. Persistent nodular lesions and allergic reactions are a concern. Also called *therapy, bee venom* and *BVT.*

therapy, behavior, *n* branch of psychotherapy that emphasizes modifying specific behaviors. Sessions include analysis of a behavior and devising ways to change it to a more desirable response.

therapy, behavioral music, *n* therapy that uses music to affect nonmusical behavior; developed from behavior modification theory to facilitate social and cognitive learning and operant conditioning.

therapy, biodynamic (bī'·ō·dī'·nam' ik the'·rə·pē), *n pr.* a mind-body–integrated therapy developed by Gerda Boyesen, a Norwegian physiotherapist; uses a variety of methods such as massage, talking, sensory awareness, and meditation to refresh the body. Also called the *Gerda Boyesen technique* or *biodynamic psychology.*

therapy, biofield, *n* any healing practice that addresses the patient's biofield, uses the biofield of the practitioner, or a combination of both. See also biofield, reiki, and therapeutic touch.

therapy, biological, n a therapeutic modality that uses the biological response modifier, part of the body's immune system, to fight disease and infection or to protect from the side effects of other treatments. Also called *biological response modifier therapy, biotherapy, BRM therapy,* or *immunotherapy.*

therapy, Block integrative nutritional (blôk˙ in˙·tə·grā˙·tiv nōō·tri˙·shə·nəl the˙·rə·pē), n a dietary system, developed by Keith Block, MD, that recommends 50% to 70% complex carbohydrates, 10% to 25% percent fat, and the remaining percentage as protein in the diet. The primary objective of this regimen is decreasing and subsequently removing dairy, refined sugars, and meat from one's diet while increasing the number of calories from complex carbohydrates such as vegetables, whole grains, and fruits. Also called *BINT.*

therapy, body-oriented, n form of psychotherapy that holds that emotions are encoded in the body as areas of restriction and tension; movement, breathing, and manual therapy are used to release such emotions.

therapy, breathing biofeedback, n a biofeedback therapy in which sensors are placed on the patient's abdomen and chest to observe and measure the rhythm, location, volume, and rate of airflow by which the patient learns deep abdominal breathing; used for respiratory conditions, hyperventilation, asthma, and anxiety.

therapy, Callahan Techniques-thought field (CT-TFT), n.pr developed by clinical psychologist Dr. Roger Callahan, therapy that draws on specific energy meridian points in a particular progression in order to eliminate the cause of negative emotions, as well as their effects on health.

therapy, Cancell, n an unconventional cancer treatment containing sodium sulfite, potassium hydroxide, nitric acid, sulfuric acid, and catechol.

therapy, cell, n a treatment for cancer in which embryonic animal cells from tissues or organs corresponding to those with the cancer are injected into the cancer patient, with the understanding that these healthy cells are incorporated into the organ, thus repairing or replacing the cancerous cells. This treatment may have side effects, including infections, serious immune responses to the foreign proteins in the cells, and death. Since 1984 the FDA has banned the importation of all injectable cell-therapy materials. Also called *cellular suspensions, cellular therapy, embryonic cell therapy, fresh cell therapy, glandular therapy, live cell therapy, organotherapy,* or *sicca cell therapy.*

therapy, Cell Specific Cancer, n.pr a treatment used for cancer, offered in the Dominican Republic, in which the client is exposed to a donut-shaped magnetic device (with an electromagnetic field weaker than in MRI) that allegedly reduces the cancer burden (i.e., destroys enough cancer cells) so that the immune system can take care of the remainder.

therapy, chelation (kē·lā˙·shən the˙·rə·pē), n **1.** removal of heavy metals, such as lead, iron, and mercury, through the use of chelating agents, usually given intravenously. **2.** the purported removal of heavy metals, plaque, and other toxins through intravenous infusion of EDTA (ethylenediaminetetraacetic acid), a synthetic amino acid and chelating agent.

therapy, cognitive, n treatment that seeks to change behavior (i.e., habits) by addressing the underlying beliefs that drive the behaviors. Comparable to and often used in concert with behavioral therapy.

therapy, cognitive behavioral, n psychotherapeutic approach used to alter thinking and behavior.

therapy, cold laser, n treatment with lasers made from helium-neon or gallium aluminum arsenide and used to treat a host of neurologic problems including carpal tunnel syndrome, migraines, arthritis, vertigo, and soft tissue injuries. Also called *low-level light therapy (LLLT)*.

therapy, colon, *n* the use of professionally administered whole-bowel enemas combined with analysis of fecal chemistry, evaluation of environmental and psychologic factors in the patient's life, and regular exercise to maintain bowel health. Based on the belief that the health of the colon is directly related to the health of the whole body and that poor colon health can manifest as a variety of illnesses. Also called *colonic hydrotherapy* or *colonic irrigation.*

therapy, color, *n* the use of color, particularly in interior furnishings and decoration, to help relieve physical and psychologic problems by rectifying imbalances in the energy flow of the body. See also feng shui.

therapy, complementary, *n* **1.** any remedy paired with another. **2.** treatment used in conjunction with and integrated with traditional Western medicine. This type of therapy is contrasted with alternative medicine, which is used independently of conventional medicine. See also therapy, adjuvant; medicine, complementary; and medicine, conventional.

therapy, cranial manipulative, *n* treatment of the tissues and fluids of the skull to correct body rhythms and induce self-healing.

therapy, craniosacral, *n* the practice of using one's hands to assess the rhythms of the tissues and fluids in the skull area and to direct those rhythms into healthful patterns. A version of cranial osteopathy sometimes conducted by nondoctors, including massage therapists and physical therapists.

therapy, creative arts, *n* the integration of artistic abilities into therapy to alleviate patients' suffering. Activities include but are not limited to drawing, painting, dancing, poetry writing, singing, and gardening.

therapy, creative music, *n* therapeutic use of improvisational music to encourage stimulation and develop-

ment of "musical intelligence," confidence, and self-actualization. Psychodynamic and humanistic theories are often used. Also called *Nordoff-Robbins improvisational music therapy.*

therapy, crystal, *n* the use of quartz crystal energy with a person's energy to facilitate a cascade of spiritual, mental, emotional, and physical changes simultaneously or following a hierarchy of cure.

therapy, dance, *n* integrative movement therapy that encourages awareness, feeling, and enhanced self-esteem. See also authentic movement.

therapy, desensitization, *n* therapy used for the prevention of serious allergic responses, in which the patient is regularly injected with increasing doses of a purified allergen to reduce the sensitivity of the immune system to that allergen.

therapy, detoxification, *n* a collection of various means for detoxification, including chelation, colonic irrigation, fasting, herbal cleansing, and nutritional cleansing. These treatments are intended to help the body's natural eliminative functions. See also chelation therapy, colon therapy, and fasting.

therapy, Di Bella, *n.pr* method used for cancer treatment that employs substances such as bromocriptine, melatonin, and retinoid solution.

therapy, differentiation, *n* cancer treatment that aims to stimulate cancer cells beyond their undifferentiated state to differentiate like normal cells to halt their uncontrolled proliferation.

therapy, digitalis, *n* the use of digitalis glycosides to increase the heart's rate of contractions and speed. This protocol can decrease the conduction speed of the atrioventricular node and create negative dromotropy, thus leading to heartbeat irregularities.

therapy, distraction, *n* approach that uses enjoyable thoughts and activities as a distraction from the pain and discomfort of disease and treatment.

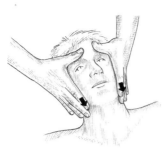

Therapy, distraction. (Chaitow, 2002)

therapy, drainage, n purging of toxins by means of low potency dosages of homeopathic remedies related to the afflicted organs. See also therapy, antihomotoxic; organ affinity; and organotherapy.

therapy, EDTA, n technique that employs intravenous transfusions containing disodium EDTA (ethylene diamine tetraacetic acid) to remove minerals, toxins, and other substances from the blood and vessels. No known risks if used properly. Also called *chelation.*

therapy, electrodermal activity (i·lek'·trō·der'·məl ak·ti'·vi·tĕ the'·rə·pē), n procedure for measuring minute amounts of perspiration that would be otherwise too subtle to detect. Sensors are placed on the palms or fingerpads of the patient and the electric current produced measures the skin conductance. Also used to treat hyperhidrosis and anxiety.

therapy, enzyme, n treatment system developed by Max Wolf, MD, in the 1930s using orally ingested enzymes derived from animals and plants to address enzyme deficiency and several illnesses.

therapy, equine, n treatment of mental and physical conditions through therapeutic interactions (e.g., riding) with horses. Also called *hippotherapy, riding therapy,* or *therapeutic riding.* See also therapy, animal-assisted.

therapy, fever, n induction of fever for healing purposes using herbal,

biological, or mechanical (e.g., hot baths) preparations. Also called *pyretotherapy.*

therapy, finger pulse, n biofeedback therapy in which the rate and force of the pulse are measured and used for controlling anxiety, hypertension, cardiac arrhythmia, and other conditions.

therapy, flotation (flō·tā'·shən the'·rə·pë), n method used in transpersonal medicine that allows an individual to attain altered states of consciousness by facilitating flotation in a saline-filled tank while sound and light are diminished or eliminated to effect physic and psychologic isolation. See also medicine, transpersonal.

therapy, frequency, n the use of specific high-frequency oscillations to destroy pathogenic organisms or cancerous cells and restore health. Also called *energoinformational therapy* or *Rife frequency therapy.*

therapy, gem, n See healing, crystal.

therapy, gene, n therapy in which genes are introduced into the patient in order to cure or treat a disease. Also called *somatic cell gene therapy.*

therapy, Gerson, n.pr an unorthodox anticancer treatment that includes a diet that comprises vegetables and fruits with nutritional supplements, liver extract injections, and coffee enemas.

therapy, Gestalt, n.pr a method of humanistic psychotherapy that examines the present emotions of the patient without consideration to the past to gain a new level of self awareness. Instead of explaining the meaning of these emotions, the therapist works with the patient to elucidate his or her own understanding of these feelings.

therapy, Gestalt art, n.pr a group-oriented, process-driven form of art therapy created by Janie Rhyne and based on the humanistic Gestalt psychology of Fritz Perls.

therapy, glandular, n a treatment in which tissue extracts of organs such as spleen, thymus, adrenal glands, or liver are used orally to help with a

T

number of conditions, including asthma, autoimmune diseases, cancer, chronic fatigue, cystic fibrosis, eczema, inflammatory diseases, low white cell count, psoriasis, rheumatoid arthritis, and other conditions.

therapy, group, *n* a form of therapy wherein people meet with each other and a therapist in order to interact and discuss their problems.

therapy, hallucinogen **(hə·lōō'·si·nō·jin the'·rə·pē),** *n* therapy that uses lysergic acid diethylamide (LSD) to decrease dependence on drugs such as alcohol or cocaine.

therapy, heat, *n* use of heat on all or part of the body to encourage hyperemia, increase circulation, facilitate sweating, and relax muscles. Used in sports and rehabilitation medicine and as a cancer treatment.

therapy, homotoxic **(hō'·mə·tôk'·sik the'·rə·pē),** *n* a form of homeopathy in which the same substance that causes an illness is also used to treat the symptoms. Also called *homeopathy, autoisopathy,* and *tautopathy.*

therapy, hormone replacement, *n* a method for treating symptoms of menopause, such as hot flashes, decreased sexual desire, vaginal dryness, sleep disorders, and mood swings by using estrogen alone or in combination with progestin.

therapy, horticultural, *n* a subcategory of nature-assisted therapy focused on gardening and horticultural activities for therapeutic benefits.

therapy, humor, *n* a means of enhancing a patient's ability to recognize, express, and enjoy humor. Used to help patients learn, express anger, relieve tensions, or manage painful emotions. See also therapy, laughter.

therapy, hyperbaric oxygen **(hī'·per·be'·rik ok''·sə·jin the'·rə·pē),** *n* therapeutic use of highly pressurized oxygen in the treatment of clostridial myonecrosis, osteoradionecrosis, skin graft healing, stroke rehabilitation, and other conditions.

therapy, hyperoxygenation, *n* a cancer treatment based on the belief that hypoxia and resulting anaerobic

metabolism promote the growth of cancerous cells. In these therapies, the patient is treated with oxygenating agents, such as germanium sesquioxide, hydrogen peroxide, or ozone. Germanium compounds can have lethal nephrotoxicity. Also called *bio-oxidative therapy* or *oxidative therapy.*

therapy, hyperthermia **(hī'·per·ther'·mē·ə),** *n* the use of heat either systemically or locally.

therapy, immunoaugmentive **(IAT)** **(i'·myə·nō·ôg·men'·tiv the'·rə·pē),** *n* Developed by Dr. Lawrence Burton, an alternative adjunctive treatment for cancer, uses four separate blood proteins and proposes improvement in immune system functioning as its mechanism.

therapy, insight-oriented, *n* psychotherapy based upon the idea that behaviors have their roots in a client's family dynamics, instinctual drives, childhood development, and genetic traits. Therapy in this vein consists of delving into these areas for information resulting in treatment of disorders.

therapy, Irlen lens, *n.pr* a treatment for scotopic sensitivity, a condition of "perceptual stress" accompanying autism and some learning disorders. In this therapy, the patient wears lenses that have been tinted to a specific color to minimize or eliminate their sensitivity.

therapy, Jacobson's Progressive Relaxation, *n.pr* a method of relaxation in which undesirable muscle tension, even if barely detectable, is systematically identified and relaxed. The eventual goal is for a state in which all undesirable tension is eliminated.

therapy, juice, *n* juices of raw fruits and vegetables administered to detoxify and provide easily assimilated concentrated nutrition.

therapy, Kelley/Gonzalez metabolic, *n.pr* cancer treatments involving dietary modifications, detoxification through coffee enemas, and nutritional and enzymatic supplementation (the Kelley variant also includes neurologic stimulation through cranial or spinal manipulation and biblically-based prayer). The treatments are tailored for each patient based on a computerized method of metabolic typing (Kelley) or analysis of the hair and blood (Gonzalez).

therapy, Kneipp, n See Kneippkur.

therapy, Koryo hand (kōr·yō), n.pr Korean microsystem of hand acupuncture that views the hand as a map for the whole body and the meridians. In this system, the middle finger is analogous to the midline of the body; the adjacent fingers represent the arms and the thumb and little finger as the legs. The posterior of the body corresponds to the dorsal surface of the hand, and the anterior corresponds to the palmar surface. Stimulation methods for these regions include pressure pellets, needles, rings, moxa, and fingertip pressure.

therapy, laughter, n the use of laughter as an aid in enhancing the patient's psychologic state. See also therapy, humor.

therapy, light, n a therapeutic modality in which disease is treated with light. The light may be natural (i.e., full-spectrum) or of specific wavelengths (e.g., colored light, low-intensity lasers, ultraviolet light). See also therapy, photodynamic and phototherapy.

therapy, low-energy emission, n treatment for insomnia in which electromagnetic fields (low amplitude–modulated) are applied directly to oral mucosa by means of a mouthpiece.

therapy, low-level light (LLLT), n treatment that employs lasers made from helium-neon or gallium aluminum; used to treat a host of neurological problems including carpal tunnel syndrome, migraines, arthritis, vertigo, and soft tissue injuries. Also called *therapy, cold laser.*

therapy, magnetic, n therapeutic application of magnets placed on the surface of the skin.

therapy, magnetic field (mag·ne'·tik fēld' the'·rə·pē), n technique in which magnets are placed on the body to treat a variety of conditions.

therapy, manner metabolic, n.pr See therapy, metabolic.

therapy, manual, n physical approaches in complementary medicine including but not limited to body work, chiropractic, tui na, and shiatsu. Therapies range from basic manual manipulations derived from osteopathy, reiki, and qi gong to energy work.

therapy, marma (mär'·mə the'·rə·pē), n in Ayurveda, massage therapy used to heal certain illnesses related to muscles, ligaments, and the nervous system. See also marmas.

therapy, medical art, n the use and making of art by patients who are physically sick or undergoing chemotherapy, radical surgery, or living with trauma to their bodies; therapeutically assists patients to process pain and death, and also facilitates restoration of health.

therapy, megavitamin, n See medicine, orthomolecular.

therapy, meridian, n a therapeutic approach that involves palpation of the acupuncture meridian systems; includes the extraordinary meridians or secondary vessels.

therapy, metabolic, n a treatment for cancer and other serious illnesses; regards the build-up of toxins as the primary cause of chronic, degenerative diseases. Specific treatments vary but typically include enemas, whole food diets, nutritional supplementation, laetrile, and glandular extracts.

therapy, microwave-resonance, n a technique that uses specific, low-intensity radiation in the microwave range to improve a variety of medical conditions. Used to treat arthritis, cerebral palsy, chronic pain, esophagitis, hypertension, neurologic disorders, and side effects of chemotherapy.

therapy, milieu (mil·yōō' the'·rə·pē), n in psychiatry, treatment that involves manipulating a patient's environment for therapeutic reasons.

therapy, monopolar direct current, n a treatment performed within a doctor's office that uses electrical current to shrink tissues. Used to treat hemorrhoids and other conditions.

T

therapy, movement, n any form of physical activity used to produce a therapeutic effect in the patient, such as exercise, dance, yoga, or martial arts.

therapy, music, n See therapy, creative music.

therapy, nature-assisted, n a therapy that uses plants, natural materials, and environment to hasten healing and improve the quality of life.

therapy, neural (nyur'·əl the'·rə· pē), n method of treatment in which an anesthetic is injected into painful areas to effect pain relief from chronic conditions.

therapy, neuroelectric (ner'·ō·ə· lek'·trik the'·rə·pē), n electrical stimulation of the mastoid region with low-level alternating current through surface electrodes. Used as a treatment for insomnia. Also called *electrosleep.*

therapy, nondirective, n professional counseling style marked by an atmosphere of help and assistance between therapist and client.

therapy, nutritional, n therapy based on the idea that an individual's health is directly related to his or her diet and nutrient intake.

therapy, oral antigen, n a method of treatment for multiple sclerosis that involves administering myelin basic protein orally. See also multiple sclerosis.

therapy, orthomolecular psychiatric (ōr'·thō·mə·lek'·yə·ler sī'·kē·a'· trik the'·rə·pē), n psychiatric treatment that provides optimal concentrations of nutrients, such as vitamins and essential fatty acids. Low concentrations in the brain of these substances are thought to cause symptoms of mental illness.

therapy, oxygen (äks'·ə·jin the'·rə· pē), n process that administers oxygen by face mask or hyperbaric chamber to relieve hypoxia associated with a variety of conditions. Possible risks include toxicity, infection, and embolism. See also therapy, hyperbaric and embolism.

therapy, ozone (ō'·zōn the'·rə·pē), n treatment that involves injecting the body with ozone or hydrogen peroxide to treat cancer, HIV/AIDS, and other degenerative conditions. Risks include infection, embolism, and hemolysis.

therapy, peloid, n treatment in which pulp (usually from lake or sea mud, peat, or other plants) is applied to the body for its therapeutic benefits.

therapy, pet, n treatment involving contact between a patient and pet (i.e., dog, cat, etc.).

therapy, phage, n treatment which uses viruses that attack only bacteria; attempts to rid the body of pathogens. Advantages of phages over antibiotics include their ability to increase in numbers and spread throughout the body as well as their potential to attack antibiotic-resistant bacteria.

therapy, photodynamic (fō'·tō·dī· na'·mik the'·rə·pē), n form of light therapy that involves injection of irradiated pigments into tissues that are then irradiated further with certain light frequencies designed to destroy cancer cells or change conditions like macular degeneration.

therapy, poetry, n reading and/or composing poetry with the intention of affecting therapeutic change or personal development. Promotes creativity, imagination, spontaneity, appreciation of beauty, and expression of emotion. See also bibliotherapy.

therapy, polarity (pō·lar'·i·tē the'· rə·pē), n approach developed by Randolph Stone; combines Eastern and Western energy modalities to release the blockages underlying disease and restore homeostasis.

therapy, positional release, n See strain/counterstain.

therapy, psychodynamic (sī'·kō·dī· na'·mik the'·rə·pē), n emotional healing method derived from psychoanalysis, the goal of which is assisting patients to identify and settle conflicts that began in childhood and remain unresolved.

therapy, pulsed electromagnetic field, n a healing technique in which a small, electronic device that delivers weak pulse signals is used to speed healing.

therapy, purification, n See Panchakarma.

therapy, reconstructive, n injection treatment for arthritis that delivers nutritional substances into the tissues surrounding the joint to increase fibroblast activity.

therapy, reflex zone, n a method of manipulative therapy applying touch to the back, feet, hands, or head to elicit therapeutic changes in reflected tissues and organs. Also called *RZT.* See also reflexology.

therapy, regenerative injection, n See sclerotherapy.

therapy, rejuvenation, n in Ayurveda, the use of specific activities, herbs, and foods for the purpose of preventing the aging process and promoting longevity.

therapy, relaxation, n a set of techniques designed to calm the body and mind to produce relaxation in response to stressful situations. Meditation, progressive relaxation, prayer, biofeedback, and self-hypnosis are common examples.

therapy, release, n therapeutic approach used in pediatric psychotherapy to treat children affected with anxiety and stress that is associated with a particular recent event.

therapy, restricted environmental stimulation, n sensory-deprivation procedure designed to produce a nonreactive state and stimulate healing.

therapy, SHEN, n a modern version of ancient hands-on healing techniques in which a practitioner works to facilitate normal flow of energy by applying light pressure to specific areas of the body. Used to relieve chronic pain and dissipate psychological distress and emotional blockage.

therapy, single remedy, n in homeopathy, treatment that uses a remedy that contains only one ingredient that most closely matches the individual's profile of symptoms.

therapy, sleep restriction, n a treatment for sleep disorders in which the patient spends only as much time in bed as is necessary for sleep (e.g., a person who only sleeps four hours every night would only be in bed for four hours, instead of tossing and turning for four hours and sleeping for four). Restriction of bed time is believed to increase the amount of the actual sleep time.

therapy, spinal manual, n encompasses a host of hands-on processes employed by chiropractors to correct spinal misalignments that are often the source of common complaints such as neck pain, back pain, and headaches. Also called *SMT.*

therapy, step, n process in which a patient is first treated with an inexpensive treatment that works for the majority of patients with that particular complaint. If that treatment fails, the patient is stepped up to a more powerful and/or expensive treatment.

therapy, stimulus control, n a treatment for sleep disorders in which the bed and bedroom are associated solely with sleeping and, if applicable, sex. If the patient is not asleep within a set time, he or she is to leave the bedroom and not return until he or she is sleepy. Regular waking times are also emphasized, regardless of the amount of sleep obtained during the night.

therapy, supportive, n branch of psychotherapy aimed at treating individuals in crisis situations. The focus is on developing tools to cope with overwhelming situations.

therapy, symptomatic (simp·tə·ma'·tĭk the'·rə·pe), n 1. therapy aimed at treating the symptoms of a condition. 2. form of acupuncture in which needles are inserted near or surrounding the area of complaint. Differs from typical acupuncture because classic acupuncture points are not used.

therapy, systems, n branch of psychotherapy with an emphasis on resolving relationship problems. Based on theory that individuals act within the family system as a whole.

therapy, thermal biofeedback, n biofeedback that measures the temperature of the skin to index blood flow changes as the vessels dilate and constrict.

therapy, thought field (*TFT*), n form of therapy used to treat psychologic problems in which the client taps on his own energy meridian points in a particular and distinct progression while recalling painful memories, thus alleviating negative emotions and the related ill effects on the client's health. TFT was developed by clinical psychologist Dr. Roger Callahan. Also called *Callahan Techniques thought field therapy.*

therapy, traditional Chinese dietary, *n* in traditional Chinese medicine, therapeutic approach that involves the consumption of specific foods to treat specific illnesses. Often done without consulting with a practitioner.

therapy, viral, n the approach of using viruses genetically modified to transmit genetic material to specific sites.

therapy, virilization, n See vajikarana.

therapy, Zoetron, n.pr See therapy, cell specific cancer.

therapy, zone, n a therapeutic scheme that divides the body into ten vertically interconnected segments, or zones, with an understanding that tension or blockage in one part of a zone is reflected in the zone as a whole.

thermal biofeedback, *n* method that teaches participants to increase or decrease temperature of their hands by feedback of signals indicating hand temperature. Has been used primarily in the treatment of headaches.

thermogenic formulas, *n.pl* stimulants found in plants; known to increase metabolism. Caffeine and ephedrine are examples. Side effects may include increased blood pressure, anxiety, heart rate, and insomnia.

thermogram (ther'·mə·gram), *n* visual record obtained by using infrared technology that shows patterns of radiated heat from the body's surface. "Hot spots" correlate with the development of tumors and other disorders.

thermotherapy (ther'·mō·the'·rə·pē), *n* the use of heat applications such as hot packs to provide soothing pain relief and increase circulation, tissue pliability, metabolism, and

relaxation. See also paraffin bath, sauna, steam room, ultrasound, and whirlpool.

theta brainwave training, *n* methodology developed by Eugene Peniston, in which he trained alcoholics to focus inwardly and experience their higher selves. See also brainwave training.

thiamin deficiency (thī'·ə·min də·fi'·shən·sē), *n* insufficient levels of thiamin in the body to support functioning, which causes beriberi.

thiamine, *n* See vitamin B_1.

thinking current, *n* the speed at which an individual's thoughts progress from one subject to the next.

thistle, blessed, *n* Latin names: *Carbenia benedicta, Cnicus benedictus, Carduus benedictus;* parts used: upper stem, dried leaves; uses: anorexia, upset stomach, dyspepsia, myrroghia, lactation; precautions: pregnancy, children; can cause nausea and contact dermatitis. Also called *cardo santo, chardon benit, holy thistle, kardobenediktenkraut, spotted thistle,* or *St. Benedict thistle.*

thistle, carline, *n* Latin name: *Carlina acaulis;* parts used: leaves, roots, seeds; uses: diuretic, diaphoretic, spasmolytic, antimicrobial, dermatosis, wounds, ulcers, tongue cancer, gallbladder disorders; precautions: pregnancy, lactation, children. Also called *dwarf carline, felon herb, ground thistle, southernwood root,* or *stemless carline root.*

thistle, milk, *n* Latin name: *Silybum marianum;* part used: seeds; uses: relieves hepatotoxicity due to alcohol, chemicals, cirrhosis, or viral hepatitis; liver cleansing, liver tonic, protects kidneys from chemotherapy agents, gallstones; precautions: pregnancy, lactation, children, drugs metabolized by P-450 enzyme. Also called *Holy thistle, Lady's thistle, Marian thistle, Mary thistle,* or *wild artichoke.*

thistle, St. Mary's, *n.pr* See thistle, milk.

thixotrophy (thik'·sə·trō'·fē), *n* phenomenon of change in connective and other gel tissues. Movement and pressure transform the solid gel-state tissue into a more liquid, malleable state.

Thompson, *n.pr* chiropractic technique in which the thrusts are applied primarily to the pelvis to adjust dysfunction. Often the complaints are related to discrepancies in the length of the patient's legs.

thoracentesis (thō'·rə·sen·tē'·sis), *n* a surgical procedure involving the creation of an opening or hole through the wall of the chest and pleural space to aspirate fluid or air as a diagnostic tool or therapeutic approach; used as a therapy for pleural effusion, which is commonly seen in patients diagnosed with bronchogenic carcinoma. The samples of fluid can be analyzed to determine the concentration of amylase, protein, and glucose and the level of erythrocytes and leukocytes, and also cultured to study microbes. Also called *thoracocentesis.*

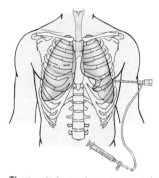

Thoracentesis. (Lewin, Heidemper, and Dirksen, 2000; Sherwood Medical, St. Louis, MO)

thoracic (thə·ra'·sik), *adj* area of the back between the neck and twelfth rib.

thoracic inlet (thō·ra'·sik in'·lət), *n* the intersection of the neck and thoracic cavity, consisting of the upper end of the sternum (the manubrium), the first thoracic vertebra, and the first ribs and their cartilages.

thoracic pump, *n* an osteopathic technique in which the thoracic cage is compressed intermittently to pro-

mote lymph flow and drainage. Also called *the osteopathic life saver.*

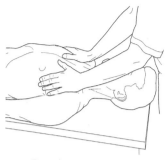

Thoracic pump. (Ward, 1997)

thoracolumbar outflow (thô'·rə·kō·lum'·bär owt'·flō), *n* catabolic system involved in preparing the body for emergencies. Also called *sympathetic nervous system.*

thorax (thōr'·aks), *n* part of the human anatomy that comprises the chamber between the diaphragm and the neck.

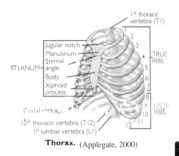

Thorax. (Applegate, 2000)

thorn apple, *n* Latin name: *Datura stramonium;* parts used: foliage, flowers, fruit, roots; uses: antiasthmatic, antiinflammatory, antispasmodic, earache, elephantiasis, motion sickness, respiratory disorders, topical pain reliever, wound healing; precautions: can cause poisoning in larger doses; abused as a recreational drug. Also called *Jimson Weed* and *stramonium.*

three heater, *n* See triple burner.

three treasures, *n* qi (energy), jing (essence), and shen (spirit). Harmony between the three treasures is indicative of a healthy individual, whereas a disruption of this balance leads to illness.

three-leaved caper, *n* Latin name: *Crataeva nurvala;* parts used: bark, leaves; uses: in Ayurveda, pacifies kapha and vata doshas, promotes pitta dosha (bitter, astringent, light, dry), antiinflammatory, demulcent, laxative, rubefacient, tonic, vesicant, antilithiatic, urinary infections, bladder and kidney stones, liver stimulant, malaria, tumors; precautions: leaves can irritate and blister skin. Also called *barna, barun,* or *varuna.*

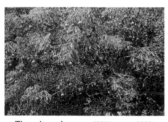

Three-leaved caper. (Williamson, 2002)

three-part yogic breath, *n* involves expansive, deep breathing that begins in the abdominals and fills the rib cage, until the air is up to the clavicle. The breath is then slowly released in the reverse order. Also called *dirgha.*

thrombocytopenia (thräm'·bō·sī'· tō·pē'·nē·ə), *n* a decrease in the number of platelets in the blood caused by either a decrease in platelet production, reduced survival of platelets, increased consumption of platelets, or splenomegaly; most common source of a bleeding disorder.

thrombosis (thräm·bō'·sis), *n* an atypical condition wherein a blood clot or thrombus forms inside a blood vessel.

thromboxane (thrôm·bôk'·sān), *n* one of a pair of compounds that effectively induces platelet aggregation.

Thuja **(thōō'·jə),** *n* parts used: twigs and leaves; uses: expectorant, antirheumatic, antiseptic, astringent, vermifuge, skin conditions; precautions: uterine stimulant, pregnancy, essential oil is *toxic.*

thunder god vine, *n* Latin name: *Tripterygium wilfordii;* part used: roots; uses: antiinflammatory reported to have some success in treating rheumatoid arthritis; precautions: leaves and flowers are highly toxic and can cause death. Also called *lei gong teng.*

thyme, *n* Latin name: *Thymus vulgaris;* parts used: leaves, flowering tops; uses: expectorant, digestive tonic, antiseptic, astringent, anthelmintic, coughs, indigestion, diarrhea, throat complaints, muscle cramps, bedwetting; precautions: none known. Also called *creeping thyme, garden thyme, mountain thyme,* or *wild thyme.*

thymectomy (thī'·mek'·tə·mē), *n* the removal of the thymus via surgical methods.

thymoleptic (thī'·mō·lep'·tik), *adj* possessing germ-eradicating properties.

thymus gland fractions, *n pl* a protein that has been used to treat HIV and other conditions.

Thymus vulgaris, *n* See thyme.

thyroid hormone (thī'·roid hōr'· mōn), *n* a combination of two hormones, triiodothyronine (T3) and thyroxine (T4), produced by the thyroid gland. These hormones are responsible for modulating basal metabolic rate and can influence blood pressure, heart rate, temperature, and weight. See also therapy, Gerson.

thyroidectomy (thī'·roi·dek'·tə· mē), *n* the removal of the thyroid gland via surgical methods as a treatment for tumors, colloid goiter, or hyperthyroidism unresponsive to antithyroid medication or iodine therapy.

tiger and lion thermie warmers (tī´·ger and lī´·ən ther´·mē wôr´·merz), *n.pl* metallic devices used to administer moxa. See also moxibustion.

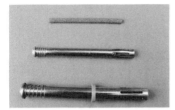

Tiger and lion thermie warmers. (Gardner-Abbate, 2001)

tikshna (tēk´·shnə), *adj* in Ayurveda, "sharp" as a guna, one of the qualities that characterizes all substances. Its complement is manda. See also gunas and manda.

***Tilia* (tē´·lē·ə)**, *n* parts used: flowers, fruits; uses: antispasmodic, nervine, indigestion, cold, colic, diuretic, mild gallbladder conditions; precautions: none known. Also called *lime flower* or *linden flower*.

time distortion, *n* the difference between objective measured time and subjective experienced time of an incident, often elicited in hypnotic states.

time modality, *n* occurring at the same or corresponding times, such as worse at night. See also modality and symptom, general.

timeless, *adj* infinite, enduring, endless.

timid, *adj* in Chinese medicine, pertaining to inadequate energy needed to face and overcome obstacles.

tincture (ting´·chər), *n* alcohol extract of herbs or other substances.

tinea pedis (ti·nē´·ə pe´·dis), *n* common fungal skin infection characterized by itching, peeling skin, and burning pain between the toes and on the soles of the feet. Also called *athlete's foot.*

Tinea pedis. (Greenberger and Hinthorn, 1993; Loren H. Amundson, University of South Dakota, Sioux Falls)

tinnitus (ti·nī´·təs), *n* a condition distinguished by a ringing sound that is heard in either one or both the ears; may be a sign of presbycusis, acoustic trauma, or an increase of cerumen that encroaches on the eardrum and occludes the external auditory canal.

***Tinospora cordifolia*, *n* See amrita.

tios´ paye (tē·ôs´ pä·ye´), *n* a Lakota Indian term for extended family, which provides the social support and material assistance for its members considered essential in health care.

tipi (tē´·pē), *n* Latin name: *Petiveria alliacea;* parts used: whole plant, root; uses: treatment of osteoarthritis and other rheumatic conditions. Also used as antifungal, antispasmodic, antipyretic, immunostimulant, sedative, abortifacient; precautions: pregnancy; individuals with hemophilia, diabetes, and hypoglycemia. Also called *anamu, apacin, huevo de gato,* and *kuan.*

tiro (tē´·rō), *n* a traditional preparation originating from Nigeria, used for cosmetic purposes and as a medicine for the eyes. It is applied to the inner surface of the eyelid, and its application and use is very similar to al kohl and surma. Tiro contains high concentrations of lead; therefore, poisoning is a potential risk associated with its application and use. See also al kohl and surma.

T

tissue affinity, *n* a homeopathic remedy that has a propensity to be attracted to and influence a certain kind of body tissue. See also disease affinity and organ affinity.

tissue salts, *n* designation for the 24 homeopathic remedies considered to be biochemic medicines. See also medicine, biochemic.

tissue texture abnormality, *n* palpable changes in tissues that signify the presence of contracture, edema, fibrosis, flaccidity, hypertonicity, vasodilation, or a combination of these conditions. Also called *TTA.* See also bogginess, ropiness, and stringiness.

tissue typing, *n* a systematic sequence of tests used to determine the compatibility between a recipient and a donor before transplantation; typing is done by identification and comparison of a series of human leukocyte antigens present in the cells.

titubation (ti′·chə·bā′·shən), *n* posture distinguished by a faltering gait while walking and a swaying motion of the trunk or head while in a sitting position. It may be an indication of cerebellar disease.

TJS-010, *n* kampo compound comprising seven herbal ingredients used to treat mental health disorders and physical complaints. Animal studies indicate anxiolytic and antidepressant effects, but human trials have not been conducted.

TL, *adj* thoracolumbar; of or relating to the torso region, specifically the chest and lower back areas.

TLC, *n* total lung capacity; the maximum amount of air the lungs can hold at peak inhalation.

TM-Sidhi program (tē em si·dhē prōō·gram), *n.pr* advanced meditation practices, including a technique called *yogic flying,* that allow a meditator to explore the deeper states of consciousness cultivated through regular practice of transcendental meditation. See also transcendental meditation and yogic flying.

toad venom, *n* a secretion from the sebaceous and parotid glands of *Bufo bufo gargarizans,* Chinese toad, which is dried and used in traditional Chinese medicine; highly toxic and only used in minute amounts. Overdose has been associated with serious, occasionally fatal cases of cardiotoxicity. Also called *ch'an su.*

tobacco, *n* Latin name: *Nicotiana tabacum;* part used: leaves; uses: relaxant, antispasmodic; induce dissolving action, diuretic, induction of vomiting, expectorant, pain, sedative, promotion of flow of saliva, rheumatism, skin conditions, scorpion stings, nausea, motion sickness, hemorrhoids; precautions: may be highly addictive; may cause nausea, vomiting, sweating, palpitations; may be toxic. Also called *cultivated tobacco, herbe à la reine, jen ts'ao, nicoziana, punche, tabac, tabac mannoque, tabaco, tabak, tabigh, tan pa ku, tanigh, toubac, tutun, yen ken, yen ts'ao,* and *yu ts'ao.*

tobacco, mountain, *n* Latin name: *Arnica montana;* parts used: flower heads and root stock; uses: helps heal bruises, sprains, surface wounds, and arthritis; precautions: blistering, inflammation, irritant to the stomach and intestines. Also called *leopard's bane* and *wolfsbane.*

tokoloshe (tō′·kŏ·lō′·shā), *n* in traditional South African healing, an evil spirit believed to cause accidents and misfortune.

tolerance, *n* a gradual decrease in the patient's response to a medicine over time; necessitates increasing the dosage to achieve the same results. See also reactivity and sensitivity.

tolle causam (tōl′·lā kŏ′·zəm), *v* to identify and treat causes; a foundational medical principle in naturopathic medicine.

tonic, *n* treatment, usually an herbal concoction, that refreshes and restores health, energy, and vitality.

tonic-clonic seizure, *n* seizure distinguished by a sudden loss of consciousness and involuntary muscle contraction that lasts for a few minutes. Persons affected may bite their tongues, clench their teeth, and lose control of bodily functions such as defecation or urination. Often the patient has no memory of the event on awakening. Also called *grand mal seizure*.

tonka bean (täng'·kə bēn'), *n* Latin name: *Dipteryx odorata;* parts used: fruits, seeds; uses: antiemetic, antinausea, aphrodisiac, possible uses in treating lymphedema and cancer; precautions: pregnancy, lactation, children, patients taking anticoagulant medications; labeled as unsafe by the FDA. Also called *cumaru, tonka seed, tonquin bean,* or *torquin bean.*

tonsillar nodes, *n.pl* lymph nodes located near the mandible at the angle of the jaw.

tonsillectomy (tôn'·sə·lek'·tə·mē), *n* surgical procedure in which the tonsils are removed, often because the inflamed tonsils interfere with swallowing or breathing. Tonsillectomies are most common in children and adolescents.

tonsillitis (tôn'·sə·lī'·tis), *n* condition characterized by inflammation of the tonsils, sore throat, swollen lymph nodes in the throat, and fever, usually caused by an infection.

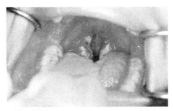

Tonsillitis. (Wong, 1999; Dr. Edward L. Applebaum, University of Illinois Medical Center)

tonus (tō'·nəs), *n* the continuous partial contraction of muscles to maintain posture and to help stabilize joints.

top notes, *n.pl* a highly volatile category of aromatic components of essential perfumes and oils that are penetrating and sharp. These are the first odors that the olfactory system perceives. See also note.

topical, *adj* pertaining to the outer surface.

topognosis (tä'·pəg·nō'·sis), *n* ability to identify the location of stimuli on the skin. Also called *topesthesia.*

tormentil (tor'·mən·til), *n* Latin names: *Geranium maculatum* L, *Potentilla erecta* L, *Potentilla tormentilla;* parts used: dried herb and rhizome; uses: antioxidant, astringent, styptic, vulnerary, tonic, diarrhea, ulcerative colitis, fever, laryngitis, pharyngitis, gums, mouth sores, hemorrhoids (topical), vaginal infections, conjunctivitis; precautions: none known. Also called *alum bloom, alumroot, American cranesbill, biscuits, bloodroot, chocolate flower, common tormentil, crowfoot, dove's foot, English sarsaparilla, geranium, old maid's nightcap, red root, septfoil, shameface, shepherd's knapperty, shepherd's knot, spotted cranesbill, storksbill, thormantle, wild cranesbill,* or *wild geranium.*

torque unwinding (tōrk' ən·wīn'·ding), *n* a technique developed by Elaine Wallace in which the body is separated into an imaginary series of overlapping or adjacent cubes that retain a memory of forces imposed by injury. Using this methodology, the practitioner can apply balanced, rhythmic pressure in a specific location that allows the residual traumatic forces to be negated by the pressure.

torr (tōr), *n* a unit of pressure equivalent to 0.001316 atmosphere; named after the physicist Torricelli. Also called *mm Hg.*

torsion, *n* **1.** motion or state of torque in which one end of an anatomical component is twisted about its longitudinal axis as the opposite end is either immobile or moves in the opposite direction. **2.** any motion around an anteroposterior axis of the sphenobasilar synchondrosis that extends outside the normal range of motion.

torsion, forward, *n* condition in which the sacrum rotates about an oblique axis so that sacral base side opposite to the axis involved glides anteriorly, producing a deep sulcus.

torsion, left-on-left (forward) sacral, *n* condition in which left rotation of the sacrum occurs about a left oblique axis.

torsion, left-on-right (backward) sacral, n condition in which left rotation occurs about a right oblique axis.

torsion, right-on-left (backward), n condition in which right rotation occurs about a left oblique axis.

torsion, right-on-right (forward), n condition in which right rotation occurs about a right oblique axis.

torsion, sacral (sa´·krəl tōr´·shən), n **1.** normal function of the sacrum, during walking and forward bending. **2.** a dysfunctional condition of the sacrum, in which twisting between the hipbones and the sacrum occurs about a diagonal axis.

torsion, SBS, n rotation of the occipital and sphenoid bones in opposing directions about an anteroposterior axis. May either be right or left, depending on which greater wing of the sphenoid bone is superior in position. Also called *sphenobasilar synchondrosis (symphysis) torsion.*

tort, n civil infractions (except for breach of contract) that result in injury entitling compensation. Includes but is not limited to trespassing, negligence, and defamation.

torticollis (tōr´·tə·kô´·lis), n spasms, usually on one side of the neck, turning the head to the side. Involves the sternocleidomastiod muscles and often the splenius, scalenes, and trapezius muscles as well. May cause vertigo. Also called *wryneck.*

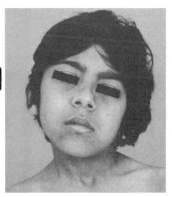

Torticollis. (Bingham, Hawke, and Kwok, 1992)

Total Body Modification Protocol, n chiropractic technique used to find the area of the body or organ that is under duress, determine the cause of the condition, and then correct the problem by restoring the nervous system to a place of balance. Focuses on how the body works to influence its structure, rather than attempting to correct the body's structure to influence its functioning, which is the basic chiropractic approach.

total load, n the sum of factors that influence an individual's life and health, including food, chemicals, microbes, psychologic factors, and other elements. Any one of these factors would not normally cause illness, but the cumulative effect of these agents may overload the functioning in an individual.

total lung capacity, n the maximum volume of air the lungs can hold.

totems (tō·təmz), n.pl in Native American culture, an Algonquin term that refers to spiritual helpers. These spiritual helpers may send messages to a patient via dreams to recommend an improved, healthier pattern of behavior. Native American healers are often contacted to act as interpreters for the dreams.

totipotency (tō´·ti·pō´·ten·sē), n ability of a cell, specifically a zygote, to develop and differentiate into a complete organism or to regenerate a body part. Also called *totipotence.*

touch for health, n a holistic approach that uses acupressure, massage, and touch for the purposes of reducing physical and mental pain, improving postural balance, and alleviating tension.

tourniquet (tur´·ni·kit), n device used to control hemorrhage by occluding the artery proximal to the area of bleeding. It should only be used in drastic situations when the injury is considered life-threatening and other treatments are deemed ineffective. It is also used to dilate veins before venipuncture.

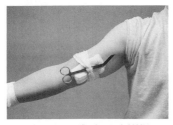

Tourniquet. (Sanders et al, 2000)

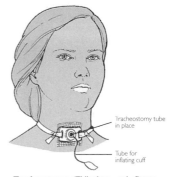

Tracheostomy. (Thibodeau and Patton, 1999)

Tracheostomy tube in place

Tube for inflating cuff

toxemia (täk·sē'·mē·ə), *n* the presence of bacterial toxins in the bloodstream. Also called *blood poisoning.*

toxemia of pregnancy, *n* condition encountered in pregnancy characterized by high blood pressure, proteinuria, and edema. May precede the onset of seizures (eclampsia). Also called *preeclampsia.*

toxicity, *n* the poisonous characteristics of a substance.

toxicity and stagnation, *n* in naturopathy, the effects of nutritional depletion including decreased metabolic functioning and buildup of chemical waste.

toxicology, *n* the discipline of examining the attributes of poisonous materials. See also drug picture.

toxin, *n* poisonous material that is synthesized or derived from an animal, mineral, or plant.

toyo igaku (tō·yō ē·gä'·kōō), *n.pr* the general term for all forms of traditional Japanese medicine, including acupuncture, shiatsu moxibustion, and kampo. See acupuncture, kampo, moxibustion, and shiatsu.

trace minerals, *n.pl* minerals needed in small amounts for optimal functioning. The list includes boron, calcium, chloride, cobalt, copper, iodine, iron, germanium, lithium, manganese, molybdenum, nickel, rubidium, selenium, strontium, tin, vanadium, and zinc.

tracheostomy (trā'·kē·äs'·tə·mē), *n* surgical procedure used to create an opening into the trachea through the neck that allows the insertion of a tube to restore normal breathing.

trachoma (trə·kō'·mə), *n* an infectious, chronic disease of the eye caused by the bacterium *Chlamydia trachomatis;* marked by pain, inflammation, an atypical sensitivity to light, and an excess secretion of tears. If the condition is not treated, blindness can eventually occur as a result of follicles that form on the upper eyelids and infiltrate the cornea. Effective therapeutic approaches include topical sulfonamides, erythromycin, and tetracycline. Surgery can repair scarred eyelids. Also called *Egyptian ophthalmia* or *granular conjunctivitis.*

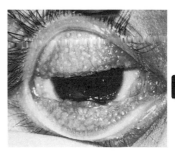

Trachoma. (Stone and Gorbach, 2000)

Trachyspermum ammi, *n* See ajowan.

traction (trak'·shən), *n* therapeutic technique that stretches the soft

T

tissues of joints and limbs by gentle pulling.

traction treatment, *n* an osteopathic procedure that uses continuous or intermittent forces to stretch the body parts being treated or to separate them along a longitudinal axis.

traditional medicine of China, *n* See China's traditional medicine.

traditional systems of health, *n.pl* the healthcare beliefs and practices that have been established by indigenous people in developing nations. Their practices often reflect the concept that human beings function as an integral part of nature and involves the use of massage, herbs, and mind/body practices, which address the physical, mental, and spiritual well-being.

Trager approach, *n.pr* founded by Milton Trager, a method of teaching clients to move in the most effortless and intuitive way possible; addresses psychological blocks to free-flowing movement and seeks to remove them to help clients live pain-free and experience release from long-standing patterns of self-imposed physical and mental limitations.

Trager psychophysical integration, *n.pr* See Trager approach.

trait, *n* a personal quality or distinct attribute of a human being, be it physical, mental, or genetic. See also constitution, diathesis, disposition, miasm, predisposition, susceptibility, and terrain.

trance, *n* an altered state of consciousness that can be natural or induced and is characterized by expanded or selected attention and awareness. Used for its therapeutic value in handling situations ranging from pain or stress management to phobia control, relaxation, and relief from nausea.

trance logic (trans' lä'·jik), *n* the alternate thinking process that enables ideas that would be paradoxical to the conscious self to peacefully coexist within the mind while in a state of trance.

trans, *pref.* Latin prefix for *across*.

transcendental consciousness (tran'·sen·den'·təl kôn'·shəs·nəs), *n* state achieved through the practice of transcendental meditation in which the individual's mind transcends all mental activity to experience the simplest form of awareness. See also meditation, transcendental.

transcendental meditation, *n.pr* a mental technique that involves the use of mantras to produce physical relaxation and increased mental alertness. See also mantra.

transcranial electrostimulation (TCES) (trans·krā'·nē·əl i'·lek·trō·sti'·myə·lā'·shən), *n* therapeutic method in which the brain is stimulated by small electric currents through the scalp; this is thought to activate endogenous opiate activity and is used to treat pain and substance abuse.

transcranial magnetic stimulation, *n* a diagnostic tool comparable to a nerve conduction study; uses a surface magnetic impulse over a client's head, and electrical stimulation over the neck, thus resulting in stimulation of the upper motor neurons and nerve tract so that the timing of electrical impulse from the brain to the muscle can be measured. Has also been used to treat neurologic conditions, such as migraine, epilepsy, insomnia, depression, and alcoholism.

transcutaneous electrical nerve stimulation, *n* a technique used for pain relief in which nerves are electronically stimulated to block transmission of pain information to the brain.

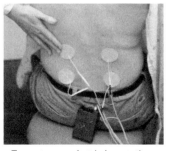

Transcutaneous electrical nerve stimulation (TES). (Ignatavicius, Workman, and Mishler, 1999)

transfer, *n* See energy exchange.

transfer factor, *n* a natural protein that is used to treat bacterial and viral diseases postulated to transfer immunity from one cell to another, thereby boosting immune function.

transference (trans·fur´·enz), *n* in psychotherapy and psychoanalysis, a client's feelings for the therapist. May be used to understand the origins of the client's emotional and psychologic problems.

transition phase, *n* in holistic nursing, the second segment of a ceremony or rite in which a person makes an effort to identify sections of his or her life that need improvement. During this segment, the person enters an unknown territory to discover himself or herself, establish aspects that are worthy and real, and verify facets of his or her life that need healing.

transitional vertebra, *n* a congenital vertebral defect in which the vertebra develops features of the adjoining region or structure—for example, lumbosacral or cervicothoracic—resulting in major postural effects on the vertebral column.

translation, *n* **1.** axial motion. **2.** transfer of information from mRNA to proteins.

transmission/scanning electron microscopy (tranz·mi´·shən/ skya´·ning i·lek´·trŏn mī´·krŏ´· skə·pē), *n* the use of focused beams of electrons to study either the surface features (i.e., scanning) or the interior structure and composition (i.e., transmission) of tiny structures.

transmitting, *v* to send and receive information, signals, and so on; allows a therapist to perceive a client's physical, emotional, and spiritual states.

transmutation (tranz´·myu·tā´· shən), *n* **1.** a mutation that results in a significant change in a species during evolution. **2.** the process of converting a chemical element into another, by nuclear decay or radioactive bombardment.

transmutation of minerals, *n* situation in which an element with a higher atomic number gradually decays and transforms into a different element with a lower atomic number.

transpersonal beings, *n.pl* according to spiritual psychology, the supernatural beings or spirits, the visits or presence from whom appear to bring about altered states of consciousness and spiritual growth, leading to therapeutic benefits.

transpersonal psychology, *n* the branch of psychology that attempts to integrate the science of psychology with the insights of various spiritual disciplines, including the role of altered states, mystical experiences, contemplative practices, and ritual for self-transcendence.

transubstantiation (tran´·səb·stan´· shē·ā´·shən), *n* **1.** a substitution of one tissue type with another. **2.** in Catholic Christianity, the doctrine that the substances of the bread and wine shared in the Eucharist (Holy Communion) are miraculously transformed into the body and blood of Christ.

transverse luo (tranz·vers´ lō), *n* in Chinese medicine, channel that serves as a connection between the main and extraordinary channels through which qi flows. See also qi.

transverse myelopathy (tranz· vers´ mī·lŏ´·pə·thē), *n* an inflammation of the spinal cord that extends across the width of the thick cord of nervous tissue; considered a potential complication of an acupuncture treatment as a result of the insertion of a needle into the paraspinal musculature that pierces the spinal cord. Sensory and motor dysfunction in portions of the trunk and extremities receiving signals from those affected nerves—at or beneath the point of insertion—is related to the condition. Motor, sensory, bowel, and sexual dysfunctions are common manifestations. Also called *TM*.

transverse plane, *n* any plane that passes through the body perpendicular to the sagittal dividing the body into superior and inferior sections. Also called *horizontal plane*.

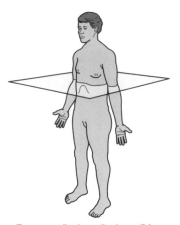

Transverse (horizontal) plane. (Salvo, 2003)

therapy applied encourages muscle movement in the direction opposite to the area of restriction, thus increasing the pain-free edge of the muscle's range of motion.

treatment, soft-tissue, *n* an osteopathic technique in which the tone of muscles and fascia is altered to increase arterial blood flow and relax connective tissue and muscle.

treatment healing system, *n* the components of an integral model of healing, which is activated when a person requests assistance for a health complaint from a professional healthcare provider. Then, diagnosis, treatment, and follow-up strategies are developed to return the individual to satisfactory health. See also homeostatic healing system, mind-body healing system, and spiritual healing system.

trauma (trä′·mə), *n* any physical or emotional injury due to sudden or violent action, exposure to dangerous toxins or profound shock.

traumatic incident reduction, *n* a meridian-based psychotherapy that involves repeated recall, or "viewing," of a memory that a client experienced as damaging. Used to help those with post–traumatic stress disorder, the sessions are nonhypnotic, one-on-one, and highly structured.

Traumeel (trô·mēl′), *n* antiinflammatory and analgesic homeopathic remedy combination that contains small amounts of belladonna, arnica montana radix, *Aconitum napellus,* chamomilla, *Symphytum officinale, Calendula officinalis, Hamamelis virginina,* millefolium, hepar sulphuris calcareum, and mercurius solubilis.

treatment, *n* **1.** a remedy for a health complaint. **2.** the administration of a therapeutic remedy.

treatment, direct, *n* an osteopathic technique in which a patient's range of motion is restored or increased by moving a body part in the direction of its restriction.

treatment, indirect, *n* an osteopathic technique in which the manual

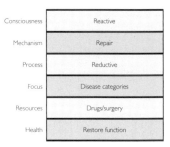

Consciousness	Reactive
Mechanism	Repair
Process	Reductive
Focus	Disease categories
Resources	Drugs/surgery
Health	Restore function

Treatment healing system. (Micozzi, 2000)

tree, *n* any woody perennial plant.

tree, bo, *n* Latin name: *Ficus religiosa*; parts used: fruits, bark, seeds, leaves, latex; uses: in Ayurveda, pacifies kapha and pitta doshas (astringent, heavy, dry), hypoglycemic, antiulcer, antiasthmatic, antitumor, antibacterial, antiprotozoal, antiviral, anthelmintic, diarrhea, dysentery, mumps, warts, earache, skin diseases; contraindications: none known. Also called *ashwattha, peepal, peepul, pipal, pippala,* or *sacred fig.*

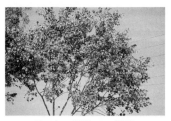

Tree, bo. (Williamson, 2002)

tree, chaste, *n* Latin name: *Vitex agnus castus*; part used: fruit (dried, ripe); uses: PMS, infertility, mastodynia, uterine bleeding, prostatitis, spermatorrhea; precautions: pregnancy, lactation, children; can cause headaches, diarrhea, stomach cramps, anorexia, depression, rash. Also called *chasteberry, gatillier, hemp tree, keuschbaum,* or *monk's pepper.*

tree, cola, *n* Latin names: *Cola nitida, Cola acuminata*; part used: seeds; uses: antidepressant, diuretic, antiinflammatory, antidiarrheal, cardiovascular disease, dyspnea, fatigue, morning sickness, migraines, wound healing; precautions: pregnancy, lactation, children; patients hypersensitive to chocolate or with gastrointestinal ulcers, ischemic heart disease, hypertension, dysrhythmias, or irregular heartbeats. Also called *bissy nut, cola nut, guru nut, kola nut, and kolanier.*

tree, European spindle, *n* Latin name: *Euonymus europaeus*; parts used: roots, seeds, leaves, fruit; uses: general health, cholagogic, gentle promotion of bowel movements, stimulation of physiologic processes, appetite, liver conditions after or accompanying fevers, induction of vomiting, skin parasites; precautions: may produce painful, watery bowel movements; may irritate intestines. Also called *common spindle tree, evonimo, igagaci, spindle bush, spindle tree,* and *wilde kardinaalsmuts.*

tree, Jaborandi **(jä·bō´·rən·dē trē),** *n.pr* Latin names: *Pilocarpus jaborandi, Pilocarpus microphyllus, Pilocarpus pinnatifolius*; part used: leaves; uses: glaucoma, diabetes, nephritis, psoriasis, eczema; precautions: patients with asthma, angle-closure glaucoma, obstructive pulmonary conditions, heart disease, kidney disease, or neurologic conditions. Also called *arruda brava, arruda do mato, Indian hemp, jamguarandi, jaurandi,* or *pernambuco jaborandi.*

tree, mango, *n* Latin name: *Mangifera indica*; parts used: fruit, seeds, pulp, bark, roots, leaves; uses: in Ayurveda, pacifies kapha and pitta doshas (astringent, light, dry), antiseptic, astringent, stomachic, vermifuge, laxative, diurectic, diarrhea, anemia, bronchitis, rheumatism; juice: tonic, heat stroke; seeds: asthma; precautions: skin and sap can cause mango dermatitis. Also called *aam* or *aamra.*

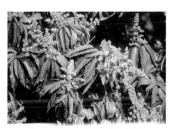

Tree, mango. (Williamson, 2002)

tree, marking-nut, *n* Latin name: *Semecarpus anacardium*; parts used: fruit, gum, oil; uses: in Ayurveda, pacifies vata dosha (light, oily, sharp, sweet, astringent), antineoplastic, immunomodulator, antiarthritic, antimicrobial, anthelmintic, hypocholesterolemic; juice: cracked skin, tumors; fruit: carminative, rubefacient, vesicant, anorexia, asthma, alopecia, ulcers, leprosy, corns, nervous conditions; precautions: allergies. Also called *bhallataka* or *bhilawa.*

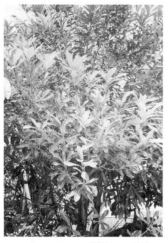

Tree, marking-nut. (Williamson, 2002)

tree, silk cotton, n Latin name: *Salmalia malabarica*; parts used: seeds, leaves, fruits, roots, flowers, gum; uses: in Ayurveda, pacifices pitta and vata doshas (sweet, heavy, dry), cardiac stimulant, astringent, diuretic, expectorant, tonic, emetic, alterative, antiinflammatory, styptic, demulcent, influenza, acute dysentery, bladder conditions, catarrh, cystitis, gonorrhea, chickenpox; precautions: none known. Also called *Bombax malabaricum, rakta-pushpa,* or *semul.*

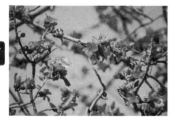

Tree, silk cotton. (Williamson, 2002)

tree, tea, n Latin name: *Melaleuca alternifolia*; parts used: oil distilled from branches, leaves; uses: topical antiseptic, insect bites, antibacterial, antiviral, antifungal, acne, eczema, psoriasis, candidiasis, gum disease; precautions: pregnancy, lactation, children; may cause skin irritation. Also called *Australian tea tree oil* or *melaleuca oil.*

tree, ti-, n See tree, tea.

trespass to the person, n inappropriate interference with another individual; proof of injury to the individual not required.

triadic type (trī·aˑ·dik tīpˊ), n in Tibetan medicine, a psychosomatic set of characteristics; the three fundamental types are chi, schara, and badahan. Establishing an individual's constitution is an important step toward diagnosis. See also chi type, schara type, and badahan type.

triage (trēˊ·äj), n a process of sorting a group of patients in a hospital or military or disaster setting to determine the immediacy of an individual's need for treatment. The type of injury or illness, the condition's severity, the level of urgency involved, the availability of medical facilities, and the likelihood of survival are the criteria used in triage.

triangle of health, n a depiction of the factors affecting human wellness in the form of a triangle; the three sides of the triangle represent structural, biochemical, and emotional components. Harmony between these three components is indicative of good health.

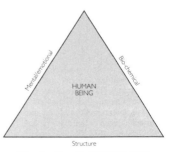

Triangle of health. (Leskowitz, 2003)

triangulation, *n* a methodological approach in qualitative research used to integrate, verify, and interpret data derived from many different sources, including interviews.

tribulus, *n* See caltrops.

Tribulus terrestris, *n* See caltrops.

trichome (trī'·kōm), *n* tiny, delicate threadlike structure located on the surface of plants.

trichomoniasis (tri'·kə·mə·nī'·ə· səs), *n* sexually transmitted disease caused by the parasitic microbe *Trichomonas vaginalis.* In men, the infection is usually asymptomatic and goes away without any intervention within a few weeks. Some men may notice a mild itching in the area of the urethra, discharge, or a mild burning sensation after ejaculation or urination. Prostatitis or epididymitis may also result as a progression of the infection. In women, the infection is generally indicated by a foul-smelling vaginal discharge that has a frothy consistency and a yellow or greenwhite color. There may be itching in the inner thigh and labia. The labia may also be swollen. Also called *Trichomonas vaginitis* or *trich.*

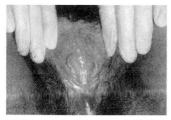

Trichomoniasis. (Monahan and Neighbors, 1998; Leonard Wolf, MD, New York)

Trichosanthes kirllowii, *n* See cucumber, Chinese.

tricuspid valve (trī·kus'·pid valv'), *n* a heart valve with three primary flaps; positioned between the right ventricle and right atrium of the heart, comprises strong fibrous tissue. It allows blood to flow from the atrium into the ventricle and tightly closes to prevent the reverse flow of the blood when the ventricle contracts. Also called *right atrioventricular valve.*

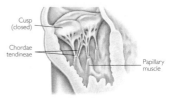

Tricuspid valve. (Mosby's Medical, Nursing & Allied Health Dictionary, ed 6, 2002)

tridosha (trē·dō'·shə), *n* in Ayurveda, the collective term for the three fundamental psychosomatic principles that sustain and regulate all psychologic and physiologic functions. Each principle in turn is a combination of two elements (mahabhutas). See also kapha, pitta, vata, and mahabhutas.

Trifolium pratense, *n* See red clover.

trigeminal neuralgia (trī·je'·mə· nəl ner·al'·jē·ə), *n* a condition in which the trigeminal facial nerve is subject to paroxysms. Presents clusters of stabbing pain that may be transient but that usually remain for hours. Caused by pressure or damage to any of the three branches of the trigeminal facial nerve.

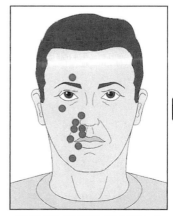

Trigeminal neuralgia: distribution of trigger zones. (Perkin, 1998)

Trillium erectum, *n* See beth root.

Trillium grandiflorum, *n* See beth root.

triphala (trē'·phä·lä), *n* in Ayurveda, a rasayana formula used to enhance youthful energy, strength, and vitality. See also rasayanas.

triple bond, *n* a covalent bond in which three valence (outer) electrons are contributed from each participating atom, which results in a total of six electrons; represented in a chemical formula by three lines that join the participating atoms. See also covalent bond.

triple burner, *n* See triple heater.

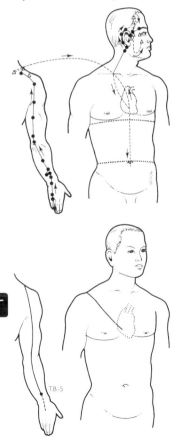

Triple burner. (Maciocia, 1989)

triple energizer, *n* in traditional Chinese medicine, one of the 12 main meridians in the body treated with acupuncture, moxibustion, or cupping. See also medicine, traditional Chinese.

***Tripterygium wilfordii* (trip·tə·rī'· jē·əm wil'·fōr·dē),** *n* part used: plant; uses: antiinflammatory, antirheumatic, eliminate toxins, relieve pruritis, ulcers of the waistband, ankylosing spondylitis, systemic lupus erythematosus, glomerulonephritis; precautions: may cause gastrointestinal distress, skin irritation, amenorrhea, leukopenia, thrombocytopenia, oligospermia, azoospermia, decrease size of testes, suppress immunity; should not be taken internally. Also called *chekiang.*

triterpenoid saponins (trī'·ter'·pə· noid sa'·pə·ninz), *n.pl* glycosides produced by plants used as foaming agents in beverages, emulsifiers, and detergents.

***Triticum repens* L.,** *n* See couchgrass.

trituration (tri·chə·rā'·shən), *n* the initial steps during the creation of homeopathic remedies based on a source material that is solid or insoluble. This source material is ground together with lactose. Further potentization of the resulting liquid can be accomplished by dissolving it in water accompanied by vigorous shaking. See also trituration, C3 and dilution.

trituration, ball-mill, *n* method in which an unspecified number of porcelain balls are homogenized in a porcelain pot with one part source material and nine parts lactose as the vehicle. See also trituration.

***trituration, C3* (sē thrē tri·chə·rā'· shən),** *n.pr* **1.** the three preliminary stages in the creation of homeopathic remedies by means of grinding source material (sometimes fresh plants) with lactose as the diluent. The degree of dilution is 3c. **2.** trituration method used by Hahnemann on all kinds of source material such as petroleum, fresh plants or their expressed juices, mercury, or other liquids. See also trituration, fresh plant.

trituration, centesimal, n grinding together 99 parts of sugar that is present in milk with one part of a homeopathic source material. Materials that are unable to be dissolved are triturated to 1/1000 (3c) before any additional suspension. See also trituration, C3; potency, centesimal; dilution; and suspension.

trituration, fresh-plant, n the creation of homeopathic remedies by means of grinding fresh plants with lactose as the diluent.

triune of life (trī'·yōōn), n concept developed by BJ Palmer; basis for modern chiropractic care according to which, life is a trinity that encompasses three united factors—intelligence, matter, and force.

tropane alkaloids (trō'·pān al'·kə·loidz), n.pl powerful substances found in several plants, including deadly nightshade, jimson weed, henbane, and European mandrake, that inhibit or block the action of acetylcholine, a neurotransmitter. Adverse effects include dry mouth, blurred vision, delirium, and drowsiness.

trophic (trō'·fik), adj relating to nutrition.

trophicity (trō'·fə·si'·tē), n the body's innate inclination to replenish its depleted supplies of nutriment.

trophotropic (trō·fə·trō'·pik), adj relating to the innate inclination for preservation and restoration of depleted nutritional supplies.

true aromatherapy product, n in the United States, the designation given by the National Association for Holistic Aromatherapy to an essential oil, thus certifying its purity standards.

true pomades, n.pl fats saturated with scent produced as a result of the maceration process to extract essential oils from plant material.

trypsin (trip'·sin), n digestive enzyme found in the stomach that breaks down protein. Also called *proteolytic enzyme,* or *proteinase.*

tryptophan (trip'·tə·fan), n an essential amino acid used in the treatment of insomnia, depression, behavioral disorders, stress, and premenstrual syndrome (PMS). Also called *L-tryptophan.*

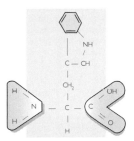

Chemical structure of tryptophan.
(Mosby's Medical, Nursing & Allied Health Dictionary, ed 6, 2002)

tsubo (tsōō·bō), n.pl mapped points on the body that correspond to and influence certain organs. Also called *acupoints.*

TT, n. therapeutic touch. See Kreiger/Kunz method.

tui na (tōō·ē nä), n a manual therapy used in traditional Chinese medicine; based on the principles of yin-yang, the five elements, and a meridian view of the body. The goal is to encourage free flow of qi by manipulating the joints, viscera, and soft tissue. See also qi.

tulsi (tōōl'·sē), n See holy basil.

tumescence (tōō'·mes·əns), n condition of being swollen or edematous.

tumorigenesis (tōō'·mə·rə·jen'·i·sis), n the process of initiation and progression of a tumor.

tuning in, v process in which a therapeutic touch practitioner centers himself or herself so as to be aligned with or "in tune" with a healing energy "frequency," so that the patient may choose to join the practitioner (tune in) and experience healing.

turmeric (tōōr'·mər·ik), n Latin name: *Curcuma longa*; part used: rhizome; uses: in Ayurveda, balances tridosha (bitter, pungent, light, dry), antioxidant, antiinflammatory, menstrual complaints, colic, dyspepsia, hematuria, flatulence, possible uses as anticancer, antiretroviral, cholecystitis, arthritis; precautions: pregnancy, lactation, children; patients with gall bladder obstructions, gallstones, peptic ulcers, bleeding disorders; those taking anticoagulant medications, immunosuppressants, NSAIDs; gastrointestinal ulcerations may occur with high dosages. Also called *curcuma, haldi, haridra, Indian saffron, Indian valerian, jiang huang, kyoo, radix, red valerian, tumeric,* or *ukon.*

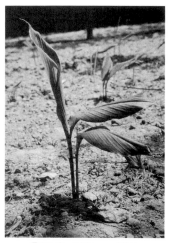

Turmeric. (Williamson, 2002)

Turnera diffusa, n See damiana.
Tussilago farfara, n See coltsfoot.
Tussilago petasites, n See butterbur.
twelve-step program, *n* group programs that treat problems such as alcoholism by completing twelve tasks. Participants gain self-acceptance and share experiences. Twelve-step programs traditionally ask members to rely on a power greater than their own.
twisting and wringing, *v* to put pressure on a part of the client's body so that the part moves simultaneously; twisting induces a unique rotation wave, whereas wringing combines twisting and squeezing. Both correct

areas of distortion and misalignment in the body.
tylophora (tī·lō·fō´·rə), *n* Latin name: *Tylophora indica;* parts used: leaves, roots; uses: antiinflammatory, antiallergic, antispasmodic; treatment for asthma, dysentery, aches and pains, respiratory conditions; precautions: patients with severe liver or kidney conditions.
Tylophora indica, n See tylophora.
type-1 movement, *n* a classification of spinal positioning in which rotation and side-bending occur in opposing directions.
type-2 movement, *n* a classification of spinal positioning in which rotation and side-bending occur in the same direction.
type-A pain, *n* deep, dull, throbbing pain that radiates into various tissues. See also sclerotome pain.
type-B pain, *n* pain that is experienced superficially and locally.
type-C pain, *n* pain experienced as a shocking sensation, often attended with feelings of weakness or paralysis, caused by compression of a nerve.
type-I somatic dysfunction, *n* **1.** in American usage, a group curvature that affects lumbar and/or thoracic vertebrae, wherein side-bending and rotation occur in opposite directions (in accordance with the first principle of physiologic motion) as the vertebral segments are in a neutral position. **2.** in French usage, a second-degree somatic dysfunction, as defined by Lovett. See also physiologic motion of the spine.
type-II somatic dysfunction, *n* **1.** in American usage, dysfunction of a single lumbar or thoracic vertebra, wherein side-bending and rotation occur in the same direction (in accordance with the second principle of physiologic motion) as the vertebra is significantly extended or flexed. **2.** in French usage, a first-degree somatic dysfunction, as defined by Lovett. See also physiologic motion of the spine.
typhus (tī´·fəs), *n* an acute infectious disease caused by *Rickettsia* species; characterized by chills, headache,

fever, and maculopapular rash. The infection spreads from infected rodents to humans via bites from fleas, lice, ticks, or mites.

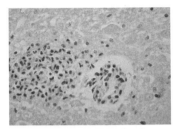

Typhus nodule in the brain. (Cotran, Kumar, and Collins, 1999)

typical associated somatic dysfunctions, *n.pl* the somatic dysfunctions that characterize psoas syndrome, including flexed dysfunctions in the upper lumbar region, sacral dysfunctions, hipbone dysfunctions, and extended dysfunctions of the fifth lumbar vertebra. See also syndrome, psoas.

typical gait, *n* the gait that characterizes psoas syndrome; the upper body totters toward the side affected by the hypertonic psoas, thus producing a swaying, waddling gait. Also called *Trendelenburg gait*. See also syndrome, psoas.

typical posture, *n* the posture typical of psoas syndrome; involves hip flexion and side bending of the lumbar region in the spine toward the direction of the hypertonic psoas muscle. See also syndrome, psoas.

tyromatosis (tī′·rō·mə·tō′·sis), *n* a process involving the degeneration of necrotic tissue into a mass that lacks a visible form; has a granular consistency and looks similar to cottage cheese. See also necrosis.

tyrosine (tī′·rə·sēn), *n* an amino acid involved in the synthesis of neurotransmitters; has other functions. Has been used to treat sleep disorders, enhance cognitive function, and alleviate symptoms of ADD. No known precautions. Also called *L-tyrosine.*

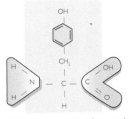

Chemical structure of tyrosine. (Mosby's Medical, Nursing & Allied Health Dictionary, ed 6, 2002)

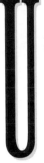

uberrimae fidei (ə·b·er·rē′·mā fi·dā′·ē), *n* utmost good faith; the expectation between parties entering into a legal agreement that all relevant information has been provided and is accurate, insofar as it influences the decision to enter the agreement and to tolerate any risk associated with the agreement.

ubidecarenone, *n* see coenzyme Q$_{10}$.

ubiquitin (yōō′·bi′·kwi·tin), *n* a 76-amino acid polypeptide from modification of histones; present in yeast and in most eukaryotic cells.

udakavahasrotas (ōō′·dä·kä·vä′·häs·rō′·təs), *n.pl* in Ayurveda, one of the thirteen kinds of srotas, or body channels, that carry fluids and water and are found in the pancreas and palate. See also srotas.

udvartana (ōōd·wär′·tə·nə), *n* in Ayurveda, body massage that uses a paste made of ground grains to cleanse the skin, improve circulation, and help weight loss.

ujjayi (ōōj·jä′·yē), *n* See ocean-sounding breath.

ulceration (əl·sə·rā′·shən), *n* the process of forming an ulcer or becoming ulcerous.

ulcerative colitis (ul′·sə·rā′·tiv kə·lī′·tis), *n* episodic, chronic autoimmune disease of the large intestine; marked by diarrhea consisting of varying amounts of pus, blood, and mucus. Also called *inflammatory bowel disease (IBD)*. See also Crohn's disease.

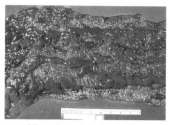

Ulcerative colitis. (Rosai, 1996)

Ulmus fulva, *n* See slippery elm.

Ulmus rubra, *n* See slippery elm.

ultramolecular, *adj* in homeopathy, a characteristic of the highest dilution of remedies. Attenuated until no molecules of the original substance are present in the solution (to the 24th decimal or 12th centesimal). Also called *submolecular.*

ultramolecular dilution, *n* See infinitesmal dose.

ultrasound, *n* **1.** a diagnostic radiology technique that uses sound waves to image internal body structures. **2.** a machine that applies heat to injured tissue to relieve pain and encourage healing. Used in physical therapy and rehabilitation.

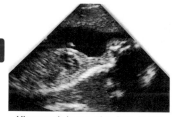

Ultrasound: image of a fetus in the second trimester. (Mosby's Medical, Nursing & Allied Health Dictionary, ed 6, 2002)

ultraviolet (UV), *n* electromagnetic radiation that has shorter wavelengths than visible light; used in chemical analytical techniques and antisepsis.

ultraviolet (UV) spectroscopy, *n* method used to measure the absorption of ultraviolet light (UV) in wavelength units to identify substances within a mixture. See also ultraviolet (UV).

uña de gato (ōō·′·nyə dä·gä·′·tō), *n* Latin name: *Uncaria tomentosa;* part used: root bark; uses: inflammation, rheumatism, gastric ulcers, tumors, dysentery, and birth control. Also popular in South American folk medicine for gastric ulcers, arthritis, and wound healing; precautions: pregnancy, lactation, autoimmune diseases, and tuberculosis. Also known as *cat's claw.*

Unani (ōō·nä·′·nē), *n* traditional healing system prevalent in the Middle East, India, Pakistan, and neighboring countries, according to which the body comprises four basic elements—earth, air, water, and fire—and four humors—blood, phlegm, yellow bile, and black bile. An equilibrium in the humors indicates good health while a disturbance in this equilibrium results in disease.

Unani Tibb, *n.pr* a system of health care found in Bangladesh, India, Pakistan, Persia, and the Middle East; based on Arabic interpretations of Galenic humoral medicine. See also Ayurveda, Galenic medicine, and humoral medicine.

Uncaria guianensis, *n* See cat's claw.

Uncaria tomentosa, *n* See cat's claw.

uncertainty, *n* **1.** principle in quantum physics; states that simultaneously knowing both the position and the momentum of a particle is impossible. **2.** the state of medical decision making for many conditions and situations.

uncommon compensatory pattern, *n* a preferred motion pattern of alternating fascia at the body's transitional areas, moving in opposite directions to those of the common compensatory pattern, classified by osteopath J. Gordon Zink.

U

uncompensated (ən·kôm'·pən·sā'·təd), *n* a clinical classification of a postural pattern in which no alterations in response to treatment occur.

uncompensated fascial pattern, *n* fascial preferences that typically occur symptomatically after some form of trauma, the motions of which fit neither the common nor the uncommon compensatory patterns. See also common compensatory pattern and uncommon compensatory pattern.

unconscious, *n* in hypnotherapy, the unconscious is viewed as sensory information not in current awareness.

underlabeling, *n* inaccurate information about a product in which the label does not list all ingredients or components contained within the product.

undirected prayer, *n* prayer that does not contain a specific request.

unguents, *n.pl* See ointments.

uniarticular (yōō'·nē·är·ti'·kyə·ler), *n* a muscle that crosses a single joint.

unicist prescribing (yōō'·nə·sist pri·skrī'·bing), *n* homeopathic practice, popular in the United Kingdom, of prescribing one remedy at a time, in single or repeated dosages. Also called *classical homeopathy.*

unidirectionality (yōō'·nē·də·rek'·shə·na'·li·tē), *n* the notion that reality is contained within an immutable, linear time-space continuum, in which past precedes present, which in turn precedes future.

uniform three-group design, *n* the fundamental basis for developing pharmacological preparations used in Tibetan medicine. Specifically, a preparation must provide the following types of components: active ingredients, ingredients altering gastrointestinal absorption, and ingredients counteracting any possible adverse effects that may develop as a result of the active ingredients.

unilateral sacral flexion, *n* condition involving a one-sided inferior sacral shear that results in a deep sulcus and an ipsilateral downward-backward inferolateral sacral angle.

unipolar design (of magnets), *n* design used in electromagnet therapies, in which a single polarity is applied to the body—either the south or the north—to activate the parasympathetic nervous system.

United States Indian Health Service, *n.pr* a federal agency within the Department of Health and Human Services that provides health services to Native Americans and Alaska Indians with the mission of raising their physical, mental, and spiritual health to the highest level.

United States Pharmacopoeia, *n.pr* **1.** the nongovernmental organization that promotes public health and safety by establishing state-of-the-art standards for medications. Also called *USP-NF.* **2.** the reference work published by this organization in which these standards may be found. In this context, it is more properly known as the *United States Pharmacopoeia* and the *National Formulary.*

unruffling and pain ridge, *v* to implement soothing outward rhythms with the hands 1 to 6 inches from the client, moving from top of the head to the feet. A healing touch process used to eliminate congestion.

unsaturated compound, *n* a chemical compound that comprises at least one double or triple bond.

upadhatus (ōō·pə·dhä·tōōs), *n.pl* in Ayurveda, secondary tissues formed as by-products during the creation of the primary tissues (dhatus). See also dhatus.

UPPP, *n* See uvulopalatopharyngoplasty.

uranium (yə·rā'·nē·əm), *n* a radioactive metal element naturally occurring in pitchblende and uraninite; prolonged exposure to uranium dust is linked to lung cancer in humans.

uremia (yōō·rē'·mē·ə), *n* the presence of increased amounts of urea and other nitrogenous waste products in blood. The condition typically results from renal failure. Also called *azotemia.*

urethrocele (yōō·rē'·thrō·cēl), *n* in females, a protrusion of a portion of the urethra and the connective tissue that surrounds it into the anterior vaginal wall. This acquired or congenital condition may be due to the

U

birthing process, obesity, or poor muscle tone. A larger protrusion may cause decreased ability to void, a certain level of incontinence, dyspareunia, or an infection of the urinary tract. Usual therapeutic approach is surgery.

Urginea maritima, *n* See squill.

urinary incontinence, *n* failure to restrain urination. Functional incontinence is due to cognitive or physical aspects that increase the difficulty of reaching a facility in time. Overflow incontinence is due to an obstruction in the urinary tract or the failure of the detrusor muscle to contract when the bladder reaches capacity. Stress incontinence is brought on by a cough, sneeze or strain, most often after childbirth in women. The therapeutic approach depends on the source of the condition; retraining the bladder, anticipatory toileting, biofeedback, medication, surgery, and exercising perineal muscles may be prescribed. See also *incontinence.*

urinary meatus (yŏŏ′·rə·nar′·ē mē′·təs), *n* the urethra's external opening.

urinary tract infection (UTI), *n* infection in one or more of the structures that make up the urinary system. Occurs more often in women and is most commonly caused by bacteria. Characteristic symptoms include frequent urination, pain when urinating, and—in severe cases—blood or pus in the urine.

urine evaluation, *n* in Tibetan medicine, a tool of diagnosis employed by practitioners to assess the presence of certain medical conditions, including chi disorder, schara disorder, and badahan disorder, in a patient's body. In particular, the practitioner uses color, odor, steam, sedimentation, and bubble formation of the urine as criteria for the evaluation. See also *disorder, chi; disorder, schara;* and *disorder, badahan.*

urolithiasis (yur′·ə·li·thē′·ə·səs), *n* stones present in the urinary tract (i.e., the kidneys, bladder, and/or urethra). Predisposing factors include dehydra-

tion and high uric acid (increased by some medications). Also called *nephrolithiasis* or *renal calculi.*

Urtica dioica, *n* See nettle.

usnea (us′·nē·ə), *n* Latin name: *Usnea barbata;* part used: entire lichen; uses: common cold, cough, sore throat, infection, an antibiotic; precautions: pregnancy, lactation. Also known as *old man's beard.*

USP, *n.pr* See United States Pharmacopoeia.

usui shiki ryoho (ōō·sōō·ē shē· kē ryō·hō), *n* another name for reiki, translated as "natural healing by the Usui method" after Dr. Mikao Usui. See also reiki.

Usui System of Natural Healing (ōō·sōō′·ē), *n.pr* a Japanese oral tradition that promotes healing through hands-on methods. Endorses the concept of reiki, or universal life energy, which may be channeled from person to person, person to plant, or person to animal.

uterine (yōō′·ter·in), *adj* pertaining to the uterus.

uterine ischemia (yōō′·tə·rin′ i· skē′·mē·ə), *n* a decrease in the supply of blood to the uterus.

uterotomy (yōō′·tə·rä′·tə·mē), *n* a surgical cut made in the uterus, as in a caesarean section.

utgo (ōōt·gō′), *n* a Seneca term used to describe a malevolent force. Native American medicine believes that disease, sorcerers, the deceased, storms, events, places, and objects can exude this evil form of energy. Simply being in the presence of this type of force can cause development of disease, pain, or discomfort.

utilization approach, *n* a naturalistic hypnosis technique, which structures the induction phase and subsequent session around the habits and personality of the patient. See also induction.

uva-ursi, *n* See bearberry.

uveitis (yōō′·vē·ī′·tis), *n* an inflammatory condition of the uveal tract of the eye, which includes the choroid, iris, and ciliary body; characterized by pain, abnormal secretion, irregular pupil shape, inflammation surrounding the cornea, accumulation of opaque deposits on the cornea, and the presence of pus within the anterior cavity. The condition can be due to infection, allergy, diabetes, trauma, skin, autoimmune, or collagen disease.

uvulopalatopharyngoplasty (yōō'·və·lō·pa'·lə·tō·fə·rin'·jō·plas'·tē), *n* surgical removal of excess palatal and pharyngeal tissues to remedy severe obstructive sleep apnea believed to be caused by obstructions in the nose or pharynx.

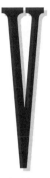

Vaccinium erythrocarpum, n See cranberry.
Vaccinium macrocarpon, n See cranberry.
Vaccinium myrtillus, n See bilberry.
Vaccinium oxycoccus, n See cranberry.
vaginal douche (va'·gə·nəl dōōsh'), *n* forcing water or another liquid into the vagina for purposes of washing or cleaning, linked to greater incidence of infections and pelvic inflammatory disease (PID).

vaginitis (va·ji·nī'·tis), *n* condition marked by vaginal inflammation and secretions. May result from yeast or a sexually transmitted disease.

vaidyas (vä·ē·dyas), *n.pl,* Ayurvedic physicians, whose practice is built on wisdom gained through cosmic consciousness as a result of religious introspection and meditation.

vajikarana (vä'·jē·kä·rä'·nə), *n* in Ayurveda, the discipline associated with promoting and producing fertility. Specifically, one of the purposes of this discipline is the protection of the following three forces crucial to life: ojas, tejas, and prana. Also called *virilization therapy.* See also ojas, tejas, and prana.

valency (vā'·len·sē), *n* the number of chemical bonds that an atom of a par-

ticular element can form, used as a measure of the chemical reactivity of that element.

valerian (və·lir'·ē·ən), *n* Latin name: *Valeriana officinalis;* parts used: rhizomes, roots; uses: anxiolytic, insomnia, nervousness; precautions: GRAS, pregnancy, lactation, children; overdose is hepatotoxic; patients with liver conditions or taking CNS depressants, MAOIs, phenytoin, warfarin. Also called *all heal, amantilla, baldrianwurzel, capon's tail, great wild valerian, herba benedicta, katzenwurzel, phu germanicum, phu parvum, setewale, setwell, theriacaria,* or *valeriana.*

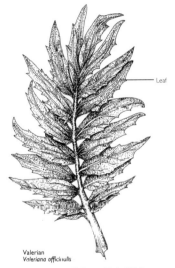
Leaf

Valerian
Valeriana officinalis

Valerian. (Skidmore-Roth, 2004)

valerian, Greek, n Latin name: *Polemonium caeruleum;* parts used: rhizome and roots; uses: spasm prevention, sedative, anxiety, sleeplessness; precautions: none known. Also called *Jacob's ladder.*

Valeriana officinalis, n See valerian.

value-centered decision making, *n* the ability of an individual or community to choose options that reflect the moral constraints by which decision makers have chosen to abide.

valvular regurgitation (val'·vyə·lər rē·gur'·ji·tā'·shən), *n* the backflow of blood during contraction of the heart; caused by a defective heart valve.

vamana (vä'·mə·nə), *n* in Ayurveda, one of the five steps of panchakarma, which refers to therapeutic vomiting induced to eliminate the mucus causing buildup of kapha; used to treat conditions related to an imbalance of kapha within the body—including chronic asthma, skin diseases, chronic cold, diabetes, chronic indigestion, obstruction of the lymphatic system, chronic sinus problems, edema, and recurring tonsillitis. See also panchakarma and kapha.

vanadium (və·nā'·dē·əm), *n* an element/mineral thought by some to be essential for health. Has been used for its antidiabetic properties. Vanadium is toxic (nephrotoxic, hepatotoxic, and teratogenic) in excess and can accumulate in tissues. Caution is advised for patients with severe kidney or liver conditions and for those taking antidiabetic medications. Also called *vanadyl sulfate* or *vanadate.*

vapocoolant sprays (va·pō·kō'·lənt sprāz'), *n.pl* topical cold application sprays. See also cryotherapy.

vapors, *n.pl* See inhalants.

varicose veins, *n* twisted and enlarged veins; can develop anywhere on the body, but feet and legs are most commonly affected. Although usually a cosmetic defect for some, it can be a source of discomfort and pain. Occasionally may indicate underlying circulatory problem. More prevalent in females than in males.

varicosis (var'·i·kō'·sis), *n* a common condition distinguished by the presence of at least one varicose vein in the legs or lower trunk. It may be due to innate defects in the walls of the veins or the valves, congestion, or increased intraluminal pressure as a result of standing for extended periods of time, pregnancy, a tumor in the abdomen, or a chronic systemic infection. See also varicosity.

varicosity (var'·i·kä'·sə·tē), *n* a condition, usually within a vein, distinguished by swelling and repetitive turns, twists, or bends.

variety, *n* **1.** diversity. **2.** an intermediate taxonomical category in biology and bacteriology. Usually synonymous with *subspecies.* See also subspecies.

varuna (vä·rōō·nə), *n* Latin name: *Crataeva nurvala;* parts used: bark, leaves; uses: in Ayurveda, pacifies kapha and vata, promotes pitta dosha (bitter, astringent, light, dry), demulcent, laxative, tonic, liver stimulant, urinary infections, kidney stones; precautions: skin irritation. Also called *Crataeva religiosa, barna, barun,* or *three-leaved caper.*

vasaka (və·sä'·kə), *n* Latin name: *Adhatoda vasica;* parts used: leaves, roots, flowers and bark; uses: in Ayurveda, pacifies kapha and pitta doshas (light, dry, bitter, astringent), respiratory ailments, childbirth, abortifacient; precautions: emetic at large doses, pregnancy. Also called *adosa* or *malabar nut.*

Vasaka. (Williamson, 2002)

vasoconstriction (vā'·zō·kən·strik'·shən), *n* state of constriction or narrowing of a blood vessel.

vasoconstrictor (vā'·zō·kən·strik'·ter), *n* a substance that narrows blood vessels by constricting the smooth muscle in the walls; increases blood pressure.

vasodilation (vā'·zō·dī·lā'·shən), *n* state of dilation or widening of a blood vessel.

vasodilator (vā'·zō·dī'·lā·ter), *n* a substance that widens blood vessels by relaxing the smooth muscle in the walls; decreases blood pressure.

vata (wä´·tə), *n* in Ayurveda, one of the three organizing principles (doshas) responsible for maintaining homeostasis. Formed by a combination of air and water, vata is involved in dynamic bodily functions, such as blood circulation, peristalsis, and elimination of food. See also doshas.

vata, apana (u·pə·nə), *n* in Ayurveda, a subdivision of the vata dosha, the influence of which is evident in the large intestine and rectum, bladder, and genitals. It promotes elimination, procreation, and menstruation, and when imbalanced, it results in constipation or diarrhea, lumbago, sexual dysfunction, and diseases of the genitourinary tract. See also doshas.

vata, prana (prä´·nə wä´·tə), *n* in Ayurveda, a subdivision of the vata dosha, the influence of which is evident in the brain, throat, heart, and lungs. It sustains respiration, cognition, memory, feeling, and perceptions; when out of balance, it contributes to respiratory, neurological, and cognitive disorders. This is the most important subdosha to keep in balance because it leads all other aspects of vata dosha, which in turn governs all three doshas. See also doshas.

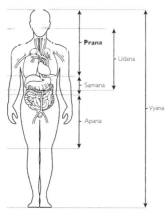

Vata, prana. (Sharma and Clarke, 1998)

vata, sama (sä·mə wä·tə), *n* in Ayurveda, ama in combination with a vata imbalance, manifesting in the form of constipation, abdominal gas, and anorexia. Remedied with pungent, digestive, carminative, and laxative herbs. See also ama, vata.

vata, samana (sä·mä·nə), *n* in Ayurveda, a subdivision of the vata dosha, the influence of which is evident in the stomach and intestines. It promotes peristalsis; when imbalanced, it results in indigestion and anorexia. See also doshas.

vata, udana (ōō·dä´·nə), *n* in Ayurveda, a subdivision of the vata dosha whose influence is evident in the lungs, throat, and navel. It sustains speaking, swallowing, and bodily energy in general; when imbalanced, it results in fatigue, speech disorders, and throat conditions. See also doshas.

vata, vyana (vē·ä·nə), *n* in Ayurveda, a subdivision of the vata dosha, the influence of which is evident in the integument, circulatory, and nervous systems. It promotes healthy circulation and the sense of touch. An imbalance of this dosha results in cardiovascular conditions and neurologic disorders. See also doshas.

vati (wä´·tē), *n* in Ayurveda, a method of medicine preparation in which herbal extracts are concentrated into pill form. Also called *gutika*.

vault hold, *n* See occiput.

vayu, *n* See vata.

VC, *n* See vital capacity.

Vedic tradition (vā´·dik trə·di´·shən), *n.pr* the religious, philosophic, and cosmologic system that has as its source the *Vedas* and *Upanishads* of India. The Vedic tradition is characterized by an emphasis on the preeminence of the subjective, in which an unmanifest field of consciousness is regarded as the fundamental reality of both the individual and the cosmos. Vedic meditation techniques are inspired by and seek the direct experience and awareness of this field.

velacione (vā·lä·sē·ō´·nä), *n* in Curanderismo, the Mexican healing system, a ritual during which candles are burned to produce supernatural results; colors and objects are believed to have vibratory power that can directly affect the patient; for instance, blue candles are burned for peace, and red candles for health or power.

velocity, *n* rate of movement (speed) in a specific direction.

venesection (ve·'nə·sek'·shən), *n* surgical cutting of a vein. Also called *phlebotomy.*

venotomy (vēn·ô·'tə·mē), *n* a procedure performed surgically in which an incision is made into a vein.

venous insufficiency (vē·'nəs in·sə·fi·'shen·sē), *n* a condition of the circulatory system distinguished by a noticeable decrease in the return of venous blood from the legs to the trunk. Edema is the first indication of the condition and is followed by ulceration, varicosity, and pain. Treatment includes correcting the underlying source of the condition, elevating the legs, and using elastic stockings.

venous plethysmography (vē·'nəs pleth'·iz·môg'·rə·fē), *n* a manometric test that measures variations in the size or volume of a limb (arm or the leg), thereby determining the change in the amount of blood in the limb.

venous pulse (vē·'nəs puls'), *n* a vein's pulse; typically palpated over the neck's external and internal jugular veins. In general, the jugular vein's pulse is measured to assess the type of the pressure wave and the pulse's pressure. This is particularly significant in individuals who have been diagnosed with a cardiac arrhythmia or a defect involving cardiac conduction. See also arrhythmia.

ventral (ven'·trəl), *adj* pertaining to the front. Also called *anterior.*

ventral respiratory group (ven'·trəl res'·pə·rəh·tōr'·ē grŏŏp'), *n* the group of neurons located in the medulla oblongata, which, although inactive during normal breathing, are activated by signals from the dorsal respiratory group during heavier breathing and in turn stimulate the muscles of forced exhalation

ventricular fibrillation (ven·tri'·kyə·ler fib'·rə·lā'·shən), *n* an arrhythmia of the cardiac muscle distinguished by the ventricular myocardium's quick depolarization; characterized by ventricular ejection and the complete absence of organized electrical activity; blood pressure falls to zero; and the individual enters a state of unconsciousness. Within 4 minutes, death may result. The immediate initiation of cardiopulmonary resuscitation accompanied by defibrillation and the appropriate dosage of medications designed to resuscitate are necessary to sustain life. Also called *VF.*

ventriculoureterostomy (ven·tri'·kyə·lō'·yŏŏ·rē'·ter·rôs'·tə·mē), *n* procedure performed surgically to direct cerebrospinal fluid into the general circulation. Typically performed in newborns, this approach is performed as an alternative to aurioculoventriculostomy to treat an obstructive form of the condition known as hydrocephalus. See also hydrocephalus.

venules (vēn'·yŏŏlz), *n.pl* small blood vessels that merge with the veins and return blood from other tissues to the heart.

***Veratrum album* (və·rä'·trəm al'·bəm),** *n* a homeopathic preparation of white hellebore, used to treat gushing diarrhea, cramps, vomiting, and cold sweat.

Veratrum viride, *n* See American hellebore.

Verbasci flos, *n* See mullein.

Verbascum thapsus, *n* See mullein.

Verbena officinalis, *n* See European vervain.

vermifugal (ver·mə·fyŏŏ'·gəl), *n* a substance that is used for eradicating intestinal worms. Also called *vermifuge.*

Veronica virginica, *n* See black root.

Veronicastrum virginicum, *n* See black root.

vertebral (ver'·tə·brəl), *adj* pertaining to the spinal column.

vertebral subluxation complex (ver'·tə·brəl sub'·lək·sā'·shən kôm'·pleks), *n* See segmental dysfunction.

vertebral unit, *n* two contiguous vertebrae and related connective, lymphatic, muscular, neural, skeletal, and vascular tissues.

vertebrobasilar insufficiency (ver'·tə·brō·bā'·zə·ler in'·sə·fi''·shən·sē), *n* a disorder caused by decrease of blood flow in the vertebral or basilar arteries due to atherosclerosis or compression placed on the external wall of the arteries. Symptoms may include loss of vision, dizziness, or nausea. Also called *VBI, vertebrobasilar circulatory disorders,* or *posterior circulation ischemia.*

vertebrobasilar system (ver'·tə·brō·bā'·zə·ler sis'·təm), *n* the three blood vessels—the two vertebral arteries and one basilar artery—located towards the back of the brain that provide about 20% of the intracranial blood supply. Also called *posterior circulation.*

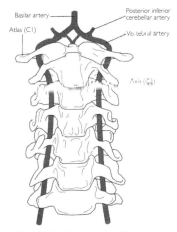

Vertebrobasilar system. (Gibbons and Tehan, 2000)

vertigo, *n* a condition in which the patient perceives the external world as spinning around him or her (objective vertigo), or the individual may feel as though he or she is revolving in space (subjective vertigo).

vesicant (ve'·sə·kənt), *n* a substance used to induce blistering.

vestige (ves'·tij), *n* an organ that has developed imperfectly and is largely considered nonfunctional. It may have provided a significant function in a more primordial type of life or during an earlier life stage. The vermiform appendix in humans is an example of a vestige.

viable, *adj* pertaining to the ability to develop, grow, and sustain the functions of life. For example, the human fetus without abnormalities is considered viable at the twenty-fourth week of gestation.

vibraciones mentales (vē·brä'·sē·ō'·nās men·tä'·les), *n.pl* in Curanderismo, the Mexican healing system, the mental vibrations that a healer may channel or harness to directly affect a person's physical or mental state.

vibrating, *v* using quivering hand motions made across the client's body for therapeutic purposes.

vibration, *n* massage technique believed to enhance nerve function by using small superficial rapid movements of the fingertips or palm.

vibrissae (vī·bri'·sā), *n pl* the thick hairs which grow inside the nostrils to help keep large particles from entering the nasal passages.

Viburnum opulus, *n* See black haw.

Viburnum prunifolium, *n* See black haw.

vicarious responsibility, *n* the indirect legal responsibility that an employer bears for the unlawful behavior of its employees while they are working.

videntes (vē·den'·tās), *n.pl* in Curanderismo, the Mexican healing system, psychics who work on the spiritual level.

vigilambulism (vi'·jə·lam'·byōō·li'·zəm), *n* a condition in which an individual performs motor actions, such as walking, in an unconscious yet waking state.

vikriti (vi·kri·tē), *n* in Ayurveda, the prevalent imbalance in dosha that is the cumulative effect of imbalances and impurities present in an individual. Ayurveda aims at rectifying vikriti to restore the deha prakriti. See also dosha and deha prakriti.

viniyoga (vē·nē·yō'·gə), *n* a methodology developed by Shri T. Krishnamacharya, which emphasizes practicing yoga based on individual needs and capacities by using asanas, pranayama, meditation, ritual, and prayer, thus leading to overall well-being.

vinpocetine (vin·pō'·sə·tēn), *n* a chemical derived from an alkaloid present in the leaves of the periwinkle plant (*Vinca minor*). Has been used as a neuroprotector to increase blood flow to the brain and to treat dementia and ischemic stroke. No known precautions, but caution is advised for patients who are taking warfarin. Also called *periwinkle.*

vinyasa (vēn·yä'·sə), *n* in Sanskrit, connecting; the sequence of a number of yoga postures in a specific way.

Viola odorata, *n* See violet.

Viola tricolor, *n* See pansy.

violet, *n* Latin name: *Viola odorata*; parts used: leaves, flowers; uses: clears mucus from lungs, eczema, inflammation of the eye, insomnia, coughs, bronchial conditions; precautions: possible contact dermatitis. Also called *sweet violet.*

vipaka (vē·pä'·kə), *n* in Ayurveda, postdigestive taste, one of the qualities used to classify foods and drugs. The three vipaka are sweet, sour, and pungent.

vipassana (vē·päs'·sä·nə), *n* a meditation practice that focuses on mindfulness.

viral hepatitis, *n* an inflammatory condition of the liver, caused by the hepatitis viruses: A, B, C, delta, E, F, G, or H. It is characterized by a general feeling of ill health, anorexia, a painful sensation near the liver, headache, jaundice, fever, darkened urine, reddish stool samples, vomit-

ing, and nausea; transmitted via blood transfusion or sexual contact. It occurs more frequently in individuals who engage in risky behavior or are infected with the human immunodeficiency virus (HIV). Treatment involves supportive measures, plenty of rest, regular regimen of vitamins and minerals, interferon and antiviral medications, and continuous monitoring of functions within the kidneys and liver. If untreated, severe cases may result in destruction of tissue, development of cirrhosis, coma, liver cancer, or possibly death.

viral load, *n* a measure of the number of virus particles present in the bloodstream, expressed as copies per milliliter. This measurement helps in treatment decisions and to monitor the efficacy of a treatment.

viral pharyngitis, *n* an inflammation of the pharynx caused by a virus. Symptoms are similar to streptococcal pharyngitis. Zinc lozenges and *Echinacea* may provide relief from symptoms and decrease the duration of the infection. See also streptococcal pharyngitis.

viranga (vē·räng'·gə), *n* Latin name: *Embelia ribes;* parts used: berries, leaves; uses: in Ayurveda, balances kapha and vata doshas (pungent, light, dry, sharp), anthelmintic, antitumor, insecticide, antimicrobial, analgesic, contraception, nervine, constipation, diuretic, worms; precautions: none known. Also called *embelia* or *vidanga.*

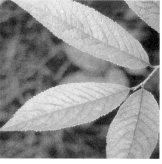

Viranga. (Williamson, 2002)

virechana (vē·rā'·chə·nə), *n* in Ayurveda, one of the five steps in the Panchakarma therapy, in which castor oil or other laxatives are administered to induce purgation after being on an empty stomach for 12 hours. See also therapy, Panchakarma.

virus, *n* the smallest living microscopic organism. Comprises nucleic acid and enclosed by a layer of protein. It only reproduces within another living organism, and viruses are responsible for a number of diseases including the common cold, influenza, and AIDS.

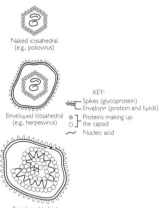

Naked icosahedral (e.g., poliovirus)

KEY:
— Spikes (glycoprotein)
— Envelope (protein and lipids)
Enveloped icosahedral (e.g., herpesvirus)
⊕ ⌐ Proteins making up
○ ⌐ the capsid
~ Nucleic acid

Enveloped helical (e.g., influenza virus)

Virus. (Ackerman and Dunk-Richards, 1991)

virya (vēr'·yə), *n* in Ayurveda, potency, one of the qualities used to classify foods and drugs; divided into eight types that are categorized in pairs: heavy-light, hot-cold, dull-sharp, and unctuous-dry.

vis medicatrix naturae (vēs' me·di·kä'·triks nä·tōō'·rā), *n* the recognition by Hippocratic physicians that life is self-healing. Used as a philosophical basis for many complementary and natural therapies.

viscera (vis'·er·ə), *n* internal organs enclosed within the cavity of the body, such as the thoracic, abdominal, endocrine, and pelvic organs.

visceral dysfunction, *n* diminished or modified mobility of the viscera and associated connective, lymphatic, neural, skeletal, and vascular tissues.

visceral manipulation (vi'·ser·əl mə·nip'·yə·lā'·shən), *n* manual therapy that incorporates gentle massage techniques applied to the organs located in the abdominal and pelvic areas.

viscerosomatic (vi'·ser·ō·sə·ma'·tik), *n.pl* areas in the paraspinal tissue that present palpable, localized, sensitive symptoms related to visceral dysfunction.

viscerotonia (vi·ser·ə·tō'·nē·ə), *n* one of the three temperaments described by WH Sheldon; characterized as relaxed, comfortable, tolerant, and gregarious.

viscosity (vis·kô'·sə·tē), *n* the degree of resistance of a liquid to flow.

Viscum abietis, *n* See mistletoe.

Viscum album, *n* See mistletoe.

Viscum austriacum, *n* See mistletoe.

vishada (vē·shä'·də), *adj* in Ayurveda, "clear" as a guna, one of the qualities that characterizes all substances. Its complement is avila. See also gunas and avila.

vishesha (vē·shä·shä), *adj* in Ayurveda, opposite; opposite elements or mahabhutas diminish a dosha. See also mahabhutas and dosha.

vision quest, *n* See Hanbleceya.

visual agnosia (ag·nō'·zhə), *n* the lack of ability to use one's sense of sight to distinguish objects even though eyesight is intact.

visual/kinesthetic dissociation, *n* an approach that is exposure-based and seeks to assist an individual's freedom from kinesthetic memories of trauma, thus enabling him or her to process the traumatic event(s) from a less invested perspective. Clients are instructed to see themselves from a vantage point above the scene, then to observe themselves in a physical level equal to the event—yet still distant enough for it to not intimidate them—whereas practitioners help them to reprocess the event from the security of the healing venue.

V

visualization, *n* structured technique in which the individual uses his or her imagination to create images of desired life changes. See also relaxation and visualization.

visualizing, *v* **1.** holding an image in one's mind. **2.** forming an image of a goal or destination in one's mind before undertaking it, so as to facilitate success.

vital capacity, *n* the maximum amount of air that can be expelled following maximum inhalation, representing the maximum breathing capacity. Used to determine the condition of the lung function.

vital force, *n* the bioenergetic aspect of living things. Some assert that qi, acupuncture, and homeopathic remedies work on this level instead of at the gross physical level.

vital spirit, *n* See energy, vital.

vitalism (vī'·təl·i·zəm), *n* doctrine that a nonphysical energy permeates all living organisms and that gives them the property of life. See also prana and qi.

vitamin, *n* an organic substance that is an essential nutrient.

vitamin A, *n* a fat-soluble vitamin found in dark-colored vegetables and fruits, meats, dairy products, and whole eggs. Has been used to treat deficiencies, viral infections, and skin disorders. Contraindicated for pregnant women (beta-carotene is recommended instead), especially those taking valproic acid and for patients taking warfarin or isotretinoin. Also called *retinol.*

vitamin B$_1$, *n* a water-soluble vitamin found in blackstrap molasses, brewer's yeast, organ meats, pork, wheat germ, and whole-grain cereals. Has been used to treat deficiencies (including those caused by loop diuretics), congestive heart failure, and Alzheimer's disease. No known precautions.

vitamin B$_2$, *n* a water-soluble vitamin found in organ meats, brewer's yeast, leafy green vegetables, mushrooms, beans, and peas. Has been used for deficiencies (including those caused by birth control pills), migraines, sickle cell anemia, and to augment

athletic performance. No known precautions.

vitamin B$_3$, *n* a water-soluble vitamin found in yeast, seeds, legumes, wild rice, and whole grains and available in three supplemental forms—niacin, inositol hexaniacinate, and niacinamide. Has been used for deficiencies (including low levels from isoniazid), high cholesterol (using niacin), intermittent claudication and Raynaud's phenomenon (using inositol hexaniacinate), osteoarthritis (using niacinamide), and diabetes (using niacinamide). High-dose niacin therapy may cause liver inflammation and is contraindicated for those with ulcers, gout, or excessive consumption of alcohol. Niacinamide is contraindicated for those taking anticonvulsant medications, and caution is advised for children and pregnant or lactating women, for whom the maximum daily dose is 35 mg. Also called *inositol hexanicotinate.*

vitamin B$_6$, *n* a water-soluble vitamin found in nutritional and brewer's yeasts, beans, seeds, wheat germ, nuts, bananas, and avocados. Has been used to maintain cardiovascular health, to remedy deficiencies—including lower levels from taking hydralazine, isoniazid, MAOIs, penicillamine, and theophylline—and to treat morning sickness, asthma, carpal tunnel syndrome, depression, seborrheic dermatitis. Is also used to prevent kidney stones and the side effects from theophylline and photosensitivity. Megadoses may cause sensory neuropathy. Supplementation is contraindicated for those taking levodopa. Caution is advised for children and pregnant or lactating women, for whom the maximum daily dose is 100 mg. May cause neuropathy at large doses. Also called *pyridoxine hydrochloride* or *pyridoxal-5-phosphate.*

vitamin B$_8$, *n* an isomer of glucose involved in the functioning of muscles, nerves, cell membranes, and fat metabolism in the liver. Has been used for depression, panic disorders, bulimia, obsessive-compulsive disorder, ADD, and Alzheimer's disease. Caution in patients with bipolar depression. Also called *inositol hexaphosphate, IP6, myoinositol,* or *phytic acid.*

vitamin B₁₂, *n* a water-soluble vitamin found in animal foods such as meat, eggs, and dairy. Has been used for deficiencies (often found in vegetarians, particularly vegans) or lower levels from colchicine, metformin, phenformin, AZT, and nitrous oxide and to treat pernicious anemia and bursitis of the shoulder. No known precautions. Also called *cyanocobalamin, hydrocobalamin,* or *methylcobalamin.*

vitamin C, *n* a water-soluble vitamin found in citrus fruits, cruciferous vegetables, leafy greens, peppers, and strawberries. Has been used to remedy deficiencies (including low levels caused by taking aspirin and birth control pills); to prevent and treat upper respiratory conditions; to prevent reflex sympathetic dystrophy, easy bruising, and skin aging; to treat high blood pressure and bedsores; and to improve behavior associated with autism. Caution in those prone to develop kidney stones, with kidney disease, excessive iron, deficient copper, or intestinal conditions and for patients taking warfarin and heparin. Caution is advised for children and pregnant or lactating women, for whom the maximum daily dose is 2000 mg. Also called *ascorbate.*

vitamin D, *n* a fat-soluble vitamin found in fatty fish and fortified dairy products and synthesized by the body via sunlight. Has been used to remedy deficiencies (including depressed levels by taking medications such as cimetidine, corticosteroids, heparin, isoniazid, phenobarbital, phenytoin, primidone, rifampin, and valproic acid), to treat osteoporosis and polycystic ovaries (in conjunction with calcium supplementation), high blood pressure, type-1 diabetes, and psoriasis. Caution in patients with hyperparathyroidism or sarcoidosis, those taking calcium channel–blocking medications or thiazide diuretics. Caution is advised for children and

pregnant or lactating women, for whom the maximum daily dose is 2000 IU (50 μg). Also called *calcipotriol (topical vitamin D₃), cholecalciferol (vitamin D₃),* or *ergocalciferol (vitamin D₂).*

vitamin E, *n* a fat-soluble vitamin found in nuts, vegetable oils, seeds, and whole grains. Has been used to remedy deficiencies and for immunomodulatory effects; to treat cataracts, cardiac autonomic neuropathy, dementia, diabetic neuropathy, painful menstruation, preeclampsia (with vitamin C supplementation), rheumatism, and type-2 diabetes. Caution for patients taking hypoglycemic medications, supplements with anticoagulant or antiplatelet effects, such as garlic, gingko, or policosanol supplements, and those undergoing chemotherapy. Caution is advised for children and pregnant or lactating women, for whom the recommended daily intake is 15 mg with a maximum daily dose of 1000 mg. Also called *alpha-tocopherol, D-tocopherol, DL-tocopherol, DL-alpha-tocopherol, tocopheryl succinate, tocopheryl acetate, D-alpha-tocopherol, D-delta-tocopherol, D-beta-tocopherol, D-gamma-tocopherol,* or *mixed tocopherols.*

vitamin H, *n* See biotin.

vitamin K, *n* a fat-soluble vitamin found in leafy greens, beans, peas, oats, and whole wheat. Has been used to remedy deficiencies (including those associated with alcoholism, Crohn's disease, diarrhea, and ulcerative colitis), osteoporosis, and menorrhagia. Pregnant women taking anticonvulsants may need to supplement vitamin K to prevent birth defects. Contraindicated for patients taking warfarin and caution with cephalosporins. Also called *menadione, menaquinone,* or *phylloquinone.*

vitamin M, *n* See folate.

vitamin P, *n* See niacin.

vivisection (vi′·və·sek′·shən), *n* the dissection of living animals to view anatomic systems.

VLF-sferics, *n.pl.* signals, produced by lightning, which fall into the very

V

low–frequency (VLF) range. Also called VLF-atmospherics.

vocational rehabilitation counselor, *n* term coined in the 1960s and 1970s for a professional who incorporates the best of psychology, social work, and nursing in an attempt to integrate psychology with traditional rehabilitation protocols.

volatile (vô'·lə·təl), *n* the ability of a substance to change from a solid or a liquid to a vapor or a gas. It provides a foundation for the categorization of aromatic components of essential perfumes and oils into top, middle, and base notes.

volatility, *n* the measure of a chemical's vapor pressure, which is the basis for its evaporation rate, boiling point and—if the chemical is flammable—its flammability.

-volemia (-vō·lē'·mē·ə), *comb* combining form that refers to the amount of plasma within the body.

volenti non fit injuria (vō·len'·tē nôn fit in·jə·rē'·ə), *n* "to the willing there is no wrong," taking full personal responsibility for exposing oneself to risk.

voluntary stress, *n* activities produce stress but also increase endorphins and challenge the participant in a positive manner (i.e., extreme sports); considered beneficial to overall health.

volvulus (vol'·vyə·ləs), *n* a condition in which a portion of the bowel slides down into its ramen. The condition is commonly due to a protrusion of a portion of the mesentery—particularly in the cecum, ileum, or the sigmoid segments of the bowel. The condition is characterized by lack of bowel sounds, nausea, vomiting, painful sensations, and a taut and swollen abdomen. If untreated, the obstructed bowel becomes necrotic and is followed by inflammation of the peritoneum and then rupture of the bowel, resulting in death.

vomer (vō'·mer), *n* the thin plow-shaped bone of the skull that forms the anterior and posterior parts of the nasal septum.

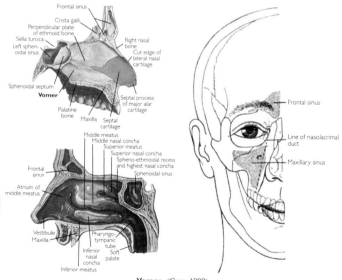

Vomer. (Gray, 1989)

v-spread, *n* an osteopathic technique (used in craniosacral therapies) that uses forces transmitted along the skull's diameter to facilitate movement in the sutures.

Vt, *n* tidal volume; the amount of air that is inhaled or exhaled during each normal respiratory cycle.

vulnerary (vəl'·nə·re'·rē), *n* a wound-healing substance.

vulval washes (vul'·vəl wä'·shez), *n.pl* the application of diluted essential oils to the female genitalia for purposes of treating infections and leukorrhea (white or greenish discharge due to inflammation of the membrane that lines the genitals).

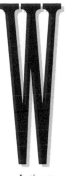

wagamama (wä·gä·mä'·mə), *n* in Japan, an emotional disorder marked by childlike behavior, emotional outbursts, lack of feelings, and negative attitude. No equivalent form of this disorder exists in North America.

wahoo (wä·hōō'), *n* Latin name: *Euonymus atropurpureus;* parts used: bark, stem, root bark, stem bark, seed; uses: heart problems, induction of strong bowel movements, stimulation of flow of bile, induction of perspiration, induction of vomiting, expectorant, general health, gall bladder dysfunction, facial sores, gynecological conditions, appetite stimulant, liver dysfunction, skin disorders, malaria, constipation, dandruff, vomiting of blood, painful urination, stomach pain; precautions: may cause intestinal irritation; may be toxic in large quantities. Also called *burning bush, eastern wahoo, Indian arrow-wood, spindle tree,* and *waahoo.*

Wakantanka (wä·kän'·tän·kä), *n* in Lakota Indian medicine, the "great spirit," creation's great mystery that represents sacred medicine.

wall germander (wäl jer·man'·der), *n* Latin names: *Teucrium chamaedrys, Teucrium officinale;* parts used: whole plant; uses: joint inflammation, rheumatism, promotion of mild bowel movements, contraction of living tissues, digestion, flow of bile, repair of the intestinal lining, regulation of secretion of glycogen and insulin, carminative, induction of perspiration, diuretic, stimulation of physiologic processes, general health, gout, weight loss, wound healing; precautions: may cause liver damage. Also called *camedrio, common germander, germander, germandree petit chene, kamaderyos,* and *yermesesi.*

walnut, *n* Latin name: *Juglans regia;* parts used: leaves, rind, seed, oil, cotyledons, bark, root bark; uses: pain, joint inflammation, contraction of living tissues, blood purification, cancer, elimination of toxins, removal of dead and diseased matter, diuretic, induction of bowel movements, stones from bladder and kidney, respiratory disease, skin conditions, stimulation of physiologic processes, constipation, chronic coughs, asthma, diarrhea, dyspepsia, dizziness, anemia, low back pain, frequent urination, weakness in legs, menstrual irregularities, precautions: may be carcinogenic. Also called *black walnut, ceviz agaci, ch'iang t'ao, common walnut, English walnut, guz, hei t'ao, hu t'ao, hu tao, jawiz, joz, noqal Parsian walnut, qoz,* and *walnoot.*

wandering sickness, *n* according to the Pima Indian healing system, disorders believed to occur because of impurities wandering into and throughout the body.

wang (wäng), *n* in traditional Chinese medicine, the first aspect of diagnosis that involves visual examination of patients—particularly their spirit, form, and bearing; the face and the head; and excreted substances. See also qie and wen. ⓦ

warm-ups, *n.pl* movements preceding an exercise regimen. Performed to increase blood circulation, release muscle tension, and increase awareness.

warranties, *n.pl* the details of a contract; considered less important than the conditions. Whereas the penalty for breach of conditions is the termination of the contract, the penalty for breach of warranties is payment of damages to the innocent party.

warrior stance, *n* biomechanically correct position from which to reach across the body and apply short transverse strokes during massage. With toes pointing forward, both feet are planted hip width apart. Also called *horse stance.*

water, *n* one of the five phases, or elements, in Chinese cosmological and medical theory, the characteristic manifestations of which include anxiety, introspection, mystery, nervousness, philosophical speculation, solitude, and truthfulness.

water, aromatic, *n* fluid prepared in a laboratory by combining distilled water with any number of essential oils; may also comprise some artificial and synthetic ingredients and in some cases, alcohol.

water, essential, *n* the end product of the process in which steam is passed through plant material to derive the benefits of the plant's essence.

water, floral, *n* the residual water from distillation carried out to extract essential oils from plant material, considered therapeutically useful and used in skin care and perfumery industries. Also called hydrosol.

water, hamamelis **(ham'·ə·me'·lis wä'·ter),** *n* liquid infused with an extract from *Hamamelis virginiana* twigs for use as an astringent. Also called *witch hazel.*

water, memory of, *n* the theoretical ability of water or water-ethanol mixes to carry information during dilution and succession.

water, prepared, *n* a product containing any number of natural and artificial ingredients; meant to resemble plain water.

water, smart, *n* theoretically, a solvent (typically water) that retains the information imprinted by the substance(s) dissolved in it. Used by some to explain the mechanism through which homeopathic remedies work.

water distillation, *n* a method for extracting essential oils from aromatic plant materials that uses steam to transfer the volatile oils. Because the plant materials are first immersed in water before being heated, some constituents are protected from being overheated. This process can take a significant amount of time, and damage may be incurred to some of the compounds.

water injection (wä'·ter in·jek'· shən), *n* therapy that involves the subcutaneous injection of sterile water over trigger points; used to effect relief from painful conditions, especially those due to myofascial trigger points.

water-soluble vitamins, *n.pl* any of a variety of substances essential to human health and function that dissolve in water, such as vitamin C and vitamin B complex. Assist important enzyme activity such as energy production from fats and carbohydrates. If excessive amounts are consumed, they are passed from the body through urine, whereas a deficiency affects growing or rapidly metabolizing tissues such as those in blood, skin, nervous system, and the digestive tract.

water-and-steam distillation, *n* a method of extracting essential oils in which water and plant materials are mixed and steam is introduced into them.

weaning, *n* the period of transition from breast feeding to eating solid foods.

weather modality, *n* the factor of weather, which modifies the behavior of a symptom that, for example, could be worse during a storm. See also modality and symptom, general.

weather sensitivity, *n* phenomenon whereby living creatures exhibit physiologic and mental changes as a result of a concurrent change in the weather.

W

web of causation, *n* the interrelationships of several factors that precipitate a particular disease.

Weber-Fechner Principle, *n.pr* principle according to which a change in a sensory stimulus is a fraction of the existing sensory load.

wei level (wā le·ʹ·vəl), *n* the outer layer of energy; comprises the main and secondary meridians. This layer relates to muscles and skin. Because it is the outermost layer, it is easily invaded by heat.

wellness, *n* the subjective perception of being optimally healthy.

wen (wən), *n* in traditional Chinese medicine, the second aspect of diagnosis that includes listening to the sounds of the body and being aware of the odors of the patient's breath, body, and excreta. See also qie and wang.

wet-sheet pack, *n* a hydrotherapy technique in which the patient is enveloped in a white sheet that has been soaked in cold water and almost completely wrung out. The patient undresses and lies down securely wrapped in the wet sheet, with two wool blankets above and below him. The treatment proceeds through four phases: the tonic stage, the neutral stage, the heating stage, and the elimination stage. Entire treatment takes 1 to 3 hours.

wet-sheet treatment, *n* a hydrotherapy technique in which patients are wrapped tightly in several layers of cold, wet sheets, followed by heavy wool blankets, and left in bed until they begin to sweat, at which point the blankets are removed and the patients are drenched with cold water.

wheal-and-flare reaction (wēlʹ -and-flerʹ rē·akʹ·shən), *n* a three-stage reaction that develops on the surface of the skin because of injury or exposure of the body to an antigen via injection. The condition is characterized by redness and swelling that results from release of histamine.

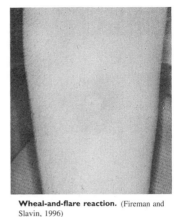

Wheal-and-flare reaction. (Fireman and Slavin, 1996)

wheatgrass, *n* a nutritional grass available popularly as juice. Wheatgrass contains large amounts of chlorophyll and other pigments. See also therapy, juice.

wheeze (wēz), *n* an atypical, high- or low-pitched sound observed during expiration; caused by an increased velocity of air being forced through a constricted passage; may be caused by inflammation, asthma, bronchospasm, or an airway obstruction by a foreign body or tumor.

whey protein, *n* soluble protein found in milk whey that has been clotted by rennin, examples of which include alpha-lactalbumin, lactoglobulin, and lactoferrin. One of the primary proteins in breast milk, whey protein is a good source of sulfur amino acids and glutamine. Also called *lactalbumin.*

whiplash, *n* sprain or strain injury occurring at the fourth/fifth cervical junction due to rapid acceleration or deceleration of the body.

whirlpool, *n* local or general hot water application characterized by forceful jets of air through the water. Used most commonly in rehabilitation to stimulate circulation and provide pain relief. See also thermotherapy.

white, *adj .* in Chinese medicine, a facial coloration indicative of either lung conditions or of an accumulation of cold energy, as in colic. See also energy, cold.

white hellebore (wīt' he·'·lə·bōr'), *n* Latin name: *Veratrum album;* parts used: root and rhizome; uses: homeopathic remedy for dysmenorrhea; Raynaud's syndrome, menstrual problems and PMS; precautions: highly toxic.

white leadwort, *n* Latin name: *Plumbago zeylanica;* parts used: roots, leaves; uses: in Ayurveda, pacifies kapha dosha (pungent, light, dry, sharp), anticancer, antifertility, antiinflammatory, antimicrobial, antioxidant, prevention of antibiotic resistance, immunomodulator, anticoagulant, abortifacient, vesicant, rheumatism, diarrhea, diuretic, skin conditions; precautions: pregnancy. Also called *chitra* or *chitraka.*

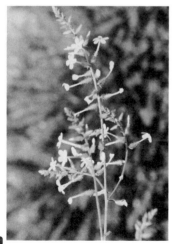

White leadwort. (Williamson, 2002)

white peony, *n* Latin name: *Paeonia lactiflora;* part used: roots; uses: spasms, antiinflammatory, pain, men-strual pain, abortion, anticoagulant; precautions: could augment activity of blood-thinning medications. Also called *bai shao yao.*

white snakeroot (wīt' snāk'·rōōt), *n* Latin name: *Eupatorium rugosum;* parts used: leaves, root; uses: ague, diarrhea, painful urination, antipyretic, kidney stones, revival of unconscious patients, treat snakebites; precautions: may cause "milk sickness" with indications of weakness, trembles, vomiting, nausea, delirium, and prostration.

white squill (wīt' skwil'), *n* Latin name: *Urginea maritima;* part used: inner scales of the bulb; uses: cardiac treatment, diuretic, expectorant, and vomit inducer; precautions: pregnant and lactating women; individuals with hypokalemia, hypertropic cardiomyopathy, or ventricular tachycardia. Also called *squill, European squill, Indian squill, red squill, sea onion,* or *sea squill.*

whole-body ablution (hōl' bä'·dē ə·blōō'·shən), *n* hydrotherapy technique in which a practitioner vigorously rubs a coarse washcloth or loofah dipped in cold water across the client's body one section at a time to create friction. The rubbing is done in sequence with the patient lying supine. Performed as a tonifying treatment. Also called *cold friction rub.*

wholeness, *n* completeness, indivisibility; a fundamental concept embraced by many healing systems that assert that all things are connected and that each is part of a singular whole. It is accepted that this singular whole is much greater than the total of all its elements. It is thought that any particular phenomena is only able to be comprehended in terms of the wholeness from which it derives.

wholism, *n* See holism.

whooping cough, *n* a bacterial disease triggered by *Bordetella pertussis.* The illness is characterized by the distinctive spasmodic cough, difficult-to-dislodge mucus, and general weakness.

wi'ikt ceya (wē'·ēkt che·yä'), *n* Lakota Indian term for an individual's capacity for selfless giving.

W

wicasa wakan (wē·kä´·sä wä´·kän), *n* in Native American medicine, a Lakota term for a holy person who communicates with the healing powers.

Wickram Experience Inventory, *n.pr* 24-item questionnaire used to measure hypnotic ability. Participants responding "true" to 18 or more of the questions are considered to have a moderate to high hypnotic ability.

wicozani (wē·chō´·zä·nē), *n* Lakota Indian term for good total health, used to describe a healthy, well-functioning tribal community.

wild black cherry bark, *n* Latin name: *Prunus virginiana;* part used: dried stem bark; uses: externally for wound healing, relaxant, antipyretic; for treating coughs, asthma, colitis, diarrhea, and dysentery; precautions: could cause death or other serious consequences. Also called *cherry bark.*

wild cherry, *n* Latin names: *Prunus virginiana, Prunus serotina;* part used: bark; uses: coughs, colds, respiratory ailments, diarrhea, astringent, bronchial sedative, possible anticancer agent; precautions: pregnancy, lactation, children; may cause respiratory depression, cardiovascular depression, low blood pressure, possible respiratory failure, teratogenic; contains cyanide compounds. Also called *black cherry, black choke, choke cherry, rum cherry,* or *Virginia prune.*

wild yam (wīld´ yam´), *n* Latin name: *Dioscorea villosa* L., part used: rhizome; uses: gallbladder conditions, rheumatism, cramps, dysmenorrhea, hormone supplementation, immunoregulator, cognitive functioning; precautions: pregnancy, lactation, children, patients with liver disease, family history of cancer (particularly breast, uterine, prostate or ovarian). Also called *colic root, Mexican wild yam,* or *rheumatism root.*

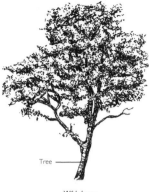

Tree

Wild cherry
Prunus serotina

Wild cherry. (Skidmore-Roth, 2004)

wild-crafted, *n* in herbal medicine, the practice of collecting medicinally beneficial plants directly from their natural habitat as opposed to cultivating them in a greenhouse or on a farm.

willow, *n* Latin name: *Salix* spp., part used: bark; uses: analgesic, antiinflammatory, general health, bursitis, antipyretic, tension headache, osteoarthritis, rheumatoid arthritis, gastrointestinal disorders; precautions: can cause allergic skin reactions, bronchospasm, stomach ulcers, nausea, or diarrhea. Also called *white willow* and *european willow.*

willpower, *n* in Tibetan medicine, a quality that accomplishes one's unfulfilled feats. Awareness, willpower, and compassion play an important role as three significant functions of the mind

W

and the intellectual patterns that correspond with chi, schara, and badahan, respectively. Awareness, willpower, and compassion also play a vital role in the development of spirituality. See awareness, compassion, chi (Tibetan), schara, badahan.

wind, *n* in traditional Chinese medicine, wind is the environmental factor that causes chaos and imbalance and is believed to be the main instigator of disease.

winter cherry, *n* See ashwagandha.

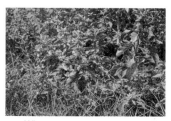

Winter cherry. (Williamson, 2002)

winter nutrition, *n* in Tibetan medicine, the adjustment of an individual's eating habits to cold weather; it is believed that the absorptive and digestive (schara and badahan) functions of the body are in balance and are prepared to meet the increased seasonal demands of supplying energy from the calories within food. It also thought that the excretory functions related to chi are decreased as a measure to further conserve energy. As a rule, individuals are instructed to consume a wide selection of foods more often, although small quantities are encouraged to continually sustain the digestive process and meet the body's nutritional needs. See also chi (Tibetan), schara, and badahan.

wintergreen, *n* Latin name: *Gaultheria procumbens;* parts used: bark, leaves; uses: topical—sore muscles and joints, neuralgia, bladder inflammation, urinary tract conditions,

prostate disease, kidney disease; precautions: pregnancy, lactation, children, patients with GERD; avoid long-term use; those taking anticoagulant medications, salicylate sensitivity; may cause potential salicylate toxicity. Also called *boxberry, Canada tea, checkerberry, deerberry, gaultheria oil, mountain tea, oil of wintergreen, partridgeberry,* or *teaberry.*

wireweed, *n* Latin name: *Polygonum aviculare;* parts used: whole plant, leaves; uses: in Ayurveda, pacifies kapha and vata doshas (bitter, pungent, light), antifibrotic, antimicrobial, antiinflammatory, hepatoprotection, anticoagulant, anodyne, tonic, vermifuge, diuretic, bronchitis, diabetes, dysentery, jaundice, malaria, bleeding disorders; precautions: overdose. Also called *anjawar, knotgrass, machoti, nasomali,* or *prostrate knotweed.*

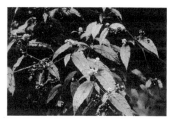

Wireweed. (Williamson, 2002)

witch hazel, *n* Latin name: *Hamamelis virginiana;* parts used: bark, leaves; uses: antioxidant, antiviral, prevention of skin aging, astringent, venous insufficiency, hemmorhoids, antiitch, antiinflammatory, gargle, oral health; precautions: pregnancy, lactation, children; harmful if ingested. Also called *snapping hazel, spotted alder, tobacco wood,* or *winterbloom.*

withania, *n* See ashwagandha.

Withania somnifera, n See ashwagandha.

without prejudice, *n* by invoking this statement, a party is asking for assurances from the other party that the information provided by them will not be used against them to their disadvantage.

Wiwang Wacipi (wē·wäng' wä·chē'·pē), *n* an Indian healing tradition, which translates to "dancing in balance in the circle of life," and includes 4 days of fasting and offering one's blood through piercing as a way of sacrifice. Also called *gazing-at-the-sun dance.*

wo'onsila (wô'·ôn·sē'·lä), *n* Lakota Indian term for compassion—the ability to have pity on another person.

wo'wableza (wô'·wä·ble·zä), *n* Lakota Indian term for understanding between different cultural or ethnic groups.

wolf's foot, *n* Latin name: *Lycopus europaeus;* parts used: flowering herb, leaves; uses: contraction of living tissue, calm nerves, hyperthyroidism, reduction of blood glucose levels, pain, sedative, heart contractions, coughs, bleeding from the lungs, menstrual irregularities, wound healing; precautions: hypothyroidism; may cause an increase in size of thyroid gland, weight loss, nervousness, tachycardia. Also called *common gipsyweed, Egyptian's herb, European bugleweed, farasyon maiy, gipsy-wort, gipsywort, gypsywort, menta de lobo, su ferasyunu, water horehound,* and *wolfspoot.*

Wolff's law, *n.pr* a law according to which biologic systems such as hard and soft tissues become distorted in direct correlation to the amount of stress imposed upon them.

wood, *n* one of the five phases, or elements, in Chinese cosmologic and medical theory, the characteristic manifestations of which include anger, assertiveness, competition, conflict, creativity, frustration, and leadership.

Woodfordia fruticosa, *n* See fireflame bush.

wopila (wô·pē'·lä), *n* Lakota Indian practice of the give-away ceremony, during which wealth was distributed

to ensure that no one person's or one family's wealth dominates others.

World Federation of Acupuncture and Moxibustion Societies, *n.pr* an international organization formed in 1987 that promotes acupuncture. It organizes worldwide symposiums and conferences, facilitates the process to gain legal status for acupuncture throughout the international community, develops educational resources, and publishes academic publications. The World Health Organization (WHO) provides guidance to the group. Also called *WFAS.*

World Federation of Chiropractic, *n.pr* an international society formed in 1988 that represents the interests of chiropractors and chiropractic associations located all over the world. The organization promotes uniformity in standards related to chiropractic research, education, and practice. It provides information related to chiropractic and world health and works to develop an informed public opinion regarding the chiropractic field. It also advocates implementing appropriate legislation for the chiropractic field. Besides its affiliations with several international and national programs, the society is aligned with the World Health Organization (WHO) and is a member of the Council of International Organizations of Medical Sciences (CIOMS). Also called *WFC.*

World Health Organization (WHO), *n* entity under the authority of the United Nations with a mission to promote the best possible health care for all the world's citizens. Sponsors educational programs that inform people about sanitation, safe water, food supply, and nutrition issues. Also actively involved in the ongoing effort to stop the spread of AIDS worldwide. See also AIDS.

worldviews, *n.pl* the implicit, organized belief systems that undergird our understanding of the world. See also sense of coherence.

wormwood, *n* Latin name: *Artemisia absinthum;* parts used: leaves, flowering shoots; uses: anthelmintic, bacteriostatic, antispasmodic, carminative, flow of bile, menstrual irregularities, febrifuge, sedative, stimulation of physiologic processes, general health, joint inflammation, digestion; nutrient absorption, anorexia nervosa, antitumor activity, wound healing, muscle sprain, gall bladder dysfunction, liver dysfunction; precautions: adolescence; may cause mental deterioration; may damage nervous system; and may be toxic in large quantities. Also called *absintalsem, absinth sagewort, absinth wormwood, absinthe, ajenjo, ajenjo oficial, common wormwood, feuilles ameres, niga-yomogi, old woman, oldman, pelin, wormwood,* and *wormwood.*

wound irrigation, *n* the use of water or medicated solution to rinse a wound or the cavity created by a wound to cleanse the region as well as remove excessive discharge and debris.

wound preparation, *n* procedures used to establish aseptic conditions before the closure of a wound. These procedures include providing anesthetic, stopping blood flow, removing hair through trimming (not shaving), irrigating and debriding the wound, and disinfecting the skin.

wound sealing, *v* moving the hands over an injury to facilitate energy gathering and then holding them above the injury for one minute.

wrap, *n* sheets or blankets, wet or dry, used to wrap the body as part of hydrotherapeutic treatment. See also hydrotherapy.

wu style (wo͞o), *n* variation of tai chi, characterized by compact movements and medium pacing.

wu xing (wo͞o zhēng), *n* in traditional Chinese medicine, the fives phases—earth, wood, metal, fire, and water.

wuweizi (wo͞o·wā·dzə), *n* Latin name: *Schisandra chinensis;* part used: fruit; uses: inflammation, liver care, asthma; precautions: none known. Also called *wurenchun.*

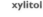

xanthosis (zan·thō′·sis), *n* **1.** a yellowish discoloration typically observed in deteriorating tissues; results from a malignant condition. **2.** an atypical condition distinguished by accumulation of yellowish fatty tissue in the reticuloendothelial system, internal organs, and skin. The condition could be related to paraproteinemia, hyperlipoproteinemia, lipoid storage disorders, or additional atypical conditions associated with adipose tissue. Also called *xanthomatosis.*

xenobiotics, *n.pl* potentially harmful, lipid-soluble chemicals that are foreign to the human body.

xenoestrogens (zē′·nō·es′·trō·gənz), *n.pl* environmental estrogens. See also phytoestrogens.

xenophobia (zē′·nō·fō′·bē·ə), *n* an irrational fear of foreigners or strangers.

xerostomia (ze′·rə·stō′·mē·ə), *n* decreased saliva secretion that causes dry mouth; may result from a disease or a drug reaction. Common side effect after radiation therapy.

xin (tsēn), *n* faithfulness and sincerity, one of five virtues in Chinese medicine, for which yi is responsible. See also yi.

xixin (shē·shēn), *n* Latin name: *Asarum heterotropoides;* part used: whole plant; uses: pain, coughing, sedation, common cold, headache; precautions: unknown.

X-signal system, *n* biologic system, separate from the nervous system; governs the way cells in a body communicate with each other. The *X* comes from the algebraic *X,* thus acknowledging unknown facets of energy flow.

xue (shwā), *n* Chinese term for points in the skin through which wind may flow.

xylitol (zī′·lə·tôl), *n* a slowly-metabolized carbohydrate used as a sugar substitute for the prevention of cavities. Has been used to prevent inflammation of the middle ear. No known precautions.

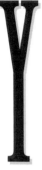

yagya (yä·ˈgyä), *n* ritual in which particular sequences from the Vedic texts are performed by pandits and are believed to remove illness and any obstacles to growth. See also pandit.

yama (yä·ˈmə), *n* personal restraints and social ethics, one of the eight limbs or paths of Patanjali yoga aimed at self-realization and self-knowledge. See also niyama, asana, pranayama, pratyahara, dharana, dhyana, and Samadhi.

yang (yang), *n/adj* the quality present, to a greater or lesser degree, in all phenomena, relating homeodynamically with yin according to the theoretic basis of Chinese medicine. Yang is like the sunny side of a mountain and is characterized as light, bright, warm, high, rising, external, active, moving, and clear. See also China's traditional medicine, pakua, traditional Chinese medicine, and yin.

yang ming (yäng ming), *n* in Chinese medicine, one of the six principal meridians through which the vital force qi flows; further subdivided into yin division (stomach) and yang division (large intestine). The balance of yin and yang components and the proper flow of qi in an individual indicate sound health. See also qi, tai yang, shao yang, tai min, shao yin, and jue yin.

yang style, *n* slowly executed version of tai chi characterized by its large movements.

yarrow (yar·ˈō), *n* Latin name: *Achillea millefolium;* parts used: dried leaves, flowers; uses: genitourinary conditions, respiratory ailments, gastrointestinal complaints, wound healing, skin conditions, eczema; precautions: pregnancy, lactation, children; those taking anticoagulant medications, high blood pressure medications, CNS depressants. Also called *bloodwort, gordaldo, milfoil, nosebleed, old man's pepper, sanguinary, soldier's woundwort, stanchgrass,* or *thousand-leaf.*

yeast infection, *n* fungal infection caused by *Candida albicans;* manifests as a superficial infection located in moist parts of the body. It affects the skin, oral mucous membranes, respiratory tract, and vagina. Rarely leads to endocarditis or a systemic infection. Also called *candidiasis.*

yeberos (ye·be·rōs), *n* folk herbalists in Latin American healing systems.

yellow dock, *n* Latin name: *Rumex crispus;* part used: roots; uses: astringent, laxative, skin irritation, blood cleanser, sore throat, antipyretic; precautions: abortifacient, pregnancy, lactation, children; patients with kidney disease, liver disease, dehydration; may cause severe electrolyte imbalance. Also called *chin ch'iao mai, curled dock, curly dock, garden patience, hualtata, hummaidh, kivircik labada, narrow dock, niu she t'ou, oseille marron, sour dock,* or *surale di bierdji.*

yellow food, *n* a motor stimulant or "pick me-up," yellow foods help to strengthen nerves, aid digestion, and ease constipation. They include bananas, papaya, mangoes, grapefruit, lemons, limes, pineapple, apples, peaches, squash, corn, and butter.

yellow jessamine (ye·ˈlō je·ˈsə·mēn), *n* Latin names: *Gelsemium sempervirens, Gelsemium nitidum;* part used: roots; uses: pain reduction, cramps or spasms, induction of perspiration, febrifuge, induction of sleep, pupil dilation, relaxation, vasodilator, neuralgia, migraine, sciatica, toothache, severe pain, meningitis; precautions: heart disease, hypotension, myasthenia gravis; can cause respiratory depression, giddiness, and double vision. Also called *carolina jasmine, carolina jessamine, evening trumpet-flower, gelsemium,*

Y

yellow jasmine, sariyasemin, wild woodbine, and *false jasmine.*

yellow lady's slipper, *n* Latin names: *Cypripedium pubescens, Cypripedium calceolus;* parts used: rhizome, roots; uses: anxiolytic, insomnia, sedative, seizure disorders, antispasmodic, antidepressant; precautions: pregnancy, lactation, children; patients with psychosis, severe anxiety disorders, severe depression, migraines, cluster headaches. Also called *American valerian, moccasin flower, nerveroot, Noah's ark, whippoorwill's shoe,* or *yellow Indian shoe.*

yerba buena (yer·bə bwā´·nə), *n* traditional name given to mint, savory, or other herbs, depending upon the local variant of Curanderismo being practiced. See also Curanderismo.

yerba maté (yer´·bə mä´·tā), *n* Latin name: *Ilex paraguariensis;* parts used: dried leaves and stems; uses: diuretic, antioxidant, vasodilator, antiobesity agent, stimulant, depression, constipation, arthritis, diabetes, gastrointestinal conditions, urinary tract complaints, kidney stones, bladder stones, cardiac insufficiency; precautions: pregnancy, lactation, children; patients with anxiety conditions, high blood pressure; may cause insomnia, restlessness, nausea, hepatotoxicity, possibly carcinogenic when used for long periods. Also called *armino, Bartholomew's tea, boca juniors, campeche, el agricultor, elacy, flor de lis, gaucho, jaguar, Jesuit's tea, la hoja, la mulata, la tranquera, lonjazo, madrugada, maté, nobleza gaucha, oro verde, Paraguay tea, payadito, rosamonte, safira, union, yi-yi,* or *zerboni.*

yerberos (yār·bā´·rōs), *n* in Curanderismo, the Mexican healing system, herbalists who treat people on the material level.

yew (yōō´), *n* Latin names: *Taxus brevifolia, Taxus baccata;* parts used: bark, branch tips; uses: the derivative taxol is used to treat metastatic cancers (particularly breast and ovarian); yew has traditionally been used for joint complaints, fever; pre-cautions: pregnancy, lactation, children; patients with liver disease, compromised immune systems; those taking antineoplastic medications; may cause low blood pressure, hepatotoxicity, thrombocytopenia, anemia, leukopenia, neutropenia. Toxic, should not be used without supervision. Also called *American yew, California yew, chinwood, globeberry, ground hemlock, Oregon yew,* or *western yew.*

yi (ē), *n* one of the five spirits. Yi is reflection and represents the capacity for verbal expression, applied thinking, and concentration and is stored by the spleen. See also five spirits.

ying level (yēng´ le´·vəl), *n* the functional, inner layer of energy that flows directly beneath the wei level and comprises the organs. It relates to the nutritive qi, which is linked with the blood. See also wei level and qi.

yin-yang (yēn-yäng), *n* governing theory behind traditional Chinese medicine; the idea that life is filled with opposite yet complementary characteristics and qualities on the physical and spiritual levels and on the macro and micro levels. The concept is that each entity can be essentially itself and its opposite; additionally, yang's seed is believed to be contained within yin. A balance of yin and yang is considered essential for good health, whereas a deficiency or imbalance in either factor can manifest as disease.

Yin-yang. (Salvo, 2003)

yoga, *n* a family of mind/body disciplines that share the goals of the integrated body and mind or the union of the self with the divine. Yogic systems are manifold, but all aim at nurturing the body through breath and posture and cultivating the mind through meditation. See also meditation.

yoga nidra (yō′·gə nē′·drə), *n* the progressive relaxation of body and mind through the cycling of awareness through the body and the release of emotional tension. Also called shavasana ("corpse pose"), which refers to the supine posture in which the yoga practitioner cultivates and integrates this relaxation.

yoga sutras, n.pl collection of aphorisms attributed to Patanjali, a second century BCE Hindu sage; systematically outlines the philosophy, practices, benefits, and ultimate goal of the discipline of yoga. Also called *yoga aphorisms of Patanjali* or *yoga sutra*.

yoga therapists (YTs), n.pl people trained in yoga methods; use stretching and breathing for therapeutic purposes. Yoga poses are assigned to patients according to their specific health concerns.

yoga, Anusara (ä·nōō·sä·rə yō·gə), *n.pr* a modern style of hatha yoga, developed by John Friend, in which one aims at controlling the body postures from the "inside out," through relaxing and opening the heart instead of brute force of will. *Anusara* means "following the heart" or "going with the flow" and is rooted in the nondual philosophy of tantra.

yoga, Ashtanga (äsh·täng′·gə yō′·gə), *n* "eight-limbed yoga," a style of hatha yoga derived from Patanjali's yoga sutras and taught by Sri K. Pattabhi Jois. In this style of yoga, breathing is synchronized with the postures, thus increasing the purifying and strengthening qualities of the yoga practice and preparing the ground for inner cultivation.

yoga, Astanga (ä·stäng′·gə yō·gə), *n.pr* See yoga, Ashtanga.

yoga, Bhakti, n a variant of yoga practice that emphasizes selfless love and devotion.

yoga, Bikram (bē′·krəm yō·gə), *n.pr* a modern style of hatha yoga developed by Bikram Choudhury. One practices a specific series of 26 postures in 105° F temperature so that muscles, ligaments, and tendons are stretched and warmed; oxygenated blood is delivered to all organs and tissues; and toxins are flushed out in the sweat.

yoga, classical, n school of yoga developed by sage Patanjali, according to which yoga represents the separation of self from ego as opposed to union with the ultimate reality although both paths lead to self-realization.

yoga, hatha (hä′·thə yō′·gə), *n* a branch of yoga that involves physical postures (asanas) and breathing exercises (pranayama) to transform and transcend the self. See also asanas and pranayama.

yoga, integral (in′·tə·grəl yō′·gə), *n.pr* practice that combines various methods of yoga, such as meditation, asanas, breathing exercises, and relaxation, for physical and spiritual well-being. See also asanas.

yoga, Iyengar (ē·yän′·gär yō′·gə), *n.pr* style of yoga developed by B.K.S. Iyengar; emphasizes the technique (refining adjustments), sequence (sequence of exercises), and timing (duration of exercises) of the asanas and pranayama with the goal of achieving physical, mental, and spiritual well-being. See also asanas and pranayama.

yoga, jñana (gin·nyä′·nə yō′·gə), *n* yoga discipline of philosophic discrimination between the real and illusory, thus leading ultimately to self-realization. See also bhakti yoga, karma yoga, and raja yoga.

yoga, karma (kär′·mə yō′·gə), *n* yoga that emphasizes selfless actions toward attainment of self-realization. See also bhakti yoga, jnana yoga, and raja yoga.

yoga, Kripalu (krē·pä′·lōō yō′·gə), *n.pr* practice of yoga with the intentions of awareness, self-acceptance, and authenticity. Physical postures, breathing techniques, relaxation, and

Y

meditation are used to increase strength, flexibility, and overall well-being.

yoga, Kundalini (kun'·dä·lē'·nē yō'·gə), *n.pr* discipline of yoga that aims at awakening the kundalini (the dormant energy at the base of the spine believed to contain all the power of consciousness) by coordinating posture, breath, chanting, and meditation.

yoga, mantra (män'·trə yō'·gə), *n* regular recitation of one or more mantras ("mind protectors," potent sounds), thus leading to self-awakening and self-transcendence. See also mantra, bhakti yoga, jnana yoga, and karma yoga.

yoga, polarity (pō·lar'·i·tē yō'·gə), *n* system of stretches combined with sound and movement used in conjunction with other treatments as part of polarity therapy. See also therapy, polarity.

yoga, raja (rä'·jə yō'·gə), *n* a classical form of yoga practiced to attain liberation.

yoga, Sivananda (sē'·vä·nän'·də yō'·gə), *n.pr* style of yoga founded by Swami Sivananda, based on the five principles of proper exercise (asanas), proper breathing (pranayama), proper relaxation (savasana), proper diet (vegetarian), and proper meditation (dhyana) toward achieving physical, mental, and spiritual well-being. See also asanas, pranayama, savasana, and dhyana.

yogic flying (yō'·gik flī'·ing), *n* a meditation practice in which the practitioner's body lifts off the ground and hops forward and the practitioner experiences exhilaration and bliss. This technique increases coherent brain function and is an aspect of the TM—Sidhi program. See also TM—Sidhi program.

yohimbe (yō·him'·bē), *n* Latin name: *Pausinystalia yohimbe;* part used: bark; uses: aphrodisiac, hallucinogen, male erectile complaints, diabetes, orthostatic hypotension; precautions: pregnancy, lactation, children; patients with kidney disease,

liver disease, high blood pressure, angina, ulcers (gastric or duodenal), bipolar depression, anxiety, schizophrenia, prostatitis; patient taking alpha-adrenergic–blocker medications, CNS stimulants, MAOIs, phenothiazines, SSRIs, tricylic antidepressants, sympathomimetic medications, tyramine, caffeine; may cause tachycardia, high blood pressure, anxiety, tremors, dysuria, nephrotoxicity. Also called *aphrodien, corynine, johimbe, quebrachine, yohimbehe, yohimbene, yohimbime,* or *yohimbine.*

yucca (yə'·kə), *n* Latin name: *Yucca schidigera;* parts used: roots, stalk; uses: antiinflammatory, arthritis, sprains, sores, dandruff shampoo, hair loss; cautions: none known.

Yucca schidigera, *n* See yucca.

yuxingcao (yōō·zhēng·tsōw), *n* Latin name: *Houttuynia cordata;* parts used: above-ground portions of plant; uses: antiinflammatory, diuretic, dysentery, infections of the urinary tract, respiratory tract swelling; precautions: none known. Also called *Houttuynia.*

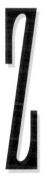

zang (tzäng), *n* Chinese term for one of two groups into which organs are classified. The liver, heart, spleen, lungs, and kidneys belong to the zang group. See also fu.

zang fu organs (zäng fōō), *n.pl* in Chinese traditional medicine, a description of the internal organ that links each to the five elements. Zang organs—including the lungs, liver, kidneys, and heart are predominantly yin and act as storage for important substances. Fu organs—including the stomach, intestines, bladder, gall bladder, and triple heater—are predominantly yang and are areas where vital fluids are in constant flux.

Zanthoxylum americanum, *n* See prickly ash.

Zanthoxylum clava-herculis, *n* See prickly ash.

ze lan (zə lən), *n* Latin name: *Lycopus lucidus;* part used: leaves; uses: traditional Chinese medicine, used to improve blood circulation, diuretic, menstrual complications, postpartum pain; precautions: none known. Also called *rough bugleweed* and *water horehound.*

zedoary (zed' ·ō·er'·ē), *n,* Latin name: *Curcuma zedoaria;* part used: rhizome; uses: condiment, digestion; relieves colic and flatulence; precautions: none known. Also called *wild turmeric, amb halad,* and *gandhmul.*

zero balancing, *n* a gentle style of massage based on the belief that there is an energetic body as well as a physical body and that injuries can affect both. Gentle pressure is used at specific points along the skeleton and musculature to return the energetic body to a state of balance within the physical body.

zhen jui (dzən djyō), *n* in Chinese meridian therapy, needle moxibustion, or acumoxa therapy.

zheng (zhēng), *n* a Chinese term for an acupuncture diagnosis achieved by thoroughly examining and interviewing a patient.

zhi (dzē), *n* 1. one of the five spirits, zhi is housed by the kidney and corresponds to will, determination, and drive; long-term memory, and information storage. 2. wisdom and trust, one of the five virtues in China; each is the virtue for which zhi is responsible. See also five spirits and five virtues.

zhi gan cao (dzē gän tsōw), *n* Latin name: *Radix glycyrrhizae uralensis;* part used: root; uses: regulation of blood glucose levels, digestive functions, metabolic functions, build strong tissue, antiinflammatory, induction of cough, sore throat, pharyngolaryngitis, secretion of throat mucosa, removal of bodily toxins, antispasmodic, duodenal and gastric ulcers; precautions: hypertension, edema. Also called *licorice root.*

zhong yao (dzəng yōw), *n* Chinese herbal medicine.

zhong yi (dzōōng yē), *n* See medicine, traditional Chinese.

zidovudine (zī·dō' ·vyōō·dēn'), *n* an antiviral drug used to treat HIV-infected patients.

zigzag approach, *n* 1. a diet in which muscle weight is gained through varying caloric intake, such as eating a reduced-calorie diet during the week and a higher-calorie diet on the weekend. The additional calories are usually consumed in the form of complex carbohydrates. 2. an approach in homeopathy in which a partial remedy is followed by another partial remedy, thus moving the patient in an irregular path to cure.

zinc, *n* an element/mineral found in meat, nuts, seeds, eggs, whole grains, and brewer's yeast. Has been used to remedy deficiencies (relatively common) and to prevent infections and to treat upper respiratory conditions, oral herpes (topical), acne, anorexia nervosa, macular degeneration, male infertility, and sickle cell anemia. Zinc is toxic when taken long-term in high doses. Caution is advised for patients taking diuretic medications, fluoroquinolones, penicillamine, and tetracyclines. Caution is advised for children and pregnant or lactating women, for whom the maximum daily intake is 40 mg. Also called *zinc sulfate, zinc gluconate, zinc citrate, zinc picolinate,* or *chelated zinc.*

zinc deficiency (zink' də·fi' ·shən·sē), *n* insufficient levels of zinc in the body to support optimal functioning. Leads to weight loss, hypogonadism in males, short stature, delayed wound healing, growth retardation, and other effects.

Z

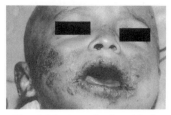

Zinc deficiency causing hemorrhagic dermatitis. (Kumar, Cotran, and Robbins, 1997)

zincum metallicum (zin′ ·kəm mə· tal′ ·li·kum), *n* a homeopathic preparation of zinc, used to treat formication, lethargy, melancholia, muscle spasms, nervous exhaustion, trembling, varicosities, weakness, and general weariness.

Zingiber officinale, *n* See ginger.

***Ziziphus jujube* (zi′ ·zə·fəs jōō′ ·jōō· bē),** *n* parts used: fruit, leaves, seed, root, plant; uses: pain, poisoning, anticancer, diuretic, irritated tissue, expectorant, sedative, respiratory disease, burns, cooling of the body, relaxant, skin conditions, facilitation of stomach action, general health, weight gain, muscular strength, stamina, liver function, immune system function, antipyretic, hair growth, strangury, vasoconstriction, blood purification, chronic fatigue, treat appetite loss, antidiarrheal, anemia, irritability, hysteria, palpitations, insomnia, night sweats, dyspepsia, wound healing, ulcers, hypertonia, nephritis; precautions: may cause angioneurotic edema. Also called *jujube, azufaifo, bedara china, Chinese date, Chinese jujube, common jujube, dara, hong zao, Indian jujube, jujube, jujubier, kan tsao, kola, liane crocs chien, liang tsao, mei tsao, nabug, nan tsao, pei tsao, perita haitiana, petite pomme, pomme malcadi, ponsere, suan tsao, ta tsao, tsao, unnab, unnap agaci, widara,* and *dazao.*

zones, *n.pl* in reflexology, areas of the body through which innate energy flows before ending in the hands or feet.

zones of irritation (ZI), *n.pl* in soft-tissue manipulation, localized areas of sensitivity in the spine, which correspond to the paraspinal acupuncture points; used to determine the manipulative direction for adjustment.

zonesthesia (zon′·es·thē′ ·zhē·ə), *n* a painful sensation of tightening or constriction, such as that felt as if a bandage is too tight, especially around the abdomen or waist. Also called *girdle sensation.*

zoonosis (zōō·ôn′ ·ə·sis), *n* a disease that originates in an animal species and is transmitted to a human host. Examples are yellow fever, rabies, equine encephalitis, leptospirosis, and possibly SARS.

zygomata (zī·gō·mä′ ·tə), *n pl* the bones of the cheek just below the eye.

zygomaticomaxillary (zī′·gō·ma′· ti·kō·mak′ ·si·le·rē), *adj* pertaining to the zygomatic bone and the maxilla.

Z

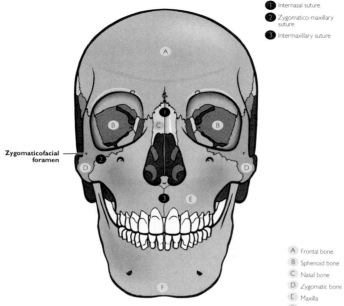

Zygomaticomaxillary. (Chaitow, 1999)

1 Internasal suture
2 Zygomatico-maxillary suture
3 Intermaxillary suture

Zygomaticofacial foramen

A Frontal bone
B Sphenoid bone
C Nasal bone
D Zygomatic bone
E Maxilla
F Mandible

Z

APPENDIX A

Acupuncture

Acupuncture originated over 4000 years ago in China. Its first definitive treatises, which included the *Huang Di Nei Jing (Yellow Emperor's Inner Classic),* were written in the second century BCE. The theory and practice of acupuncture evolved during the Chinese dynasties. From China it spread into areas under Chinese control and influence, such as Japan and Korea. Traveling European explorers and merchants eventually came into contact with acupuncture and carried it back to Europe.

In the first half of the nineteenth century, many European and American physicians experimented with acupuncture, but it did not gain wide acceptance in European medicine (outside of France) until the 1950s. In the United States, acupuncture spread from Chinatowns across the country into the mainstream of American medicine, especially after *New York Times* journalist James Reston described his experiences with postsurgical acupuncture anesthesia in China. In 1994 the FDA stopped regarding acupuncture needles as experimental devices, and in November 1997, the National Institutes of Health officially recognized the therapeutic efficacy of acupuncture for certain conditions.

Acupuncture's method of action depends on whom you ask. Traditional acupuncture visualizes the body as being covered in a lattice of about 70 *meridians,* or conduits, which transmit *qi* (pronounced "chi"), or vital energy. These meridians are dotted with over 1500 potential needling sites, or *acupoints.* Pain and disease arise when these channels are blocked and the qi stagnates; acupuncture functions by opening the meridian, thus allowing the qi to resume its normal course. To increase qi stimulation, needling is often accompanied by manual manipulation of the needles and/or *moxibustion,* the burning of moxa (powdered mugwort leaves) on or near an acupoint. This approach to acupuncture predominates among classical practitioners

The other dominant view is that of medical acupuncture (sometimes called *neuroanatomic acupuncture*), which situates traditional acupuncture practices within a theoretical biomedical and neuromuscular framework. In this view the efficacy of acupuncture is attributed primarily to its role in stimulating components of the circulatory, electromagnetic bioinformational, lymphatic, muscular, and nervous systems and in production of endogenous pain relievers.

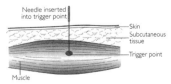

Muscle with trigger point—insertion of needle. (Campbell, 2002)

469

Variations of these two philosophical frameworks include five-element acupuncture, auriculotherapy, Korean hand acupuncture, Vietnamese acupuncture, Japanese acupuncture, French energetics acupuncture, and electroacupunture. Acupuncture treatments have also been expanded to include technological innovations such as electrical, ultrasound, and laser-stimulation of acupoints.

As of 2000, 36 states and the District of Columbia required licensure for acupuncture practice by nonphysicians. Certification from the NCCAOM (National Certification Commission for Acupuncture and Oriental Medicine) is accepted by a majority of those states. More than 50 schools in the U.S. provide certifiable training in acupuncture, and many also offer accredited master's degree programs in acupuncture. For physician practitioners, several states require registration, certification, and/or proof of formal training (typically at least 200 hours). The American Academy of Medicine Acupuncture (AAMA) offers this training and certification, as does Medical Acupuncture for Physicians, a program through the Office of Continuing Medicine Education at UCLA's School of Medicine; several other universities also offer courses.

Aromatherapy

Essential oils derived from plants have served as therapeutic agents for at least 6000 years. There is evidence of their use on every continent except Antarctica. Modern medicinal use of essential oils started in France in the years before World War II. Jean Valnet (a doctor), Maurice Gattefosse (a chemist), and Marguerite Maury (a surgical assistant) used essential oils such as thymol as antiseptics and to promote healing.

Because the olfactory center of the brain is integrated with both the memory and emotional centers, the effects of scent on emotional and physical health are evident. Essential oils can also have therapeutic benefit when they are absorbed into the bloodstream through the skin, as in massage. Different essential oils have distinct effects on the mind and body, and the effects of essential oils also differ widely in different species within a given plant genus.

Use of aromatherapy is usually categorized in one of four ways: in *esthetic aromatherapy,* oils are used because their fragrance is pleasant; *holistic aromatherapy* generally alleviates stress and augments relaxation techniques; *environmental fragrancing* is often used in commercial settings to alter or enhance moods; and *clinical aromatherapy* targets specific clinical therapeutic results. The means of delivering aromatherapy also vary; oils can be dispensed through a vaporizer or burner and inhaled, emulsified and added to a bath, used in compresses, or combined with oils to complement massage.

As of 2000, neither a national certification program nor an examination program in aromatherapy existed. No requirements for certification or accreditation existed. Although professional aromatherapy organizations (the National Association of Holistic Aromatherapy is the largest) exist, no national governing body oversees them.

Source used: CCRCAAM.

Ayurveda

Ayurveda, the traditional healthcare system of India, is translated as "science or knowledge of life" and is thought to have originated as long as 5000 years ago. Three classic texts that have informed all subsequent writing, research, and practice describe the basic theories and principles of Ayurveda: *Caraka Samhita* (1500 BCE), *Ashtang Hrdyam* (CE 500), and *Sushrut Samhita* (CE 300–400).

Ayurvedic philosophy begins with the notions that illness arises naturally from disharmony between a person and the environment, that disease really begins when one's true nature as spirit is forgotten, and that symptoms are for the body's communication of this disharmony. Ayurvedic physicians view human beings, diseases, and remedies individually as a unique mixture of qualities of nature (such as light, heavy, cold, hot, stable, mobile, sharp, dull, moist, dry, subtle, gross, dense, flowing, soft, hard, smooth, rough, and cloudy or clear). Additionally, each person comprises a combination of three *doshas* (vata, pitta, and kapha), five elements (ether—space, air—motion, fire—heat, water—flow, earth—solidity), seven *dhatus* or tissues, and many *strotas* or channels.

After assessing a patient and the presentation of an illness, an Ayurvedic physician prescribes a six- to twelve-month program that may include *five sense therapies* (special diet, color or sound therapy, aromatherapy, and massage), *pancha karma* (the five actions) for detoxification and rejuvenation, and yoga *asanas* and meditation to calm the mind.

Training programs in Ayurveda are offered in several states, but complete clinical training that includes an internship is offered only at the California College of Ayurveda in Grass Valley, California. None of the 50 states provides licensing at this time for Ayurvedic physicians; many associations, however, are forming to remedy this situation. In India and in several Asian countries, dozens of Ayurveda colleges offer training five to six years beyond high school.

Sources used: CCRCAAM, ECAAM.

Biofeedback

Although low-technology self-regulatory techniques have existed for millennia, as evinced in the meditative and yogic disciplines of India and China, modern *biofeedback* and *biofeedback therapy* are relatively new disciplines. In the 1960s, several scientists independently developed instruments capable of monitoring subtle physiological changes and feeding this information back to the subject. With the refinements of these inventions, the new science of biofeedback was born. The term *biofeedback* was first used at a 1969 conference organized by EEG innovator Barbara Brown. At that same conference the Biofeedback Research Society was formed. In 1976 this organization became the Biofeedback Society of America, and in 1988 the name was changed once more—this time to the Association for Applied Psychophysiology and Biofeedback (AAPB). Today biofeedback is used therapeutically by a variety of practitioners, and it also serves as an adjunct to many disciplines.

Biofeedback therapy uses technologies to amplify and feed back an individual's typically unconscious physiologic processes, such as heart rate or blood pressure, so that the individual may recognize these processes and develop intuitive, voluntary control over them. In many cases the nature of this control remains poorly understood, and most participants in biofeedback research and therapy describe it as more like an intuitive skill than an act of conscious volition. In short, biofeedback is seen as a useful mind-body tool in which physiologic responses to stressors are brought into the subject's conscious awareness so that they may be moderated, reduced, or transformed, thus restoring the body's healing homeostasis. Although not essential to biofeedback, patients often learn relaxation exercises and breathing techniques to facilitate biofeedback treatment.

Many professionals—including dentists, hypnotherapists, marriage counselors, primary care physicians, psychotherapists, stress management counselors, and substance abuse counselors—use biofeedback therapy as an adjunct treatment. It has been used to treat conditions such as epilepsy, pain, headaches, high blood pressure, incontinence, attention deficit disorder, and neuromuscular dysfunctions. Biofeedback therapy is also valued for its role in encouraging self-confidence, enhancing quality of life, and cultivating inner resources and skills (e.g., pain management or stress management).

As of 2000, no licensing requirements were established for biofeedback, but a practitioner should be licensed to practice in his or her healthcare profession (if applicable) and should be certified in clinical biofeedback. The Biofeedback Certification Institute of America (BCIA) grants four-year certifications to those applicants with bachelor's degrees in approved fields and who have formally trained for a minimum of 200 hours in biofeedback therapy. Applicants must have passed written and practical examinations. Legal recognition of biofeedback varies from state to state; each state has its own biofeedback society under the national aegis of the AAPB.

Sources: CCRCAAM, 32-40; ECAM, 410-425.

Bodywork

In the last 100 years, many new bodywork modalities have appeared in the United States. Some developed out of dance and movement therapies; others are second-generation, created by students of early-century teachers; and a number are the work of intuitive self-healers. The better-known approaches include the Alexander Technique, Aston-Patterning, Bowen Technique, craniosacral therapy, the Feldenkrais Method, Hellerwork Structural Integration, Bonnie Prudden Myotherapy, Rolfing Structural Integration, Rosen Method, and the Trager Approach.

Although emphases vary from one therapy to the next, all bodywork modalities share some general philosophies. The habits of the mind and patterns of emotional expression and thought play a very large role in physical health. Physical habits—ingrained over time through characteristic posture, responses to trauma, or repetitive work and exercise movements—can also greatly

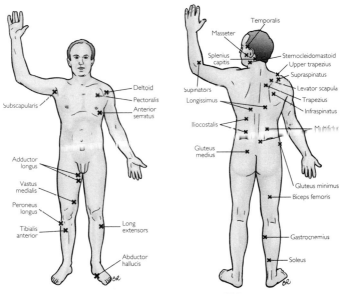

Common trigger points. (Fritz, 2004)

influence physiologic and mental function. Bodywork massage techniques, mobilizations, and exercises are designed to repattern dysfunctional habits, support self-healing mechanisms, increase awareness, and integrate all the parts of the self.

Problems treated successfully by these therapies include repetitive strain injuries, symptoms of developmental disabilities, respiratory conditions, pain, and stress-related disorders. Additionally, clients report improved coordination, posture, stamina, energy, flexibility, and ease of movement.

Training ranges from seminars covering several weekends to programs providing up to 3000 clinical hours of experience and is offered by institutes and certified teachers throughout the country. Some training is only available to licensed healthcare providers for use as an adjunct therapy. Certification is available to most practitioners—but not necessarily in every part of the country.

APPENDIX F

Chiropractic

Chiropractic therapy began in 1895 when Daniel David Palmer began to develop his techniques of spinal adjustment. Chiropractors' clinical rationale and lexicon evolved separately from that of allopathic medicine, and the differences between the two practices were emphasized.

The principles of *vitalism* that emerged in the late nineteenth century influenced many early writings on chiropractic therapy. Shunning surgery and medications, chiropractors use hands-on methods to realign the skeletal structure, thereby catalyzing the innate recuperative powers of the body, improving function, and reducing painful symptoms.

Chiropractors treat patients with skeletomuscular dysfunctions and complaints of head, neck, or back pain with the application of *adjustments* to lesions of the spine called *subluxations*. "The subluxation in its simplest form is a local, uncontrolled mechanic response to spine environment loads that manifest clinically as a set of symptoms" (CCRCAAM, 311). The adjustments are made with directed, controlled force on the affected area(s) to improve physiologic function. Chiropractors emphasize early intervention, and the desired results depend upon the condition of the soft tissue that has been stressed. Currently, successful collaborative efforts in treating musculoskeletal dysfunction have been made; more clinical research into the efficacy of chiropractic techniques is underway.

Numerous CCE-accredited (Council on Chiropractic Education) and CCE-monitored chiropractic colleges train students who have at least sixty semester hours (including sciences) upon entering the program. Every state has a state licensing board for chiropractors. These use either state or NDCE-administered (National Board of Chiropractic Examiners) examination(s). Additionally, chiropractors may be credentialed by HMOs, PPOs, or IPAs.

Source: CCRCAAM.

Energy Medicine

The term *energy medicine* refers to a large number of contemporary therapies with roots in ancient Asian, European, and Native American traditions. Energy medicine involves moving energy or spirit to effect healing. Modern modalities include light therapy, magnetic therapy, qi gong, reiki, therapeutic touch (TT), color therapy, quartz crystal therapy, pulsing electromagnetic fields (PEMFs), and millimeter wave therapy. Diagnostic tools such as electrocardiograms, magnetocardiograms, electroencephalograms, and magnetoencephalograms are examples of energy used in conventional medicine.

The many modalities of energy healing share some basic concepts. Practitioners assert—and studies affirm—that energy fields exist "within and around the human body, and these fields are vitally important to the health of the organism" (*Energy Medicine in Therapeutic and Human Performance,* 1) and, further, that humans can sense and modify the flow of energy to increase their own health and vitality. Mechanisms are currently unknown but may involve alteration of cellular calcium flux and cell function.

Energy practitioners use their hands and hearts to facilitate health and well-being. A growing body of evidence suggests that some energy healers' hands can project pulsing electromagnetic fields that correspond in frequency and strength to those of clinical devices currently being developed to catalyze tissue repair. Because emotions such as love, anger, and grief affect the electromagnetic frequencies produced by the heart and conducted throughout and around the body, many schools and teachers emphasize the importance of cultivating a relaxed, caring attitude.

Specific illnesses treated with reported success include allergies, arthritis, hypertension, injuries (resulting in injury repair), pain, chronic fatigue syndrome, gastrointestinal complaints, female health concerns, and stress. Research on energy medicine is, however, in its infancy.

The many modalities of energy medicine constitute adjunctive training for licensed health care practitioners, martial artists, and others. No credentialing or licensing is available, and no national standards exist, although individual organizations do provide promotion and education services.

Source: *Healing, Intention, and Energy Medicine,* ed. Wayne B. Jonas & Cindy C. Crawford (2003).

Environmental Medicine

Environmental medicine is an approach to health care that developed in the 1960s in response to increased complex, chronic health concerns. In the environmental medical model, organisms are understood as constantly adjusting to their changing surroundings; this active interplay between the organism and its environment is considered *homeodynamic* (in contrast to homeostatic) *functioning*. Because an organism's surroundings may destabilize its healthy homeodynamic function, the environment is not viewed as essentially benign but is instead recognized as a source of various stressors, including chemicals, radiation, electromagnetic fields, dietary substances, noise, and pathogens, among others.

Environmentally triggered illnesses (ETI) are defined as those conditions resulting from compromised homeodynamic functioning; environmental medicine seeks to recognize, manage, and prevent these illnesses. These three goals are reached by a variety of means, such as patient education, specific therapeutic diets and detoxification regimes, nutritional supplementation, immunotherapies, environmental changes, and allopathic medicines.

Most practitioners of environmental medicine are medical doctors or doctors of osteopathy licensed to perform all aspects of a comprehensive treatment plan. The American and International Boards of Environmental Medicine (ABEM/IBEM) have developed a Core Curriculum of Environmental Medicine upon which is based the continuing medical education program in environmental medicine currently provided by the American Academy of Environmental Medicine (AAEM). The ABEM and IBEM provide board certification to physicians trained in the core curriculum.

Source: CCRCAAM.

The Health Insurance Portability and Accountability Act (HIPAA) of 1996

The Health Insurance Portability and Accountability Act (HIPAA) of 1996 was signed into law by President Bill Clinton on August 21, 1996. Conclusive regulations were issued on August 17, 2000, to be instated by October 16, 2002. HIPAA requires that the transactions of all patient healthcare information be formatted in a standardized electronic style. In addition to protecting the privacy and security of patient information, HIPAA includes legislation on the formation of medical savings accounts, the authorization of a fraud and abuse control program, the easy transport of health insurance coverage, and the simplification of administrative terms and conditions.

HIPAA comprises three primary areas, and its privacy requirements break down into three types: privacy standards, patients' rights, and administrative requirements.

1. Privacy Standards. A central concern of HIPAA is the careful use and disclosure of protected health information (PHI), which generally is electronically controlled health information that can be distinguished individually. PHI also refers to verbal communication, but the HIPAA Privacy Rule is not intended to hinder necessary verbal communication. The United States Department of Health and Human Services (USDHHS) does not require restructuring, such as soundproofing, architectural changes, and so forth, but some caution is necessary when exchanging health information by conversation.

An Acknowledgment of Receipt Notice of Privacy Practices, which allows patient information to be used or divulged for treatment, payment, or healthcare operations (TPO), should be procured from each patient. A detailed and time-sensitive authorization can also allow the healthcare professional to release information in special circumstances other than TPOs. A *written consent* is also an option. Healthcare professionals can disclose PHI *without* acknowledgement, consent, or authorization in very special situations, for example, perceived child abuse, public health supervision, fraud investigation, or law enforcement with valid permission (i.e., a warrant). When divulging PHI, a healthcare professional must try to disclose only the *minimum necessary* information to safeguard the patient's information as much as possible.

It is important that healthcare professionals adhere to HIPAA standards because healthcare providers (as well as healthcare clearinghouses and healthcare plans) who convey *electronically* formatted health information via an outside billing service or merchant are considered *covered entities.* Covered entities may be dealt serious civil and criminal penalties for violation of HIPAA legislation. Failure to comply with HIPAA privacy requirements may result in civil penalties of up to $100 per offense with an annual maximum of $25,000 for repeated failure to comply with the same requirement. Criminal penalties resulting from the illegal mishandling of private health information can range from $50,000 and/or one year in prison to $250,000 and/or 10 years in prison.

2. Patients' Rights. HIPAA allows patients, authorized representatives, and parents of minors, as well as minors, to become more aware of the health information privacy to which they are entitled. These rights include but are not limited to the right to view and copy their health information, the right to dispute alleged breaches of policies and regulations, and the right to request alternative forms of communicating with their healthcare professional. If any health information is released for any reason other than TPO, the patient is entitled to an account of the transaction. Therefore healthcare professionals must keep accurate records of such information and provide them when necessary.

The HIPAA Privacy Rule determines that the parents of a minor have access to their child's health information. This privilege may be overruled—for example, in cases of suspected child abuse or parental consent to a term of confidentiality between the healthcare professional and the minor. The parent's rights to access his or her child's PHI also may be restricted in situations when a legal entity, such as a court, intervenes and when a law does not require a parent's consent. For a full list of patient rights provided by HIPAA, be sure to acquire a copy of the law and to understand it well.

3. Administrative Requirements. Complying with HIPAA legislation may seem like a chore, but it does not need to be so. One should become appropriately familiar with the law, organize the requirements into simpler tasks, begin compliance early, and document progress in compliance. An important first step is evaluating the current information and practices of your office.

Healthcare professionals will need to write a *privacy policy* for their office, a document that details for their patients the office's practices concerning PHI. Understanding the role of healthcare information for your patients and the ways in which they handle the information while they are visiting the office are useful. Train your staff; ensure that they are familiar with the terms of HIPAA and your office's privacy policy and related forms. HIPAA requires that designation of a *privacy officer*, a person in the office who will be responsible for applying the new policies in your office, fielding complaints, and making choices involving the minimum necessary requirements. Another person with the role of *contact person* will process complaints.

A *Notice of Privacy Practices*—a document detailing the patient's rights and the healthcare office's obligations concerning PHI—also must be drafted. Further, any role of a third party with access to PHI must be clearly documented. This third party is known as a *business associate* (BA) and is defined as any entity that, on behalf of the healthcare professional, takes part in any activity that involves exposure of PHI.

The main HIPAA privacy compliance date, including all staff training, was April 14, 2003, although many covered entities that submitted a request and a compliance plan by October 15, 2002, were granted one-year extensions. Contact the local branch of your healthcare professional association for details.

Healthcare professionals should prepare their offices ahead of time for all deadlines, which include preparing privacy polices and forms, business associate contracts, and employee training sessions.

Web sites that may contain useful information about HIPAA include the following:

- USDHHS Office of Civil Rights
  www.hhs.gov/ocr/hipaa
- Work Group on Electronic Data Interchange
  www.wedi.org/SNIP
- Phoenix Health
  www.hipaadvisory.com
- USDHHS Office of the Assistant Secretary for Planning and Evaluation
  http://aspe.os.dhhs.gov/admnsimp/

Sources: *HIPAA Privacy Kit;* http://www.azhha.org.

Homeopathy

Homeopathy began in Germany when the physician Samuel Hahnemann published his discussions and observations of a healing system he called the law of similars in *Organon of the Medical Art* (1810). Hans Graham, a homeopathic physician, arrived in the United States in 1825; Constance Hering followed in 1844. Together they founded the American Institute of Homeopathy (AIH), the oldest nationwide medical organization still active in the United States. The American homeopathy movement thrived; a number of classic texts were written and greatly influenced homeopathic practice. Among them are *Kent's General Repertory* (James Tyler Kent), *Encyclopedia of Pure Materia Medica* (Timothy F. Allen, MD), and *Guiding Symptoms* (Constance Hering). The practice of homeopathy declined in the early twentieth century as a result of changes in allopathic medicine, including the discovery of antimicrobials and suppression of homeopathic practice, only to enjoy resurgence of popularity beginning in the 1970s. The use of computerized repertory programs, the over-the-counter availability of most remedies and the perceived efficacy of homeopathic medicine have made it the second most popular healthcare system worldwide.

Several concepts underlie homeopathic research and practice. One is Hahnemann's law of similars, which states that any substance that causes certain symptoms will cure those same symptoms. The substances are tested by *provings*—that is, they are administered in microdoses to healthy volunteers who are evaluated over time for any subjective or objective changes or symptoms. The substances used and symptoms discovered are written in repertories that can be accessed by homeopathic physicians researching the best remedy for a patient. Homeopathic physicians are interested in comprehending and treating the totality of symptoms—that is, their physical, mental, emotional, lifestyle, and inherited attributes. Homeopaths view them as the body's attempt to heal itself and as windows into the nature of the illness. Homeopathic doctors prescribe the lowest possible dose to effect stimulation of innate healing capacities. Finally, Hering's law states that symptoms move in the reverse order of their initial appearance and that disease moves from more to less vital organs during the curative process—from the center to the surface, for instance.

Microdose remedies are prepared with a technique called potentization, involving *serially agitated dilution* steps to create dilutions so minute that sometimes none of the molecules from the original substance can be measured. Plant, animal, mineral, or disease substances are diluted in distilled water, pharmaceutical alcohol, or lactose and are used directly, pressed into tablets, or sprayed onto sugar pills. Clinical evidence for the efficacy of microdoses is accumulating; however, the mechanism of action remains speculative. Homeopathic philosophy holds that "disease exists on a dynamic or energetic level before the appearance of measurable and observable changes" (*Essentials of*

Complementary and Alternative Medicine, 475); thus the effectiveness of microdoses may be on an energetic level.

Two primary styles of homeopathy, classical and clinical, are practiced widely. Classical homeopaths prescribe a single remedy for all the symptoms while clinical homeopaths use a remedy mixture or series to address a specific condition. These combination medicines account for 85% of all over-the-counter remedies. There are five major components of classical patient evaluation: initial interview, physical examination and diagnostics, data analysis, prescription, and regular follow-ups.

Homeopathic remedies have been used to treat infections, injuries, neuromuscular conditions, allergies, psychologic disturbances, gastrointestinal disorders, and many other illnesses.

Many schools train students in homeopathy, and the CHC (Council on Homeopathic Certification) leads a certification movement. Only three states—Nevada, Arizona, and Connecticut—license homeopathic doctors, although physicians can hold licenses in other states. Worldwide, homeopathy is taught in medical schools and is recognized by governments in Europe, India, and South America.

Sources: ECAAM, CCRCAAM.

Hypnotherapy

Cross-cultural and cross-temporal examples of hypnosis abound, (e.g., the Oracle at Delphi, *I-Ching,* and hypnosis by shamans). The secular nature and approach to modern hypnosis was developed initially by Anton Mesmer. Mesmer called his discovery *animal magnetism,* and his name lives on in the terms *mesmerism* and *mesmerize.* Other people associated with the development of hypnosis are Esdaile (hypnotic surgical anesthesia), Braid (facilitating acceptance of hypnosis by the medical community), Charcot (healing hysteria), Hull (defining hypnosis as a psychologic study), and Erickson (incorporation into everyday psychologic practice). Hypnotherapists can generally be categorized as either *authoritarian* (or paternal), or *Ericksonian* (or maternal), based on their conceptions of the roles of therapist and patient.

The use of hypnosis as an adjunct to various psychologic and emotional therapies (such as cognitive behavior therapy) is believed to improve their efficacy. Hypnosis can also aid in the treatment of a wide range of physical conditions; examples include habit alteration, chronic pain, AIDS, warts, and possibly obesity and diabetes mellitus.

No generally accepted standards for hypnotherapy licensing and practice exist. Although the federal government does not regulate hypnotherapy, some states do require official or academic credentials. Moreover, board certifications are available through the American Boards of Dental, Medical, or Psychological Hypnosis (ABDH, ABMH, or ABPH). These three boards provide certifications for licensed practitioners in their respective disciplines. The American Society of Clinical Hypnosis, located in Des Plaines, Illinois, provides information about certified practitioners.

Latin American Medicine

No standardized healing systems like those in India or in China exist in Latin America. Instead healing practices vary depending upon the cultures, peoples, geographic location, and local history in which they are embedded. Generally speaking, however, the current traditional medical systems of Latin America originate with the contact between the indigenous Aztec and Mayan peoples and their respective European conquerors; these systems tend to share such sources as Spanish Catholicism, humoral medicine, early European ideas about witchcraft, indigenous spiritual beliefs, and herbalism.

In Mexico (and areas with significant populations of Mexican immigrants) the system of traditional ethnomedicine is known as *curanderismo,* and its practitioners, typically women, are known as *curanderas.*

Within these myriad systems, illness is understood as resulting from—variously—imbalances in the heat and cold of the bodily humors, discordant social or spiritual relationships, displacement of parts of the physical or spiritual body, offended spiritual entities, and past sins. Such etiologies may overlap so that a condition may be diagnosed as having multiple causes, only some of which are recognizable as such within the biomedical model of disease and health care. Little distinction is made between physical, emotional, mental, or spiritual problems, and many of the conditions treated in Latin American medicine, such as *susto, empacho,* and *mal de ojo,* have no counterpart in biomedicine; they are referred to as *culture-bound syndromes.* These conditions are treated with herbs, hot/cold modifications to diet and behavior, spiritual interventions, rituals, and manipulative techniques.

Curanderas and their male counterparts, *curanderos,* find themselves called to the vocation, often after overcoming their own difficult illnesses. Visits to healers are very informal, often occurring on a first-come, first-served basis in the healer's home. Because of the folk nature of these ethnomedical systems, no licensing requirements or official certifications exist.

Source: CCRCAAM.

APPENDIX M

Magnetic Field Therapy

Magnets have been used throughout history, possibly as long ago as 200 BCE. in China, when a branch of acupuncture used magnetic fields. D'Arsonval used a strong electromagnetic field in a wired electric cage around a subject's head in 1896. In 1965, Barker used electromagnetic stimulation across a person's brain. Magnetic field therapy has enjoyed a range of uses since the 1970s in Russia, Eastern Europe, and Japan and since 1996 in North America and Western Europe as well.

Magnetic fields, when applied, influence a person's physiological state. Reported alterations, as described by Pawluk include, "1) vasodilation; 2) analgesic action; 3) antiinflammatory action; 4) spasmolytic activity; 5) healing acceleration; and 6) antiedema activity." The applied fields are generally either electromagnetic (static fields) or pulsed (time-varied fields).

No license is required for magnetic field practitioners as of 2000. The North American Academy of Magnetic Therapy spreads awareness of this field of therapy and seeks to develop a credentialing process. The FDA is involved in certifying magnetic field devices available through licensed professionals. Further research and regulations concerning their use are needed and are likely in the future.

Source: CCRCAAM.

Massage Therapy

Massage therapy is a very old medical technique; evidence exists for its use in China over 4000 years ago. Hippocrates, the "father of medicine," believed massage to be something with which the "physician must be acquainted."

Modern massage therapy began in Sweden with *medical gymnastics* and *Swedish movement cure,* two terms coined by Per Henrik Ling (1776–1839) to describe an integrated system of massage and exercise that he developed. Brother physicians George and Charles Taylor brought Ling's system to America from Sweden in the 1850s. Many physicians subsequently adopted massage techniques into their practice.

With the emergence of biomedicine and new technologies in the early twentieth century, time-intensive massage duties were given to nurses or assistants and later dropped from medicine altogether in many cases. A small number of therapists continued to offer massage therapy until the 1970s, when popular interest in alternative therapies, stress reduction, and health maintenance revitalized the field.

A major philosophy underlying the application of massage is *vis medicatrix naturae,* or catalyzing the self-healing ability of the body to maintain or increase health and well-being. The soft-tissue manipulation techniques used to accomplish this include active and/or passive movements and varying degrees of fixed or moving pressure. All systems, particularly the musculoskeletal, nervous, and circulatory, are affected. Both the scientific component of anatomy and physiology and the artistic component of sensitive touch are vitally important. Sensitivity allows the therapist to determine the appropriate amount of pressure to use, gives the therapist important information about the body of an individual, and conveys a caring attitude to the massage recipient.

Massage is reported to increase circulation, reduce stress, relax tense or contracted muscles, tone flaccid muscles, improve sleep and digestion, ease depression, increase flexibility, and reduce pain. It has been used for treating stress, lymphedema, fibromyalgia, tension headaches, osteoarthritis, repetitive stress disorders, and soft tissue injuries. Massage also facilitates responses in premature and addicted infants. Practitioners of some styles of massage—including Swedish, deep tissue, sports, neuromuscular, and manual lymph drainage—work directly on the skin, often using oil or lotion to reduce friction. Other styles of a more subtle nature are worked through the clothing of the patient. These include acupressure, shiatsu, cranialsacral, and zero balancing therapies.

Currently, 29 states and the District of Columbia license massage therapists; most require a minimum of 500 hours of training and an examination. A national certification program begun in 1992 was inaugurated by the NCBTMB (National Certification Board for Therapeutic Massage and Bodywork) and adopted by many states. Numerous accredited schools throughout the country offer basic education and advanced training.

Sources: CCRCAAM, ECAAM.

APPENDIX O

Native American Medicine

Native American medicine is a name given to the variety of healing practices, rituals, beliefs, and traditions in which the indigenous inhabitants of the American continent engaged for at least 12,000 years. The diversity, particularity, and uniqueness of these practices, originating as they do from approximately 500 distinct nations ("tribes"), cannot be overstated. However, shared values and beliefs are incorporated into the definition of Native American medicine.

Themes common to Native American healing traditions include the recognition that humanity is an integral part of the whole natural order, that spirit infuses all things (so that all things are alive), and that energies are real and have an impact—potentially both helpful and harmful—on health and well-being. Disease is not seen as something that merely happens; instead disease results from spiritual imbalances, which are in turn caused by a person's thoughts, feelings, words, and deeds. Thus the role of the healer is to restore balance to the spirit and hence to the body, emotions, and mind. Generally speaking, Native treatments may include the application of *sweat lodge* ceremonies; sacred pipe ceremonies; smudging with dried herbs; unruffling with feathers; and the use of rattles, herbs, drums, singing, cleansing with mud, laying on of hands; vision quests; and dream interpretation.

Native American healers, *medicine men* and *women,* may be shamans, herbalists, singers, ritualists, or some combination thereof. Typically they have suffered and recovered from some form of illness; their particular illnesses constitute their areas of expertise. Every reservation has at least one such medicine man or woman—larger Nations often have *medicine societies*—but formal medical associations as such do not exist. Moreover, most Nations have a *medicine family,* or clan, in which the healing traditions are preserved. Training as a healer often begins in middle age, but each Nation and medicine family, clan, or society has its own particular protocols. Healing education is based on oral transmission from healer to apprentice (nothing is written down or passed on to the public as that is thought to weaken the medicine), and such apprenticeships often last 10 to 20 years.

Sources: CCRCAAM, ECAM.

APPENDIX P

Naturopathic Medicine

Naturopathic medicine, or *naturopathy*, was founded in the United States in the early 1900s by two men, Dr. Benedict Lust, a German immigrant and student of Father Kneipp's hydrotherapy *(Kneippkur)*, and Dr. Robert Foster. Naturopathy originally comprised an eclectic host of practitioners, most of whom avoided heroic medicine and subscribed to some form of vitalism. In 1956 the National College of Naturopathic Medicine was founded in Portland, Oregon, and the countercultural movements of the 1960s reawakened interest in alternative healing philosophies and practices, including naturopathy. Naturopathic medicine has been especially successful in the Pacific Northwest, and the nationwide resurgence of interest in complementary and alternative medicine should facilitate its future growth.

Naturopathic medicine is a complete philosophy of health and way of life. The philosophical basis of naturopathy may be summarized in the following seven key points:

1. The body has the innate tendency to maintain health and well-being *(vis medicatix naturae)*.
2. Disease is caused by a multitude of factors; as such, the whole person—not simply the disease—must be treated.
3. The symptoms of a disease indicate the body's healing process, and suppression of symptoms without removing the cause of the disease does more harm than good *(primum no nocere,* "first do no harm").
4. The cause of the illness must be diagnosed and treated, instead of merely addressing symptoms.
5. Cultivating healthful habits and preventing illness are the foundations of good health.
6. The doctor's primary task is as a teacher, establishing a trusting relationship with patients, educating and empowering them to take charge of their health.
7. Establishing optimum health and well-being—rather than fighting disease—is the primary goal of the naturopathic physician.

Naturopathic physicians use a variety of techniques and therapies to maintain and optimize health. These include clinical nutrition, phytotherapy, homeopathy, acupuncture, oriental medicine, massage, manipulation, hydrotherapies, relaxation therapies, body-mind exercises, minor surgical procedures, midwifery, and natural childbirth procedures. They do not perform heroic medicine and refer patients in need of such treatments (e.g., major surgeries, medical emergencies) to their allopathic and/or osteopathic colleagues.

As of this writing, Alaska, Arizona, Connecticut, Hawaii, Kansas, Maine, Montana, New Hampshire, Oregon, Utah, Vermont, and Washington, as well as Puerto Rico and the U.S. Virgin Islands, license naturopathic medical practice. Licensure requires graduation from a four-year naturopathic medical program at one of four accredited (or accreditation-pending) naturopathic medical schools in the U.S. These programs consist of two years of basic medical sciences, two years of naturopathic philosophy and techniques, and 1500 clinical hours.

Sources: CCRCAAM, ECAM.

APPENDIX Q

Orthomolecular Medicine

The rationale for orthomolecular medicine originated in the 1920s, when nutrients began to be used in clinical situations. Although megadoses of nutrients had been in therapeutic use since 1950, the term "orthomolecular" did not appear until 1968. Two-time Nobel Prize winner Dr. Linus Pauling then authored a paper in which he used the term to describe the "correct" (*ortho* in Greek) amounts of nutritional substances needed to maintain optimal health.

Orthomolecular medicine has as its philosophical foundation the principle of *biochemical individuality,* which recognizes that the range of optimal nutrient intake may vary between individuals by as much as 700%. Moreover, many health problems are believed to be related to *subclinical deficiencies,* or situations in which a patient's intake of particular nutrients is low yet not manifested in classic deficiency signs and symptoms. Nutritional assessments, including laboratory tests, gauge the patient's nutrient intake and accompany standard physical examinations. Orthomolecular physicians treat many of the same conditions, including psychiatric conditions, as their conventional counterparts, but the approach to diagnosis and treatment differs significantly; megadoses of needed nutrients usually are prescribed instead of pharmaceuticals.

Though most conventional *cum* orthomolecular physicians are self-trained, standard naturopathic medical education strongly emphasizes the nutritional component of health care. Moreover, the American Holistic Medical Association, the American College for Advancement in Medicine, the International Society of Orthomolecular Medicine (in Canada), and the Universidad de Guadalajara (in Mexico) present regular seminars on the topic. As of 2000, no licensing requirements or certification programs in the United States for practitioners of orthomolecular medicine existed.

Source: CCRCAAM.

Osteopathic Medicine

In 1892, Dr. Andrew Taylor Still founded the American School of Osteopathy, where he taught his methods of diagnosis and treatment through manipulation and palpation. Instead of awarding MD degrees, Still insisted on granting DO (Doctor of Osteopathy) degrees to distinguish his students and their medical training. A pharmacological component was added to osteopathic practices in the 1940s. The contributions of James Jealous (embryological approach), Robert Fulford (percussion hammer), Frank Chapman (reflex points), Lawrence Jones (strain/counterstrain), and Fred Mitchell, Jr. (10-step screening exam) have broadened the scope of osteopathic medicine. Osteopathic physicians currently practice the same forms of medicine and surgery as their MD counterparts do, often with little emphasis on Still's manipulative techniques.

In modern osteopathic medicine, pharmacologic, biologic, and physical sciences join together to improve a person's overall health and to prevent or cure disease. Palpatory diagnosis—checking tissue texture, asymmetry, restriction of motion, and tenderness—is the initial phase of osteopathic medicine. Palpation of the musculoskeletal structure, in conjunction with other, more conventional medical techniques and practices, improves the patient's condition.

Osteopaths are licensed physicians under the U.S. Department of Education and are required to pass national board exams for state certification in a given specialty. The National Board of Osteopathic Medicine administers the exams in three parts over six days. Several states have specific exams only for doctors of osteopathy (DO); whereas other states use American Medical Association (AMA) boards in conjunction with American Osteopathic Association (AOA) boards for licensing DOs.

Source: CCRCAAM.

494

Reflexology

Evidence exists in a papyrus scene for the use of zone therapy (the precursor to reflexology) by ancient (2500 BCE) Egyptian physicians. Before spreading through Europe, zone therapy was practiced by Chinese doctors and Native American healers from several tribes. Dr. William Fitzgerald (1872–1942), the founder of modern zone therapy, was familiar with both the European and "Red Indian" practices. Dr. Joe Shelby Riley studied numerous therapies, including zone therapy, and used it in his practice. Dr. Riley's own therapist, Eunice Ingham (1879–1974), developed reflexology and shared self-help techniques through her teaching and several popular books with work continued by her nephew, Dwight Byers. Mildred Carter's book *Helping Yourself with Foot Reflexology* has brought greater recognition to the practice of reflexology.

Reflexology assists the body in correcting, strengthening, and reinforcing itself. Reflex areas or zones located on specific points of the feet or hands correspond to various glands, organs, or systems of the body. Stimulation of these areas through manipulation and focused pressure techniques helps the body achieve a parasympathetic healing state by activating electromagnetic energy along meridian lines and through the nervous system. Reflexologists normalize tender spots and gritty deposits under the skin that may indicate system disharmony or energy blockages.

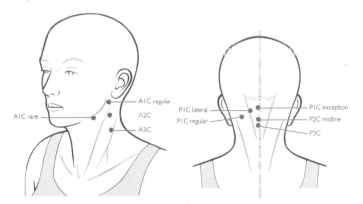

Location of left-sided tender points. Right-sided tender points are located at mirror-image positions. *A*, Anterior; *P*, posterior. (Chaitow, 2002)

495

Reported benefits of reflexology include relaxation and stress reduction, circulation enhancement, and natural physiologic regulation. As a complementary therapy, reflexology has been used in the treatment of chronic fatigue syndrome; allergies; ear, lung, and bladder infections; digestive and sleep disorders, stress, chronic pain, and labor and delivery.

Currently, no formal credentialing for reflexologists exists. Certifications are received from individual schools offering programs ranging from 100 to 1000 hours of coursework and internship.

Source: CCRCAAM.

APPENDIX T

Relaxation Therapies

Relaxation therapies are diverse methods for tapping into the body's innate *relaxation response.* First identified by Dr. Herbert Benson in the early 1970s, the relaxation response is the physiologic counterpoint to the flight-or-flight response, and it is characterized by balanced autonomic nervous system function; increased alpha and theta brainwave activity; and increased feelings of calmness, confidence, and centered well-being. Although this term and the beneficial physiologic syndrome it describes were not systematically investigated as such until the 1970s, its reality has been understood for millennia. Many civilizations, including those of India and China, have cultivated relaxation response using a wide variety of meditative disciplines and techniques.

Techniques for eliciting the relaxation response are manifold. They include disciplines discussed in other appendices, such as biofeedback and yoga. Specific relaxation therapies may be classified in terms of three general techniques, although in practice these techniques overlap: *refocusing techniques, conscious breathing/meditation,* and *body awareness.* Refocusing techniques are cognitive tools that allow a person to reframe a given situation and to reinterpret it supportively; in other words, individuals are able to read and respond to the story of their lives differently, in a more relaxed, less anxious manner.

Conscious breathing, an element of many meditative and contemplative practices (including some forms of prayer), turns the attention away from anxious mental chatter and toward the constant of the breath. (This exercise may or may not be accompanied by the repetition—silently or aloud—of sacred syllables, words, or phrases.) Body awareness involves the focusing of conscious attention on the felt sensations of the body and expansion of awareness beyond normal waking ego consciousness.

No formal credentials or licensures in relaxation therapies currently exist, although courses in specific methods are offered through many professional seminars and conferences and at some colleges and universities. Meditation techniques and centering prayer can also be learned through a variety of spiritual and religious organizations.

Source: CCRCAAM.

Spiritual Healing and Subtle Energy Medicine

As with many other alternatives to conventional Western medicine, spiritual healing has existed in various forms throughout history. For example, in ancient Greece, Pythagoras linked body and soul to effect healing; early Christians believed in spiritual healing, and Mary Baker Eddy's Christian Science is a modern variant; white witches healed with magical powers; Paracelsus in the Middle Ages believed in auras with luminous sidereal second bodies and souls; and Hawaiian Kahuna healers linked spiritual forces to healing. The nineteenth and twentieth centuries saw the promulgation of energy therapies by Karl von Riechenbach in Germany and Wilhelm Reich in America, as well as the concept of the reality of the unconscious by Freud and Jung. A plethora of branches of spiritual healing exist.

The basic concept of spiritual healing is that an individual practitioner or a group focuses on appealing to or channeling energetic or spiritual forces for healing. Use of the link between the corporeal body and the soul of a being is the foundation of spiritual healing. Some prominent examples of energy or spiritual healing and subtle energy medicine are shamanism, prani, bioenergy healing, Qi gong, reiki, therapeutic touch, healing touch, polarity therapy, SHEN therapy, and laying on of hands.

Although spiritual healing and subtle energy medicine lack detrimental side effects and can complement other therapies, no licensing schemes for them exist in America (as of 2000). However, certifications and/or training classes are available for some branches of subtle energy medicine—for example, the International SHEN Therapy Association and Healing Touch. In some nations spiritual healing guidelines and professional organizations are regulated branches of complementary medicine, as in Holland and England.

Tibetan Medicine

Tibetan medicine developed over many centuries. It has its roots in the Tibetan Bön tradition; Buddhist philosophy; and Ayurvedic, Chinese, and Greek medicine. From the seventh to the ninth centuries of the common era, the Tibetan Empire extended from Samarkand and part of China in the north to the plain of the Ganges in the south, and it was ruled by three consecutive kings: Song-tsen Gam-po, Ti-song De-tsen, and Rolpa-chon.

The second of these Tibetan kings, Ti-song De-tsen, invited Padmasambhava, a Buddhist teacher, to Tibet. Since that time, Buddhist philosophy has played a profound role in Tibetan medicine. A medical convention held at Samye (CE 755–797) brought renowned physicians traveling from Greece, Persia, India, Afghanistan, Kashmir, East Turkestan, Nepal, and China to translate their medical works into Tibetan. In addition many Tibetan teachers influenced the development of Tibetan medicine. These include sTon-pa gShen-rab (c. 1000 BCE), Dung-gi Thor-cog (150 BCE), and Elder gYu-thogYon-tan mGon-po or "Excellent Protector" (c. CE 700–900).

Tibetan medicine historically has been taught in monasteries and, since the eighth century, in some colleges. In 1959 the Tibetan Medical Institute at Dharamsala, India was founded under the leadership of His Holiness Dalai Lama. Tibetan medicine is currently practiced in Tibet, Mongolia, the Buryat Republic of Russia, St. Petersburg, North India, Europe, and the United States.

Numerous traditions and lineages exist that, while holding common core concepts and using central texts, differ in their practical applications. One core concept is the *triadic theory,* the idea that the interactions of three interdependent essential elements, *chi* (with a meaning different from the Chinese concept), *schara,* and *badahan,* determine the nature of everything perceived. *Chi* is space, a supportive element that corresponds to the skeleton, cell membranes, and mind and body systems responsible for introducing nutrition and for elimination. The corresponding taste pair is pungent-sweet.

Schara is energy, and it corresponds to organs or systems that distribute nutrients, such as upper gastrointestinal tract, liver, cardiovascular system, nervous system, and energy channels. The corresponding taste pair is bitter-salty. *Badahan* is the element that secures and protects. It corresponds to systems that absorb nutrition (adipose, lungs, brain, immune system), and the paired taste is sour-astringent. The elements exist in a spiritual, mental, and physical balance that, in the absence of physical symptoms, are believed to characterize optimal health.

The various lineages of this discipline recognize the important role that psychologic and spiritual well-being play in health and place an emphasis on personal responsibility in maintaining it. In addition to taking personal responsibility for proper nutrition, lifestyle habits, seasonal adjustments, and awareness of predispositions, the individual must invest the time and effort to cultivate objective compassion, or peacefulness, and the wisdom that allows communication between the *empiric soul* and the absolute (nonmaterial) soul. The *empiric soul,* key to the psychospiritual aspect of Tibetan medicine, consists of the mind, the attributes of the mind (ego, intellect, memory, and emotions), and the senses (sound, touch, vision, taste, and smell).

Medical diagnosis is made in the morning—when the patient is rested and fasting. It includes visual assessment and determination of constitutional type *(chi, schara, badahan),* inquiry into specific complaints, pulse reading, and urine evaluation. The physician is interested in restoring balance ("alleviating the out-of-range function") through the use of nutritional therapy, herbs, and minerals, paying particular attention to the taste. Therapeutic massage is used on the abdomen, spine, neck, and head during treatments to regulate the energy channels or subtle body, removing blockages and restoring function. Finally the patient must also address the *empiric soul* to promote healthy mental and emotional "digestion" and proper spiritual communication with the absolute soul.

No certification or licensing currently exists in the United States.

Source: ECAAM.

Traditional Chinese Medicine (TCM)

Traditional Chinese medicine (TCM), a coherent healing system, developed over several thousand years. Many classic texts articulate the philosophy and practices of Chinese medicine. These include the *Yellow Emperor's Inner Classic (Huang Di Nei Jing)*, by unknown authors, (200 BCE); *Treatise on Febrile and Miscellaneous Diseases (Shang Han Za Bing Lun)*, Zhang Zhongjing (CE 150–219); *Divine Husbandman's Classic of Materia Medica (Shen Nong Ben Cao Jing)*, unknown authors, (CE 25–220); and the *Grand Materia Medica (Ben Cao Gang Mu)*, Li Shizhen (CE 1578). Official training schools existed in China over many dynasties, but most practitioners learned through apprenticeships and family practices. Since the 1950s, colleges and universities sponsored by the government have gradually been established. Their curriculum is typically 50% TCM and 50% Western medicine.

Mind, body, and spirit are seen as an integrated whole, connected and vitalized by *qi*, one of the five major components of the TCM system. According to some authorities, the five are: *qi* (vital life force), blood, body fluid, *zang fu* (organ systems), and the body's energy system (*Jing* and *Luo*— meridians and collaterals). Others list blood and body fluid with *qi, jing,* and *shen* (mind or psyche), also known as the three treasures. The organ systems themselves correspond to the five elements: liver—wood, heart—fire, spleen—earth, lung—metal, and kidney—water. Optimal health is viewed as a state of balance among the various components, symbolized by the *yin-yang* image.

According to TCM three types of factors contribute to the disharmony that causes disease to manifest. There are external or climatic factors (wind, cold, damp, fire and heat, dryness, and summer heat, wind); internal physiologic factors (anger, joy, melancholy, worry, grief, fear, fright in excess, or want); and miscellaneous constitutional or lifestyle factors.

Diagnostic examinations typically involve visual assessment of the *shen* and various physical characteristics, including the tongue. Examinations also include auscultation, or listening to the patient's speaking voice; evaluation of body odors; interviewing for related information; and palpation of the pulse, hands, feet, and abdomen. Treatments lasting up to several weeks are tailored to the unique diagnosis of the patient and are designed to return the whole person back into a pattern of harmony. This is accomplished, for instance, by cooling excess heat or tonifying deficiencies. Treatments may include acupuncture, use of herbs, moxibustion, massage *(tui na),* movement and breathing exercises *(tai chi* and *qi gong),* food therapy, or lifestyle modification.

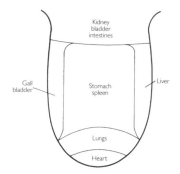

Correspondence of tongue areas to organs. (Maciocia, 1989)

Chinese medicine is claimed to be effective as a preventive and as a first line of defense against illness. It is also used for various conditions including hepatitis, infections, allergies, uterine fibroids, diabetes, sleep disorders, back pain, asthma, stress, prostate cancer, infertility, arthritis, addictions, and muscle spasms.

In the United States requirements for licensure vary from state to state, though generally students must graduate from an accredited school and pass a state board or National Certification Commission Exam (administered by the National Certification Commission for Acupuncture and Oriental Medicine). About 50 accredited schools in the United States offer programs ranging from 2 to 4 years in length. Most of the more challenging schools require completion of 60 undergraduate semester units before entering the TCM program and completion of a minimum TCM program of 3 years.

Sources: CCRCAAM, ECAAM.

APPENDIX X

Yoga

Yoga originated in India and may be as old as 6000 years. Classic texts including *the Vedas* (1000 BCE) and *The Bhagavad Gita* (CE 400) mention yoga (translated as "yoke" or "union"). It is considered to have become a mature tradition with the composition of *The Yoga Sutras* by Patanjali in 300 BCE. Yoga was brought to the United States by Swami Vivkananda in the 1890s and introduced through lectures on meditation for spiritual practice. BKS Lyengar's *Light on Yoga,* a modern classic text that features yoga postures, or *asanas,* was published in 1966.

Yoga developed as an integrating spiritual practice with many health benefits. The four paths are *Bhakti,* or the path of devotion; *Karma,* or the path of right action; *Jnana,* or the path of knowledge and realization; and *Hatha,* the path of meditation. Though they seem distinct, the four paths tend to reinforce each other and are thus ideally practiced together. Additionally, there are eight limbs (*ashtanga*) or techniques: *yama* (restraint), *niyama* (observances), *asanas* (postures), *pranayama* (breath control), *pratyahara* (withdrawal of the senses), *dharana* (concentration), *dhyana* (meditation), and *samadhi* (bliss). Many styles of yoga have emerged in the United States in recent years, developed by master teachers, though all are based on *hatha.*

The diligent and open practice of meditation, *asanas,* and *pranayama* calms the mind, eases depression, tones and strengthens the muscles and organs, increases circulation, soothes the nervous system, and reduces pain. Clinical studies that are underway demonstrate efficacy in treating back pain, hypertension, obsessive-compulsive disorder, reproductive disorders, respiratory conditions, and sleep disorders.

Yoga instructor training is monitored by individual schools, but seeks a movement seeks to standardize the credentialing process. A teacher should have a daily personal practice as well as in-depth knowledge of anatomy and physiology, *asanas, pranayama*, meditation, proper diet, and the history and philosophy of yoga.

Source: CCRCAAM.

Illustration Credits

Beresford-Cooke C: *Shiatsu theory and practice,* ed 2, London, 2003, Churchill Livingstone.

Buckle J: *Clinical aromatherapy: essential oils in practice,* ed 2, St Louis, 2003, Churchill Livingstone.

Campbell A: *Acupuncture in practice: beyond points and meridians,* Oxford, UK, 2001, Butterworth-Heinemann.

Carreiro JE: *An osteopathic approach to children,* London, 2003, Churchill Livingstone.

Cassidy CM: *Contemporary Chinese medicine and acupuncture,* New York, 2002, Churchill Livingstone.

Chaitow L: *Cranial manipulation theory and practice: osseous and soft tissue approaches,* Edinburgh, UK, 1999, Churchill Livingstone.

Chaitow L: *Palpation and assessment skills: assessment and diagnosis through touch,* ed 2, Edinburgh, UK, 2003, Churchill Livingstone.

Chaitow L, Bradley D, Gilbert C: *Multidisciplinary approaches to breathing pattern disorders,* Edinburgh, UK, 2002, Churchill Livingstone.

Chaitow L, DeLany J, Dowling D: *Modern neuromuscular techniques,* ed 2, Edinburgh, UK, 2003, Churchill Livingstone.

Chaitow L, Wilson E, Morrissey D: *Positional release techniques,* ed 2, Edinburgh, UK, 2002, Churchill Livingstone.

Chirali IZ: *Traditional Chinese medicine: cupping therapy,* Edinburgh, UK, 1999, Churchill Livingstone.

Clarke S: *Essential chemistry for safe aromatherapy,* Edinburgh, UK, 2002, Churchill Livingstone.

Coughlin P, editor: *Principles and practice of manual therapeutics,* New York, 2002, Churchill Livingstone.

Cross JR: *Acupressure: clinical applications in musculo-skeletal conditions,* Oxford, UK, 2000, Butterworth-Heinemann.

Freeman LW, Lawlis GF: *Mosby's Complementary & alternative medicine: a research-based approach,* St Louis, 2001, Mosby.

Fritz S: *Mosby's Fundamentals of therapeutic massage,* ed 2, St Louis, 2000, Mosby.

Gardner-Abbate S: *The art of palpatory diagnosis in Oriental medicine,* Edinburgh, UK, 2001, Churchill Livingstone.

Gibbons P, Tehan P: *Manipulation of the spine, thorax, and pelvis: an osteopathic perspective,* Edinburgh, UK, 2000, Churchill Livingstone.

Leskowitz E, Micozzi MS: *Complementary and alternative medicine in rehabilitation,* New York, 2003, Churchill Livingstone.

Lowe WW: *Orthopedic massage: theory and technique,* Edinburgh, UK, 2003, Mosby.

Lu S, Mao S (translator): *Handbook of acupuncture in the treatment of nervous system disorders,* London, 2002, Donica Publishing.

Maciocia G: *The foundations of Chinese medicine: a comprehensive text for acupuncturists and herbalists,* Edinburgh, UK, 1989, Churchill Livingstone.

Malvo SG: *Massage therapy: principles and practice,* ed 2, St Louis, 2003, Saunders.

McCarthy M: *Lymphatic therapy for toxic decongestion: selected case studies for therapists and patients,* London, 2003, Churchill Livingstone.

Micozzi MS, editor: *Fundamentals of complementary and alternative medicine,* ed 2, St Louis, 2001, Mosby.

Mosby's Medical, nursing, and allied health dictionary, ed 6, St Louis, 2002, Mosby.

Novey DW: *Clinician's Complete reference to complementary/alternative medicine,* St Louis, 2000, Mosby.

Oschman JL: *Energy medicine: the scientific basis,* Edinburgh, UK, 2000, Churchill Livingstone.

Payne RA: *Relaxation techniques: a practical handbook for the health care professional,* ed 2, Edinburgh, UK, 2000, Churchill Livingstone.

Petty NJ, Moore AP, editors: *Neuromusculoskeletal examination and assessment: a handbook for therapists,* ed 2, St Louis, 2001, Saunders.

Pizzorno JE, Jr, Murray MT, editors: *Textbook of natural medicine,* ed 2, Edinburgh, UK, 1999, Churchill Livingstone.

Rakel D, editor: *Integrative medicine,* Philadelphia, 2003, Saunders.

Rankin-Box DF, editor: *Nurses' Handbook of complementary therapies,* Edinburgh, UK, 1995, Churchill Livingstone.

Scott J, Barlow T: *Herbs in the treatment of children: leading a child to health,* St Louis, 2003, Churchill Livingstone.

Sharma H, Clark C: *Contemporary Ayurveda: medicine and research in Maharishi Ayur-Veda,* New York, 1998, Churchill Livingstone.

Skidmore-Roth L: *Mosby's Handbook of herbs & natural supplements,* St Louis, 2001, Mosby.

Standish LJ, Calabrese C, Galantino ML: *AIDS and complementary alternative medicine: current science and practice,* New York, 2002, Churchill Livingstone.

Tiran D: *Clinical aromatherapy for pregnancy and childbirth,* ed 2, Edinburgh, UK, 2000, Churchill Livingstone.

Williamson EM, editor: *Major herbs of Ayurveda,* London, 2002, Churchill Livingstone.

Bibliography

Acknowledgment is made to the authors and publishers of the following publications used for reference sources by the author:

Beresford-Cooke C: *Shiatsu theory and practice: a comprehensive text for the student and professional,* Edinburgh, UK, 2003, Churchill Livingstone.

Birch SJ, Felt RL: *Understanding acupuncture,* Edinburgh, UK, 1999, Churchill Livingstone.

Campbell A: *Acupuncture in practice: beyond points and meridians,* New York, 2001, Butterworth-Heinemann.

Carlston M, editor: *Classical homeopathy: medical guides to complementary and alternative medicine,* St Louis, 2003, Churchill Livingstone.

Carreiro J: *An osteopathic approach to children,* St Louis, 2003, Churchill Livingstone.

Cassidy CM: *Contemporary Chinese medicine and acupuncture,* St Louis, 2002, Churchill Livingstone.

Chaitow L: *Cranial manipulation theory and practice: osseous and soft tissue approaches,* Edinburgh, UK, 1999, Churchill Livingstone.

Chaitow L: *Modern neuromuscular techniques,* Edinburgh, UK, 1996, Churchill Livingstone.

Chaitow L: *Muscle energy techniques,* London, 2001, Churchill Livingstone.

Chaitow L, Bradley D, Gilbert C: *Multidisciplinary approaches to breathing pattern disorders,* London, 2002, Churchill Livingstone.

Chaitow L, DeLany J: *Clinical application of neuromuscular techniques, volume I: the upper body,* London, 2000, Churchill Livingstone.

Chirali IZ: *Cupping therapy: traditional Chinese medicine,* London, 1999, Churchill Livingstone.

Clarke S: *Essential chemistry for safe aromatherapy,* Edinburgh, UK, 2002, Churchill Livingstone.

Clavey S: *Fluid physiology and pathology in traditional Chinese medicine,* Edinburgh, UK, 2003, Churchill Livingstone.

Coughlin P: *Principles & practices in manual therapeutics,* St Louis, 2002, Churchill Livingstone.

Cross JR: *Acupressure and reflexology in the treatment of medical conditions,* London, 2001, Butterworth Heinemann.

Dimond B: *The legal aspects of complementary therapy practice: a guide for health care professionals,* Edinburgh, UK, 1998, Churchill Livingstone.

Dorland's Illustrated medical dictionary, ed 30, Philadelphia, 2003, Saunders.

Ernst E, editor: *Complementary & alternative medicine: a desktop reference,* St Louis, 2001, Mosby.

Freeman LW, Lawlis GF: *Mosby's Complementary and alternative medicine: a research-based approach,* St Louis, 2000, Mosby.

Fritz S: *Mosby's Fundamentals of therapeutic massage*, ed 3, St Louis, 2004, Mosby.

Gallagher RM, Humphrey FJ: *Osteopathic medicine: a reformation in progress*, St Louis, 2001, Churchill Livingstone.

Gardner-Abbate S: *The art of palpatory diagnosis in Oriental medicine*, Edinburgh, UK, 2001, Churchill Livingstone.

Gibbons P, Tehan P: *Manipulation of the spine, thorax, and pelvis: an osteopathic perspective*, Edinburgh, UK, 2000, Churchill Livingstone.

Jonas WB, Chez RA, editors: *Definitions and standards in healing research: First American Samueli Symposium, alternative therapies*, 9(3), 2003.

Jonas WB, Levin JS, editors: *Essentials of complementary and alternative medicine*, Philadelphia, 1999, Lippincott Williams & Wilkins.

Leskowitz E: *Complementary and alternative medicine in rehabilitation*, St Louis, 2003, Churchill Livingstone.

Lett A: *Reflex zone therapy*, Edinburgh, UK, 2000, Churchill Livingstone.

Loo M: *Pediatric acupuncture*, Edinburgh, UK, 2002, Churchill Livingstone.

Maciocia G: *Foundations of Chinese medicine: a comprehensive text for acupuncturists and herbalists*, Edinburgh, UK, 1989, Churchill Livingstone.

Maciocia G: *Obstetrics and gynecology in Chinese medicine*, Edinburgh, UK, 1998, Churchill Livingstone.

Maciocia G: *The practice of Chinese medicine: the treatment of diseases with acupuncture and Chinese herbs*, Edinburgh, 1994, Churchill Livingstone.

Mann F: *Reinventing acupuncture*, Edinburgh, UK, 2000, Butterworth Heinemann.

McCarthy M: *Lymphatic therapy for toxic congestion: selected case studies for therapists and patients*, Edinburgh, UK, 2003, Churchill Livingstone.

Micozzi M: *Fundamentals of complementary and alternative medicine*, ed 2, St Louis, 2001, Churchill Livingstone.

Mills S: *Principles and practice of phytotherapy: modern herbal medicine*, Edinburgh, UK, 2000, Churchill Livingstone.

Mosby's Medical, nursing, & allied health dictionary, ed 6, St Louis, 2002, Mosby.

Novey DW: *Clinician's Complete reference to complementary/alternative medicine*, St Louis, 2000, Mosby.

Oleson T: *Auriculotherapy manual: Chinese and western systems of ear acupuncture*, Edinburgh, UK, 2003, Churchill Livingstone.

Oschman J: *Energy medicine: the scientific basis*, St Louis, 2000, Churchill Livingstone.

Payne RA: *Relaxation techniques: a practical handbook for the health care professional*, Edinburgh, UK, 2003, Churchill Livingstone.

Petty NJ, Moore AP: *Neuromusculoskeletal examination and assessment: a handbook for therapists*, Edinburgh, UK, 2001, Churchill Livingstone.

Price S, Price L: *Aromatherapy of health professionals*, ed 2, Edinburgh, UK, 1999, Churchill Livingstone.

Salvo S: *Massage therapy: principles and practice*, ed 2, Philadelphia, 2003, WB Saunders.

Schnyer, R: *Acupuncture in the treatment of depression: a manual for practice and research*, Edinburgh, UK, 2001, Churchill Livingstone.

Scott J: *Herbs in the treatment of children: leading a child to health,* Edinburgh, UK, 2003, Churchill Livingstone.

Sharma H, Clark C: *Contemporary Ayurveda: medicine and research in Maharishi Ayur-Veda,* Edinburgh, UK, 1998, Churchill Livingstone.

Standish L, Calabrese C, Galantino ML: *AIDS and complementary & alternative medicine: current science and practice,* St Louis, 2002, Churchill Livingstone.

Sun P, editor: *The treatment of pain with Chinese herbs and acupuncture,* Edinburgh, UK, 2002, Churchill Livingstone.

Temes R: *Medical hypnosis: an introduction and clinical guide,* Edinburgh, UK, 1999, Churchill Livingstone.

Tietao D: *Practical diagnosis in traditional Chinese medicine,* Edinburgh, UK, 1999, Churchill Livingstone.

Tiran D, editor: *Clinical aromatherapy for pregnancy and childbirth,* Edinburgh, UK, 2000, Churchill Livingstone.

Weintraub M, editor: *Alternative and complementary treatment in neurologic illness,* St Louis, 2001, Churchill Livingstone.

West Z: *Acupuncture in pregnancy and childbirth,* Edinburgh, UK, 2001, Churchill Livingstone.

Williamson EM: *Major herbs of Ayurveda,* Edinburgh, UK, 2002, Churchill Livingstone.

Xu L: *Chinese materia medica: combinations and applications,* Beijing, 2002, Donica Publishing.

Yifan Y: *Chinese herbal medicines: comparisons and characteristics,* Edinburgh, UK, 2002, Churchill Livingstone.

Zhou ZY: *Clinical manual of Chinese herbal medicine and acupuncture,* Edinburgh, UK, 1997, Churchill Livingstone.

Websites Referenced

http://137.222.110.150/calnet/DeepNeck/page3.htm
http://1stholistic.com
http://207.188.144.45/education/jyotisha.html
http://207.188.144.45/products/ayurvedic_herbs.html
http://216.251.241.163/semdweb/InternetSOMD/ASP/1531453.asp
http://ahna.org
http://ajp.psychiatryonline.org
http://allergies.about.com
http://alternativehealing.org
http://apu.sfn.org
http://assessments.ncspearson.com
http://blswww.grc.nia.nih.gov
http://bmj.bmjjournals.com
http://bob.nap.edu
http://bodd.cf.ac.uk
http://botanical.com
http://brindedcow.umd.edu
http://cancer.gov/
http://cancernet.nci.nih.gov
http://cancerweb.ncl.ac.uk/

http://consensus.nih.gov
http://cpmcnet.columbia.edu
http://d77423.u37.smartfunction.net
http://dermatology.about.com
http://dict.die.net
http://dictionary.reference.com
http://dietary-supplements.info.nih.gov
http://digestive.niddk.nih.gov
http://distance.stcc.edu
http://education.yahoo.com
http://en2.wikipedia.org
http://ericae.net
http://essentialoil.com
http://gate8.com
http://grants1.nih.gov
http://hbotofaz.org
http://health.yahoo.com
http://healthchoice.net
http://herb.damo-qigong.net
http://herbsforhealth.about.com
http://holisticonline.com
http://homeopathyworld.com
http://honey.bio.waikato.ac.nz
http://howstuffworks.lycoszone.com
http://hsc.usf.edu
http://it.uku.fi
http://jcem.endojournals.org
http://kidney.niddk.nih.gov
http://kidshealth.org
http://library.med.cornell.edu
http://library.thinkquest.org
http://lonestar.texas.net
http://mathworld.wolfram.com
http://medlib.med.utah.edu
http://www.med.umich.edu
http://memory.ucsf.edu
http://muscle.ucsd.edu
http://my.clarins.com
http://my.webmd.com
http://nccam.nih.gov
http://notes.utk.edu
http://odphp.osophs.dhhs.gov
http://pages.prodigy.net
http://pediatrics.about.com
http://physics.uwa.edu.au
http://praxis.md
http://preventionpartners.samhsa.gov
http://rife.org
http://schools.naturalhealers.com

http://serendip.brynmawr.edu
http://skepdic.com
http://sportsmedicine.about.com
http://steinschwitzbad.de
http://stress.about.com
http://superstringtheory.com
http://swmi.net
http://tcm.health-info.org
http://the-atlantic-paranormal-society.com
http://two.not2.org
http://uk.gay.com
http://uscneurosurgery.com
http://users.cell2000.net
http://vm.cfsan.fda.gov
http://wfas.acutimes.com
http://whatis.techtarget.com
http://womenshealth.about.com
http://www.1hpi.com
http://www.1stchineseherbs.com
http://www.1uphealth.com
http://www.3ho.org
http://www.7hz.com
http://www.aacp.uk.com
http://www.aafp.org
http://www.aaimedicine.com
http://www.aamc.org
http://www.aaom.org
http://www.aap.org
http://www.aapb.org
http://www.aboutrhinoplasty.com
http://www.academyofosteopathy.org
http://www.acaom.org
http://www.acupuncturetoday.com
http://www.acuxo.com
http://www.adta.org
http://www.aegis.com
http://www.aids.org
http://www.aidsinfonyc.org
http://www.akse.de
http://www.alexandertechnique.com
http://www.allergycontrol.com
http://www.alltm.org
http://www.alternativemedicine.com
http://www.alternative-medicine-info.com
http://www.alternativementalhealth.com
http://www.ama-assn.org
http://www.amerchiro.org
http://www.american.edu/
http://www.americanheart.org

http://www.amershamhealth.com/
http://www.amsa.org
http://www.andrew-may.com
http://www.aniwaya.org
http://www.anu.edu.au
http://www.anusara.com
http://www.aoa-net.org
http://www.aoa-net.org/Publications/glossary202.pdf
http://www.apa.org
http://www.apitherapy.org
http://www.apta.org
http://www.aromaweb.com
http://www.ars-grin.gov
http://www.arthritis.org
http://www.arttherapy.org
http://www.asch.net/index.htm
http://www.ashtanga.com
http://www.askdrbrent.com
http://www.astaxanthin.org
http://www.aston-patterining.com
http://www.astro.ufl.edu
http://www.auburn.edu
http://www.autism.org
http://www.aworldofacupuncture.com
http://www.ayurveda.com
http://www.ayurveda-herbal-remedy.com
http://www.ayurvedic.org
http://www.bachcentre.com
http://www.b-and-t-world-seeds.com
http://www.bartleby.com
http://www.bbc.co.uk
http://www.bccancer.bc.ca
http://www.bcia.org
http://www.behavenet.com
http://www.beyondveg.com
http://www.bikramyoga.com
http://www.biocompare.com
http://www.biofield.arizona.edu
http://www.biomedcentral.com
http://www.biomed2.man.ac.uk
http://www.biopulse.org
http://www.bloodjournal.org
http://www.bluecloud.org
http://www.bmulligan.com
http://www.bodymindcentering.com
http://www.bodysoulspiritexpo.com
http://www.bodyved.com
http://www.boger-boenninghausen.com
http://www.books.md

http://www.botanical.com
http://www.botany.uwc.ac.za
http://www.braintuner.com
http://www.braindictionary.com
http://www.brainydictionary.com
http://www.brainplace.com
http://www.breathwork.com
http://www.brianmac.demon.co.uk
http://www.bu.edu
http://www.buyindies.com
http://www.cacr.ca
http://www.calmspirit.com
http://www.cancer.gov
http://www.cancer.org
http://www.cancerguide.org
http://www.cc.nih.gov
http://www.cc200.com/branches/chiro/acupuncture.htm
http://www.cdc.gov
http://www.cdc.gov/nceh/lead/CaseManagement/Appendixes.pdf
http://www.centeringprayer.com
http://www.chedu.org
http://www.chappellhealth.com
http://www.chinesemedicinesampler.com
http://www.chiro.org
http://www.chirobase.org
http://www.chiroweb.com
http://www.chisuk.org.uk
http://www.chpus.com
http://www.christianscience.org
http://www.circlesofrhythm.com
http://www.cl.utoledo.edu
http://www.clevelandclinicmeded.com
http://www.cmbm.org
http://www.cmedicines.com.hk
http://www.cnme.us
http://www.coedu.usf.edu
http://www.cognitiveliberty.org
http://www.compmed.umm.edu
http://www.consegrity.com
http://www.convertit.com
http://www.coxtechnic.com
http://www.cranialacademy.com
http://www.craniosacraltherapy.org
http://www.csp.org
http://www.csuchico.edu
http://www.cyberbohemia.com
http://www.dailyreadings.com
http://www.daily-vitamins.com
http://www.deancoleman.com

http://www.deeptissue.com
http://www.dharma-haven.org
http://www.diabetes.org
http://www.Dictionary.com
http://www.doctorshealthsupply.com
http://www.dralexvasquez.com
http://www.dr-dom.com
http://www.drbob4health.com
http://www.drlam.com
http://www.drfeder.com
http://www.drrcdwood.com
http://www.drugdigest.org
http://www.drz.org
http://www.dr-perkins.com
http://www.duj.com
http://www.dyspareunia.org
http://www.egregore.com
http://www.ehealthconnection.com
http://www.ehendrick.org
http://www.elajmd.com
http://www.emedicine.com
http://www.emergentmind.org
http://www.encyclopedia.com
http://www.endtime.org
http://www.energyschool.com
http://www.entcolumbia.org
http://www.eosinophilia-myalgia.net
http://www.epa.gov
http://www.erowid.org
http://www.fallingbostel.de
http://www.fao.org
http://www.fasthealth.com
http://www.fda.gov
http://www.findarticles.com
http://www.fitnesslynn.com
http://www.floehandbones.com
http://www.focusing.org
http://www.food-allergy.org
http://www.foodproductdesign.com
http://www.fsmb.org
http://www.fsu.edu
http://www.futureceuticals.com
http://www.gastricbypass.org
http://www.gastromd.com
http://www.gdvusa.org
http://www.gem-systems.com
http://www.gerd.com
http://www.google.com
http://www.graciesplace.net

http://www.gsdl.com
http://www.hannasomatics.com
http://www.hanp.net
http://www.hardinessinstitute.com
http://www.healing4u.com
http://www.healer.ch/Chakras-e.html
http://www.health.gov
http://www.health.state.mn.us
http://www.healthandage.com
http://www.healthpromotionjournal.com
http://www.healthpyramid.com
http://www.healthsystem.virginia.edu
http://www.healthwatcher.net
http://www.healthworks.fsnet.co.uk
http://www.healthy.net
http://www.heartmath.com
http://www.herbalgram.org
http://www.herbalgram.org
http://www.herbalists.on.ca
http://www.herbaltransitions.com
http://www.herbasin.com
http://www.herbsmd.com
http://www.herbnet.com
http://www.hernia.org
http://www.hhchealth.com
http://www.himalayahealthcare.com
http://www.hippocrates.com
http://www.hmrtec.com
http://www.holistic-online.com
http://www.holographic.org
http://www.homeoint.org
http://www.homeopathicdoc.com
http://www.homoeopathyclinic.com
http://www.hopkins-gi.org
http://www.hort.vt.edu
http://www.hyperdictionary.com
http://www.hpus.com
http://www.iahp.org
http://www.iarp.org
http://www.ibiblio.org
http://www.icakusa.com
http://www.icmart.org
http://www.ifst.org
http://www.ihs.gov
http://www.iiom.net
http://www.indian-creek.net
http://www.indiangyan.com
http://www.info.gov.hk
http://www.intelihealth.com

http://www.internetpharmacyservices.com
http://www.ish.unimelb.edu.au
http://www.issels.com
http://www.issseem.org
http://www.itg.uiuc.edu
http://www.jamierosanna.com
http://www.judoinfo.com
http://www.judythweaver.com
http://www.k-12stanford.edu
http://www.kiiko.com
http://www.kundaliniyogacenter.com
http://www.lab.anhb.uwa.edu.au
http://www.labtestsonline.org
http://www.labthermics.com
http://www.lalecheleague.org
http://www.lamaze-childbirth.com
http://www.largocanyon.org
http://www.lbl.gov
http://www.lef.org
http://www.levity.com
http://www.lifesci.ucsb.edu
http://www.lime.ki.se
http://www.llewellynencyclopedia.com
http://www.logan.edu
http://www.lucidity.com
http://www.lung.ca
http://www.macular.org
http://www.madrasibaba.org
http://www.maharishi.co.uk/mak.htm
http://www.mantra-meditation.com
http://www.manomedica.com
http://www.mapi.com
http://www.maripoisoncenter.com
http://www.martrix.org
http://www.massagetoday.com
http://www.massteacher.org
http://www.masterworksinternational.com
http://www.mayoclinic.com
http://www.mbmi.org
http://www.mckinley.uiuc.edu
http://www.mdheal.org
http://www.med.miami.edu
http://www.med.umich.edu
http://www.medem.com
http://www.medhelp.org
http://www.medical-acupuncture.co.uk
http://www.medicinenet.com
http://www.medicomm.net
http://www.medscape.com

http://www.medterms.com
http://www.memantine.com
http://www.mentalhealth.com
http://www.mentalhealthandillness.com
http://www.mercksource.com
http://www.mirasol.net
http://www.mja.com.au
http://www.mouritz.co.uk
http://www.mskcc.org
http://www.mult-sclerosis.org
http://www.musictherapy.org
http://www.mycustompak.com
http://www.myofascial-release.com
http://www.myshamanicvision.com
http://www.mythos.com
http://www.naropa.edu
http://www.nass.co.uk
http://www.naturalhealthcourses.com
http://www.naturalhealthnotebook.com
http://www.naturalhealthservice.org
http://www.naturalhealthvillage.com
http://www.naturedirect2u.com
http://www.naturopathic.org/about/aanp.html
http://www.ncbi.nlm.nih.gov
http://www.nccam.nih.gov
http://www.nci.nih.gov
http://www.ncvhs.hhs.gov
http://www.nemsn.org
http://www.networkofminds.com
http://www.neuroskills.com
http://www.newadvent.org
http://www.next-wave.org
http://www.nhlbi.nih.gov
http://www.nhsia.nhs.uk/
http://www.nhsplus.nhs.uk
http://www.niaid.nih.gov
http://www.niams.nih.gov
http://www.nida.nih.gov
http://www.niehs.nih.gov
http://www.nih.gov.
http://www.ninds.nih.gov
http://www.nlm.nih.gov
http://www.nmrhca.state.nm.us
http://www.noetic.org
http://www.nof.org
http://www.notsodailynews.com
http://www.nutraceuticalalliance.com
http://www.nutritionfocus.com
http://www.objectrelations.org

http://www.ongleyonline.com
http://www.online-ambulance.com
http://www.orthopaedic.ed.ac.uk
http://www.osteo.org
http://www.osteopathy.org
http://www.paam.net
http://www.pdrhealth.com
http://www.peripatus.gen.nz
http://www.ph.ucla.edu
http://www.phd.msu.edu
http://www.philosophypages.com
http://www.phm.umds.ac.uk
http://www.pitt.edu
http://www.positivehealth.com
http://www.ppatp.org
http://www.psiresearch.org
http://www.psychiatrictimes.com
http://www.psychosomaticmedicine.org
http://www.psychosynthesis.org
http://www.pubmedcentral.nih.gov
http://www.pulsemans.com
http://www.pureliquidgold.com
http://www.purplesage.org.uk
http://www.qimaster.com
http://www.quackwatch.org
http://www.qualitychineseherbs.com
http://www.radiologyinfo.org
http://www.rain-tree.com
http://www.ranchovista.org
http://www.rareearth.org.
http://www.raysahelian.com
http://www.reflexology-usa.org
http://www.regetox.med.ulg.ac.be
http://www.reikiassociation.org
http://www.repetitive-strain-injury.com
http://www.rice.edu
http://www.richmond.edu/~allison/glossary.html
http://www.rls.org
http://www.rochester.edu
http://www.rockefeller.edu
http://www.rosedaleclinic.co.uk
http://www.rxmed.com
http://www.sahajayoga.org
http://www.santosha.com
http://www.selegiline.com
http://www.selfgrowth.com
http://www.selfmastery.com
http://www.shareguide.com
http://www.shentherapy.info

http://www.shiatsutherapy.ca
http://www.shodor.org
http://www.siib.org
http://www.simillimum.com
http://www.sjogrens.com
http://www.sleepdisorderchannel.net
http://www.sodbrennen-welt.de
http://www.sofea.co.uk
http://www.soulempowerment.com
http://www.soulfulliving.com
http://www.specialtouch.info
http://www.spinesolver.com
http://www.st.kufm.kagoshima-u.ac.jp
http://www.stanleykrippner.com
http://www.statsoftinc.com
http://www.strengthcats.com
http://www.sublux8.com
http://www.summerfieldhousepractice.co.uk
http://www.syntonicphototherapy.com
http://www.taichifinder.co.uk
http://www.tcmbasics.com
http://www.terrachrista.com
http://www.tftrx.com
http://www.thaiyoga.com
http://www.the-cma.org.uk
http://www.thesaurus-dictionary.com
http://www.theosophy-nw.org
http://www.tiscali.co.uk
http://www.tm.org
http://www.toacorn.com
http://www.touch4health.com
http://www.trainair.co.uk
http://www.treff-raum-espaciotime.com
http://www.ugr.es
http://www.uiowa.edu
http://www.uktherapists.com
http://www.usp.org
http://www.vh.org
http://www.viable-herbal.com
http://www.vitacost.com
http://www.vivendodaluz.com
http://www.webhealthcentre.com
http://www.webref.org
http://www.wfc.org
http://www.whale.to
http://www.whitehousedrugpolicy.gov
http://www.who.int
http://www.wholefoods.com
http://www.wholehealthmd.com

http://www.wholehealthnow.com
http://www.whyvitamins.com
http://www.womens-menopause-health.com
http://www.wordreference.com
http://www.wordspy.com
http://www.worldchiropracticalliance.org
http://www.wound-healing.net
http://www.yahooligans.com/reference/gray/index.html.http://www.nlpinfo.com.
http://www.yogamovement.com
http://www.yourskin.co.uk
http://www.youthstrugglingforsurvival.org
http://www.yrec.org
http://www2.merriam-webster.com
http://www3.mdanderson.org
http://x-rts.com
http://yalenewhavenhealth.org